# Food Safety
## Theory and Practice

Paul L. Knechtges, MS, PhD, REHS

Visiting Assistant Professor
East Carolina University
Greenville, North Carolina

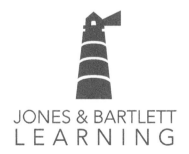

JONES & BARTLETT
LEARNING

*World Headquarters*
Jones & Bartlett Learning
5 Wall Street
Burlington, MA 01803
978-443-5000
info@jblearning.com
www.jblearning.com

Jones & Bartlett Learning books and products are available through most bookstores and online booksellers. To contact Jones & Bartlett Learning directly, call 800-832-0034, fax 978-443-8000, or visit our website, www.jblearning.com.

Substantial discounts on bulk quantities of Jones & Bartlett Learning publications are available to corporations, professional associations, and other qualified organizations. For details and specific discount information, contact the special sales department at Jones & Bartlett Learning via the above contact information or send an email to specialsales@jblearning.com.

**DISCLAIMER**
Trade names or manufacturers' names are used in this book as examples only. This usage does not constitute an endorsement, either expressed or implied, by the author or the author's affiliations.

Some images in this book feature models. These models do not necessarily endorse, represent, or participate in the activities represented in the images.

**Production Credits**
Publisher, Higher Education: Cathleen Sether
Senior Acquisitions Editor: Shoshanna Goldberg
Senior Associate Editor: Amy L. Bloom
Associate Marketing Manager: Jody Sullivan
Production Director: Amy Rose
Senior Production Editor: Renée Sekerak
Production Assistant: Sean Coombs
V.P., Manufacturing and
    Inventory Control: Therese Connell
Artist and Photo Researcher: Carolyn Arcabascio
Composition: Auburn Associates, Inc.

Cover Images: Stalks of wheat © Alekcey/ShutterStock, Inc.;
    Chicken inspection, Courtesy of Keith Weller/USDA ARS;
    Dairy factory © Vasily Smirnov/ShutterStock, Inc.; Fresh eggs
    © Alexander Bark/ShutterStock, Inc.; Dinner at restaurant
    © wrangler/ShutterStock, Inc.; *Salmonella* typhimurium,
    Courtesy of Janice Haney Carr/CDC; Tree spores,
    Courtesy of Keith Weller/USDA ARS
Printing and Binding: Edwards Brothers Malloy
Cover Printing: Edwards Brothers Malloy
Cover Design: Scott Moden

**Library of Congress Cataloging-in-Publication Data**

Knechtges, Paul L.
    Food safety : theory and practice / Paul L. Knechtges.
        p. ; cm.
    Includes bibliographical references and index.
    ISBN-13: 978-0-7637-8556-7 (pbk.)
    ISBN-10: 0-7637-8556-3 (pbk.)
    1. Food--Safety measures.  2. Food contamination—Prevention.  I. Title.
    [DNLM: 1. Food Safety. 2. Food Contamination—prevention & control. WA 695]
RA601.K54 2012
363.19'2—dc23
                                                                          2011019355
6048

Printed in the United States of America

17  16  15  14  13     10 9 8 7 6 5 4 3

# Dedication

*In memory of my grandmother, Mrs. Rena Castelow,
and my Uncle "Pete" Castelow.*

*To Marilyn, your encouragement and patience were
invaluable and allowed me to complete this project on time.*

# Contents

# Preface

My interest in food safety stems from my experiences and the changes that I've observed in the food supply over the years. Having spent my teenage years living and working on family farms, I learned firsthand about raising crops and livestock for subsistence and the market. When I started working in public health many years later, I was responsible for the inspection of food service facilities at military installations in three states and the District of Columbia. At that time, the emphasis was upon using inspection checklists and promoting good sanitary practices during food preparation. Later, when I was assigned overseas and responsible for the safety of food supplies for deployed troops, I learned the importance of safety management and sanitary practices throughout the entire food supply chain. It also became apparent that the agricultural and food processing industries had changed dramatically since my days of working on the farm, which made safety management of the food supply much more challenging. To meet these complex challenges, the concepts of risk analysis and the adoption of food safety management tools became essential. One of the most important food safety management tools to become widely adopted was the Hazard Analysis and Critical Control Point (HACCP) system.

When I was first asked to teach a graduate level course in food safety to environmental health students, I surveyed the published food safety textbooks. Many outstanding textbooks were available on particular topics in food safety, but I could not find a textbook that provided a comprehensive overview of food safety. Specifically, I desired a textbook with a "farm-to-fork" perspective that also explained the scientific basis and public health rationale for food safety standards. In addition, I wanted a book that covered biological, chemical, and physical agents of foodborne diseases. After several years of teaching, I decided to write an introductory textbook on food safety. The amount of information on various food safety topics was overwhelming. Despite the fact that I started with a detailed outline, I was constantly faced with deciding which details to include or exclude from the manuscript during my research. Overall, I believe this textbook covers critically important topics and organizes them in a manner to facilitate teaching students who are, or who may become, food safety professionals.

Each chapter in this textbook begins with a complete set of learning objectives and ends with an extensive list of references and other useful resources. The references and resources can be used to develop case studies and also for additional research. By design, the writing style is concise and to the point, and the textbook serves as a central reference for students and instructors. Figures and tables are used throughout the text to assist students in understanding important concepts related to food safety. Chapters are arranged in a logical order and build upon information provided in the preceding chapters. The first three chapters introduce the student to the history of food safety and the agents of foodborne diseases. The fourth chapter introduces the student to the fundamental principles of food safety. Chapter 5 provides an overview of important engineering controls and technology for food safety, which have become indispensable to controlling hazards in the modern food industry. In keeping with current trends, Chapter 6 is devoted to the risk and hazard analysis of foods, including the principles of the HACCP system. To provide students with an appreciation of the value and limitations of food testing, an overview of laboratory and analytical methods is provided in Chapter 7. Finally, Chapter 8 pulls together the topics from previous chapters into a farm-to-fork perspective regarding safety management of the food supply.

The *Code of Federal Regulations* (CFR) is also frequently cited parenthetically in this book. The format used is "title-CFR-part and subpart" (e.g., 21 CFR 120.1). Regulations sometimes change as a result of the rule making process, and the contents and/or part numbers may be different from those originally cited in this book. Therefore, the student is encouraged to learn how to navigate online versions of the CFR in order to find the most up-to-date regulatory requirements. This provides a valuable learning opportunity for the student. At the time this book went into production, President Obama signed into law the Food Safety Modernization Act, heralded as the most comprehensive revision of food safety laws in over 70 years. Undoubtedly, new regulations will emerge as a result of this statute over the next several years, and instructors and students will need to use the Internet to access current food safety regulations.

# Acknowledgments

I am extremely grateful for the guidance and quality of education provided to me many years ago by the professors of the Environmental Health Program at East Carolina University. Dr. Bernard Kane was particularly influential in helping me to understand and comprehend the principles of sanitary microbiology and food sanitation.

I would like to thank the federal employees who helped me locate key information necessary for this book. In particular, I am grateful for the help of those assigned to the Economic Research Service of the U.S. Department of Agriculture (USDA), the National Center for Environmental Health of the U.S. Centers for Disease Control and Prevention (CDC), and the Center for Food Safety and Applied Nutrition of the U.S. Food and Drug Administration (FDA).

Many of the figures and tables used in this book were obtained or adapted from U.S. government agencies such as the CDC, USDA, FDA, the U.S. Government Accountability Office (GAO), and the U.S. Environmental Protection Agency (EPA). Furthermore, the work of all those cited as references in this book is greatly admired and appreciated. You have made lasting contributions to food safety research, practice, and education.

Finally, thank you to the following reviewers for their valuable feedback on the manuscript: Ed G.M. van Klink, DVM, PhD, Agr, Dipl. ECVPH, University of Minnesota; JoAnna Foegeding, Distance Education Coordinator, Department of Food, Bioprocessing, and Nutrition Sciences, North Carolina State University; Dr. John Orta, RD, FADA, California State University, Los Angeles; and Pera Jambazian, DrPH, MS, RD, California State University, Los Angeles.

# CHAPTER 1

# History and Overview of Food Safety

## LEARNING OBJECTIVES

1. Briefly describe the early history of foodborne diseases, and recognize important events and times in history that contributed to food safety.
2. Explain how the canning industry revolutionized food preservation, and describe the new hazards introduced into the food supply during the early days of canning.
3. Describe the history of milk consumption and why milk became a major source of several diseases in the late nineteenth and early twentieth centuries.
4. List the solutions to controlling food hazards in the canning and dairy industries, and explain how these transformed canned food and dairy products into some of the safest foods in the marketplace today.
5. List and describe the major events leading to development of the meat packing industry and its regulation by the federal government.
6. Describe the primary methods used by meat inspectors throughout much of the twentieth century, and explain the limitations of these methods.
7. Explain how most foodborne hazards associated with the consumption of molluscan shellfish are intimately linked to the environment.
8. List the key events and describe the history of regulating chemicals in the U.S. food supply.
9. Describe the events that led to more comprehensive regulation of pesticide exposures, particularly in foods.
10. Provide examples of food safety practices implemented throughout the food supply chain that made a difference in the rates of foodborne diseases.
11. Describe the historical and current roles of epidemiology in the recognition and control of infectious and foodborne diseases.
12. Explain how disease surveillance contributes to food safety.
13. Explain why the reported number of foodborne illnesses represents only a fraction of the total number in the population.

14. List and describe the basic steps to investigating a foodborne illness outbreak.
15. List the different categories of foodborne diseases, and recognize the types of etiologic agents responsible for these different foodborne diseases.
16. Recall estimates on the total number of foodborne illnesses in the United States, and explain why precise numbers are difficult to derive.
17. Recall estimates on the burden of foodborne illnesses in terms of economic costs.
18. Explain why the burden of foodborne illnesses is important to estimate in terms of morbidity, mortality, and costs.
19. List and describe current and future trends that will influence the practice of food safety.
20. Define food safety, and describe the roles of various disciplines involved with food safety.

## HISTORICAL ASPECTS OF FOOD SAFETY

The availability and nutritional adequacy of food have been driving forces of human evolution and civilization. Prior to the domestication of plants and animals, some 12,000 to 10,000 years ago, humans lived an existence as hunters and gatherers. Survival of a group or tribe of people depended on the relative abundance of wild animals and plants and the ability of its members to hunt and gather the fauna and flora, respectively. People often lived a nomadic existence, following the migration of animals or moving during seasonal changes in the weather. Scholars generally believe the domestication of plants and animals occurred gradually over millennia through a series of accidents or subconscious behavior until, at some point, humans consciously manipulated other forms of life to their advantage and survival (Zeder 2006). The adoption of agriculture and the domestication of plants and animals reduced the need for nomadic lifestyles among groups of people. Communities of humans became more permanent and grew larger, allowing skilled craftspersons to barter or sell their services in exchange for the necessities of life—principally food. Eventually, as agriculture flourished and produced larger food surpluses, these communities grew into cities that furthered the pursuits of government, art, and technology for which human civilization is known.

With the adoption of agriculture and a relatively reliable source of food, civilization came to face new challenges to human survival. Among these challenges were communicable diseases, a leading cause of death in the history of city dwellers. Although humans have long suffered from parasites with which they have coevolved, the domestication of animals allowed some variants of parasites and other pathogens to be transmitted from animals to humans (Cox 2002; Diamond 1999). Furthermore, ancient people were ignorant of disease causation, and they unknowingly created environmental conditions that facilitated the transmission of communicable diseases. Specifically, disease transmission was enhanced by poor protection and contamination of food and water, accumulation of human and animal wastes, thriving populations of rats and other disease vectors, poor hygiene, and overcrowded conditions. Larger food surpluses also facilitated expeditions of travelers to explore, colonize, and trade in other lands and to conduct military campaigns. These travelers often exported diseases to other regions of the world and returned home with new diseases. It would take millennia before science, engineering, and the concepts of public health enlightened people about the causes and control of diseases.

In early historical writings, it is not easy to ascertain a distinction between foodborne diseases and other diseases (e.g., waterborne, vectorborne, person-to-person). Anthropologists and other scientists attempt to deduce or infer the types of foodborne diseases people in early civilizations suffered from, but the physical evidence is very limited. Using available information, Morton Satin wrote a popular book on the impact of foodborne diseases on human history (Satin 2007). Apparently, ancient humans were exposed to a number of foodborne hazards ranging from parasitic diseases to chronic toxicity caused by heavy metals such as lead. These hazards provide possible explanations for several events in recorded history. Tales of witchcraft and demonic possession, for example, may actually have been behaviors resulting from the consumption of toxins produced by several molds that grow in food grains. These toxins can cause multiple symptoms and several types of diseases when consumed in sufficient quantities, including hallucinations and bizarre behavior. Lead toxicity, which can manifest as many different health problems, also afflicted people throughout history. In ancient Rome, lead was used in water pipes and cooking and eating vessels, and Romans used lead-containing syrup to sweeten wines. Mental impairment associated with neurotoxicity from ingesting lead is often credited for the demise of the Roman aristocracy, eventually leading to the downfall of the Roman Empire.

Although most food contamination was either unintentional or accidental, foods were also purposely contaminated throughout history. One purpose was to poison individuals or political leaders, that is, commit murder or assassination. Another purpose was to swindle individuals who purchased foods in an act known as economic adulteration. Adulterants, inedible or innutritious ingredients, were added to increase the weight or change the appearance of foods, making them more appealing or disguising or hiding inferior quality, such as meats from diseased animals. Sometimes, food adulterants were toxic, and the greedy act of economic adulteration had serious health consequences. To discourage adulteration of foods, over the centuries governments instituted laws forbidding it that often were backed up with harsh or even cruel punishments. Yet, despite a long history of laws and punishments, the problem of economic adulteration persisted through the centuries. Although less common today, unscrupulous individuals and companies still commit economic adulteration. A recent example of this practice is the adulteration of Chinese infant formula with melamine, an industrial chemical that is toxic in sufficient concentrations (Food Safety and Inspection Service [FSIS] 2009). This tragic event resulted in kidney disease among 50,000 Chinese children, including 16,000 hospitalizations and at least six deaths.

During the eighteenth and nineteenth centuries, science greatly advanced the understanding and knowledge about the causation of diseases. The greatest leap forward is known as the golden age of microbiology, dating from about 1860 to 1920 (Weeks 2008). During this time, the germ theory of disease was espoused, and scientists actively competed to identify the causative agents of infectious diseases. Along with these advancements came new culturing and staining methods for microbial cells, which greatly expanded laboratory testing capabilities (Guardino 2005). At the same time, methods to destroy or reduce microbial populations were being developed and refined. Among them was a mild thermal treatment later called pasteurization, named after its developer, Louis Pasteur. This and other microbial control technologies, such as food canning and refrigeration, were greatly improved in the late nineteenth and early twentieth centuries (see Table 1-1). Although initially developed to preserve foods and their freshness, the benefits of these technologies in foodborne disease prevention also became apparent. Heat treatments kill bacterial pathogens or reduce their populations in potentially contaminated foods, and refrigeration retards the growth of bacterial pathogens in foods during transport and storage.

**Table 1-1** Key Historical Events in Food Safety

| Year | Event |
| --- | --- |
| 1804 | Nicholas Appert opens the first vacuum bottling plant in France, predecessor to the canning industry. |
| 1825 | Patent granted in United States for preserving food in tin cans. |
| 1862 | Louis Pasteur develops a mild thermal process to prevent the spoilage of wine and beer, later called "pasteurization." |
| 1873 | First successful refrigerator compressor is developed in Sweden. |
| 1874 | Pressure-cooking "retort" was invented for canning operations. |
| 1882 | First commercial pasteurization equipment is manufactured in Germany. |
| 1893 | Recommendations are made to certify and pasteurize milk to prevent milk-borne diseases. |
| 1905 | Upton Sinclair publishes his book *The Jungle*, raising public awareness of unwholesome meat packing practices. |
| 1906 | Pure Food and Drug Act and Meat Inspection Act are passed by the U.S. Congress. |
| 1908 | Pasteurization of milk becomes compulsory in Chicago. |
| 1916 | Piggly Wiggly opens in Memphis, Tennessee, becoming the first self-service grocery store, forerunner of the modern supermarket. |
| 1917 | Frozen foods become available at retail. |
| 1920s | Household refrigerators with freezer compartments become commercially available. |
| 1921 | First White Castle fast-food hamburger restaurant opens in Wichita, Kansas. |
| 1923 | Clarence Birdseye invents a method for rapid freezing of foods and later sells it to a food company. |
| 1923 | Botulism Retort Cook Method/Standard for safe canning is adopted by industry. |
| 1925 | National Shellfish Certification Program is established. |
| 1927 | U.S. Public Health Service's milk ordinance and code is published, forerunner of the current Grade A Pasteurized Milk Ordinance. |
| 1930 | Quick-frozen foods (vegetables, fruits, seafood, meats) are first sold to the public. |
| 1934 | *Restaurant Sanitation Regulations* are proposed by the U.S. Public Health Service in cooperation with the Conference of State and Territorial Health Officers and the National Restaurant Code Authority. This is the predecessor of the current Food Code published by the U.S. Food and Drug Administration. |
| 1938 | Food, Drug, and Cosmetic Act is passed by the U.S. Congress, replacing the obsolete 1906 law. |
| 1942 | Collection of national surveillance data on nontyphoid salmonellosis is started. |
| 1947 | Federal Fungicide, Insecticide, and Rodenticide Act is passed by U.S. Congress. |
| 1950 | Approximately 80% of farms and 90% of urban homes in the United States have a refrigerator. |
| 1950 | The Association of State and Territorial Health Officers authorizes a council to annually determine which diseases should be "notifiable" or reportable to federal health authorities. |
| 1952 | Forerunner of the current *Morbidity and Mortality Weekly Report (MMWR)* is published. |
| 1954 | Swanson makes its first frozen TV dinner. |

| | |
|---|---|
| 1954 | Miller Pesticide Amendment delineates procedures to set safety limits for pesticides on raw agricultural commodities. |
| 1958 | Food Additives Amendment: Manufacturers of new food additives must establish safety. Delaney Clause added to ban food additives that cause cancer in laboratory animals. List of substances generally recognized as safe (GRAS) first published by FDA in the *Federal Register*. |
| 1960 | Color Additive Amendment requires manufacturers to establish safety of coloring agents added to foods, drugs, and cosmetics. |
| 1962 | "Potentially hazardous food" (PHF) is defined as perishable food that supports rapid and progressive growth of infectious or toxigenic microorganisms. |
| 1982 | Interstate Shellfish Sanitation Conference is established to foster and promote shellfish sanitation and safety in cooperation with the National Shellfish Sanitation Program. |
| 1996 | Landmark rule on Pathogen Reduction/Hazard Analysis Critical Control Point (HACCP) Systems is issued by USDA to meat processors. |
| 1996 | Food Quality Protection Act passed by U.S. Congress requiring stricter standards and safety reviews for pesticides residues on food and feed crops. |
| 2005 | "Temperature controlled for safety" (TCS) food is used as an equivalent and transition term for PHF in the *Food Code*. |

During the twentieth century, the preservation of foods using industrial canning and refrigeration/freezing technologies had a significant impact on American consumption patterns. In 1900, more than 60% of the U.S. population was considered rural, with some areas being nearly all rural or consisting only of small towns (U.S. Census Bureau 2010). Families often had gardens for fresh vegetables, and processing and preserving fresh foods at home were common activities. With the exception of certain meats and grains, local farmers produced foods for nearby populations, thus limiting the need to transport foods long distances. As farmers became more productive using new agricultural technologies, and the availability of foods became greater, foods could be stored and transported farther using canning, refrigeration, and freezing technologies. The new food processing technologies, along with changing social norms and higher family incomes, coincided with a shift in American consumer demand for more processed and convenience foods (Morrison, Buzby, and Wells 2010). Americans also began adding different foods to their diets. Changing consumer demand, in turn, influenced the development of new food production and processing technologies, and this ultimately influenced the nature of potential hazards in the U.S. food supply.

## The Canning Industry

An example of how food production and processing technologies can change the nature of food hazards is best illustrated by the retort canning process. In 1804, Nicholas Appert opened the first vacuum bottling plant in France to boil and hermetically seal meats and vegetables in jars (Fellows 2009). Napoleon Bonaparte had offered a prize to anyone who could find a way to preserve foods for soldiers and sailors during long military campaigns as an incentive for this accomplishment. Just a few years later, Appert's work became the basis for similar processes that used iron or tin-plated canisters (i.e., cans) instead of glass jars (Satin 2007). These canning processes were successfully used to preserve foods, despite the fact that the underlying reasons for preventing spoilage were not yet understood. These reasons would not be revealed until the golden age of microbiology, when it was determined that the destruction of spoilage microorganisms was responsible. Nonetheless, with enhancements in production capability, food canning became a thriving industry that started in the mid-1800s and continues today.

The heating process in canning killed many common pathogenic microorganisms, but early canning techniques also introduced at least two unanticipated hazards to the food supply. The first is botulism, a deadly disease caused by toxins produced from a spore-forming bacterium called *Clostridium botulinum*. Botulism was not a new disease to humanity, but the conditions necessary for the formation of botulinum toxins were enhanced by the canning process. *C. botulinum* is a common soil-dwelling bacterium frequently encountered in vegetable and animal products. To grow and produce botulinum toxins, however, this bacterium requires anaerobic and low-acid conditions. Whenever these conditions do not exist, *C. botulinum* forms tough and dormant structures called spores, which can even withstand boiling temperatures. For many years, canning was done at boiling temperatures, allowing *C. botulinum* spores to survive. With non-acidic foods and anoxic conditions in cans, *C. botulinum* spores could germinate and produce their deadly toxins in the food product. The spores of *C. botulinum* can be destroyed at temperatures above boiling, but pressurization is required to achieve these temperatures. In 1874, a pressure-cooking "retort" was invented that raised temperatures above boiling and reduced the time necessary for canning operations (Fellows 2009). But the identification of *C. botulinum* had not yet occurred, and the relationship between temperature, canned foods, and botulism was not understood. This changed in 1897 when *C. botulinum* was described following a foodborne outbreak in Belgium (Centers for Disease Control and Prevention [CDC] 1998).

Poor canning practices were not uncommon in the early twentieth century. Some commercial operations and many home canners did not use retorts or pressure cookers. And if a retort canning process was not carefully controlled, the cans may not have been adequately heated to destroy *C. botulinum* spores. During and following World War I, several epidemics of botulism in the United States raised public awareness about unsafe commercial canning practices (Tauxe and Esteban 2007). The canning industry subsequently funded research on safe canning methods, and in 1923, the industry adopted the *botulism retort cook* method as a standard (Tauxe 2002). Over the course of the twentieth century, commercially canned products developed a reputation of being very safe, with the majority of reported botulism cases from 1950 through 1996 associated with home-processed foods (CDC 1998). However, following an outbreak of botulism in 1973 from commercially canned vichyssoise soup, which was determined to be caused by defects in the cans, the U.S. government codified canning standards into federal regulations (Tauxe and Esteban 2007).

A second hazard introduced by the canning process is contamination of foods with the heavy metal lead. For many years, the seams of tin cans were sealed with lead-based solder. In many cases, the lead content of the solder exceeded 50%, and poor construction or sloppy applications of solder allowed contact with the food inside, causing the lead to leach into the foods—especially if the food was acidic (Satin 2007). The toxic effects of lead are very much dose-dependent, and researchers believe that high lead levels in canned foods in the early years of canning contributed to several maladies. Over the years, manufacturers employed several strategies to reduce the amount of lead exposure from canned foods, including coating the inside of cans with enamel. Other sources of lead (e.g., lead paint chips and leaded gasoline) were also identified as contributors to lead exposure. During the 1980s, several research studies identified subclinical effects on the cognitive development of children and fetuses from very low levels of lead exposure. Consequently, the Centers for Disease Control and Prevention (CDC Advisory Committee on Childhood Lead Poisoning Prevention 2007) lowered the blood lead levels of concern in children to 10 micrograms per deciliter (μg/dL). Canning manufacturers voluntarily began eliminating lead solder in cans, and over the decade of the 1980s, the percentage of food cans with lead solder decreased from more than 90% to approximately 6% (Mushak and Crocetti 1990). In an effort to further reduce lead exposures from foods, the U.S. Food and Drug Administration (FDA) banned the use of lead-soldered cans in 1995.

## The Milk and Dairy Industry

Milk and dairy products, such as cheese, have been a part of human diets in many societies for millennia. The first cows were probably domesticated for meat purposes around 8,000 to 10,000 years ago, but it was probably several thousand years later before milk was harvested from cows and other animals for human consumption (Ajmone-Marsan, Garcia, Lenstra 2010; Loftus et al. 1994). The key turning point in milk consumption was natural selection for the lactase gene in human populations, which permitted humans to digest the lactose sugar in milk (Burger et al. 2007). Those who do not possess the lactase gene suffer from a condition called lactose intolerance after consuming dairy products. Those with the lactase gene were able to incorporate milk in their diets, adding a rich source of calcium and energy. The lactase gene is geographically prevalent among people with a history of dairy farming and herding. Over time, milk and dairy products became a major food group in the diets of Western societies.

Milk was also an ideal vehicle for transmitting pathogenic microorganisms, some responsible for serious and deadly infectious diseases. Contamination of milk with pathogens occurred through direct contact with surfaces in the environment, particularly on the farm or from human contact, and pathogens were excreted in the udders of infected animals. This contamination hazard was exacerbated when bacterial pathogens rapidly multiplied in unrefrigerated milk. With its neutral pH, ample nutrients, and moisture, milk is an ideal growth medium for bacteria. When milk was produced and consumed locally from local farms or family-owned cows, milk-borne diseases were not widely reported. However, as cities grew and the demand for milk became greater, dairies became larger operations, and milk was shipped longer distances and in greater quantities. All of these factors probably contributed to the contamination of milk, growth of bacterial pathogens, and wider dissemination of milk-borne diseases.

The significant role that milk played in the transmission of infectious diseases was recognized in the late nineteenth and early twentieth centuries. Contaminated milk was implicated in epidemics of typhoid fever, diphtheria, tuberculosis, severe streptococcal infections, brucellosis, Q fever, dysentery, and many other diseases (Steele 1954; Tauxe and Esteban 2007). At the time, mortality from infectious diseases was exceptionally high in the cities, and although unsafe water supplies were probably responsible for most enteric disease deaths, milk was believed to play an important role in childhood mortality. And childhood mortality was very high in the cities. From 1890 to 1892 in New York City, for example, more than one-third of all deaths occurred in children younger than 2 years old (Waserman 1972).

The campaign to provide safe milk to children in cities is often credited to a pediatrician named Dr. Henry L. Coit. After the death of his infant son, Dr. Coit embarked on a project to protect children from unsafe and unhygienic milk, and in 1893 he proposed a plan to produce "Certified Milk" (Waserman 1972). This plan entailed a medical commission to establish standards for the hygienic (i.e., sanitary) production of milk, and the conduction of inspections and performance of milk testing. Around the same time, another solution was promoted by the co-owner of Macy's Department Store in New York: pasteurization of milk (Tunick 2009). Over the next two decades, research was conducted on methods to produce safe milk, and debate ensued over the benefits of certification versus pasteurization of milk (CDC 1999). Several municipalities encouraged and even mandated the pasteurization of milk. Finally, in 1923, an officer in the U.S. Public Health Service combined the two processes of certification and pasteurization (Tauxe and Esteban 2007). In 1924, the U.S. Public Health Service produced a voluntary *Standard Milk Ordinance* to assist state and local milk control agencies (Food and Drug Administration [FDA] 2009a). In 1927, a code was added to the ordinance to assist in determining satisfactory compliance with the ordinance. This ordinance with the code is the forerunner of the current *Grade "A" Pasteurized Milk Ordinance* (FDA 2009a).

Over the next several decades, pasteurization techniques were further improved, and pasteurized milk was widely promoted over raw milk across the United States, making a tremendous impact on the safety of milk supplies. For example, in 1938, approximately 25% of all food- and waterborne disease outbreaks were associated with milk (FDA 2009a; LeJeune and Rajala-Schultz 2009). Today, milk is considered one of the safest foods available, accounting for less than 1% of all foodborne illness outbreaks (FDA 2009a). And most of the milk-borne disease outbreaks that occur nowadays are associated with the consumption of raw milk or postpasteurization contamination of dairy products (Oliver, Jayarao, Almeida 2005). Although the disease risks of raw milk are greater compared with pasteurized milk, some consumers still prefer raw milk and/or dairy products made from raw milk. Many states have instituted standards for raw milk producers, but the risks of raw milk still remain greater compared with pasteurized milk (Oliver, Boor, et al. 2009).

## The Meat Packing Industry

In the United States, prior to the Civil War, pork was the principal meat that was packed and shipped for sale. Fresh-cut pork could be easily preserved using various salt compounds, whereas beef and mutton did not preserve as well using these methods (Azzam and Anderson 1996). Instead, most cattle and sheep were herded or "driven" to sites for slaughter and meat packing near the points of sale. This began to change just before, during, and after the Civil War with the westward expansion of people and railroads. With railroads, livestock could be shipped greater distances in a shorter period of time for less cost. Larger and more centrally located stockyards, slaughter plants, and meat packing houses began to emerge. With the introduction of refrigerated railcars in the

1870s, dressed carcasses and packed meat could be shipped longer distances without spoilage, allowing meat packers to move farther west from the East Coast. The development of electricity and artificial refrigeration in the 1880s was another great leap forward for the industry. Prior to this time, packing houses could operate only during the cold months. After the introduction of refrigeration, meat packing houses could operate year-round. The midwestern United States became the major location for stockyards, livestock slaughter, meat packing, and shipping around the country.

For the most part, federal government oversight of meat safety was virtually nonexistent until 1884, when President Chester Arthur signed an act that established the Bureau of Animal Industry (FSIS 2007). The primary function of this new bureau was to prevent diseased animals from becoming human food, but with only 20 employees and a small budget, the bureau's mission was overreaching. During this era, competition in the meat industry was escalating, and many states attempted to ban beef from the Midwest because it was not subjected to local inspections. The Supreme Court, however, overturned the state laws in 1890 (Wade 1991). Around the same time, the United States was exporting livestock and other animal products to foreign countries, but the foreign countries were imposing stringent restrictions on U.S. imports. To better compete in foreign trade, an inspection act was approved in 1890 and later amended in 1891. Under the act, and at the request of meat packers or foreign governments, inspections and certifications were performed for exports of salted pork, bacon, livestock, and cattle destined for slaughter when the meat was to be exported (FSIS 2007). Microscopic examinations were also conducted on exported pork products to certify that they were free of trichinae, a type of microscopic worm that becomes encysted in the muscle tissues of pigs. By 1900, federal inspectors were working in 149 packing houses in 46 cities (Wade 1991).

The public still voiced concerns about the quality and safety of meat products from packing houses. This concern reached a pinnacle when a book titled *The Jungle* by Upton Sinclair was published in the year 1905. Mr. Sinclair had visited Chicago's Packinghouse district to research his book about the capitalistic exploitation of workers and the blind pursuit of profits (Wade 1991). But it was his grotesque descriptions of unsanitary conditions and the adulteration of meat products that captured the attention and lead to the outrage of the American public. People were horrified by the heretofore unknown preparation and handling of their meats. The resulting furor spurred federal investigations and congressional action. In 1906, Congress passed and President Theodore Roosevelt signed the Federal Pure Food and Drug Act and the Federal Meat Inspection Act (Hinderliter 2006). Among its provisions, the Federal Pure Food and Drug Act prohibited the addition of ingredients to foods that would "substitute for the food, conceal damage, pose a health hazard, or constitute a filthy or decomposed substance" (FDA 2009b). The Bureau of Chemistry (forerunner of the U.S. Food and Drug Administration, or FDA) was charged with administering the provisions of this law. Under the Federal Meat Inspection Act, inspections became mandatory for preslaughter livestock and for every postmortem carcass. This act also authorized the Bureau of Animal Industry to set federal standards for sanitary operations of slaughterhouses, and it granted access by the bureau's inspectors to monitor and enforce these standards. By 1907, the Bureau of Animal Industry had grown to more than 2,200 inspectors and was responsible for monitoring approximately 700 facilities (FSIS 2006). This bureau would eventually become the Food Safety and Inspection Service (FSIS) under the U.S. Department of Agriculture (USDA).

In 1906, nearly all the tests performed on meats during inspections were organoleptic (Hinderliter 2006). In other words, the tests of the meat were based on the inspector's senses of sight, smell, and touch. The only scientific tool used for meat inspection was the microscopic examination of pork carcasses for trichinae, but this practice was completely abandoned by the year 1907 (Wade 1991). The rationale for abandoning this practice was that thorough cooking of meat made it safe, so there was no need to conduct the tests. Whereas organoleptic tests of meats can identify several animal diseases and detect some parasites, they are ineffective in detecting contamination with pathogenic microorganisms and chemicals. Nonetheless, the organoleptic tests remained the meat inspector's primary tools for most of the twentieth century. As diseased animals became less of a problem over the years, the inspector's focus changed to detecting filth and fecal contamination during the slaughter process (Institute of Medicine [IOM] 2003). At the same time, classical milk-borne and waterborne diseases declined, and other foodborne diseases associated with meat and poultry products such as salmonellosis began to emerge (Foster 1997).

A major turning point in the meat inspection process occurred following a large foodborne disease outbreak in 1993, resulting in hundreds of cases and hospitalizations—including several deaths (Bell et al. 1994). The disease was traced to a fast-food restaurant chain that served hamburgers contaminated with a bacterium called *E. coli* O157:H7. The source of contamination was determined to be the beef itself, and contamination was spread by the meat mixing and grinding operations. Prior to the outbreak, traditional meat inspections failed to identify *E. coli* O157:H7 in the beef, and the *E. coli* O157:H7 bacteria were not destroyed in the hamburgers because of insufficient cooking. This incident highlighted how the combination of unsafe practices throughout the food supply chain can culminate in large and distributed outbreaks. In 1996, the USDA proposed regulations requiring meat processors to implement a food safety management tool called the Hazard Analysis and Critical Control Point (HACCP) system. In addition, certain meat and poultry processors were required to perform laboratory testing to detect fecal bacteria (i.e., generic *E. coli*), *E. coli* O157:H7, and *Salmonella* and to verify the effectiveness of the HACCP system.

Throughout much of the twentieth century, the control of foodborne infections from meat products emphasized cooking. Indeed, the risks of most foodborne infections can be minimized by good food preparation and cooking practices. But the most effective food safety strategies emphasize controls throughout the food supply chain. This is exemplified by the control of trichinellosis (or trichinosis) over the last century. Several species of trichinae are capable of causing trichinellosis, but the most common species associated with pork products is *Trichinella spirilis*. As described earlier, trichinae are parasitic worms whose larvae encyst themselves in the muscle tissues of pigs. When undercooked pork containing these larvae is consumed by humans, the larvae are released by stomach acid and pepsin and invade the mucosa of the small intestine, where they molt several times before becoming adult worms (National Agricultural Library [NAL] 2010). These worms then migrate into the lumen of the small intestine to mate, and the gravid female then reinvades the intestinal mucosa. After several days, the female begins to shed larvae that enter the lymphatic system. From the lymphatic system, the larvae enter the bloodstream and travel to several tissues, causing a variety of disturbances. Larvae that reach striated muscle tissue become encysted in the muscle. A variety of signs and symptoms appears over the course of several weeks, and cardiac and neurologic complications may occur, sometimes leading to death from myocardial failure. Berton Roueche provides an excellent literary description of a trichinellosis outbreak in his short story *A Pig from Jersey* (1988).

American swine were infected with trichinae in the year 1900 at a rate exceeding 2.5% (Namminga 1998). This is why many European countries imposed import bans on American pork products until the federal government could certify them trichinae-free (Wade 1991). Many Americans became infected from eating undercooked pork products during the early twentieth century. As late as the 1940s, an estimated 16% of the U.S. population had trichinellosis (Wright, Kerr, Jacobs 1943). Efforts to reduce trichinae infections involved breaking the parasite's life cycle on the farm, treatment of pork products, and surveillance of human trichinellosis cases. Pork producers, in cooperation with the USDA, formed a trichinae-free program that emphasized changes in feeding and husbandry practices. The most important preventive measures were not allowing pigs to be fed uncooked garbage and excluding rodents (hosts of trichinae) from pig-rearing areas. Federal regulations also required treatment of certain pork-containing products to destroy trichinae (9 CFR 318.10). Reported human cases of trichinellosis dropped over the twentieth century, and during 2002–2007, only 66 cases of trichinellosis were reported to the Centers for Disease Control and Prevention (Kennedy et al. 2009). Of those cases where the source of trichinae was identified, only 19% were associated with consuming pork. The remaining cases were associated with nonpork sources, most often from consuming bear meat.

## Shellfish Sanitation, Environmental Contamination, and Food Additives/Adulterants

Shellfish are considered a gastronomic delicacy in the Western world, and an important source of protein in many parts of the world, particularly in coastal villages and fishing communities. In the late nineteenth and early twentieth centuries, public health officials in America and Europe were concerned about numerous outbreaks of disease from eating raw oysters, clams, and mussels. This concern moved to the forefront of public attention in 1924, when a large outbreak of typhoid fever swept across the United States among those who consumed oysters taken from sewage-contaminated waters (Tauxe and Esteban 2007). With more than 1,500 reported cases and 150 deaths in 12 cities, this outbreak alarmed the public and resulted in a loss of consumer confidence in the safety of shellfish. In response, the Surgeon General of the U.S. Public Health Service called a Conference on Shellfish Sanitation in 1925, where prevention principles and controls were formulated and incorporated into the National Shellfish Certification Program (Interstate Shellfish Sanitation Conference [ISSC]/FDA 2007). The purpose of the program was to prevent illnesses from fresh and fresh-frozen molluscan shellfish (oysters, clams, mussels, and scallops) by encouraging standardized regulations and industry practices among the states. The program was renamed the National Shellfish Sanitation Program (NSSP), and in 1982, the Interstate Shellfish Sanitation Conference (ISSC) was formed from participating states, industry representatives, FDA, and other federal agencies. The ISSC still functions today, providing a forum for state regulatory officials to establish uniform guidelines for shellfish safety (ISSC/FDA 2007).

Foodborne diseases from molluscan shellfish epitomize the relationship between the environment, pollution, and food safety. Molluscan shellfish are filter feeders that actively pump water through their bodies to strain plankton and particles. Along with concentrating the plankton, the molluscan shellfish can also concentrate pathogenic microorganisms from the water. If the shellfish beds are located in waters polluted with sewage, they will accumulate and concentrate the pathogens in significant quantities. The risks of infection are increased several-fold when these shellfish are consumed raw or partially cooked. Indeed, many outbreaks of infectious diseases have been associated with the consumption of raw or undercooked shellfish (Huss, Ababouch, Gram 2004; IOM 1991). Pathogens known to be transmitted by shellfish include certain aquatic bacteria (e.g., *Vibrio* species), enteric bacterial pathogens, and viruses. In 1988 in Shanghai, China, more than 290,000 people contracted hepatitis A after consuming clams harvested from sewage-polluted waters; this was the largest ever recorded foodborne illness outbreak (CDC 1990; Huss et al. 2004).

Control measures for shellfish-borne infectious diseases include sanitary surveys and bacteriologic testing of shellfish harvesting waters, along with sanitary handling and processing procedures (ISSC/FDA 2007). For aquatic bacteria such as *Vibrio* species, sanitary surveys of shellfish harvesting waters are less effective because these bacteria are free-living in the environment. Nonetheless, management plans based on water temperatures and other parameters, along with disease surveillance for human cases, are used to minimize the risks of acquiring *Vibrio* infections.

Shellfish are also sources of exposure to a variety of toxic substances. Certain algae in the aquatic environment are capable of producing a variety of marine toxins. These toxins may accumulate in the aquatic food chain and enter the human food supply with seafood. Molluscan shellfish are especially efficient at concentrating toxigenic algae and their toxins. Depending on the type and amount of toxins in the shellfish tissues, intoxication syndromes can range in severity from gastrointestinal disturbances to neurotoxicity—including "memory loss, paralysis and death" (Huss et al. 2004). Unlike with infectious agents, cooking the shellfish has very little effect on the marine toxins. Although shellfish intoxication syndromes have been known for centuries, the frequency of marine toxins in shellfish and other fish have increased over the decades, primarily because human activities have increased the nutrient loading of local waters. This contributes to the growth of toxigenic algae and events known as "harmful algal blooms" (Glibert et al. 2005), characterized by a population explosion of algae accompanied by an obvious decline in water quality (e.g., eutrophication, red tide). Prevention of shellfish intoxication syndromes from an environmental perspective is challenging. Under the NSSP, the FDA and ISSC recommend a Marine Biotoxin Contingency Plan consisting of an early warning system and bans or limitations on shellfish harvesting, along with other interventions (ISSC/FDA 2007).

Environmental pollution with industrial chemicals and metals is another problem that affects the safety of the human food supply in general—and shellfish in particular. Many environmentally persistent chemicals eventually become part of the sediments in waterways and coastal areas. Because molluscan shellfish are benthic organisms, meaning they live in or on the seabed, they are directly exposed to chemicals and metals in the sediments. Besides being in close proximity to chemical pollutants, shellfish are prone to accumulate environmentally persistent chemicals and metals in their tissues, a process called bioaccumulation. The most infamous case of shellfish and seafood toxicity from industrial pollutants is the mercury poisoning of residents of a fishing city in Japan called Minimata. From 1938 until 1968, a factory dumped wastewater containing methylmercury into the local bay, where it bioaccumulated in the local shellfish and finfish. The residents consumed the tainted seafood over the years, resulting in thousands of birth defects and at least 1,784 deaths. The poisoning permanently affected at least 10,000 people (Imamura, Ide, Yasunaga 2007). This tragedy underscores the importance of regulating environmental pollution to protect the human food supply.

## Regulating Chemicals in the Food Supply

Chemicals enter the food supply either deliberately, unintentionally, or unavoidably. Deliberate addition of chemical substances to human food has occurred for millennia. The primary reasons have been for preservation, flavor, taste, or to impart other desirable characteristics on the foodstuff. As mentioned previously, deliberate addition of chemical substances may also occur for purposes of economic adulteration. In these cases, the consumer usually does not know what adulterant has been added to the food item, and the manufacturer or retailer obviously does not want to reveal the unwanted or substandard ingredient (i.e., adulterant). During the nineteenth century, as food processing became more industrialized, adulteration of foods and beverages became a widespread practice. At that time in the United States, federal legislation covering food adulteration was minimal, and individual states were responsible for legal control of food quality and adulteration (Satin 2007). This began to change around 1870 with a growing public concern over adulterants and the desire for pure foods. Legitimate food manufacturers were also concerned about adulteration because unscrupulous manufacturers could outcompete them by selling inferior food products at lower costs. All of this attention led to the testing of foods for contamination by the Bureau of Chemistry of the USDA in 1883 (Tauxe and Esteban 2007). The new leader of this bureau and testing program was a professor of chemistry, Dr. Harvey W. Wiley.

Under the leadership and direction of Dr. Wiley, the Bureau of Chemistry was relentless in its testing of foods for chemical additives. Dr. Wiley had a personal bias that chemical additives were unnecessary adulterants of foods (FDA 2009b). He even went so far as to have groups of young men voluntarily eat foods containing various chemical additives to test their effects. The press dubbed this group the "Poison Squad" (Satin 2007). Although considered unethical by today's human use standards, the work done by Dr. Wiley and the Poison Squad helped capture the public's and Congress's attention about the problems of food adulteration. Like a perfect storm, Dr. Wiley's work and crusade for pure foods, along with Upton Sinclair's novel *The Jungle*, culminated in congressional action early in the twentieth century.

Starting in 1879, nearly 100 bills had been introduced in Congress to regulate food and drugs, but the Federal Pure Food and Drug Act of 1906 was the first comprehensive legislation finally passed (FDA 2009b). In honor of Dr. Wiley, the legislation was also called the Wiley Act. Along with his contributions to the chemical safety of foods, Dr. Wiley also contributed to food safety by hiring microbiologists who helped transform the canning, egg, and refrigeration industries (Meadows 2006). Unfortunately, Dr. Wiley encountered many conflicts over commercial interests and bureaucratic infighting (Satin 2007). He resigned in 1912 but left the bureau with a much larger staff and budget. Nonetheless, because of the shortcomings of the 1906 Pure Food and Drug Act, the bureau encountered many difficulties with enforcement. In 1913, the act was amended to require that the contents of foods be clearly marked on the outside of the package, that is, labeled. Still, loopholes existed in the legislation that allowed companies to get around food adulteration standards. For example, a product called BRED-SPRED was marketed like jam or jelly, even though it was made from coal tar, grass seed, and other miscellaneous ingredients (Meadows 2006). Because the product was not explicitly called a jam or jelly and had a distinctive name, it was not legally considered adulterated or a misbranded product.

With a changing scope of mission, the Bureau of Chemistry was renamed in 1927 and again in 1930 to its current name, the U.S. Food and Drug Administration (FDA). In 1933, after years of problems with enforcing standards to protect the public from unsafe food and drug products, the new FDA recommended to Congress an overhaul of the outdated 1906 act (Meadows 2006). But legislative battles ensued for 5 years before another act was passed. The precipitating event for a new law was an epidemic of paralysis and deaths from an elixir adulterated with an industrial chemical by the trade name of Lindol, also known as TCOP (tri-ortho-cresyl phosphate). Approximately 107 people, many of them children, died from this tainted elixir, and as many as 50,000 to 100,000 people suffered some degree of paralysis (Meadows 2006; Satin 2007). The new law was called the Federal Food, Drug, and Cosmetic (FD&C) Act of 1938. It gave the FDA unprecedented authority to regulate drugs, and it closed loopholes that permitted abuses in food packaging and quality (FDA 2009b). Furthermore, the FD&C Act established a legal mandate for enforceable food standards, and it permitted the setting of safe tolerances for certain toxic or poisonous substances. Other important provisions of the law were authorizations for factory inspections and the use of injunctions as enforcement tools. Over the years since it was first enacted, the FD&C Act has been amended many times. Eventually, the agency responsible for administering the law (FDA) was transferred from USDA to its current organizational location under the U.S. Department of Health and Human Services (DHHS).

As the rates of cancer increased dramatically in the 1930s and 1940s, the public became increasingly concerned about new chemical additives and other ingredients or contaminants in foods, which of course resulted in congressional actions (Fortin 2009). The Federal Insecticide, Fungicide, and Rodenticide Act (FIFRA) was passed in 1947. Among the mandates of FIFRA were requirements for product label registration of pesticides, and the pesticide manufacturer became responsible for the burden of documenting the safety and efficacy of its products. A few years later, in 1950, the Delaney Committee started a congressional investigation into the safety of various chemicals in foods and cosmetics. The committee's report, issued in 1952, stated that chemicals were being produced at an increasing rate and that existing laws were inadequate to protect the public from unsafe chemicals used as food additives. The report did acknowledge that many chemicals were genuinely needed with the food supply (Hutt 2002). The Delaney Committee's report had a strong influence on the introduction of legislation by Congress over the next 8 years.

During this time, three pieces of legislation were critically important to the premarket evaluation and approval of chemical substances affecting the food supply (Hutt 2002). The first was the Miller Pesticide Amendment of 1954. This legislation authorized the establishment of safe tolerances for pesticides on raw agricultural commodities and certain processed foods. It also required premarket safety and efficacy testing of pesticides.

The second critically important legislation was the Food Additives Amendment of 1958. Under this amendment, the safety of new food additives must be established by the manufacturer prior to marketing, and FDA must grant premarket approval of new food additives. However, for substances with approval and use prior to the amendment (1938–1958), and substances with a known history of safe use, premarket approval was considered unnecessary. Legally, these substances were not considered as food additives per se, but instead became known as prior-sanctioned substances and generally recognized as safe (GRAS) substances. The amendment also made the distinction between direct food additives and indirect food additives; the former were added or incorporated directly into the food, whereas the latter were considered contamination of food from contact with the surfaces of packaging, equipment, and other objects. In retrospect, the most controversial provision of the amendment was called the Delaney Clause. This provision basically required the banning of all substances capable of causing cancer in laboratory animals. As analytical tests for chemicals became much more sensitive, and the complexity of cancer biology became better understood, the Delaney Clause became an anachronism. For example, minute traces of chemicals carcinogenic to animals (not necessarily humans) may be detected in foods, but they may be considered lower risk compared with other naturally occurring carcinogens.

The third critically important legislation for premarket evaluation and approval of chemical substances in foods was the Color Additives Amendment of 1960. Unlike other food additives, color additives and preservatives had been regulated in the United States since 1900, when Congress passed the Color and Preservatives Act of 1900 (Hutt 2002). Mostly because of historical reasons and a Supreme Court decision, the 1960 amendment did not include a general exclusion for color additives similar to the GRAS substances. In other words, manufacturers of food colorings must demonstrate the safety of any and all color additives and petition FDA for premarket approval. The Delaney Clause also applied to color additives, meaning that any color additive was generally banned if demonstrated to cause cancer in laboratory animals.

Starting in the early 1940s and lasting until the late 1970s, an unprecedented increase in agricultural productivity known as the Green Revolution occurred (Parayil 2003). This was achieved by research and development that produced new pesticides, fertilizers, strains of crops, and other technologies and methods. With the Green Revolution, the rate of pesticide discovery, development, and application figuratively "exploded" during the 1940s and 1950s (Klass 2005). But greater pesticide usage also had its critics. In 1962, Rachael Carson's book *Silent Spring* raised public awareness about the risks of pesticide use and was credited with helping to start the modern environmental movement. Over the next 10 years, public concerns and environmental activism helped drive federal action to control toxic chemical exposures—especially pesticides. The FIFRA was amended in 1964 to close several loopholes in the original piece of legislation. Under an Executive Order by President Nixon, the U.S. Environmental Protection Agency (EPA) was established in 1970, and nearly all the federal environmental regulatory activities of the United States were transferred to EPA. In 1972, responsibility for the pesticides program was transferred from USDA, FDA, and other agencies to EPA with further amendments to FIFRA and the FD&C Act. Yet, to this day, three federal agencies (EPA, USDA, and FDA) continue to share various degrees of responsibility for pesticide residues in foods.

The next landmark legislation to affect the regulation of pesticide residues in foods was the Food Quality Protection Act (FQPA) of 1996. Under this act, EPA was directed to develop and implement regulations to protect the food supply from unreasonable risks of pesticide residues. Unlike earlier legislation, the FQPA required a complete overhaul of pesticide and food safety laws. Some of the provisions included stricter safety standards, especially for infants and children, and an evaluation of aggregate and lifetime (cumulative) risks of pesticides with common mechanisms of toxicity. Furthermore, the FQPA required all existing pesticide tolerances in foods be reevaluated within 10 years of the act. With respect to pesticide tolerances, the FQPA defined the term *safe* as "a reasonable certainty that no harm will result from aggregate exposure to the pesticide chemical residue, including all anticipated dietary exposures and all other exposures for which there is reliable information" (Public Law 104-170 of August 3, 1996). Essentially, the FQPA rendered the Delaney Clause of 1958 obsolete. To assist EPA with risk assessments of pesticide residues, USDA was directed to conduct food consumption surveys, collect pesticide usage data for U.S. agriculture, and collect monitoring data for pesticide residues in raw and processed agricultural commodities.

## EPIDEMIOLOGIC INVESTIGATIONS AND SURVEILLANCE

### Origins and Contributions of Epidemiology

Since the earliest days of civilization, certain individuals were astute observers of events associated with prosperous or disastrous consequences for their society. This included the occurrence of disease and death from practices, places, and contact with elements in their environment. Hippocrates (460–377 BCE) of ancient Greece was the first to record his theories of disease occurrence, dismissing supernatural explanations; he also created the terms *endemic* and *epidemic* to distinguish between the relative occurrence of disease in a population (Nelson and Williams 2007). An endemic disease is one that always seems to be present in a population, whereas an epidemic disease may be detectable in a population, but it sometimes occurs in greater numbers or frequency during certain times. Over the centuries that followed, prevailing theories of disease causation were rooted in cultural and religious beliefs of the times. The scientific method had to be adopted before the emergence of the discipline now called epidemiology.

Modern epidemiology as a distinct discipline was developed in the mid-nineteenth century amid widespread infectious diseases in Europe and North America. An epidemiological society was established in London in 1850, and the first book to use the term *epidemiology* was published in 1873 (Rosen 1973). At first, the principal focus of epidemiology was on infectious diseases, but its scope broadened in the late twentieth century to include chronic diseases and determinants of health related to social and behavioral factors, as well as the study of injury prevention. According to the American Epidemiological Society, *epidemiology* is defined as "the study of disease distribution and the determinants of health and disease risk in human populations" (2011). Today, epidemiologists are participants in virtually all efforts to study and control disease and injury, including measuring the benefits and costs of disease or injury interventions. To this end, the definition of epidemiology offered by CDC is somewhat broader: "The study of the distribution and determinants of health-related states or events in specified populations, and the application of this study to the control of health problems" (Dicker et al. 2007).

As the term *epidemiology* implies, the origins of the discipline are rooted in the study of epidemics, that is, an increase of diseases above the expected number in a specific population over period of time. A synonymous term often used for a localized epidemic is an *outbreak* (Dicker et al. 2007). The investigation of epidemics/outbreaks in the late nineteenth and early twentieth centuries rapidly advanced knowledge and understanding of infectious disease transmission. Epidemiology systematically identified the risk factors and determinants of infectious diseases in a population. With additional knowledge of pathogens gained during the golden age of microbiology, health practitioners could more precisely diagnose patients with an infectious disease, and epidemiologists could put together a theoretical framework for disease causation. Diseases could then be classified by the principal modes of transmission (e.g., waterborne, foodborne, vectorborne, person-to-person), and interventions could be designed to break the chain of transmission.

Identification of the etiologic (i.e., causative) agent of a foodborne disease outbreak permits a much better understanding of the epidemiology. However, epidemiologists are capable of identifying common factors in outbreaks without necessarily identifying the etiologic agent. In fact, before the germ theory of disease arose, epidemiologists developed profound insights into the contagious nature of infectious diseases, albeit incomplete or flawed knowledge limited their ability to control many of these diseases effectively (Nelson and Williams 2007). But even in the twenty-first century, with all its knowledge and technology, the etiologic agents of many foodborne disease outbreaks remain unidentified. This is one reason for the distinction between foodborne illnesses and foodborne diseases. An *illness* is a condition of being unwell without necessarily an understanding of the etiology and biology of the condition (Helman 1981). In contrast, a *disease* is a condition that has been diagnosed by a physician with an understanding of the etiology and biology. Thus, a foodborne illness outbreak involves cases where an etiologic agent has not been identified and/or the underlying biology is not fully understood, whereas a foodborne disease outbreak involves diagnosed cases with identification of the etiologic agent(s). Although technically incorrect, the terms *foodborne illness* and *foodborne disease* are often used interchangeably.

An important revelation from early epidemiologic investigations was the role of human disease carriers in foodborne disease transmission. The first established case of an asymptomatic and healthy carrier of typhoid fever in the United States was a woman by the name of Mary Mallon. During the years of 1900–1907 and 1915, while working as a cook, Ms. Mallon was responsible for infecting at least 47 people with typhoid fever, with at least 3 deaths (Leavitt 1996). Typhoid fever was a notorious killer in the nineteenth and early twentieth centuries. With the introduction of urban sanitation and water filtration/chlorination, typhoid fever began to wane but nonetheless remained an important public health threat. Following a typhoid fever outbreak at a rented summer home in Long Island, New York, the owners hired a Ph.D. sanitary engineer by the name of George Soper to investigate the source of the outbreak. Using a process of elimination and field epidemiologic investigations, Dr. Soper developed a strong suspicion that a cook, Ms. Mallon, was responsible for a series of typhoid fever outbreaks in different homes.

Dr. Soper had a reputation of being arrogant and overbearing, and after Ms. Mallon refused to provide him with samples of her feces, urine, and blood for laboratory testing, he recruited assistance from the New York City Health Department (Leavitt 1996). A physician and health inspector by the name of Dr. S. Josephine Baker implored Ms. Mallon to provide specimens for laboratory testing, and when she again refused, Ms. Mallon was forcibly taken to the hospital by the police. After finding high levels of the bacteria responsible for typhoid in her feces, Ms. Mallon was kept isolated from society in a bungalow for several years. While being held against her will, Ms. Mallon was subjected to specimen collection for routine laboratory testing, where it was determined that she did not consistently shed the typhoid bacteria. She was released in 1910 after agreeing never to work again as a cook. Unfortunately, after an outbreak of typhoid fever among the staff of a hospital in 1915, Ms. Mallon was discovered working under an alias as a cook at the hospital. Following this incident, Ms. Mallon was kept in isolation until her death in 1938.

During Ms. Mallon's first period of detention and isolation, a tabloid-style article published by a newspaper in 1909 dubbed her "Typhoid Mary" (Leavitt 1996). This publication unfairly characterized Mary Mallon as a villain, and the moniker "Typhoid Mary" would from then on connote an unclean and deadly woman. In reality, Ms. Mallon was a victim of prejudice and poor judgment by all those involved in handling the case. Many typhoid carriers had been identified during Ms. Mallon's detention and isolation, yet she was the only person to be detained against her will for so long. Over the years since Ms. Mallon's initial case and into the current century, epidemiologic investigations have discovered infected food workers as the source of many foodborne illness outbreaks, particularly those caused by enteric viruses. With knowledge gained from these investigations and microbiological research, sanitary and hygienic practices have been developed to minimize the risk of disease transmission from food workers. Nonetheless, food workers still continue to be a significant source of foodborne infections (Grieg et al. 2007).

## Public Health and Disease Surveillance

A function closely related to epidemiology that developed over many years is disease and public health surveillance. According to CDC, *surveillance* "is the ongoing, systematic collection, analysis, interpretation, and dissemination of data regarding a health-related event for use in public health action to reduce morbidity and mortality and to improve health" (German et al. 2001). The origins of disease surveillance can be traced back to the plague or "Black Death" of the fourteenth and fifteenth centuries, when ships were inspected to detect cases of plague, and quarantine was imposed on travelers from plague-infected areas (Declich and Carter 1994). Over the next 400 years, various systems for collecting and tabulating morbidity and mortality data were implemented. In the nineteenth century, leaders such as Sir Edwin Chadwick and William Farr of England and Lemuel Shattuck of Massachusetts fully recognized the value of using surveillance for public health policies. In the twentieth century, the concept of surveillance was greatly expanded, and the methods of data collection, analysis, and dissemination were greatly advanced (Declich and Carter 1994; Thacker 2010). Today, in the early twenty-first century, information technology and the Internet have facilitated disease reporting, analysis, and dissemination in a manner that would have been unimaginable 100 years ago.

Prior to 1925, the reporting of disease morbidity in the United States was limited to the individual states. National reporting of disease morbidity was spurred by a severe poliomyelitis epidemic in 1916 and the influenza pandemic of 1918–1919 (Thacker 2010). Surveillance of the foodborne diseases typhoid fever and botulism started in the early twentieth century, and the national collection of nontyphoid salmonellosis data started in 1942 (Tauxe and Esteban 2007). In 1949, the National Office of Vital Statistics published weekly statistical reports at the national level, and the forerunner of the currently published *Morbidity and Mortality Weekly Report (MMWR)* was started in 1952 (Thacker 2010). The CDC gained responsibility for publishing the *MMWR* in 1961, and this publication has since become widely read by health professionals and public health practitioners across the nation and around the world. Readers consider it a timely, authoritative, objective, and useful source of scientific information and guidance on public health issues, including the reporting of foodborne disease outbreaks and surveillance information.

The legal requirements for reporting diseases and other conditions rest at the individual state level, and differences exist between states' lists of reportable diseases and conditions. However, starting in 1950, the Association of State and Territorial Health Officials (formerly Officers, ASTHO) authorized an annual conference or council of epidemiologists to decide which diseases should be reported to federal public health authorities. These lists of nationally notifiable infectious and noninfectious diseases/conditions are periodically updated by the council, and CDC compiles and maintains disease reports. Many of the notifiable infectious diseases are transmitted by multiple modes (foodborne, waterborne, etc.). Among the nationally notifiable diseases potentially transmitted by foods are botulism, salmonellosis, hepatitis A, listeriosis, shiga toxin-producing *E. coli*, shigellosis, trichinellosis, and vibriosis, along with several historically important foodborne diseases (e.g., brucellosis, Q fever, typhoid fever).

Surveillance systems are designed and used for many purposes (Thacker 2010). A particularly important purpose is the detection of epidemics. An unusual increase in disease cases or laboratory tests in a surveillance system can alert local and federal authorities to a potential public health problem. This typically leads to a more focused collection of data and an epidemiologic investigation. Public health officials have detected many point-source outbreaks of foodborne illnesses and diseases using several surveillance systems. Epidemiologists can also use data from surveillance systems to generate hypotheses for further epidemiologic and laboratory research, which can elucidate the risk factors and causes of diseases and outbreaks. Another important purpose of surveillance systems is characterization of the history, distribution, and spread of diseases. Such information is useful for measuring the effectiveness of control and prevention strategies. For example, the effectiveness of programs to reduce or eliminate a particular pathogen in the food supply should be reflected in the reported incidence and outbreaks of the corresponding disease.

The actual number of foodborne illnesses and diseases in the United States each year is not accurately reflected in surveillance systems because the vast majority of foodborne illnesses are never reported to local, state, and/or federal agencies. There is a variety of reasons for this shortcoming. Figure 1-1 illustrates the difficulty of capturing foodborne illness and disease data. A great many foodborne illnesses cause either self-limiting or nonfatal conditions, typically diarrhea, vomiting, and other signs and symptoms related to gastroenteritis. For conditions that resolve themselves in a few days, ill people frequently do not visit medical treatment facilities (i.e., bottom of pyramid in Figure 1-1). If individuals do seek medical attention, the illness may be misdiagnosed, or the health care practitioner may not identify a specific etiology. Sometimes the latter occurs because a specimen is not submitted to the clinical laboratory, or the patient is no longer shedding the pathogen, or the clinical laboratory does not identify/confirm the specific pathogen with its battery of tests. Finally, the clinical laboratory may not submit a report to the surveillance authority, especially for diseases that are not considered reportable or notifiable.

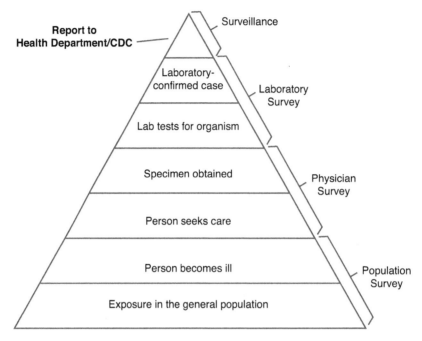

**Figure 1-1** Burden of Illness Pyramid. *Source:* Courtesy of CDC

In general, cases of foodborne illnesses are more likely to be reported when they cause severe illness or death, or when an unusual number of cases occur in a particular period of time and place, that is, an outbreak. Among the people suffering from a foodborne disease, a certain percentage will experience more severe consequences that require medical intervention, while others will suffer only minor symptoms. The reasons for such differences include different doses of the etiologic agent, different levels of susceptibility and resistance by the individuals, and a number of other variables. Highly susceptible individuals are more vulnerable to severe outcomes from a foodborne disease. They include the very old, very young, immunocompromised persons, pregnant women, and others. Even with hospitalizations and deaths, foodborne diseases are frequently misdiagnosed and likely underreported (Mead et al. 1999). With large foodborne illness outbreaks, disease cases are more likely to be recognized and reported because epidemiologic investigations have alerted clinicians and raised suspicion for particular diseases.

### Steps Involved with Foodborne Illness Outbreak Investigations

Epidemiologic investigation of foodborne illness outbreaks is historically the role of local, state, and federal public health agencies. A *foodborne illness outbreak* is defined by CDC as two or more people suffering the "same illness from the same contaminated food or drink" (CDC 2009a). Outbreaks of foodborne illness can range greatly in size and distribution of cases. Local outbreaks typically involve a common meal or food item from a common place in the local community. Larger outbreaks can occur as part of an event attended by many people, or they can be part of an extended or distributed outbreak across the state or nation from the distribution of food items. Although foodborne illness outbreaks capture the attention of public health officials and the press, in reality, the majority of illnesses acquired from foods do not involve outbreaks, or they are not detected as part of an outbreak (Mead et al. 1999). These nonoutbreak cases of food-borne illness are called sporadic cases. Foodborne transmission of sporadic cases is difficult or impossible to prove using rigorous scientific methods. Nonetheless, based on circumstantial evidence and existing knowledge of foodborne diseases and transmission, sporadic cases are judged to be very common occurrences.

The following paragraphs describe the basic steps involved in investigating a foodborne illness outbreak. At this point in the book, the description is cursory because the student needs to acquire additional knowledge from later chapters to appreciate fully the nuances of conducting an outbreak investigation. Additional training resources and tutorials on outbreak investigations are provided at the end of this chapter in the References and Useful Resources sections.

For most foodborne illness outbreaks, a team of professionals is assembled to conduct the investigation. A typical team consists of an epidemiologist, microbiologist or laboratory professional, environmental health specialist or sanitarian, and a physician/clinician to diagnose cases. Depending on the scope and magnitude of the suspected outbreak, the team may be augmented with regulatory compliance officers/inspectors, statisticians, veterinarians, chemists, toxicologists, and other specialists. Generally, the expertise on the team should represent the three major components of the investigation process: (1) epidemiology, (2) laboratory, and (3) environmental (Michigan Department of Agriculture [MDA] 2010). When a suspected outbreak occurs across several jurisdictions, the team may find it necessary to coordinate with and/or include other state and federal agencies. With some local jurisdictions involving smaller outbreaks, the team epidemiologist may be remotely located, and the local health department may be responsible for conducting the investigation. In these situations, established protocols and a good communication network will facilitate the investigation. Timely investigations are important to gathering the necessary information and samples, to identify the source(s) of the outbreak, and to implement controls to prevent further cases.

Figure 1-2 illustrates the basic steps involved in an investigation of a foodborne illness outbreak. These steps are not necessarily sequential, and several steps may proceed simultaneously and often in an iterative fashion. The obvious first step is detecting and ascertaining that an outbreak has occurred. Surveillance systems, consumer complaints, informal reports from health care facilities, and formal reports of reportable or notifiable diseases from physicians and/or laboratories can alert the investigative team to an outbreak. As soon as possible, the physician should verify diagnosis. The clinician should describe cases of clinical illness, and the team should collect specimens from the patients for laboratory analysis. Standardized forms for clinical personnel are very helpful in ensuring that the team collects the type, frequency, and duration of signs and symptoms. The team should also collect additional demographic information on age, sex, race, and occupation of patients. Laboratory identification of the etiologic agent(s) from patient specimens is very important, but sometimes the microbiologist cannot isolate a pathogen or other agent. If the laboratory professional isolates a pathogen, additional subtyping of the pathogen strain is desirable, and this may require sending the culture to a state or federal laboratory.

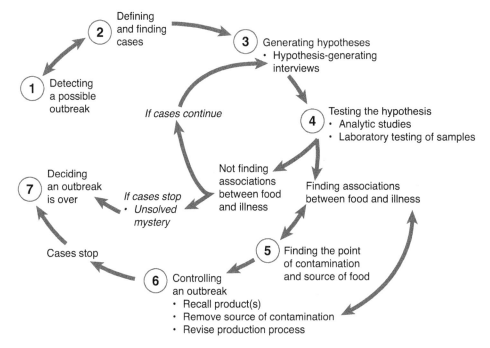

**Figure 1-2** Steps in a Foodborne Outbreak Investigation. *Source:* Courtesy of CDC

Following detection of a potential outbreak, the team should seek additional cases associated with the outbreak. This starts with establishing a definition for what constitutes a case. Based on the available clinical information, time frame, and geographic locations, cases may be defined as either possible or confirmed. Clinical information for a case definition includes characteristics of the illness such as signs, symptoms, clinical laboratory findings, and confirmation of the etiologic agent through laboratory analysis, if possible. The investigative team should restrict case definitions to suspected time frames and geographic locations of the outbreak to avoid adding nonoutbreak or sporadic cases. Sharing information with other regional, state, or federal agencies will assist in determining whether the outbreak is more widely distributed. With the case definition, the team can find additional cases through surveillance systems, physicians' offices, emergency rooms, clinical laboratories, group surveys, and other sources. Contacting and providing these other organizational entities with the case definition helps to alert them to the outbreak and aids in scrutinizing cases for possible inclusion and notification.

As cases are identified, the team must maintain records on each for review and analysis. At the same time, the epidemiologist can use the identified cases to plot an epidemic curve and/or to pinpoint locations on a map for determining the locales or spread of illnesses. This can help verify the existence of an epidemic or outbreak. Early interviews of a few cases may help identify a possible source of the outbreak, but it is best to generate hypotheses on the mode of transmission to minimize reinterviews of the cases, which saves valuable time and effort later. Investigators should approach the problem of solving the outbreak with an open mind. Several modes of transmission by pathogens are possible, and several routes of exposure to chemical toxicants or toxins are possible. By generating plausible hypotheses about the mode of transmission, the team can better structure interviews of cases to identify the potential source(s) of the etiologic agent. If a foodborne illness is suspected, interviews should focus questions on foods eaten in the 72 hours before the onset of symptoms because most people do not have reliable recall beyond 72 hours (MDA 2010). For suspected diseases with longer incubation periods, the investigators should query cases about the foods eaten, but the best available information may be limited to places where foods were consumed. Prior to the interviews, the team should develop an outbreak-specific questionnaire to ensure all relevant questions are asked and to record the results of the interviews.

On the basis of timing, places, and persons associated with the illnesses, the initial hypotheses can be refined or new hypotheses can be generated. If a particular source or place is suggested by the data, reinterviews of cases may be necessary, and information about specific foods may be needed. With the suspected location and/or foods identified, an environmental investigation is necessary to collect food samples for laboratory analysis and to find the point of contamination and source of the food. In many cases, unless kept as leftovers, the suspect food is no longer available for testing, and reconstruction of the food handling and preparation practices is necessary to identify risk factors. Old menus and diagramming the work flow are helpful in a retrospective examination of food handling/preparation practices. For some foodborne diseases, an infected food worker may be involved, and additional interviews and clinical referrals by the local health authority may be necessary.

With sufficient epidemiologic information strongly supported by laboratory and food data, formal hypothesis testing using statistical tests may be unnecessary to determine the source of the outbreak (World Health Organization [WHO] 2008). However, formal hypothesis testing or analytical epidemiology may be necessary where data are lacking or key questions remain unanswered. With several statistical tests, the epidemiologist can estimate the relative risks of different variables associated with the foodborne illness outbreak. On the basis of the investigation and/or hypothesis testing, control measures can be implemented immediately to prevent further cases or recurrences of outbreaks. If a particular food item is associated with the illnesses among several different facilities or establishments, a traceback investigation may be necessary to find the original source of the item in the food supply chain. This may lead to food recalls by the company or issuance of public education messages to protect consumers. If the food or foods are associated with a particular food service or retail food establishment, several actions may be necessary to protect public health. These may involve closing the facility, cleaning and sanitizing equipment, retraining the food handlers and managers, and implementing additional control measures. Last, the investigators should write a final report of the outbreak investigation and share it with other public health authorities. The report may provide the basis of several actions later, and in a broader context, a report or publication contributes to knowledge in the field of public health and food safety.

## CLASSIFICATION OF FOODBORNE DISEASES AND ETIOLOGIC AGENTS

Twenty-first-century epidemiologists have the benefit of hindsight and knowledge when examining past and present food safety problems. Current knowledge about foodborne diseases and food safety is the accumulation and amalgamation of contributions from many disciplines over many years. But the food supply in this modern era is still changing and becoming increasingly complex, and new foodborne pathogens and other hazards continue to emerge. For this reason, it is helpful to lay out a classification scheme for foodborne diseases and etiologic agents. There are many different ways to classify foodborne diseases and etiologic agents based on the perspectives of the discipline involved. Several of these classification schemes are discussed further in later chapters. For now, however, the classification scheme presented here is designed to provide the student with a broad overview. This classification scheme is limited to acute and subchronic foodborne diseases. In other words, it is limited to those foodborne diseases that produce clinical signs and symptoms within hours, days, or weeks. Certainly, chronic or long-term diseases such as cancer are important, but the etiology of these diseases is much more complex and difficult to ascertain, particularly considering the milieu of natural and synthetic ingredients found in foods and the nonfood exposures of people to toxicants. Chapter 3 discusses several important toxicants of some chronic diseases, and Chapter 6 describes how exposure standards to toxicants in foods are derived.

Contaminated food is known to transmit or cause more than 200 different diseases (Bryan 1982). The etiologic agents of these foodborne diseases are biological, chemical, or physical in nature. Figure 1-3 illustrates the relationship between the classification of foodborne diseases and etiologic agents. People use the term *food poisoning* colloquially to describe all foodborne diseases, but this is misleading because food poisoning represents only one possible category of foodborne disease. Poisonings or intoxications occur as the result of ingesting chemicals, toxins, allergens, or radionuclides. Toxins represent a special type of toxic substance because they are produced biochemically by living organisms. A great variety of toxins are in the natural world, and these toxins may enter the food chain from within the tissues of certain food animals or plants, or they may be produced by toxigenic microorganisms that contaminate foods. By contrast, synthetic and nonbiologically produced chemicals can originate from a variety of sources. If present in sufficient quantities, chemical substances can cause adverse health effects when consumed. The types of adverse health effects depend on the chemical structures of the substances and the quantity consumed (i.e., dose). Some toxins and chemicals are enterotoxic, causing a toxic response in the gastrointestinal tract, while others are neurotoxic or affect other organs and systems.

Allergens may or may not be classified as toxic chemicals or toxins. Some individuals experience adverse responses to substances that are innocuous to most other people. These responses are commonly referred to as food allergies. But not all such reactions are true allergies. Some reactions are actually food intolerances, which are hypersensitive reactions to a food or ingredient without involvement of the immune system. Most food intolerances are inherited or acquired deficiencies in metabolism. A commonly encountered form of these conditions is lactose intolerance, where the individual lacks the gene for lactase, an enzyme needed to digest lactose in milk.

Radioactive elements called radionuclides occur naturally as well as are produced by human activity. If radionuclides contaminate the food chain, they can become internalized in humans through ingestion. Depending on the type of radionuclide, internalization can cause a spectrum of health problems. Radionuclides associated with human activity include discharges from nuclear power plants or from past nuclear weapons testing. Another source of human-activity radionuclides is from wastes generated by industrial, medical, and research organizations. In most regions of the world, naturally occurring radionuclides in the food chain are below levels of concern to human

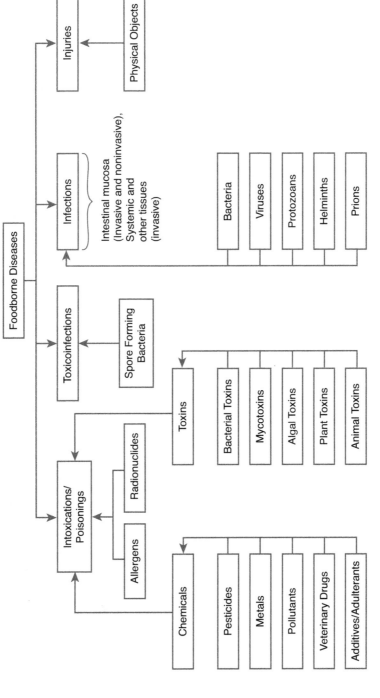

**Figure 1-3** Classification of Foodborne Diseases and Etiologic Agents. *Source:* Adapted from Bryan FL. 1982

health. But human activities may also concentrate naturally occurring radioisotopes to unnaturally high levels in materials such as sludge, petroleum wastes, mining wastes, and other materials.

Infections with pathogenic microorganisms and parasites represent the most common and important type of foodborne disease. Most foodborne infections involve the gastrointestinal tract, where the pathogens colonize and may invade the mucosa and underlying tissue. Under certain circumstances and with particular pathogens, the infection may spread to other organs and become systemic. Pathogens are broadly classified as bacteria, viruses, protozoans, and helminths (worms). Over the past few decades, an additional type of pathogenic agent has been recognized: the prion. Unlike other pathogens, prions are not living organisms. Instead, prions are corrupt (i.e., misfolded) proteins that have the ability to corrupt other proteins when consumed. The result is the formation of plaques in tissues of the central nervous system that cause a multitude of neurologic problems, eventually leading to death. The best-known prion disease is bovine spongiform encephalitis (BSE), also known as mad cow disease.

Another type of foodborne disease is partly an infection and partly an intoxication—called a toxicoinfection. This is caused by certain soil-dwelling bacteria that are capable of forming spores, a tough cellular structure that can resist harsh environmental conditions. When consumed in sufficient numbers, certain spore-forming bacteria of the genus *Clostridium* and *Bacillus* can release toxins into the lumen of the intestinal tract without colonizing the intestinal mucosa. The toxins are then absorbed by the intestines, where they may exert their toxic effects or may be transported to other organs via the bloodstream.

Injury from sharp or hard objects in foods is another potential hazard. Physical objects from a variety of sources may contaminate foods. During the harvesting of crops, stones can become collected with grains and vegetables. Bone fragments may be left in boneless meat or meat dishes during processing or preparing. Metal fragments in the form of shavings, screws, or similar items may contaminate foods during processing. Glass fragments and slivers of glass can contaminate foods from poor quality jars or broken light bulbs. All of these aforementioned items and other objects cause harm when ingested by consumers, sometimes resulting in very serious injuries.

Knowledge about the relative importance of different etiologic agents of foodborne illnesses and diseases comes mostly from reported outbreaks and surveillance systems. Over the course of the twentieth century, the relative importance of different foodborne diseases has changed dramatically. Food safety measures implemented over the first half of the twentieth century greatly reduced foodborne disease transmission of typhoid fever, brucellosis, trichinellosis, and septic sore throat. In the latter half of the twentieth century, new foodborne diseases and etiologic agents began to emerge, and the incidence of some infrequently reported foodborne diseases began to increase. Many reasons account for this change, but changes in the production and processing of foods and preferences of consumers have been most influential. For example, intoxication (a.k.a. food poisoning) from enterotoxins produced by the bacterium *Staphylococcus aureus* was the leading foodborne disease in the 1960s and 1970s (Bergdoll and Wong 2006). At that time, the majority of reported cases were associated with large outbreaks from point sources in the highly productive food industry. Although staphylococcal intoxications still remain very common, especially in noncommercial settings and in sporadic cases, large outbreaks associated with the food industry have dramatically decreased. Reasons for this reduction are attributed to better attention to sanitation, temperature controls, and engineering controls.

Figure 1-4 illustrates the percentages of foodborne disease or illness outbreaks by etiology based on mean annual reported outbreaks in the United States for the years 2001–2005 (CDC 2009b). Viruses represented the largest known category of etiologic agents (30%) during this time frame, followed closely by bacterial etiologies (28%). Interestingly, for 32% of all reported outbreaks, the etiology was unknown, that is, it was neither confirmed nor suspected. This proportion of outbreaks with an unknown etiology represents a substantial decrease compared to the previous 20 years. During the years 1983–1987, the percentage of outbreaks with an unknown etiology was 62% (Bean et al. 1990). For outbreaks with confirmed or suspected etiologies, comparisons between years in the number of outbreaks are difficult to interpret, primarily because of variations in the states' outbreak detection, investigation, and reporting practices (CDC 2009b). Nevertheless, the change in reported viral etiologies from the 1980s to the current time is remarkable. In the mid-1980s, viruses were confirmed as the etiologic agent in approximately only 2% of outbreaks (Bean et al. 1990). The change in the reported proportion of viral etiologies is probably a combination of at least two factors. First, better viral diagnostic tests are available to identify the etiology (Lynch et al. 2006). Second, the number of outbreaks from viral etiologies (specifically the norovirus) has actually increased (CDC 2009b).

The lack of warning properties of an etiologic agent in foods is the most difficult aspect of food safety. If food has a foul smell, bad taste, or unappealing appearance, people are unlikely to consume it. This aversion to disgusting materials is instinctual and probably helped primitive and ancient humans to avoid disease from contact with feces, decaying bodies, and other sources of

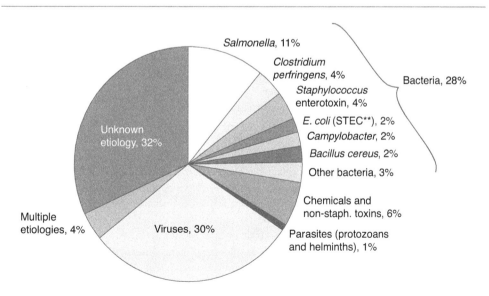

**Figure 1-4** Percentage of Reported Foodborne Disease Outbreaks and Outbreak-Associated Illnesses by Etiology Based on Mean Annual Totals,* United States, 2001–2005. *Source:* Data from CDC

infection (Curtis, Aunger, Rabie 2004). Unfortunately, the presence of pathogenic microorganisms, toxins, or toxic chemicals in foods is rarely associated with warning smells or appearances. The only way to know for sure that a contaminant exists is either by laboratory testing of the food or by confirming a foodborne illness outbreak. For reasons that are discussed in Chapter 7, laboratory testing has limitations when used to screen foods and to detect etiologic agents. And for obvious reasons, waiting for a foodborne illness outbreak to occur is undesirable because the primary goal of food safety is to prevent foodborne illnesses and diseases. Consequently, food safety is very dependent on the establishment of standards with respect to the production, processing, handling, and preparation of foods. The public health rationale for these standards is based on historical knowledge, epidemiologic data, and/or laboratory research. Standards help with judging whether or not foods are considered safe.

## THE BURDEN OF FOODBORNE ILLNESSES AND TRENDS IN FOOD SAFETY

### Measuring the Burden of Foodborne Illnesses

Because the actual incidence or prevalence of foodborne illnesses cannot be directly measured using existing surveillance systems, indirect methods of estimating them have been developed. Dr. Paul S. Mead and his colleagues conducted a widely and frequently cited estimate of foodborne illnesses in the United States (Mead et al. 1999). Using multiple surveillance systems and other sources, the authors compiled and analyzed information to estimate the number of foodborne illnesses, hospitalizations, and deaths that occur in the United States each year. Based on their estimates, a total of 76 million illnesses, 325,000 hospitalizations, and 5,000 deaths occur each year in the United States from foodborne sources. Remarkably, of the total estimates, approximately 62 million illnesses (82%), 265,000 hospitalizations (82%), and 3,200 deaths (64%) are attributed to unknown etiologic agents. This suggests that the causes for the majority of foodborne illnesses, hospitalizations, and deaths are never definitively determined.

The United States and several other countries have undertaken a number of other initiatives to estimate the actual incidence and burden of foodborne illnesses (Flint et al. 2005). Each of these initiatives has unavoidable methodologic issues that limit interpretation of the study results. Perhaps the greatest issue is the multimodal means of pathogen transmission. Many common foodborne pathogens can also be transmitted by water, objects (e.g., fomites), and person-to-person contact. Unless associated with an outbreak, an illness or disease cannot be definitively attributed to foodborne transmission. Another issue is related to common or overlapping signs and symptoms of diseases. This issue is more problematic with self-reported illness surveys or syndromic surveillance, where certain signs and/or symptoms experienced by individuals are presumed to represent a particular disease and/or mode of transmission. Chapter 2 covers the significance of clinical signs and symptoms with infectious diseases in greater detail.

A common symptom with most—but not all—foodborne illness outbreaks and sporadic disease cases is diarrhea, and to a lesser extent vomiting or nausea (American Medical Association [AMA] et al. 2004). Researchers have conducted several surveys on the rates of acute diarrheal illness or disease (ADI) among segments of the U.S. population, and then they applied multipliers to the figures to derive rates of ADI across the nation. In one of the most recent studies, surveys were conducted of populations in the catchment area of a clinical laboratory–

based surveillance system called FoodNet (Jones et al. 2007). From 1997 to 2003, four separate population-based telephone surveys were conducted to determine the rate of ADI in the population. A combined total of 52,840 interviews were conducted during the study period. Efforts were made to exclude from analysis the respondents with an underlying chronic disease for which diarrhea is a common symptom (e.g., colitis, irritable bowel syndrome). The definition of ADI was also restricted to individuals who had experienced three or more loose stools with a 24-hour period, and for whom the diarrhea either lasted longer than one day, or the diarrhea impaired daily activities. Results of this study indicate that the average monthly prevalence of ADI in the population ranged from 4.5% to 5.2%, with an overall weighted prevalence of 5.1% (Jones et al. 2007). Furthermore, those with the highest rates of ADI were children younger than 5 years old. Among those with ADI, 33.8% also experienced vomiting, and 19.5% and 7.8% visited a medical doctor and were treated with antibiotics, respectively. Considering the conservative definition of ADI, and that the estimates represent the average monthly prevalence, these statistics suggest ADI is a significant burden on the U.S. population and the health care system.

Researchers presume that a large proportion of ADI cases in the United States is associated with foodborne transmission. This presumption is based partly on the safety of U.S. water supplies. In the past, during the late nineteenth and early twentieth centuries, drinking water was the most common source of diarrheal diseases in the United States. Municipal water supplies are now required by law to be treated and monitored for contamination. Smaller drinking water disease outbreaks still occur, but most of these occur outside the jurisdiction of a water utility (Yoder et al. 2008). For cases of ADI where infectious agents were identified, the proportion attributed to foodborne transmission can be estimated from a combination of literature reviews, historical outbreak data, and expert opinion. Although this proportion can vary from 1% to 100% for different infectious agents, an overall flat rate of 36% has been used to estimate the proportion of all ADIs attributed to foodborne transmission in the United States (Mead et al. 1999).

Much less is known about the proportion of illnesses or diseases attributed to foodborne sources in lesser developed countries because disease surveillance systems and epidemiologic investigation capabilities are severely limited. Statisticians base most estimates on rates of clinical diseases regardless of the sources or modes of transmission. The World Health Organization (WHO) estimates that 2.5 billion cases of diarrhea or ADI occur each year among children younger than 5 years old, with an estimated 1.5 million deaths, which actually represents a decline from 5 million deaths just two decades earlier (United Nations Children's Fund [UNICEF] and WHO 2009). Diarrhea is second only to pneumonia as the top killer of young children in the lesser developed world. The primary pathogens that cause ADI in children of lesser developed countries include those commonly associated with foodborne diseases, but a large percentage (~23%) of the enteric pathogens are unknown or undetermined (Lanata, Mendoza, Black 2002). Because unsafe water supplies and other modes of transmission are frequently encountered in lesser developed countries, the proportion of these pathogens transmitted by foods cannot be reliably estimated. Nonetheless, one estimate is that 70% of all diarrheal episodes are caused by foodborne transmission (Kaferstein 2003).

To better estimate the burden and costs of foodborne illnesses in the world, WHO has established the Foodborne Disease Burden Epidemiology Reference Group (FERG). Unlike previous initiatives, the primary purpose of FERG is to estimate the burden of acute and chronic foodborne diseases caused by important pathogens, parasites, and chemicals (WHO 2006). A strategic framework for the program has been established and is currently being implemented. The first part of the strategy involves reviewing diseases transmitted by foods and other modes to assess what proportion are probably foodborne. Another part of the strategy involves the development of research tools for individual countries to estimate their own burdens of foodborne disease. The ultimate goal is for individual countries to monitor their burden of foodborne diseases and use this information to develop public health policies and food safety standards. This information will also be shared with WHO to provide a global perspective on the burden of foodborne diseases.

Why measure the burden of foodborne illnesses? The burden is important to know in setting priorities to control specific foodborne diseases and in developing public health policies to manage the risks of foodborne illnesses. Morbidity and mortality statistics associated with foodborne illnesses provide a measure of burden in terms of human suffering. However, economists and public policymakers prefer to express the burden of foodborne illnesses in terms of costs, which provides a common denominator for comparing the disease burden against the resources necessary to reduce it. This type of comparison is called cost–benefit analysis (or benefit–cost analysis) and is particularly helpful in weighing the benefits to society against the costs of new food regulations. Determining the costs of foodborne illnesses is complicated by the distribution of expenses across society. These costs may include doctor visits, medications, hospitalizations, loss of household income, loss of worker productivity, and other direct and indirect costs. Pain and suffering are also important and may affect personal productivity and lifestyle, but it is difficult to assign costs to such intangibles. Other significant costs are encountered in the food industry, when foodborne illness outbreaks prompt food recalls, law suits, and consumer avoidance (i.e., loss of sales) of the company's food products.

Most foodborne illnesses are usually considered mild and self-limiting compared to other medical conditions. But this is not the case with all foodborne illnesses. More recently, the field of public health has recognized that even common foodborne illnesses can have serious and chronic sequelae (i.e., secondary conditions or complications) that affect several organs and systems. Among the known sequelae are Guillain-Barre syndrome, hemolytic uremic syndrome (HUS) and other kidney damage, irritable bowel syndrome, paralysis and neurologic complications, reactive and rheumatoid arthritis, and premature death (Buzby and Roberts 2009; Kaferstein 2003). Estimating the costs of sequelae from foodborne illnesses is problematic because a condition may not be easily recognized as a consequence of foodborne illness. Using available epidemiologic data and economic models, researchers can estimate costs for a number of foodborne diseases (see USDA website in the Useful Resources section). One recent model estimates the costs for *E. coli* O157:H7 infections based on the degree of severity of different cases (Buzby and Roberts 2009). For a single hospitalized case of *E. coli* O157:H7 infection, the average cost is estimated at $6,922. For a single hospitalized case of *E. coli* O157:H7 infection where the patient suffers HUS and dies, the average cost is a staggering $6,963,826.

At the national level, the estimated costs of foodborne illnesses vary greatly. One author estimates the average annual cost of all foodborne illnesses in the United States is $1.4 trillion (Roberts 2007), and this estimate does not include the disease sequelae, suggesting that the real costs may be even higher (Buzby and Roberts 2009). A more moderate estimate was done in 1995 for only six bacterial pathogens and one parasite associated with foodborne diseases (Buzby and Roberts 1997). Adjusting for inflation in 2009 dollars, the estimated costs of these six foodborne diseases alone in the United States range from $8.6 billion to $46.4 billion. Another estimate of health-related costs from all foodborne illnesses in the United States is $152 billion, with a possible range from $40.0 billion to $264.8 billion (Scharff 2010). Whatever the exact costs, it is clear that foodborne illnesses inflict a tremendous burden on the U.S. economy. This is particularly important from the standpoint of public policy and establishing regulatory standards for food safety. Under a Presidential Executive Order, all proposed regulations in the United States that could have an annual effect of more than $100 million on the economy must receive a benefit–cost analysis (Buzby and Roberts 2009).

## Current and Future Trends That Influence Food Safety

From the historical perspective provided earlier, it is apparent that changes in agricultural production, food processing and distribution, environmental pollution, population demographics, and consumer preferences are important influences on the types of hazards encountered in the food supply and the occurrence of foodborne illnesses. Changes continue to occur in the twenty-first century and will undoubtedly present new challenges to ensuring a safe food supply. At the agricultural production level (i.e., the farm), changes in growing crops and raising livestock have created new ecological niches for pathogens and introduced new agricultural chemicals. Vegetables have become increasingly contaminated in the field with enteric pathogens, and studies have determined that many of these pathogens may survive in the plants through a process called internalization (Beuchat 2006; Buck, Walcott, Beuchat 2003). The contamination and survival of pathogens in fresh produce has contributed to several highly publicized foodborne illness outbreaks in recent years (Mandrell 2007).

Infections of livestock with zoonotic pathogens (i.e., can also infect humans) have changed over the past several decades. New strains of pathogens have emerged and continue to do so, some with greater virulence (disease-causing ability) and antibiotic resistance (Oliver, Patel, et al. 2009; Tauxe 2002). Factors contributing to the emergence of these new foodborne pathogens include industrial production of animals and the use of antibiotics for growth purposes. The introduction of new pathogenic strains of microorganisms into herds and flocks is also facilitated by international trade of animals for breeding purposes. And contaminated animal feed has spread infections to livestock that enter the human food supply. For example, the spread of bovine spongiform encephalitis (BSE, or mad cow disease) among cattle was facilitated by both international trade and the contamination of feedstuff with prions (CDC 2004). Similarly, international trade and contaminated feed contributed to the infection of chickens around the world with *Salmonella* (Molbak, Olsen, Wegener 2006).

Consumer preferences drive many changes in the food supply. Of all consumer preferences, convenience is an overarching desire of most Americans. During 1971–2007, the percentage of American food budgets spent on "eating out" grew from approximately 26% to nearly 42% (Economic Research Service [ERS] 2008). In addition, more than half of the foods purchased for home preparation and consumption nowadays are packaged, processed, and convenience foods

(Morrison et al. 2010; Sloan 2008). But American consumers still demand freshness and good tastes with their foods. This has led food manufacturers to offer a variety of convenience products known as "minimally processed foods" (Fellows 2009). These foods are not treated with harsh processes that damage organoleptic and nutritional properties. Consumer demand for year-round freshness has also spurred more interstate shipments and the importation of foods. All of the consumer-driven changes mentioned previously present new challenges to food safety.

When eating outside of the home or purchasing carryout, the consumer depends on the food safety practices of retail food establishments. Approximately 52% of the reported foodborne illness outbreaks are associated with retail food establishments, including restaurants, hotels, cafeterias, and delicatessens (Jones and Angulo 2006). Retail food establishments usually prepare foods in large quantities for large numbers of people. And although most food safety hazards can be minimized or controlled at the food preparation stage, a simple omission or momentary lapse in food safety practices can result in a large foodborne illness outbreak across the community. The development and enforcement of food safety standards for retail food establishments rest principally with state and local governments. To promote uniformity across the states, the U.S. Public Health Service and FDA have recommended a series of model regulations and ordinances since 1934; the current model is known as the Food Code and has grown in complexity to longer than 600 pages (FDA and Public Health Service [PHS] 2009). With an increasing number of consumers "eating out" and more complicated food safety regulations, state and local governments are challenged to inspect all retail food establishments regularly and to enforce the regulations, especially in an era of decreasing government resources.

Changes in food processing have several implications with regard to food safety. With more processed and packaged foods available, a contaminated ingredient may be incorporated into numerous products and distributed around the country (or globe). This may result in foodborne illness outbreaks that are more distributed and not "clustered" geographically, and multiple contaminated products mean the identification and recall of these products will be extremely difficult. This situation occurred with a nationwide outbreak of salmonellosis involving contaminated peanuts, which were provided by one supplier to more than 200 companies with 3,900 peanut-containing products (Wittenberger and Dohlman 2010). Another safety aspect of food processing is with minimally processed foods. Because these food products are not subjected to harsh treatment processes, the destruction of pathogens is less assured, and multiple controls known as the "hurdle concept" must be applied to minimize the hazards of pathogens (Gorris 2000). To ensure these foods are safely processed, food safety management tools such as the Hazard Analysis and Critical Control Point (HACCP) system are becoming mandatory.

Americans demand year-round availability of certain seasonal fresh foods. These foods include various fruits, vegetables, and seafood. The food industry has responded by shipping foods across the country and importing foods from foreign countries. Transporting foods longer distances offers the opportunity for contamination and other unsafe handling practices. Recently, federal standards were proposed for the transport of foods (FDA 2010). Importation of foods is another way to meet consumer demand, and often at less cost to the consumer. The importation of foods into the United States has steadily increased over the past two decades. In 2005, the aggregate share of U.S. foods that were imported was 15% by volume (Jerardo 2008). Some food commodities constituted a much higher share. For fish and shellfish, fruits and nuts, and vegetables, the proportion of imported foods by volume was 79%, 32%, and 13%, respectively. With imported foods, U.S. officials do not directly oversee the conditions under which the food products are produced and handled, and point-of-entry inspections during importation do not always identify potential hazards. Among the hazards of greatest concern are pesticide residues and pathogenic microorganisms. The expanding global trade of food leaves all countries universally vulnerable to foodborne diseases from the country of origin (Tauxe et al. 2010). This represents yet another pathway for the introduction of new foodborne pathogens. The importation and distribution of foods also make it more difficult to detect and control foodborne illness outbreaks caused by pathogens and adulterated foods.

A trend in consumer preferences over the last two decades has created rapid growth in the "organic" foods market. The term *organic* in this context generally applies to foods that have been grown, harvested, and processed with very little or no use of synthetic chemicals. Retail sales of organic foods have increased from $3.6 billion in 1997 to $21.1 billion in 2008 (Dimitri and Oberholtzer 2009). To help assure consumers that organic foods meet consistent and uniform standards, the National Organic Program under USDA manages a program for developing standards and requirements for certifying organic food production and handling operations; these standards and requirements are codified in the federal regulations (7 CFR 205). A National List of Allowed Synthetic and Prohibited Non-Synthetic Substances is contained in the regulations. Organic foods are produced without the use of animal hormones or antibiotics, petroleum-based fertilizers, most conventional pesticides, sewage sludge fertilizer, genetically modified materials, or irradiation. Natural materials are generally considered allowable for organic foods production and handling. For example, animal manure can be used as fertilizer in organic farming operations, despite the fact that animal manure may contain numerous zoonotic pathogens that could contaminate crops if not properly managed (Institute of Food Science and Technology [IFST] 2009). Organic foods are also just as vulnerable as other foods to contamination with pathogens from various environmental sources and food handlers. Thus, although consumers may feel assured that fewer synthetic chemical residues are detectable in organic foods, simply designating or labeling foods as organic does not decrease the risks of transmitting pathogens, nor does it reduce the risks of toxins produced by bacteria or fungi. Consumers of organic foods may need to be educated about the risks of pathogenic or toxigenic microorganisms and how to reduce these risks.

Changes in the demographics of a population have relevance to food safety in several ways. The most important change is the proportion of people who are highly susceptible to foodborne diseases. In the United States, approximately 39.5 million people are older than 65 years, and this number of older people is expected to double over the next 20 years (IOM 2010). In general, older people are more susceptible to acquiring infections from certain pathogens, and they are much more likely to experience serious health outcomes from foodborne infections and intoxications. Other groups considered at high risk of foodborne illnesses include pregnant women, young children and infants, and those who are immunocompromised because of pharmacological therapy or other diseases (e.g., HIV infection). Approximately 20 million children younger than 5 years live in the United States, and approximately 63% of these children are kept in some sort of regular child care arrangement (Laughlin 2010). Some estimate that 20% of the U.S. population is included in the high-risk category for foodborne illnesses (Gerba, Rose, Haas 1996; Kendall et al. 2003).

Providing an added level of food safety for this high-risk population is challenging, particularly if they consume foods prepared in retirement homes, hospitals, or child care facilities.

New and emerging technologies will greatly affect food safety strategies and practices in the future. First, new food processing technologies will be introduced to preserve or treat foods with minimal damage to quality. Some processing technologies, such as food irradiation, will provide an added measure of food safety (Tauxe 2001), while other processing technologies may increase the risks of foodborne illnesses—unless the technology is carefully assessed and integrated into the food supply system. New food processing technologies, ingredients, and packaging may also introduce new chemical hazards into foods (Jackson 2009). Genetically modified organisms (GMOs) will become increasingly important to meeting the increasing global demand for food supplies, but the potential risks posed by GMOs are difficult to assess fully, and many consumers may reject GMO foods. Finally, new laboratory and field testing methods will make a big impact on food safety. New nucleic acid testing methods can provide more accurate and rapid identification of pathogens from patients and in foodstuffs. This will greatly aid in identifying etiologic agents of foodborne diseases, thus providing better knowledge about the burden of different foodborne diseases. New testing technologies will also aid in protecting the food supply by increasing the capabilities and feasibility of screening foods for contamination.

A thorny problem that will challenge individual countries and the global community is balancing issues of food security, food safety, and food defense. *Food security* is a term long used to describe whether a country has sufficient food to avoid starvation and meet dietary energy needs. Following a World Food Summit in 1996, the definition of food security was expanded to include sufficient, safe, and nutritious food that will meet "dietary needs and food preferences for a healthy and active life" (Pinstrup-Andersen 2009). This definition implies several levels of food security. For study purposes, people are considered food insecure if they consume less than 2,100 calories per day per person (Shapouri et al. 2010). Food insecurity has declined overall in the world, but the projected number of food insecure people in 2010 is estimated at 882 million (Shapouri et al. 2010). While some regions of the world have seen decreases in food insecurity, other regions, especially in sub-Saharan Africa, have seen an increase in food insecurity. It is also projected over the next decade that the aggregate level of food insecurity will decrease by only 1% (Shapouri et al. 2010). The principal challenge in the future will be providing a sufficient and safe food supply to meet the needs and preferences of a growing world population.

Food safety is intrinsically linked with food security because the provision of food safety comes with a cost. Americans have the luxury of an ample food supply with a high standard of food safety, though 14.6% of households in the United States are considered food insecure sometime during the year (Nord, Andrews, Carlson 2009). The ability of a country to produce or import food to alleviate food insecurity can be hindered by excessive food safety standards. Additionally, overly strict food safety regulations and treaties can stifle innovation to produce larger quantities of food at less cost. Differences in national food standards is another concern because developed countries may sell (or dump) substandard or unsafe foods in lesser developed countries. A suggested solution to this dilemma is the right mix of policies and international standards to ensure foods in global trade are safe, yet they allow entrepreneurship and innovation by the food industry (Council for Agricultural Science and Technology [CAST] 1998). Among the international organizations that develop food standards for adoption by countries is the Codex Alimentarius Commission, an organization that is considered the single greatest reference point for international food standards (Food and Agriculture Organization [FAO] and WHO 2006).

To avoid confusion with the concept of food security, the term *food defense* is used to describe the protection of foods against deliberate contamination (Monke 2007). As discussed earlier, foods have been intentionally adulterated or contaminated for centuries to cause harm to someone or a group of people. The motivations for such acts range from murder to causing fear and furthering a political agenda (i.e., terrorism). Over the past several decades, the threat of terrorism has increased in countries around the world. Food represents a vulnerable target and a highly effective vehicle for disseminating harmful biological, chemical, or radiological agents to large segments of the population. In addition, the introduction of new plant or animal diseases into U.S. agriculture can result in severe economic losses and raise serious concerns about food productivity and safety. Deterring and thwarting efforts to contaminate foods deliberately are more difficult compared with controlling other food safety hazards. Considering the complexity of the food supply chain, effective food defense measures will be a major challenge to implement in the coming years. In the future, food safety professionals will likely be involved with implementing and managing food defense programs.

## DEFINING FOOD SAFETY

Despite the fact that food safety and improved nutrition are considered some of the greatest public health achievements of the twentieth century (CDC 1999), very few satisfactory definitions of food safety can be found in regulations or other documents. A term that is often used interchangeably with food safety is *food sanitation*. The origins of *sanitary* come from the Latin words *sanitas* (healthy) and *sanus* (healthy, sane). Over the past century, the definition of sanitation has changed and expanded to include many environmental aspects of disease prevention. According to Marriott and Gravani (2006), sanitation "is an applied science that incorporates the principles of design, development, implementation, maintenance, restoration, and/or improvement of hygienic practices and conditions." By extension, food sanitation is an applied science that incorporates the preceding principles into the hygienic and healthful handling of foods, usually for the purposes of eliminating or reducing the levels of disease-causing microorganisms. Sanitation is the foundation of ensuring a safe and wholesome food supply. By comparison, food safety is a broader umbrella-like term that encompasses sanitation and other sciences and preventive measures.

To derive a working definition of food safety, a good starting point is to define the words *food* and *safety*. The Codex Alimentarius Commission defines *food* as "any substance, whether processed, semi-processed or raw, which is intended for human consumption, and includes drink, chewing gum and any substance which has been used in the manufacture, preparation or treatment of 'food' but does not include cosmetics or tobacco or substances used only as drugs" (Codex Alimentarius Commission 2010). The definitions of safety have changed somewhat over the decades and vary with different organizations and sources. One of the most important developments with safety and health sciences is the incorporation of risk analysis. Risks can never be completely eliminated in any human endeavor, but they can be reduced through design and/or practices. Therefore, the definition of safety should include the term *risk*. According to the American Society of Safety Engineers, *safety* is "That state for which the risks are at an acceptable level, and tolerable in the setting being considered" (American Society of Safety Engineers [ASSE] 2009). From the definitions quoted here, the following definition of food safety is derived.

Food safety is the state of acceptable and tolerable risks of illness, disease, or injury from the consumption of foods. It is achieved through policies, regulations, standards, research, engineering designs and technology, surveillance and monitoring, and other applicable measures to reduce the risks or control hazards in the food supply chain. This includes all food and prefood materials, starting with agricultural production and continuing through harvesting, processing/manufacturing, storage, distribution, handling, preparation, and any other activities up to the point of consumption, that is, the "farm-to-fork" continuum. The level of acceptable and tolerable risks from the consumption of foods is determined through a process called risk analysis, which is discussed in greater detail in Chapter 6.

For the purposes of this book, food safety does not include nutritional adequacy or quality losses of foods, such as spoilage, loss of nutrients, oxidation, and other chemical or biological changes resulting in undesirable characteristics. These issues are certainly important with foods, but the scope of this text is limited primarily to the risks of illness, disease, and injury from biological, chemical, and physical agents that contaminate foods. For most food technologists and engineers, *food protection* is more a inclusive term for describing food safety, preservation, and quality—including protection against the loss of nutrients and the maintenance of color, taste, texture, aroma, and other desirable characteristics. Whereas many food quality issues are culturally relative and dependent on consumer preferences, food safety is a universal expectation among all consumers, albeit the level of acceptable risk may differ among consumers.

Modern food safety is a multidisciplinary field. Specialists and subspecialists are required to address the multitude of potential hazards encountered. Physicians are critical to the diagnosis and treatment of patients, understanding the pathology of foodborne diseases, and alerting public health authorities of notifiable/reportable diseases. Clinicians and nutritionists may also council patients and high-risk individuals about food safety practices. Veterinarians play a pivotal role in animal health and in defining the relationship between animal health and foodborne disease. Many veterinarians are also directly involved with other food safety and food defense activities. Microbiologists are essential to the laboratory identification of pathogens in patient specimens and in foods; research to determine the conditions of survival, growth, and destruction of pathogens and microbial toxins in foods; and the development of laboratory methods and technologies. Toxicologists and chemists are necessary to define the relationship of toxicant levels in foods and adverse health effects and to conduct and develop new methods for laboratory analysis of chemicals in foods. Engineers and physical scientists determine parameters in the food environment that contribute to the spread of diseases, and they design equipment and systems to reduce the risks of foodborne diseases. Attorneys and legislators develop laws and enforcement tools for food safety. Environmental health specialists or sanitarians are involved in many aspects of food safety, including inspections, training, outbreak investigations, enforcement, and related activities. Epidemiologists are critically important to investigating foodborne illness outbreaks, but they also integrate the contributions of other disciplines to identify the determinants of foodborne diseases and to help assess the effectiveness of intervention/prevention strategies.

## REFERENCES

Ajmone-Marsan P, Garcia JF, Lenstra JA. 2010. On the origin of cattle: How aurochs became cattle and colonized the world. *Evol Anthropol* 19:148–157.

American Epidemiological Society. 2011. Mission. Available from: http://americanepidemiologicalsociety.org/cms2/view.htm/67/1135/Mission.

American Medical Association, American Nurses Association-American Nurses Foundation, Centers for Disease Control and Prevention, Center for Food Safety and Applied Nutrition, Food and Drug Administration, Food Safety and Inspection Service, US Department of Agriculture. 2004. Diagnosis and management of foodborne illnesses: A primer for physicians and other health care professionals. *MMWR Recomm Rep* 53(RR-4):1–33.

American Society of Safety Engineers. 2009. *Prevention through design guidelines for addressing occupational risks in design and redesign processes.* Report nr ASSE TR-Z790.001-2009. Des Plaines, IL: American Society of Safety Engineers. Available from: http://www.asse.org.

Azzam AM, Anderson DG. 1996. *Assessing competition in meatpacking: Economic history, theory, and evidence.* Report to Packers and Stockyards Programs, Grain Inspection, Packers and Stockyards Administration, USDA. Contract No. 53-6395-2-128. Report nr GIPSA-RR 96-6. Available from: http://archive.gipsa.usda.gov/pubs/packers/rr96-6.pdf.

Bean NH, Griffin PM, Goulding JS, Ivey CB. 1990. Foodborne disease outbreaks, 5-year summary, 1983–1987. *MMWR CDC Surveill Summ* 39(1):15–57.

Bell BP, Goldoft M, Griffin PM, Davis MA, Gordon DC, Tarr PI, Bartleson CA, Lewis JH, Barrett TJ, Wells JG. 1994. A multistate outbreak of Escherichia coli O157:H7–associated bloody diarrhea and hemolytic uremic syndrome from hamburgers. The Washington experience. *JAMA* 272(17):1349–1353.

Bergdoll MS, Wong ACL. 2006. Staphylococcal intoxications. In: *Foodborne Infections and Intoxications.* 3rd ed. Rieman HP, Cliver DO, eds. Amsterdam: Academic Press.

Beuchat LR. 2006. Vectors and conditions for preharvest contamination of fruits and vegetables with pathogens capable of causing enteric diseases. *British Food Journal* 108(1):38–53.

Bryan FL. 1982. *Diseases transmitted by foods (classification and summary).* Atlanta, GA: Public Health Service, Centers for Disease Control and Prevention, U.S. Department of Health and Human Services.

Buck JW, Walcott RR, Beuchat LR. 2003, January 21. Recent trends in microbiological safety of fruits and vegetables. *Plant Health Progress.* doi:10.1094/PHP-2003-0121-01-RV.

Burger J, Kirchner M, Bramanti B, Haak W, Thomas MG. 2007. Absence of the lactase-persistence-associated allele in early neolithic Europeans. *Proc Natl Acad Sci U S A* 104(10):3736–3741.

Buzby JC, Roberts T. 2009. The economics of enteric infections: Human foodborne disease costs. *Gastroenterology* 136(6):1851–1862.

Buzby JC, Roberts T. 1997. Economic costs and trade impacts of microbial foodborne illness. *World Health Stat Q* 50(1–2):57–66.

Centers for Disease Control and Prevention. 2009a. Foodborne Outbreak Investigations. Atlanta, GA: U.S. Centers for Disease Control and Prevention. Available from: http://www.cdc.gov/outbreaknet/investigations/.

Centers for Disease Control and Prevention. 2009b. Surveillance for foodborne disease outbreaks—United States, 2006. *MMWR* 58(22):609–615.

Centers for Disease Control and Prevention. 2004. Bovine spongiform encephalopathy in a dairy cow—Washington State, 2003. *MMWR* 52(53):1280–1285.

Centers for Disease Control and Prevention. 1999. Achievements in public health, 1900–1999: Safer and healthier foods. *MMWR* 48(40):905–913.

Centers for Disease Control and Prevention. 1998. *Botulism in the United States, 1899–1996. Handbook for epidemiologists, clinicians, and laboratory workers.* Atlanta, GA: U.S. Centers for Disease Control and Prevention.

Centers for Disease Control and Prevention. 1990. Foodborne hepatitis A—Alaska, Florida, North Carolina, Washington. *MMWR* 39(14):228–232.

Centers for Disease Control and Prevention Advisory Committee on Childhood Lead Poisoning Prevention. 2007. Interpreting and managing blood lead levels < 10 microg/dL in children and reducing childhood exposures to lead: Recommendations of CDC's Advisory Committee on Childhood Lead Poisoning Prevention. *MMWR Recomm Rep* 56(RR-8):1–16.

Codex Alimentarius Commission. 2010. *Codex Alimentarius Commission procedural manual.* 19th ed. Rome, Italy: Joint Food and Agricultural Organization/World Health Organization (FAO/WHO) Food Standards Programme.

Council for Agricultural Science and Technology. 1998, June. *Interpretive summary: Food safety, sufficiency, and security.* Ames, IA: Council for Agricultural Science and Technology.

Cox FE. 2002. History of human parasitology. *Clin Microbiol Rev* 15(4):595–612.

Curtis V, Aunger R, Rabie T. 2004. Evidence that disgust evolved to protect from risk of disease. *Proc Biol Sci* 271 Suppl 4:S131–S133.

Declich S, Carter AO. 1994. Public health surveillance: Historical origins, methods and evaluation. *Bull World Health Organ* 72(2):285–304.

Diamond J. 1999. *Guns, germs, and steel.* New York: W. W. Norton.

Dicker RC, Coronado F, Koo D, Parrish II RG. 2007. Glossary of epidemiology terms. Atlanta, GA: U.S. Centers for Disease Control and Prevention. Available from: http://www.cdc.gov/excite/library/glossary.htm.

Dimitri C, Oberholtzer L. 2009. *Marketing U.S. organic foods: Recent trends from farms to consumers.* Economic Information Bulletin Number 58. Washington, DC: Economic Research Service, U.S. Department of Agriculture.

Economic Research Service. 2008. Diet quality and food consumption: Food away from home. Washington, DC: U.S. Department of Agriculture. Available from: http://www.ers.usda.gov/Briefing/DietQuality/FAFH.htm.

Fellows PJ. 2009. *Food processing technology: Principles and practices.* 3rd ed. Cambridge, England: Woodhead Publishing Limited.

Flint JA, Van Duynhoven YT, Angulo FJ, DeLong SM, Braun P, Kirk M, Scallan E, Fitzgerald M, Adak GK, Sockett P, et al. 2005. Estimating the burden of acute gastroenteritis, foodborne disease, and pathogens commonly transmitted by food: An international review. *Clin Infect Dis* 41(5):698–704.

Food and Agriculture Organization and World Health Organization. 2006. *Understanding the Codex Alimentarius.* 3rd ed. Rome, Italy: Joint FAO/WHO Food Standards Programme.

Food and Drug Administration. 2010. *Guidance for industry: Sanitary transportation of food.* Washington, DC: U.S. Department of Health and Human Services. Available from: http://www.fda.gov/Food/GuidanceComplianceRegulatory Information/GuidanceDocuments/default.htm.

Food and Drug Administration. 2009a. *Grade "A" pasteurized milk ordinance (2009 revision).* Rockville, MD: U.S. Public Health Service/U.S. Food and Drug Administration.

Food and Drug Administration. 2009b. *FDA's Origin & Functions.* Washington, DC: U.S. Department of Health and Human Services. Available from: http://www.fda.gov/AboutFDA/WhatWeDo/History/Origin/default.htm.

Food and Drug Administration and Public Health Service. 2009. *Food code 2009.* College Park, MD: U.S. Department of Health and Human Services. Available from: http://www.fda.gov/Food/FoodSafety/RetailFoodProtection/Food Code/FoodCode2009/default.htm.

Food Safety and Inspection Service. 2009, May. *FSIS testing results for melamine in retail meat and poultry products.* Washington, DC: U.S. Department of Agriculture. Available from: http://www.fsis.usda.gov/PDF/Testing_Results_ Melamine_May2009.pdf.

Food Safety and Inspection Service. 2007. About FSIS: Agency history. Washington, DC: U.S. Department of Agriculture. Available from: http://www.fsis.usda.gov/About_Fsis/Agency_History/index.asp.

Food Safety and Inspection Service. 2006. Celebrating 100 Years of FMIA. Washington, DC: U.S. Department of Agriculture. Available from: http://www.fsis.usda.gov/About_FSIS/100_Years_FMIA/index.asp.

Fortin ND. 2009. *Food regulation: Law, science, policy, and practice.* Hoboken, NJ: John Wiley.

Foster EM. 1997. Historical overview of key issues in food safety. *Emerg Infect Dis* 3(4):481–482.

Gerba CP, Rose JB, Haas CN. 1996. Sensitive populations: Who is at the greatest risk?. *Int J Food Microbiol* 30:113–123.

German RR, Lee LM, Horan JM, Milstein RL, Pertowski CA, Waller MN, Guidelines Working Group Centers for Disease Control and Prevention (CDC). 2001. Updated guidelines for evaluating public health surveillance systems: Recommendations from the Guidelines Working Group. *MMWR Recomm Rep* 50(RR-13):1,35; quiz CE1-7.

Glibert PM, Anderson DM, Gentien P, Graneli E, Sellner KG. 2005. The global, complex phenomena of harmful algal blooms. *Oceanography* 18(2):136–147.

Gorris LG. 2000. Hurdle technology. In: *Encyclopedia of food microbiology.* Vols. 1–3. Robinson RK, ed. London: Elsevier. Available from: http://knovel.com/web/portal/browse/display?_EXT_KNOVEL_DISPLAY_bookid=1870&VerticalID=0.

Greig JD, Todd EC, Bartleson CA, Michaels BS. 2007. Outbreaks where food workers have been implicated in the spread of foodborne disease. Part 1. Description of the problem, methods, and agents involved. *J Food Prot* 70(7):1752–1761.

Guardino RF. 2005. Early history of microbiology and microbiological methods. In: *Encyclopedia of rapid microbiological methods*. Vol. 1. Miller M, ed. River Grove, IL: DHI Publishing.

Helman CG. 1981. Disease versus illness in general practice. *J R Coll Gen Pract* 31(230):548–552.

Hinderliter J. 2006. From farm to table: How this little piggy was dragged through the market. *USFL Rev* 40:739–767.

Huss HH, Ababouch L, Gram L. 2004. *Assessment and management of seafood safety and quality*. FAO Fisheries Technical Paper 444. Rome, Italy: Food and Agriculture Organization of the United Nations.

Hutt PB. 2002. Regulation of food additives in the United States. In: *Food additives*. 2nd ed. Branen AL, Davidson PM, Salminen S, et al., eds. New York, NY: Marcel Dekker.

Imamura T, Ide H, Yasunaga H. 2007. History of public health crises in Japan. *J Public Health Policy* 28(2):221–237.

Institute of Food Science and Technology. 2009, November. *Organic foods*. London: Institute of Food Science and Technology.

Institute of Medicine. 2010. *Providing healthy and safe foods as we age: Workshop summary*. Washington, DC: National Academies Press.

Institute of Medicine. 2003. *Scientific criteria to ensure safe food*. Washington, DC: National Academies Press.

Institute of Medicine. 1991. *Seafood safety*. Washington, DC: National Academy Press.

Interstate Shellfish Sanitation Conference and Food and Drug Administration. 2007. *National shellfish sanitation program guide for the control of molluscan shellfish, 2007 revision*. Washington, DC: U.S. Department of Health and Human Services.

International Union of Food Science and Technology. 2009, September. *Organic food*. IUFoST Scientific Information Bulletin. Ontario, Canada: International Union of Food Science and Technology. Available from: http://iufost.org/sites/default/files/docs/IUF.SIB.Organic.Food.pdf.

Jackson LS. 2009. Chemical food safety issues in the United States: Past, present, and future. *J Agric Food Chem* 57(18):8161–8170.

Jerardo A. 2008. What share of U.S. consumed food is imported? *Amber Waves* 6(1):36–37.

Jones TF, Angulo FJ. 2006. Eating in restaurants: A risk factor for foodborne disease? *Clin Infect Dis* 43(10):1324–1328.

Jones TF, McMillian MB, Scallan E, Frenzen PD, Cronquist AB, Thomas S, Angulo FJ. 2007. A population-based estimate of the substantial burden of diarrhoeal disease in the United States; FoodNet, 1996–2003. *Epidemiol Infect* 135(2):293–301.

Kaferstein FK. 2003, September. *Food safety as a public health issue for developing countries*. 2020 Vision Briefs. Focus 10, Brief 2 of 17. Washington, DC: International Food Policy Research Institute (IFPRI). Available from: http://www.ifpri.org/sites/default/files/publications/focus10_02.pdf.

Kendall P, Medeiros LC, Hillers V, Chen G, Di Mascola S. 2003. Food handling behaviors of special importance for pregnant women, infants and young children, the elderly, and immune-compromised people. *J Am Diet Assoc* 103(12):1646–1649.

Kennedy ED, Hall RL, Montgomery SP, Pyburn DG, Jones JL, Centers for Disease Control and Prevention. 2009. Trichinellosis surveillance—United States, 2002–2007. *MMWR Surveill Summ* 58(9):1–7.

Klass AB. 2005. Bees, trees, preemption and nuisance: A new path to resolving pesticide land disputes. *Ecology Law Quarterly* 32:763–820.

Lanata CF, Mendoza W, Black RF. 2002. *Improving diarrhoea estimates*. Geneva: World Health Organization.

Laughlin L. 2010. *Who's minding the kids? Child care arrangements: Spring 2005/Summer 2006*. Report nr P70-121. Washington, DC: U.S. Census Bureau.

Leavitt JW. 1996. *Typhoid Mary: Captive to the public's health*. Boston, MA: Beacon Press.

Lejeune JT, Rajala-Schultz PJ. 2009. Food safety: Unpasteurized milk: A continued public health threat. *Clin Infect Dis* 48(1):93–100.

Loftus RT, MacHugh DE, Bradley DG, Sharp PM, Cunningham P. 1994. Evidence for two independent domestications of cattle. *Proc Natl Acad Sci U S A* 91(7):2757–2761.

Lynch M, Painter J, Woodruff R, Braden C, Centers for Disease Control and Prevention. 2006. Surveillance for foodborne-disease outbreaks—United States, 1998–2002. *MMWR Surveill Summ* 55(10):1–42.

Mandrell RE. 2007. Fruits and vegetables that make you sick. "What's going on?" *Microbiology Today* 34(8):112–115.

Marriott NR, Gravani RB. 2006. *Essentials of food sanitation*. 5th ed. New York, NY: Springer Science + Business Media. [AU: please provide page number/s for quote]

Mead PS, Slutsker L, Dietz V, McCaig LF, Bresee JS, Shapiro C, Griffin PM, Tauxe RV. 1999. Food-related illness and death in the United States. *Emerg Infect Dis* 5(5):607–625.

Meadows M. 2006, January–February. A century of ensuring safe foods and cosmetics. *FDA Consumer Magazine* Centennial Edition.

Michigan Department of Agriculture. *Training program for the professional food service sanitarian. Module 7: Foodborne illness investigations.* Lansing, MI: State of Michigan. Available from: http://www.michigan.gov/documents/MDA_mod_07_21297_7.html.

Molbak K, Olsen JE, Wegener HC. 2006. Salmonella infections. In: *Foodborne infections and intoxications.* 3rd ed. Rieman HP, Cliver DO, eds. Amsterdam: Academic Press.

Monke J. 2007. *CRS report for Congress. Agroterrorism: Threats and preparedness.* Report nr Order Code RL32521.Washington, DC: Congressional Research Service.

Morrison RM, Buzby JC, Wells HF. 2010. Guess who's turning 100? Tracking a century of American eating. *Amber Waves* 8(1):12–19.

Mushak P, Crocetti AF. 1990. Methods for reducing lead exposure in young children and other risk groups: An integrated summary of a report to the U.S. Congress on childhood lead poisoning. *Environ Health Perspect* 89:125–135.

Namminga K. 1998, September. *Trichinosis prevalence from farm to table.* Report nr ExEx 14046. Brookings, SD: College of Agriculture and Biological Sciences, South Dakota State University/U.S. Department of Agriculture. Available from: http://pubstorage.sdstate.edu/AgBio_Publications/articles/ExEx14046.pdf.

National Agricultural Library. 2010. *Trichinella: A focus on Trichinella—updated version.* Washington, DC: U.S. Department of Agriculture. Available from: http://fsrio.nal.usda.gov/nal_web/fsrio/fsheet.php?id=230.

Nelson KE, Williams CFM. 2007. Early history of infectious disease: Epidemiology and control of infectious diseases. In: *Infectious disease epidemiology: Theory and practice.* 2nd ed. Nelson KE, Williams CFM, eds. Boston, MA: Jones & Bartlett.

Nord M, Andrews M, Carlson S. 2009. *Household food security in the United States, 2008.* Report nr ERR-83. Washington, DC: U.S. Department of Agriculture.

Oliver SP, Boor KJ, Murphy SC, Murinda SE. 2009. Food safety hazards associated with consumption of raw milk. *Foodborne Pathog Dis* 6(7):793–806.

Oliver SP, Jayarao BM, Almeida RA. 2005. Foodborne pathogens in milk and the dairy farm environment: Food safety and public health implications. *Foodborne Pathog Dis* 2(2):115–129.

Oliver SP, Patel DA, Callaway TR, Torrence ME. 2009. ASAS centennial paper: Developments and future outlook for preharvest food safety. *J Anim Sci* 87(1):419–437.

Parayil G. 2003. Mapping technological trajectories of the green revolution and the gene revolution from modernization to globalization. *Research Policy* 32(6):971–990.

Pinstrup-Andersen P. 2009. Food security: Definition and measurement. *Food Sec* 1:5–7.

Roberts T. 2007. WTP estimates of the societal costs of US food-borne illness. *Am J Agr Econ* 89(5):1183–1188.

Rosen G. 1973. An American epidemiologist views his discipline. *Yale J Biol Med* 46:1–2.

Roueche B. 1988. *The medical detectives.* New York, NY: Truman Talley Books.

Satin M. 2007. *Death in the pot.* Amherst, NY: Prometheus Books.

Scharff RL. 2010. *Health-related costs from foodborne illness in the United States.* Washington, DC: Produce Safety Project at Georgetown University. Available from: http://www.producesafetyproject.org/admin/assets/files/Health-Related-Foodborne-Illness-Costs-Report.pdf-1.pdf.

Shapouri S, Rosen S, Peters M, Baquedano F, Allen S. 2010. *Food security assessment, 2010–20.* Report nr GFA-21.Washington, DC: U.S. Department of Agriculture.

Sloan AE. 2008. What, where, and when America eats: State-of-the-industry report. *Food Technology* 62(1): 20–29.

Steele JH. 1954. Milk sanitation, communicable disease, and public health. *Public Health Rep* 69(11):1065–1073.

Tauxe RV. 2002. Emerging foodborne pathogens. *Int J Food Microbiol* 78(1–2):31–41.

Tauxe RV. 2001. Food safety and irradiation: Protecting the public from foodborne infections. *Emerg Infect Dis* 7(3 Suppl):516–521.

Tauxe RV, Doyle MP, Kuchenmuller T, Schlundt J, Stein CE. 2010. Evolving public health approaches to the global challenge of foodborne infections. *Int J Food Microbiol* 139 Suppl 1:S16–28.

Tauxe RV, Esteban EJ. 2007. Advances in food safety to prevent foodborne diseases in the United States. In: *Silent victories: The history and practice of public health in twentieth-century America.* Ward JW, Warren C, eds. New York, NY: Oxford University Press.

Thacker SB. 2010. Historical background In: *Principles and practice of public health surveillance.* 3rd ed. Lee LM, Teutsch SM, Thacker SB, et al., eds. New York, NY: Oxford University Press.

Tunick MH. 2009. Dairy innovations over the past 100 years. *J Agric Food Chem* 57(18):8093–8097.

United Nations Children's Fund and World Health Organization. 2009. *Diarrhoea: Why children are still dying and what can be done.* Geneva: WHO Press.

U.S. Census Bureau. 2010. *2010 statistical abstract: Historical statistics.* Washington, DC: U.S. Census Bureau. Available from: http://www.census.gov/compendia/statab/2010/2010edition.html.

U.S. Food and Drug Administration. 2009. *FDA History Parts I–V.* Washington, DC: U.S. Food and Drug Administration. Available from: http://www.fda.gov/AboutFDA/WhatWeDo/History/Origin/ucm054819.htm.

Wade LC. 1991. The problem with classroom use of Upton Sinclair's *The Jungle. American Studies* 31(2):79–101.

Waserman MJ. 1972. Henry L. Coit and the certified milk movement in the development of modern pediatrics. *Bull Hist Med* 46(4):359–390.

Weeks BS. 2008. *Microbes and society.* 2nd ed. Sudbury, MA: Jones & Bartlett.

Wittenberger K, Dohlman E. 2010. *Peanut outlook: Impacts of the 2008–09 foodborne illness outbreak linked to* Salmonella *in peanuts.* Report nr OCS-10a-01.Washington, DC: U.S. Department of Agriculture.

World Health Organization. 2008. *Foodborne disease outbreaks: Guidelines for investigation and control.* Geneva: WHO Press.

World Health Organization. 2006. *WHO consultation to develop a strategy to estimate the global burden of foodborne diseases: Taking stock and charting the way forward.* Geneva: WHO Press.

Wright WH, Kerr KB, Jacobs L. 1943. Studies on trichinosis, XV. Summary of the findings of *Trichinella spiralis* in a random sampling and other samplings of the population of the United States. *Public Health Reports* 58(35):1293–1327.

Yoder JS, Hlavsa MC, Craun GF, Hill V, Roberts V, Yu PA, Hicks LA, Alexander NT, Calderon RL, Roy SL, et al. 2008. Surveillance for waterborne disease and outbreaks associated with recreational water use and other aquatic facility-associated health events—United States, 2005–2006. *MMWR Surveill Summ* 57(9):1–29.

Zeder MA. 2006. Central questions in the domestication of plants and animals. *Evol Anthropol* 15(3):105–117.

## USEFUL RESOURCES

Centers for Disease Control and Prevention. Food Safety Information. http://www.cdc.gov/foodsafety/

Centers for Disease Control and Prevention. *Foodborne Outbreaks Investigations.* Table of Contents. http://www.cdc.gov/outbreaknet/investigations/

Centers for Disease Control and Prevention. Foodborne Outbreak Online Database: Search OutbreakNet by year, state, location, and etiology. http://wwwn.cdc.gov/foodborneoutbreaks/

Centers for Disease Control and Prevention. How to Investigate an Outbreak. http://www.cdc.gov/EXCITE/classroom/outbreak/index.htm

Centers for Disease Control and Prevention. *Morbidity and Mortality Weekly Report (MMWR).* Important publications on current (and past) disease outbreaks and trends, including foodborne diseases. http://www.cdc.gov/mmwr/

Centers for Disease Control and Prevention. OutbreakNet Team: Outbreak Surveillance Data, including by year and etiology, Foodborne Illness A–Z, National Outbreak Reporting System (NORS). http://www.cdc.gov/foodborneoutbreaks/index.htm

Foodprocessing.com. http://www.foodprocessing.com/index.html

FoodSafety.gov. Gateway to federal food safety information. http://www.foodsafety.gov/

Harmful Algae. Distribution of HAB in the U.S. http://www.whoi.edu/redtide/page.do?pid=14898

Institute of Food Technologists. http://www.ift.org/

Interstate Shellfish Sanitation Conference. http://www.issc.org/

Michigan Department of Agriculture. Training Program for the Professional Food Service Sanitarian. Module 7: Foodborne Illness Investigations. http://www.michigan.gov/documents/MDA_mod_07_21297_7.html

National Agricultural Statistics Service. Charts and Maps. http://www.nass.usda.gov/Charts_and_Maps/index.asp

U.S. Department of Agriculture. Economic Research Service. Foodborne Illness Cost Calculator. http://www.ers.usda.gov/Data/FoodborneIllness/

U.S. Environmental Protection Agency. Agriculture: Pesticides. http://www.epa.gov/agriculture/tpes.html

World Health Organization. Food Safety. *Foodborne Disease Outbreaks: Guidelines for Investigation and Control.* http://www.who.int/foodsafety/publications/foodborne_disease/fdbmanual/en/

CHAPTER **2**

# Foodborne Infectious and Microbial Agents

## LEARNING OBJECTIVES

1. Describe the Tree of Life and explain the differences between prokaryotic (procaryotic) and eukaryotic (eucaryotic) cell types.
2. Name and describe the main taxonomic categories of microorganisms and the important foodborne pathogens in each category.
3. Briefly describe how microorganisms acquire new traits, and how these traits contribute to their survival and pathogenicity.
4. Discern the differences between foodborne illnesses, diseases, infections, toxicoinfections, intoxications, and poisonings.
5. Describe the steps in the cycle of parasitism and infection, and define key terms used in the processes of the cycle.
6. Describe common signs and symptoms of diseases caused by foodborne pathogens and, in general terms, the mechanisms of pathogenicity involved.
7. Identify factors or circumstances that may increase pathogen virulence or reduce host resistance to a foodborne infection.
8. Explain the importance of serotyping and other classification schemes for the identification and control of pathogens in foods, particularly for the genera *Escherichia* and *Salmonella*.
9. For each important foodborne pathogen, identify the major food groups most often associated with the disease(s) it causes.
10. List the important bacterial pathogens that cause foodborne illnesses, and identify their common and unique reservoirs and/or sources of food contamination.
11. Name the viruses that are most frequently transmitted by foods, and explain how foods are most likely contaminated with these viruses.
12. List important protozoans that may be transmitted by foods, and identify their primary reservoirs.
13. Describe the sources of parasitic helminths in foods and their relationships to humans and animals.

14. Understand the nature of prions and the diseases they cause, and explain how they may enter the human food chain.
15. Differentiate between emerging and contemporary foodborne diseases, and give examples of how various factors contribute to the emergence of foodborne diseases.

## TYPES OF INFECTIOUS AND MICROBIAL AGENTS

The oldest and most adaptable forms of life on earth are microorganisms. They occupy every part of the biosphere, the theoretical boundaries of life extending several miles above and below the earth's surface. Over the course of 3.8 billion years of evolution, microorganisms have adapted to survive under very diverse environmental conditions, and they have developed complex microbial communities and ecosystems. Furthermore, these adaptations have been essential to the evolution and survival of other organisms such as plants and animals. The relationships of microorganisms with plants and animals are frequently symbiotic. This may include mutualism, commensalism, and/or parasitism. The principal differences between these three types of symbiotic relationships are related to the differences in benefits between the organisms. With mutualism, both species (e.g., plant/animal and microorganism) benefit somehow by the relationship, whereas with commensalism, one species benefits from the relationship, while the other species neither benefits nor is harmed by it. In contrast, parasitism is where one species (e.g., microorganism) benefits and the other species (e.g., plant or animal) is somehow harmed by the relationship.

The adaptation of microorganisms to environmental conditions results in some becoming pathogenic (i.e., able to cause disease) in plants and animals. These adaptations can be measured in two general time frames: (1) millions of years, resulting in the creation of totally new species; and (2) days and years, leading to new variants in a species or strain (Groisman and Casadesus 2005). The underlying mechanisms of such microbial adaptations are in the genes, specifically from changes in the coding and/or regulatory control of DNA (or RNA in the case of certain viruses). The genetic makeup of microorganisms is variable and subject to rapid change by a number of different mechanisms. And because under ideal conditions the reproduction/multiplication time of most microorganisms is measured in minutes, genetically new populations of microorganisms can evolve in a short time, at least compared with the evolution of more complex organisms. These new variants and strains of microorganisms may be endowed with genes to survive new environments (including in foods or within human hosts), develop resistance to antibiotics, or become increasingly pathogenic. Additional information about DNA and the genes of pathogens is presented later in Chapter 7.

Despite the vast number of microbial species on earth, a relatively small number are pathogenic to animals—including humans. The pathogenic agents of greatest concern in foods are taxonomically classified as bacteria, viruses, fungi, protozoa, helminths, and prions. Except for the viruses and prions, these organisms are represented in the Bacteria and Eucaryota domains of the phylogenetic Tree of Life, depicted in Figure 2-1. Although this classification scheme is speculative, it is based on the sequencing of nucleic acids (ribosomal RNA) and regarded as more relevant in terms of phylogeny than simple phenotypic characteristics. In recent years, more than 70 phylum-level bacterial lines have been identified, but only about 7 phyla contain human pathogens (Pace 2008). The phyla with human pathogens are also represented by a large body of scientific literature that includes phenotypic characteristics derived from microscopy and culturing studies. Before the advent of gene sequencing, phenotypic characteristics were the sole basis for the taxonomic classification of microorganisms, and such characteristics still remain important in the identification and understanding of microorganisms and their pathogenicity.

The taxonomic classification of microorganisms is debatable among scientists and scholars, particularly at the phyla and class levels. Nevertheless, the classification of microorganisms is important for reasons other than scientific curiosity, a fact that will become increasingly apparent in the practice of food safety. In general, an agreed-upon classification system permits the precise identification of foodborne pathogens, which in turn assists in the epidemiology of foodborne diseases and the development of prevention strategies for food safety.

## Bacteria

The bacteria are single-celled microorganisms that represent a major domain on the theoretical Tree of Life. They are diverse and ubiquitous microorganisms with genetic identities and phenotypic characteristics that distinguish them from the other domains. Their cellular composition and structures are "prokaryotic" in nature. Prokaryotic cells are characterized by the absence of a

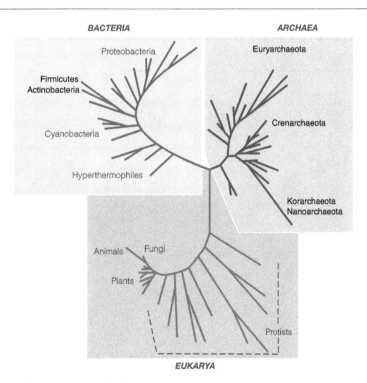

**Figure 2-1** The Phylogenetic Tree of Life*

nuclear membrane and organelles, presence of a cell wall, division by binary fission, and other characteristics exhibited in Figure 2-2. In addition to a circular DNA chromosome, bacteria have circular snippets of DNA called plasmids in their cytoplasm that may also confer traits such as resistance to antibiotics, expanded metabolic functions, and greater pathogenicity. The chromosome and plasmids can be inherited by successive generations of bacteria (called vertical transfer). Furthermore, the plasmids and chromosomal DNA may be transferred between bacterial cells (called horizontal transfer) by processes known as transformation and conjugation. Transformation involves the uptake of DNA by a viable bacterial cell from one that has ruptured. Conjugative transfer of DNA occurs between bacterial cells through appendages called pili. A third means of DNA transfer between bacterial cells is called transduction and involves bacteriophages, that is, viruses that infect bacterial cells.

Bacterial cells have a variety of morphologies, or shapes. The shapes of greatest concern in food safety are the bacillus (rod), coccus (sphere), and spiral. Cell sizes of bacteria (see Figure 2-3) can range from an extremely small 0.2 μm to a relatively large 750 μm (Schulz and Jorgensen 2001). The bacterial cell sizes most encountered with food safety range close to the rod-shaped *Escherichia coli*, about 1 μm in width and 2 μm in length. The individual coccus of *Staphylococcus aureus* is about 0.6 μm in diameter, though this bacterium is usually associated with larger grape-like clusters of cocci. External cellular structures such as the flagellum are not present in all bacteria, and the biochemical composition of the cell walls and capsules can vary among different species. Researchers can use these different characteristics to identify and classify bacterial species or strains. More details on such characteristics are provided later for individual species of food

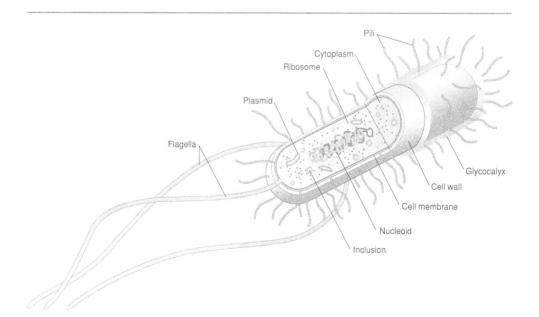

**Figure 2-2** Idealized Prokaryotic Cell Structure

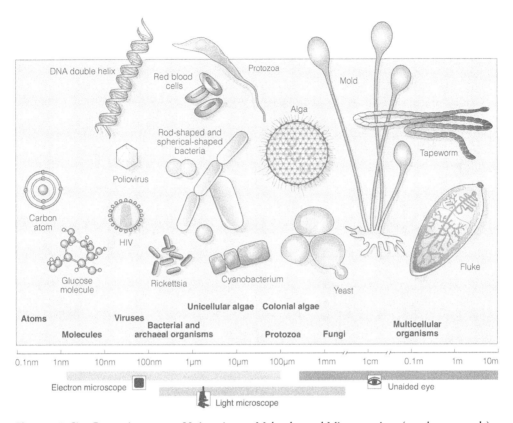

**Figure 2-3** Size Comparison among Various Atoms, Molecules, and Microorganisms (not drawn to scale)

safety importance. For now, some important bacterial species and their taxonomic classifications are listed in Table 2-1.

Various species of bacteria have different requirements for growth in terms of nutrients, temperature ranges, moisture content, and oxygen availability. All of these requirements are important with regard to food safety, in particular for destroying or controlling the growth of bacteria. The bacteria that can grow under full oxygen conditions are called aerobes, whereas bacteria that can grow only under anoxic conditions are called obligate anaerobes. Species that can grow with or without the presence of oxygen are facultative. A few species such as *Campylobacter jejuni* are microaerophilic, meaning they can use oxygen only under reduced conditions (<21% oxygen). Bacteria are also categorized by their temperature growth ranges and optima: psychrophilic (~4°C optimum), mesophilic (~39°C optimum), and thermophilic (~60°C optimum). Water availability to bacteria is determined not only by the amount of $H_2O$, but by the osmotic effect of solutes (e.g., salts and sugars) dissolved in the water. With the exception of some species, most bacteria of food safety concern are not very tolerant of high osmotic conditions.

**Table 2-1** Taxonomic Classification of Important Foodborne Bacterial Pathogens

| Phylum | Class | Order | Family | Genus | Species |
|---|---|---|---|---|---|
| Proteobacteria | Epsilonproteobacteria | Campylobacterales | Campylobacteraceae | *Campylobacter* | *jejuni* |
| | Gammaproteobacteria | Aeromonadales | Aeromonadaceae | *Aeromonas* | *hydrophila* |
| | | Enterobacteriales | Enterobacteriaceae | *Escherichia* | *coli* |
| | | | | *Salmonella* | *enterica* <br> *bangori* |
| | | | | *Shigella* | *sonnei* <br> *dysenteriae* <br> *flexneri* <br> *boydii* |
| | | | | *Yersinia* | *enterocolitica* |
| | | Vibrionales | Vibrionaceae | *Vibrio* | *parahaemolyticus* <br> *vulnificus* <br> *cholerae* |
| Firmicutes | Bacilli | Bacillales | Bacillaceae | *Bacillus* | *cereus* |
| | | | Listeriaceae | *Listeria* | *monocytogenes* |
| | | | Staphylococcaceae | *Staphylococcus* | *aureus* |
| | | Lactobacillales | Streptococcaceae | *Streptococcus* | *pyogenes* |
| | Clostridia | Clostridiales | Clostridiaceae | *Clostridium* | *botulinum* <br> *perfringens* |

*Source:* Compiled from Garrity GM, Lilburn TG, Cole JR, Harrison SH, Euzeby J, Tindall BJ. 2007. Taxonomic outline of the bacteria and archaea, release 7.7 March 6, 2007. Michigan State University Board of Trustees. Available from: http://www.taxonomicoutline.org/

The family Enterobacteriaceae is arguably the most important group of bacteria in food safety. This family consists of approximately 44 genera and 176 species, many of them living symbiotically within the intestines of animals as commensal microorganisms (Brenner and Farmer 2005). However, several species are enteric pathogens that are frequently responsible for foodborne disease outbreaks and are also detected in clinical samples from patients with infections. Whereas most Enterobacteriaceae can thrive within intestinal tracts of animals, some species also survive and multiply in the environment. This makes them problematic because of possible food contamination. On the other hand, nonpathogenic Enterobacteriaceae are useful sanitary indicators for food safety. A few species have evolved to live solely in the environment (including plants, soil, and water) and have less value as sanitary indicators. Additional information about the classification of Enterobacteriaceae and their use as sanitary indicators is provided in a Chapter 7.

## Viruses

Viruses must have access to a host cell to replicate and propagate. In other words, they are obligate intracellular parasites. This is because viruses are essentially nucleic acids (DNA or RNA) packaged in proteins that form a capsid (Figure 2-4) and have neither the molecular machinery nor the resources necessary for metabolism and independent replication. Yet, viruses are the most prolific and abundant microorganisms on earth. Viruses accomplish this feat by infecting host cells and exploiting their metabolism and resources to replicate and disseminate to new host cells. The nucleic acid packaged in the virus directs the host cell to divert its energy and resources to serve the virus's needs. Viruses have a very specific range of hosts, and they have preferences for certain cell types within a multicellular host. Virtually every organism is a host to some viruses, but the virus must have the correct proteins for access to the host cell and the correctly encoded nucleic acids to direct the host cell's activity.

The classification of viruses is challenging because they are not "living" in the same sense as other microorganisms, and they vary greatly in structure, nucleic acid content, and hosts. Two schemes for virus classification are employed: (1) the Baltimore Classification, named after the Nobel Prize Winner David Baltimore; and (2) the International Committee on Taxonomy of Viruses (ICTV), established in the early 1990s to standardize virus taxonomy. The Baltimore Classification scheme assigns viruses to groups on the basis of nucleic acid structure and other characteristics, whereas the ICTV scheme attempts to assign viruses using taxon structures similar to cellular organisms (e.g., species, genus, family, subfamily, and order). To avoid confusion, the classification of viruses is discussed as necessary in a later section on foodborne viruses.

## Protozoans

The protozoans are located under the domain of Eucarya on the phylogenetic Tree of Life. These organisms, as well as the others under the domain Eucarya, are characterized by eukaryotic cells. As illustrated in Figure 2-5, eukaryotic cell structures have many differences from prokaryotic cells, including the presence of a membrane-bound nucleus, a cytoskeleton, and other structural and chemical differences. A single kingdom does not adequately categorize all protozoans. The principal reason is the extreme diversity of these eukaryotic microorganisms, being neither

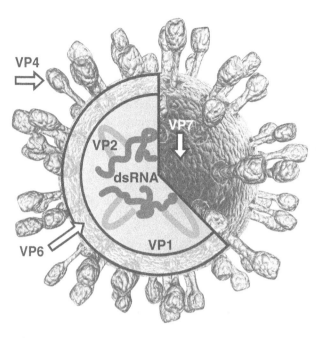

**Figure 2-4**  Diagram of a Rotavirus. *Source:* Photo © Psim/Dreamstime.com. *Note:* Double-stranded RNA (dsRNA) virus. Viral structural proteins are represented by VP1 through VP7.

animals (Animalia), plants (Plantae), nor fungi (Fungi). In the recent past, protozoans belonged to a single kingdom called Protista that seemed like the default category for eucaryotes. Under this conventional scheme, the protozoans were further classified using simple but useful criteria such as morphology, motility, host ranges, geographic distribution, and types of diseases caused. The advent of sophisticated molecular techniques that can reveal phylogenetic relationships has placed the classification of protozoans into a state of flux, leading to scientific debates about their interrelationships.

Regardless of the issues with protozoan taxonomy and phylogenetics, certain characteristics in terms of their pathogenesis and relevance to food safety can be generally described. Protozoans are unicellular organisms, most motile, with eukaryotic characteristics. Their morphologies differ among genera and species, and the protozoan morphology can also change during certain stages in their life cycle. One stage involves the development of cysts that can survive harsh environmental conditions. Most protozoans are free-living in the environment, while some also require multiple hosts to complete their life cycles. They reproduce by either binary fission or sexual fusion of cellular forms called gametes. Larval forms of the protozoan develop in animals called intermediate hosts, whereas the adult forms sexually reproduce in animals called definitive hosts. The active feeding stages of protozoans are usually called trophozoites. In most cases, the stage ingested from contaminated food is the cyst, and the stage that causes human disease is the trophozoite.

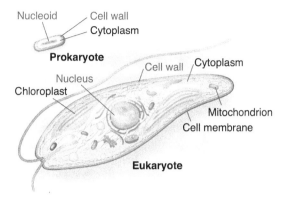

**Figure 2-5** Differences Between Prokaryotic and Eukaryotic Cells

## Fungi

The fungi represent a kingdom under the domain of Eucarya. Fungi reproduce through the development of either sexual or asexual spores that are easily and ubiquitously disseminated by the wind. Unlike bacterial spores, fungal sexual spores are not very resistant to heat. Fungal vegetative cells are more closely related to animals than plants and other microorganisms, and their morphology can be either unicellular or multicellular with filamentous threads called hyphae. When hyphae grow and overlap, they form visible tufts called mycelium. In their unicellular form, fungi are referred to as yeasts, while the filamentous forms are called molds when visible to the naked eye. Mushrooms are actually fungi where the mycelium differentiates into a fruiting body called a basidiocarp.

Although fungi are essential to life on earth as decomposers, only a relatively few are pathogenic to animals—including humans. These infections (called mycotic infections) and diseases (called mycoses) are rarely acquired from food, except in circumstances where the host is severely immunocompromised. Like animals, fungi are heterotrophic (i.e., must feed on preformed organic material), but unlike animals, fungi digest their food extracellularly with exoenzymes. Therein lies the primary hazard associated with fungi in foods: Many of the substances produced by fungi are inherently toxic, collectively called mycotoxins. These substances can contaminate foods. In the case of edible fungi such as mushrooms, toxic substances may be found within the basidiocarp. The toxic hazards associated with fungi in foods are discussed further in a section on mycotoxins in Chapter 3.

## Helminths

The term *helminths* is used to describe a broad variety of parasites colloquially called worms. The classification of helminths varies greatly among textbooks, and some of the phyla encompassed by the term *helminth* are phylogenetically distant from one another in the Tree of Life. Three phyla of helminths are important to food safety:

1. Phylum Plathyhelminthes, commonly known as cestodes, flatworms, or tape worms
2. Phylum Nematoda, commonly known as nematodes or roundworms
3. Phylum Annelida, including the commonly known trematodes or flukes

The helminths differ from protozoans by their size and complexity of biology. Helminths are multicellular organisms. Adults of most helminth species are macroscopic, capable of being seen without a microscope, though several helminth stages of development can be microscopic, for example, the egg and larval stages. Helminths usually have complex life cycles involving multiple intermediate and/or definitive hosts, and they have organ systems that permit functions such as sexual reproduction, sometimes as hermaphrodites. In lesser developed countries, the population is heavily burdened by these parasitic worms, whereas developed countries such as the United States have largely controlled helminth infections in human populations. However, the opportunity for reemergence of helminth infections always exists, either from lax food safety practices, international travel, and/or importation of unsafe foods.

## Prions

At one time, viruses were thought to be the smallest and simplest infectious agents. This changed with the discovery of prions. Essentially, prions are rogue proteins that can be transmitted through the consumption of prion-infected animals. Once consumed, these prions corrupt other proteins by inducing protein misfolding. This results in plague formation within critical neurologic tissues and organs such as the brain. The most infamous example in recent years is bovine spongiform encephalopathy, otherwise known as BSE or "mad cow disease." Several types of prions in other animals have been identified that pose a potential threat to the food chain of humans.

## FOODBORNE INFECTIONS VS. INTOXICATIONS, A.K.A. POISONING

Chapter 1 briefly introduced the difference between a foodborne "illness" and "disease." More specifically, *disease* is a condition that has been diagnosed by a clinician with a specific understanding of the etiology and biology involved. On the other hand, the term *illness* is more subjective and implies a person is "unwell" without necessarily knowing the causes or understanding the biology (Helman 1981). By extension of logic, a *foodborne illness* happens whenever a person feels sick after consuming food items, whereas a *foodborne disease* is a specific and confirmed case of disease (with a known etiology) associated with the ingestion of food.

In simplest terms, a foodborne infection is the establishment of a host–parasite relationship where the parasite entered the host by the ingestion of food. In contrast, foodborne intoxication results from an acutely toxic dose of a chemical substance in the food. The chemical substance may be a biological toxin produced by a microorganism, an inherent toxin in the tissues of a food animal or plant, or a toxicant in the environment, including food containers. The differences between foodborne infections and intoxications are discussed later in more detail.

Laypersons and the popular press sometimes refer to foodborne illnesses as "food poisoning." This colloquial term does not properly convey the etiology and prevention of a foodborne disease—or even whether it is an infection or intoxication. Yet, the term is often used and is misleading, making it difficult to educate the public about good food safety practices. For food safety professionals, the distinction between the various terms is important to understand the causes and prevention of foodborne illnesses and diseases.

Over the years, a condition called a toxicoinfection has been recognized. This term is used to describe disease from microorganisms producing toxins in the lumen of the gut after being consumed—as opposed to foodborne intoxications where the toxin is preformed in the food prior to consumption. Several bacteria are known to cause toxicoinfections and are covered in this chapter.

## Basic Pathogenesis of Foodborne Infections

To understand foodborne infections, it is necessary to understand basic infectious disease transmission and pathogenesis (i.e., origin and development of disease). First, in the strictest biological sense, an infection is a symbiotic relationship between a parasite and host. When the nature of this relationship causes harmful changes in the host, an infectious disease develops. Thus, the term *infection* describes the establishment of a host–parasite relationship, whereas *disease* is when the parasite causes clinical manifestations in the host. In such cases, a parasite is also called a *pathogen*.

Quite often, bacteria are not referred to as parasites because they are rarely obligate parasites, that is, they do not always require a host to survive and reproduce. In fact—depending on the species—a great number of pathogenic bacteria can also survive and multiply outside of a host under favorable environmental conditions for various periods of time. These survival characteristics allow some pathogens to be foodborne rather than being transmitted solely through person-to-person contact. Health professionals typically use the term *parasite* for protozoans and helminths because these organisms are often obligate parasites (though some are free-living or remain viable in foods), and they possess a complex unicellular or multicellular biology similar to animals.

As illustrated in Figure 2-6, the cycle of parasitism and infection can be described in three general steps:

1. Access to the host
2. Establishment and pathogenesis (leading possibly to a carrier state or disease pathology)
3. Egress and further transmission of pathogens

### Access to the Host

Before a pathogen can gain access to a host, it must be transmitted from a reservoir or other source. A reservoir is part of the pathogen's normal habitat, where it can reproduce and sustain species survival while awaiting an opportunity for transmission to a host. Several modes of transmission exist: person-to-person contact, consumption of contaminated food and water, handling of fomites (inanimate objects), vectors (other organisms), and through the air from aerosols or droplets. These modes of transmission are not necessarily mutually exclusive for most pathogens,

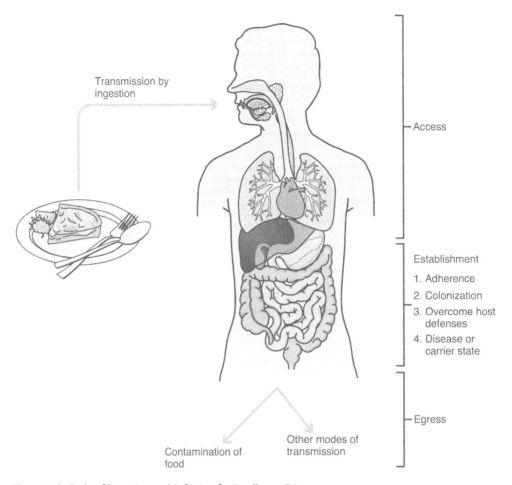

**Figure 2-6**  Cycle of Parasitism and Infection for Foodborne Disease

including the foodborne pathogens, and may involve a chain of transmission. For example, sputum or sneezing from an infected food handler can contaminate servings of food to further spread infection. Similarly, a rodent (vector) can transmit a pathogen by contaminating foodstuffs with feces and urine. And inanimate objects such as contaminated utensils and unclean dishes can facilitate communicable disease transmission among a population. Likewise, with certain infections, an initial case of foodborne infection can also spread through a population by person-to-person transmission.

Pathogen access to a host can occur through several transmission routes or portals of entry: inhalation, oral, ocular, through the skin (e.g., cuts, needles, bites), and sexual contact. Obviously, for food safety, the oral or ingestion route is the utmost concern. The majority of foodborne pathogens need to access the gastrointestinal tract to cause disease, but a few only need to access the mucous membranes, for example, the agent of strep throat (*S. pyogenes*). To gain access to the gastrointestinal tract, a pathogen must survive passage through the extremely acidic environment of the stomach, which has a normal pH range of 1 to 5, and the presence of digestive enzymes such as pepsin. Several factors can help a pathogen while passing through the harsh environment of the stomach. One factor is the protective effects of food. Pathogens suspended in lipophilic vehicles are protected to various degrees from the killing effectiveness of an acid barrier (Todd et al. 2008b). Foods such as ice cream and fat-laden desserts provide good vehicles for pathogen protection. Several species of pathogens also have an acid tolerance response (ATR) for short periods of time; this is an adaptive response involving the production of specialized proteins that prevent cellular damage from environmental stress (O'Driscoll, Gahan, Hill, 1996). Such short-term adaptive responses are driven by molecular signals that turn on or off in response to environmental conditions. As discussed earlier, these responses have evolved in microorganisms as a result of selection pressures that favored strains with such molecular mechanisms.

### Establishment and Pathogenesis

Establishment of an enteric pathogen requires its adhesion and colonization to the single layer of cells in the intestine called the mucosal epithelium, depicted in Figure 2-7. Several pathogen and host factors collectively determine whether adhesion and colonization will be successful. Among the host factors are barriers such as secreted mucins and other compounds that form a mucous layer and also provide an antimicrobial effect (Boirivant and Strober 2007). Other host factors include innate immune responses involving cytokines (signaling molecules), lymphocytes that can pass into the intestinal lumen, and a network of lymphatic vessels and nodes in the lamina propria, the mucosal layer of various cells under the epithelium (Magalhaes, Tattoli, Girardin 2007). Unlike adaptive immunity that requires prior exposure to the pathogen, the responses by innate immunity provide a relatively rapid and broad barrier for the epithelium.

Before an enteric pathogen can successfully adhere to and colonize the intestine, it must possess specialized biomolecular "traits." Adherence to the mucosal epithelium involves the binding of specialized proteins (and other molecules) on the pathogen called adhesins with receptors that span the cell membranes of the epithelium. In bacteria, most adhesins are associated with hairlike appendages protruding from the cell wall called fimbriae; these structures are sometimes referred to as pili when describing the intercellular transfer of nucleic acids (Pizarro-Cerda and Cossart 2006). The adhesins are typically associated with the apical end of the fimbriae, and the protein structure of adhesins can be different for certain species or strains of bacteria. This is important because protein structure determines the specificity and strength of binding to a receptor on the epithelial cell membrane.

An important barrier to pathogen adhesion and colonization is an extremely large population of commensal microorganisms (approximately $10^{14}$ bacteria) that reside in the gut, collectively called the microbiota. These microorganisms colonize both the lumen and the mucosal epithelium. They confer benefits to the host in terms of development and digestion, but more important, they protect the intestine from pathogens by a phenomenon called microbial interference or colonization resistance (Stecher and Hardt 2008). In essence, this phenomenon results from the

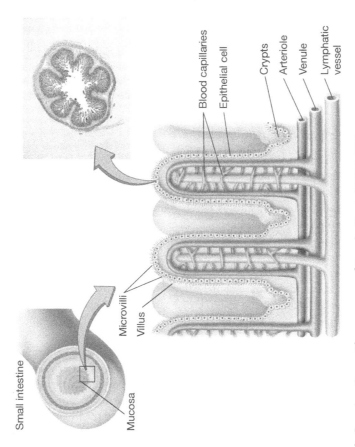

**Figure 2-7** Anatomy of the Intestine. *Source:* Photo courtesy of Douglas Burrin/USDA ARS

microbiota outcompeting enteric pathogens for space and nutrients within the microbial ecology of the intestine. At the biomolecular level, a complex set of mechanisms is involved among the pathogens, microbiota, and host. Some of these biomolecular mechanisms have been described in great detail, while others are not fully understood (Magalhaes et al. 2007).

Various species of the gut microbiota also possess adhesins for colonizing the mucosal epithelium, thus creating competition for pathogens to access the epithelium. Pathogens outcompete the microbiota in a number of ways. One way is for the pathogen's adhesins to possess a unique protein structure that preferentially binds with different receptors on the surface of the epithelium (Viswanathan, Hodges, Hecht 2009). Evidence also exists that gut inflammation can disrupt colonization resistance of the microbiota; pathogens can circumvent multiple biomolecular processes involved with colonization resistance as well (Stecher and Hardt 2008). Finally, it is well established that reduction of commensal bacteria in the gut by preexisting disease or certain exposures (e.g., radiation and antibiotic therapy) can lead to an increased risk of enteric infections and to more severe cases of infection.

Colonization by the pathogens is necessary to increase their numbers. Several species of bacterial pathogens can develop an attachment matrix called a biofilm. Actually, this matrix is not a uniform film but rather a heterogeneous mixture of bacterial cells and organic and inorganic components (Donlan 2001). Through an intercellular communication process called quorum sensing, certain pathogens can induce a colony of bacteria to produce substances for biofilm development. Biofilms offer several distinct advantages for a pathogen: (1) They provide resistance to the host immune system; (2) they provide protection against antimicrobial agents; (3) they provide an environment to exchange DNA among the pathogens; and (4) they provide a protective matrix for detachments of pathogens to colonize other parts of the body (Donlan and Costerton 2002). The importance of biofilms is discussed again later with regard to sanitation and environmental surfaces.

Pathogens must overcome the immune defenses of the host before, during, and after colonization. This is accomplished by any of several tactics involving evasion, subversion, and/or exploitation of the host's innate and acquired immunity (Finlay and Falkow 1997). One tactic is the development of biofilms discussed previously. Most tactics involve biomolecular interactions that circumvent the host immune system. For example, pathogens can disguise themselves by attaching proteins on their surfaces that mimic host proteins, causing the host's antigen-recognition mechanisms to be fooled. Other mechanisms involve secretion of compounds that enzymatically degrade or destroy the host's immune components and interfere with the molecular signaling processes. The most common pathogen tactic is antigenic variation, often by a new strain of pathogen. By changing the antigens on their surfaces (Figure 2-8), pathogens can escape recognition by the host's immune system, or at least make the recognition process less efficient.

After successful colonization by a pathogen (i.e., infection), the host can suffer disease or become an asymptomatic carrier. Incubation periods can vary before any signs and symptoms appear (Figure 2-9). The most common affliction is gastroenteritis, a general term used to describe irritation or inflammation of the gastrointestinal tract. The signs and symptoms of gastroenteritis caused by different foodborne pathogens tend to overlap one another. According to the list in Table 2-2, the predominant sign is diarrhea.

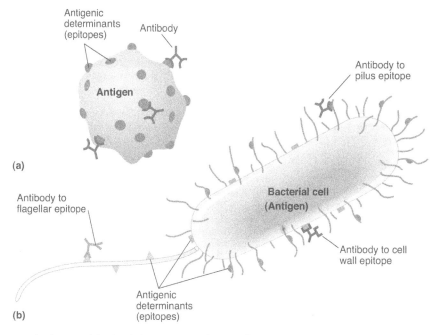

**Figure 2-8** Antigens and Antigenic Determinants (Epitopes)

The internal lining of the intestine has exquisitely evolved to maximize its surface area and to facilitate nutrient absorption, while also maintaining an electrolyte balance between the lumen contents and surrounding tissues. These important functions are primarily dependent on the mucosal epithelium. When an imbalance occurs between the absorption and secretion of ions

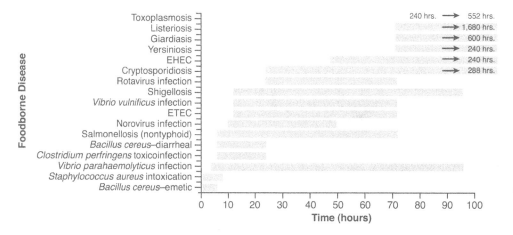

**Figure 2-9** Incubation Ranges for Selected Foodborne Diseases. *Source:* Data from Heymann, 2008

Table 2-2 Signs and Symptoms of Gastroenteritis from Foodborne Infections

| Disease | Nausea or Vomiting | Diarrhea (Type) | Cramps or Pain | Fever | Other Signs, Symptoms |
|---|---|---|---|---|---|
| Campylobacteriosis | P | P-bloody[c] (inflammatory) | P | P | — |
| EHEC[a] infection | P | P-severe-bloody[c] (inflammatory) | P | P/A | — |
| ETEC[b] infection | P/A | P-watery (noninflammatory) | P | A | — |
| Salmonellosis (nontyphoid) | P | P (inflammatory) | P | P | — |
| Shigellosis | A | P-mucus[c]-blood[c] (inflammatory) | P | P | — |
| Cholera | P | P-profuse watery (noninflammatory) | A | A | Severe dehydration |
| Yersiniosis | P | P (inflammatory) | P | P | Appendicitis-like |
| Listeriosis | P/A | P/A | A | P | Muscle aches Flu-like Bacteremia |
| Cryptosporidiosis | A | P-watery (noninflammatory) | P | P-slight | May be relapsing |
| Giardiasis | A | P (noninflammatory) | P | A | Gas |
| Norovirus infection | P | P (noninflammatory) | P | P | Myalgia Headache |
| Rotavirus infection | P | P-watery (noninflammatory) | P | P-low grade | Lactose intolerance |

Note: P = usually present; A = usually absent; P/A = may be present or absent.
[a] Enterohemorrhagic *E. coli.*
[b] Enterotoxigenic *E. coli.*
[c] May or may not be this type of diarrhea.
*Source:* Compiled from AMA et al. 2004 and Navaneethan and Giannella 2008.

and solutes by the epithelial cells, excessive water moves into the lumen, resulting in diarrhea (Viswanathan et al. 2009). Although several conditions can lead to diarrhea, the most common preventable causes are enteric pathogens—including foodborne pathogens. Two major syndromes of diarrhea are recognized: (1) noninflammatory diarrhea and (2) inflammatory diarrhea (Navaneethan and Giannella 2008).

Pathogens that alter the permeability of the mucosal epithelium to ions and solutes without significant inflammation or mucosal damage cause noninflammatory diarrhea. This typically involves pathogen adherence to and colonization of the small intestine. With this type of diarrhea, the mucosal epithelium is rarely invaded by the pathogen, except for viruses, which use a method called endocytosis. The primary mechanism for noninflammatory diarrhea is the production of target-specific exotoxins by the pathogen. Exotoxins are proteins released by pathogens that modify or destroy host cellular structures such as membranes, extracellular matrices, or other intracellular targets. Toxin structures may consist of two or more subunits and/or involve multiple molecular interactions. By altering transporter proteins and ion channels in the mucosal epithelium, some exotoxins cause diarrhea without inflammation (Navaneethan and Giannella 2008). The toxin's structure, mechanism of action, and pathogenesis are often important to classifying and identifying a strain of pathogen. Toxins that actively affect the gastrointestinal tract are collectively called enterotoxins.

As the term implies, inflammatory diarrhea is caused by molecular products from an acute inflammatory reaction of the intestinal mucosa. One cause of inflammation is the invasion of the intestinal mucosa by the pathogens. A few pathogens may actually pass through the mucosa into the bloodstream and affect other organs (e.g., *Salmonella* spp. and *Listeria monocytogenes*). The invasiveness of pathogens is enhanced by compounds appropriately called invasins. Another cause of inflammation is the production of exceptionally noxious toxins by the pathogens called cytotoxins, which severely damage host cells and induce inflammatory diarrhea (Navaneethan and Giannella 2008). Some particularly virulent pathogens cause inflammatory diarrhea by both invasiveness and the production of toxins.

Over the past few decades, research and follow-up on acute foodborne infections have revealed latent or chronic aftereffects called sequelae among a small percentage of victims (Rees et al. 2004). Among these conditions are neurologic disorders; inflammatory diseases of the bowel and joints, such as colitis and arthritis; kidney and vascular damage; and other gastrointestinal disorders (Lindsay 1997). These chronic conditions can appear weeks or years after the acute infection and may last for many years after onset, possibly leading to premature death. The particular species and strains of pathogens, along with host predisposition, can play a role in the risk of sequelae.

An important concept associated with foodborne infection (and infectious diseases in general) is the nature of pathogen virulence and host resistance. Simply stated, virulence is the capacity of a given pathogen to produce disease. Conversely, resistance is the capacity of a given host to resist disease. Virulence and resistance can be viewed abstractly as a battle between pathogens and hosts with an array of different weapons available to each one. For the pathogen, the arsenal of weapons includes adhesins, invasins, toxins, antigenic factors, dissemination to other tissues, antibiotic resistance, and molecular signals for immune system circumvention. These virulent properties or capabilities of the pathogen are referred to as virulence factors, and they are the products of specific sets of genes within the pathogen's DNA.

For the host, the defensive weapons can be classified as either nonspecific host resistance or specific host resistance. The most important defense within the realm of nonspecific host resistance is the health and nutritional status of the host. A healthy and well-nourished host is better equipped to defend against and eliminate a pathogen. On the other hand, preexisting disease and/or malnourishment can negatively affect everything from immune system function to the microbiota of the intestine. Certain drugs and medications can also have the same effect. The specific host resistance includes the synthesis of immunoglobulins and/or the development of cellular immunity. Much of the specific host resistance is determined by the host's genes. Low host resistance is equivalent to host susceptibility to infection. Both nonspecific and specific host resistance can be affected by age, with the very young and very old being most susceptible to infections because of either undeveloped (younger) or diminished (older) host resistance.

A related and important concept to food safety is the infectious dose or infective dose of a pathogen. In theory, this is the minimum number of pathogens (of a specific strain and species) necessary to cause an infectious disease in a host. However, a review of literature on infective dose does not reveal a formal definition in any medical texts (Johnson 2003). The difficulties with trying to determine an infective dose for a pathogen are numerous. Foremost, the variability associated with pathogen virulence and host resistance is huge—especially when different strains of pathogens and the heterogeneous makeup of human hosts are taken into account. Experiments to determine infective dose using similar strains of pathogens and inbred animals still yielded great variability, and the results could not be extrapolated to humans (Johnson 2003). It has been hypothesized that much of this variability can be explained by the biomolecular mechanisms of pathogenesis, but research has not adequately tested this hypothesis (Schmid-Hempel and Frank 2007).

Although extreme variability hinders establishment of an infective dose for pathogens, epidemiologic studies of foodborne illness outbreaks have provided estimates for several pathogens. Despite the shortcomings of determining infective doses, these estimates do convey the relative virulence of foodborne pathogens in healthy individuals. Furthermore, the concept of infective dose is helpful in risk assessments and determining acceptable levels of pathogens in foods (Teunis, Nagelkerke, Haas 1999). It is important to remember that infective doses can be much lower for very young or senior people, and many medical conditions or concurrent exposures, some discussed earlier, can lower host resistance and hence the infective dose.

### Egress and Transmission

The final step of the parasitism and infection cycle is egress and transmission: leaving the primary host to infect other hosts. The principal means of egress for foodborne pathogens is through defecation, usually diarrhea, and sometimes vomiting. Other body fluids may also be contaminated with the more invasive pathogens. To a great degree, inducing diarrhea is a survival mechanism for enteric pathogens because it provides the pathogens with an opportunity to leave the host in greater numbers, increasing the chances of transmission and access to other hosts. The number of pathogens expelled commonly ranges from $10^5$ to $10^9$ infectious cells or viral particles per milliliter (mL) or gram (g) of feces, sometimes as high as $10^{11}$ cells or particles per mL or g (Todd et al. 2008b).

During the incubation and convalescent phases of a disease, when a host may not exhibit disease symptoms, large numbers of pathogens can still be shed in the feces. These hosts are incubatory and convalescent carriers of disease-causing microorganisms, capable of contaminating foodstuffs and transmitting the disease to others. In situations where individuals have a great resistance to a pathogen, they can become subclinically or asymptomatically infected for indefinite periods of time. These individuals apparently do not suffer from disease but remain disease carriers capable of shedding the pathogen and transmitting it to others. They are referred to as asymptomatic carriers. The first confirmed case of an asymptomatic carrier was the villanized Mary Mallon, a.k.a. Typhoid Mary, discussed in Chapter 1. Since then, it is an established fact that a great number of asymptomatic disease carriers exist, both in human and animal populations. Disease carriers are not easily identified but are extremely important considerations in food safety.

## FOODBORNE BACTERIAL AGENTS

### Pathogenic *Escherichia coli*

News reports about outbreaks caused by *Escherichia coli* have caused grave concern among consumers and public health officials over the past few decades. Despite the notoriety that has become associated with *E. coli*, this species of bacterium usually resides peacefully within our intestines as part of the microbiota. The strain or serotype of *E. coli* determines its virulence and pathogenicity. Simply stating that *E. coli* is a hazard without stipulating a strain or serotype is a failure to understand the complexity of this bacterium's interaction with a host. The various schema used to classify *E. coli* must be introduced to better understand this phenomenon. Before this can be done, however, some definitions about the differences within a bacterial species must be provided.

Within any designation of a species, a certain amount of biological variation is expected. A strain of bacterium is a group that has distinct physiologic and/or biochemical characteristics in common but different from other groups within a species. Such groupings have traditionally been phenotypic (observed properties) based on biochemical testing, but recent advances in DNA sequencing (i.e., genomics) may eventually redefine the concept of strains and species (Konstantinidis, Ramette, Tiedje 2006). A serotype or serovar is "a group of intimately related microorganisms distinguished by a common set of antigens" (Medline Plus, Merriam-Webster Medical Dictionary). An antigen is any chemical substance, either alone or attached to another molecule, capable of evoking an immune response. The result of this immune response is the production of specialized proteins called antibodies that will bind to specific sites on the antigenic molecules called determinants or epitopes (see Figure 2-8). In the case of bacteria such as *E. coli*, components of the cell wall, flagellum, and capsule contain molecules capable of evoking an immune response. The antigenic molecules of the cell wall are lipopolysaccharides, while the flagellar antigens are proteins; capsular antigens are most often polysaccharides. The structural configuration and chemical composition of these antigenic molecules may vary greatly, and each variation can elicit production of highly specific antibodies. The antigens are classified by location using the letters O, H, and K for the cell wall, flagellum, and capsule, respectively (Figure 2-10). More than 200 O-type antigens and about 30 H-type antigens have been recognized for the bacterium *E. coli* (Kaper, Nataro, Mobley 2004). Serotype groupings often encompass strains of bacteria and vice versa, that is, common antigens may overlap with several observed physiologic properties. For example, the notorious serotype *E. coli* O157:H7 also has several different strains.

The pathogenic *E. coli* strains are further classified by properties such as their virulence factors, disease syndromes and pathology they cause, and by different effects they have on cell cultures. Table 2-3 summarizes the classification of pathogenic *E. coli* using this scheme. The table does not include the pathogenic *E. coli* responsible for extraintestinal diseases. Of the six groups, the Enterohemorrhagic *E. coli* (EHEC) strains are most important in North America, the United Kingdom, and Japan (Kaper et al. 2004). The EHEC strains most responsible for outbreaks

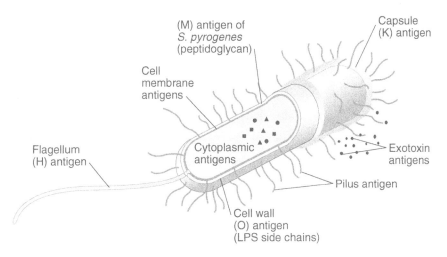

**Figure 2-10** The Various Antigens Possible on a Bacterial Cell

belong to serotype *E. coli* O157:H7 (Figure 2-11), which has been identified in many serious foodborne disease outbreaks and food recalls in the United States. Only 20% of *E. coli* O157:H7 cases are assumed to be associated with outbreaks; the majority of cases (80%) are sporadic, that is, not associated with outbreaks (Mead et al. 1997).

Foodborne disease outbreaks of *E. coli* O157:H7 have been linked to beef more than any other single food (Figure 2-12). Among beef products, ground meat represents the greatest risk of disease. The disease risk from hamburger was modeled and quantitatively related to multiple factors, but the following factors were predicted to have the greatest influence on risk: (1) concentration of *E. coli* O157:H7 in cattle feces; (2) host susceptibility, greatest with children and others with weakened resistance; and (3) the degree of beef carcass contamination with *E. coli* O157:H7 (Cassin et al. 1998). Risk mitigation strategies were also modeled, and the preventive measures with the greatest influence on reducing disease risk were the following: (1) temperature storage control to limit microbial growth (80% risk reduction), (2) preslaughter screening of cattle (46% risk reduction), and (3) consumer cooking practices (16% risk reduction). Other meats have also been linked to *E. coli* O157:H7 outbreaks, and in recent years, an increasing number of outbreaks have been associated with vegetables and fruits. The contamination of produce most likely results from poor manure waste management, contaminated water runoff, and/or livestock access to fields and harvest sites. Farm workers and equipment could also be a source of contamination.

A 1993 outbreak was a landmark event for EHEC infections, bringing attention to the problems of contaminated meat—and the seriousness and sometimes fatal consequences of infection. Among the 501 confirmed *E. coli* O157:H7 cases, 151 people (31%) were hospitalized, and 45 (9%) suffered from hemolytic uremic syndrome (HUS); 3 children also died (Bell et al. 1994). All EHEC strains produce toxins consisting of A and B subunits that are similar to those of *Shigella* species, the causative agents of bacillary dysentery. Consequently, the EHEC toxins are called

**Table 2-3** Classification of Pathogenic *E. coli* Strains

| Pathogenic Strains | Clinical Features | Virulence Factors and Pathology | Reservoirs and Transmission |
|---|---|---|---|
| Enterohemorrhagic *E. coli* (EHEC) (includes *E. coli* O157:H7) | Bloody diarrhea. May have sequelae such as hemolytic uremic syndrome (HUS). | Affects the large intestine; produces large quantities of Shiga-like toxins. All toxins consist of A and B subunits. Effacement of microvilli occurs after attachment. | Cattle are the primary reservoir, but other animals and humans may be sources. Most often transmitted by contaminated foods. Low infective dose: $10–10^2$ colony forming units (CFUs). |
| Enteroinvasive *E. coli* (EIEC) | Acute dysenteric-type diarrhea, bloody or nonbloody. | Strains generally do not produce enterotoxins, but they invade and multiply in the colonic epithelium. | Humans are the established reservoir. Limited evidence suggests foodborne transmission. |
| Enteropathogenic *E. coli* (EPEC) | Acute, watery diarrhea with mucus. May be persistent and severe among infants, whom are predominantly affected. | Strains generally do not produce enterotoxins. After localized colonization of the intestinal mucosa, they cause attachment-effacement lesions. | Humans are the established reservoir. Transmission occurs mostly from infant formula and foods, fomites, and hands. |
| Enterotoxigenic *E. coli* (ETEC) | Profuse, watery, and noninflammatory diarrhea. Often self-limiting in adults but can be persistent and severe in children. | Colonizes the small intestine but does not invade the intestinal cells. Produces one or two enterotoxins, which are categorized into two groups: heat-labile toxins (LT) and heat-stabile toxins (ST). | Strains are very species-specific for hosts. Humans are the reservoir for human ETEC disease. Major cause of diarrhea in lesser developed countries, including traveler's diarrhea. Contaminated food and water are primary modes of transmission. Infective dose is $10^8–10^{10}$ CFUs in adults. |
| Enteroaggregative *E. coli* (EAEC) | Watery diarrhea with mucus, seen mostly in infants and children. Infections may be asymptomatic. | Adheres to intestinal epithelium with a characteristic biofilm incorporating aggregations of bacteria and mucus. One or two enterotoxins may be produced. | Humans are probably the reservoir. Recognized as an important cause of infant diarrhea among lesser developed countries. Food and water are probably the main modes of transmission. |
| Diffuse-Adhering *E. coli* (DAEC) | Watery diarrhea with mucus in toddlers and preschool children. | Little is known about the virulence and pathology, except for the characteristic pattern of adherence to HEp-2 cells in culture. | Little is currently known about the reservoirs and mode of transmission. Occurs mostly in lesser developed countries. |

*Source:* Compiled from Kaper et al. 2004, Heymann 2008, Donnenberg and Nataro 2000.

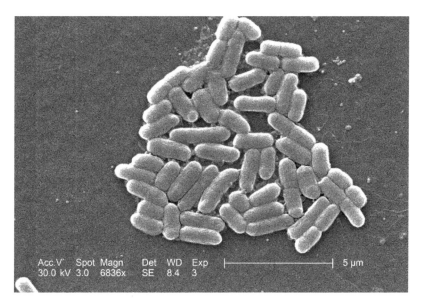

**Figure 2-11** Scanning Electron Micrograph of *E. coli* O157:H7 Bacteria. *Source:* Courtesy of Janice Haney Carr/CDC

Shiga-like toxins. After intimate attachment of EHEC to the epithelial cells, the toxin's B subunit binds to the host cell membrane, and the entire toxin is internalized by endocytosis. Once inside the host cell cytoplasm, the A subunit of the toxin interferes with protein synthesis by binding to certain ribosomes. For some victims, the shiga-toxins become attached to receptors on white blood cells and travel to other organs, including the kidneys, brain, and pancreas. Once transported to distant organs, the toxins bind more strongly to the organ's cells and become transported into the cytoplasm, where they interfere with protein synthesis and cause cellular injury and death. In the case of HUS, the formation of blood clots and the destruction of red blood cells in the small vessels of the kidney lead to renal injury or failure. Children are particularly susceptible to HUS.

The Enteroinvasive *E. coli* (EIEC) strains generally do not produce enterotoxins and are distinct from other pathogenic *E. coli* because they enter and multiply in colonic epithelial cells and further invade adjacent epithelial cells in a manner similar to another invasive bacterium called *Shigella*. The result is cell and tissue damage leading to voluminous diarrhea, either bloody or nonbloody. The Enteropathogenic *E. coli* (EPEC) also generally do not produce enterotoxins, but they cause diarrhea by producing lesions on the intestinal mucosa. Entero-toxigenic *E. coli* (ETEC) adhere to and colonize the small intestine by fimbrial colonization factors. Once attached, the ETEC produce one or two enterotoxins that cause the cellular damage and diarrhea. The last two categories of pathogenic *E. coli* (EAEC and DAEC) are not well understood, but they seem more important in lesser developed countries and/or with infant diarrheal diseases.

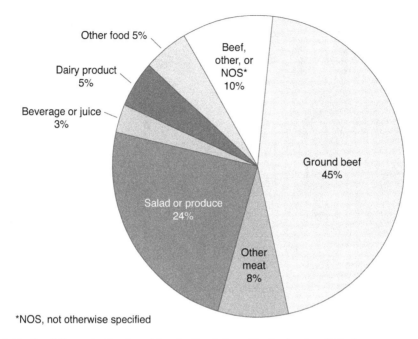

*NOS, not otherwise specified

**Figure 2-12**   Food Categories Implicated in 267 *E. coli* O157:H7 Outbreaks—U.S. from 1990–2006. *Source:* Data from: Center for Science in the Public Interest

Human carriers are the primary reservoirs of non-EHEC infections and probably play a significant role in food and water contamination. Most non-EHEC infections are presumed to be endemic in the lesser developed countries, but the investigation and publication of outbreaks in these countries are lacking to make any scientific conclusions (Todd et al. 2008b). Compared with EHEC infections, the infective doses of non-EHEC infections are considerably higher, around $10^6$ to $10^8$ colony-forming units (CFUs). This suggests that foods must either become heavily contaminated or be kept at unsafe temperatures to allow pathogen growth and multiplication. The pathogens EIEC and ETEC are often associated with enteric infections known as Traveler's Diarrhea, a syndrome attributed to those who visit foreign countries and return home ill. Foodborne outbreaks of non-EHEC have been documented in the United States, but many of them involved imported foods (Naimi et al. 2003).

Figure 2-13 illustrates the foodborne transmission of pathogenic *E. coli*.

### *Salmonella* Species and Serotypes

The name *Salmonella* has become commonplace in the vocabularies of many Americans because of unfortunate and highly publicized outbreaks of salmonellosis. In fact, the number of reported salmonellosis cases has been increasing worldwide, ironically more among the developed

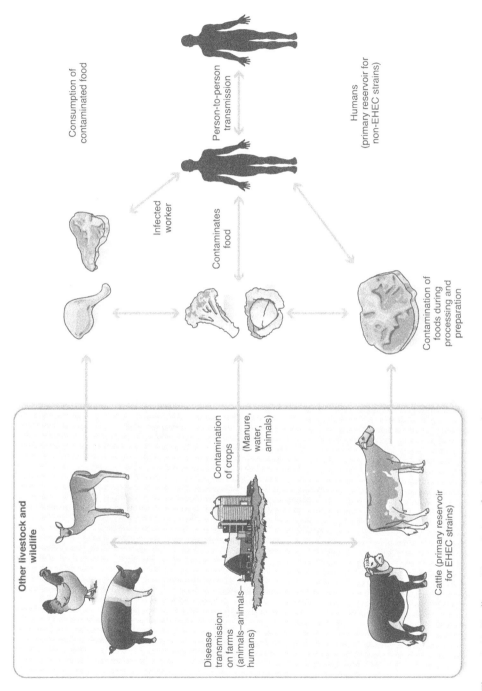

**Figure 2-13** Foodborne Transmission of Pathogenic *E. coli* Strains

or industrialized countries; it was one of the first diseases classified as an emerging infection. The name *Salmonella* originated with a veterinarian, Dr. Daniel Elmer Salmon, whose research assistant discovered the bacterium in 1885. Since that time, more than 2,500 serotypes (or serovars) of *Salmonella* (Figure 2-14) have been recognized (Centers for Disease Control and Prevention [CDC] 2008). Despite this great number of serotypes, the genus consists of only two species: *S. enterica* and *S. bangori*. The species *S. enterica* consists of six subspecies (see Table 2-4) and includes most serotypes involving animal and human infections. For the unenlightened, the naming convention for *Salmonellae* can be confusing. Nevertheless, taxonomic classification and serotyping are very important to salmonellosis control, so the topic needs to be introduced.

The naming of *Salmonella* serotypes is done by international agreement but is still evolving (Brenner et al. 2000). *Salmonellae* are first grouped by O antigen similarities and then further classified based on their H antigens. Additional classification can be pursued using antimicrobial resistance, phage typing, plasmid profiling, and other methods. In the early years of *Salmonella* research, a species or serotype was named after the disease it caused or for the animal from which it was isolated. In later years, a serotype was named after the place from where it was first isolated, a dubious honor if associated with a salmonellosis outbreak. Naming convention is such that the genus, species, and subspecies names are italicized, and the serotype names are not italicized but capitalized, that is, *S. enterica* ssp. *enterica* ser. Typhimurium. For convenience, it is acceptable to use only the genus and serotype; for example, *Salmonella* Typhimurium is an acceptable alternative.

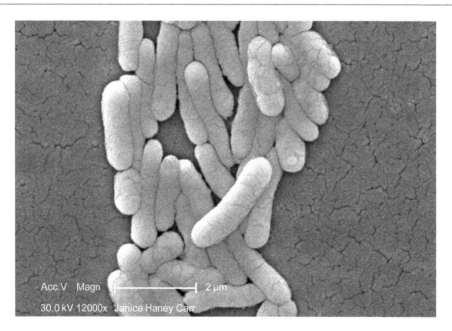

**Figure 2-14** Scanning Electron Micrograph of *Salmonella Typhimurium. Source:* Courtesy of Janice Haney Carr/ CDC

**Table 2-4** Subspecies of *S. enterica* and Serotyping Designations

| Serotyping Designation | Salmonella enterica *Subspecies* |
|---|---|
| I | *Salmonella enterica* ssp. *enterica* |
| II | *Salmonella enterica* ssp. *salamae* |
| IIIa | *Salmonella enterica* ssp. *arizonae* |
| IIIb | *Salmonella enterica* ssp. *diarizonae* |
| IV | *Salmonella enterica* ssp. *houtenae* |
| VI | *Salmonella enterica* ssp. *indica* |

*Source:* CDC, 2003.

For the purposes of consistency and international health, the Centers for Disease Control and Prevention (CDC) has adopted the Kaufman-White scheme for serotype designation. In this scheme, serotypes are designated using a standardized formula, albeit in many cases the serotype names are still used (CDC 2003). The formula designation begins by specifying the subspecies using the Roman numeral shown in Table 2-4 (for serotyping purposes, the species *S. bangori* is designated by Roman numeral V). Next, the O and H antigens are listed using the following formula and format:

Subspecies O antigens: Phase 1 H antigen: Phase 2 H antigen

Unlike the *E. coli* serotyping, the O antigens are designated as numbers (some may still use letters), and the H antigens can be designated as numbers, letters, or an alphanumeric combination. The O and H antigens may have several factors overlapping with a particular serotype; in these cases, the factors are separated by commas, and if an H phase is absent, it is designated by a hyphen (-). Following are a couple of examples using the formula designation (see CDC 2008 for additional information):

| Serotype Name Convention | Serotype Formula Designation |
|---|---|
| *S. enterica* spp. *enterica* ser. Typhimurium (or *Salmonella* Typhimurium) | I 4,5,12:i:1,2 |
| *S. enterica* spp. *enterica* ser. Enteritidis (or *Salmonella* Enteritidis) | I 9,12:g,m:- |

Based on pathogenicity, an important historical and clinical distinction is made between two designated classes of salmonellosis: Typhi and non-Typhi salmonellosis. The serotypes *S. enterica* ssp. *enterica* ser. Typhi (or *S.* Typhi) and *S. enterica* ssp. *enterica* ser. Paratyphi (or *S.* Paratyphi) are responsible for the serious diseases of typhoid fever and paratyphoid fever, respectively. The historical significance of typhoid fever was introduced in Chapter 1. This disease is systemic and characterized by fever, headache, and a number of other signs and symptoms with varying degrees of severity, depending on the virulence of a particular strain and the patient's resistance. Unlike most other enteric diseases, typhoid fever causes constipation more often than diarrhea. Before antibiotics were widely available, the case-fatality rate of typhoid fever was 10% to 20%, but with proper antibiotic therapy, the case-fatality rate drops below 1% (Heymann 2008).

In the twenty-first century, typhoid fever occurs mostly in lesser developed countries, and it is considered endemic in regions of Asia, Africa, and Latin America. In endemic regions, cases of typhoid fever can often be mild or asymptomatic and without systemic involvement. This makes the control of disease transmission very difficult because of unwary human carriers. Human typhoid fever is associated exclusively with human carriers and usually with contaminated food or water, particularly in areas with poor sanitation, raw milk, and untreated water. Paratyphoid fever is generally milder compared with typhoid fever. Several special serotype designations have been established (A, B, and C) for *S.* Paratyphi, but all serotypes of paratyphoid fever have a similar clinical presentation. The geographical occurrence and transmission of paratyphoid fevers are also similar to typhoid fever.

Outbreaks or cases of *Salmonella* infections not caused by *S.* Typhi or *S.* Paratyphi are generally referred to as "non-Typhi" salmonellosis (henceforth referred to simply as salmonellosis). The infective dose of non-Typhi *Salmonella* varies greatly with the serotype and host resistance, with a range as wide as $10^1$ to $10^9$ CFUs (Todd 2008b). The infection process for *Salmonella* serotypes occurs relatively rapidly. After ingestion, the bacilli colonize sites on the epithelium of the intestine, and within a manner of minutes, they invade cells of the intestinal mucosa, where they rapidly multiply. The preferential sites of involvement include the ileum, appendix, and right colon (Lamps 2003). In approximately 2% of cases, the bacteria invade the bloodstream (septicemia) and other organ systems. Among the signs and symptoms of enteric disease are diarrhea, fever, vomiting, and abdominal cramps. Toxins have been implicated in the disease process, but they have been difficult to isolate and study. In most cases, treatment involves supportive care and possibly rehydration and electrolyte replacement. Although the disease is usually self-limiting, severe cases can mimic ulcerative colitis or Crohn disease, and extraintestinal cases may require specific antibiotic therapy. However, the use of antibiotics in mild cases is believed to contribute to antibiotic-resistant strains. The convalescent carrier times can be quite prolonged, lasting months and possibly a year in some cases. This underscores the importance of medical clearance and good personal hygiene among food workers who have recently recovered from salmonellosis.

Clinicians now recognize several possible sequelae associated with salmonellosis that appear after acute infection has been resolved. One prominent aftereffect is postinfectious irritable bowel syndrome (PI-IBS), which is prevalent an average 15% among those who have recovered from an intestinal infection (Smith and Bayles 2007). The signs and symptoms of PI-IBS can be intermittent and include abdominal pain, diarrhea, fever, and other conditions, sometimes resulting in abdominal abscesses. The other bacteria also often associated with foodborne disease outbreaks and PI-IBS are species of *Campylobacter* and *Shigella*. Another possible sequela associated with postsalmonellosis is an autoimmune disease known as Reiter's syndrome (Lindsay 1997). This condition results when the body's immune system attacks its own tissues. The symptoms often include arthritis, eye irritation, urinary tract problems, and other symptoms. These symptoms usually occur within 3 weeks following the infection.

Compared with other pathogens in the family Enterobacteriaceae, the reservoirs of *Salmonella* encompass a greater variety of warm- and cold-blooded animals. Isolates of *Salmonella* have been cultured from the intestinal tracts of domestic and wild birds, hoofed animals, cats, dogs, rodents, reptiles, and even insects. Animal-to-human contact frequently causes transmission of salmonellosis. For foodborne transmission of salmonellosis, animals used for meat are the most important, though any animal (e.g., pests) that contaminates food-contact surfaces may be a source of foodborne transmission. Most outbreaks of salmonellosis have been traced to red meats, poultry, eggs, and unpasteurized milk products. Beef has been implicated most often in individual outbreaks, but chickens and eggs combined represent the most frequent transmission vehicles of salmonellosis, and they are major contributors to the salmonellosis pandemic (Molbak, Olsen, Wegener 2005). International trade has transported infected breeding fowl and eggs to other geographic areas, and the scope of contamination problems increased with transformation of the poultry industry into one of higher production and volume. Another contributing factor is the contamination of chicken feed with *Salmonella*. The result is inoculation of uninfected birds and the spread of infection among the flocks. Eggs were implicated in 80% of the reported outbreaks in the United States by *Salmonella* Enteritidis from 1985 through 1999 (Patrick et al. 2004). Risk modeling of eggborne S. Enteritidis infections (including sporadic and unreported cases) for the year 2000 was estimated to be between 81,535 and 276,500 cases (Schroeder et al. 2005).

Although most cases of salmonellosis are linked to meat and poultry products, the two largest outbreaks of salmonellosis in the United States were caused by contaminated dairy products. In 1985, pasteurized milk from a dairy in Illinois was somehow cross-contaminated with raw milk. This resulted in more than 16,000 culture-confirmed salmonellosis cases by an antibiotic-resistant strain of S. Typhimurium (Ryan et al. 1987). The total number of cases was estimated to be nearly 200,000 people. At that time, it was the largest reported outbreak of salmonellosis, as indicated by the spike in Figure 2-15. The exact source of S. Typhimurium was never definitively determined, but evaluations of the dairy plant operations revealed several opportunities for contamination of the pasteurized milk with raw milk. The largest reported outbreak of salmonellosis to date occurred in 1994 from contaminated ice cream. In this outbreak, an estimated 224,000 persons were infected with S. Enteritidis (Hennessy et al. 1996). Investigators of the outbreak concluded that the ice cream was contaminated with S. Enteritidis from pasteurized ice cream premix. The premix was transported in tank trailers previously used to carry nonpasteurized liquid eggs, the most likely source of S. Enteritidis. This incident highlighted the importance of cross-contamination in salmonellosis and the need for safety management of the entire food supply chain.

Whereas the majority of salmonellosis cases are associated with foods of animal origin, an increasing number of outbreaks have been linked to fruits, vegetables, and processed products. Outbreaks have been associated with produce such as alfalfa sprouts, tomatoes, peppers, cantaloupes, and lettuce (Beuchat 2006). Furthermore, *Salmonella* contamination has been detected in a great variety of fresh produce items, including cabbage, cauliflower, cilantro, parsley, green onions, strawberries, and many others (Buck, Walcott, Beuchat 2003). In February 2009, an outbreak of *Salmonella* Saintpaul involving 228 cases from 13 states was traced to contaminated alfalfa sprouts (CDC 2009d). Previous outbreaks since 1995 have also been linked to

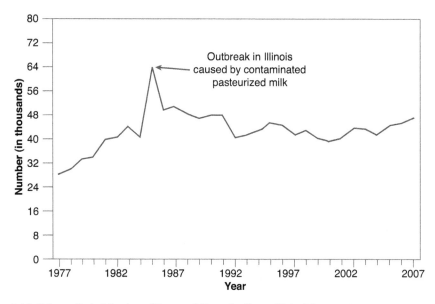

**Figure 2-15** Salmonellosis. Number of Reported Cases, by Year—United States, 1977–2007.
*Source:* Courtesy of CDC, 2009.

lightly cooked or raw alfalfa sprouts. Products like alfalfa seeds can be contaminated from poorly managed manure, contaminated runoff or irrigation water, fecal matter from uncontrolled domestic or wild animals, and improperly cleaned and maintained farm equipment. Sometimes plants can internalize pathogens like *Salmonella* within their seeds or other edible parts. This suggests that simply washing a vegetable or fruit may not be adequate for prevention of the disease.

*Salmonella* contamination has also been found in various processed foods. Products such as orange juice, snack foods, and peanut butter are just a few examples. Often a single ingredient can be contaminated with *Salmonella* and subsequently contaminate multiple products. An outbreak in 2009 of *S.* Typhimurium in peanut butter and other peanut-containing products is an example of "ingredient-driven" outbreaks (CDC 2009c). As of April 20, 2009, a total of 714 cases of salmonellosis from 46 states were reported to the CDC in this outbreak. Along with bulk containers of peanut butter, other products associated with this outbreak included peanut-containing items like snack crackers, cookies, cakes, pies, brownies, cereal, ice cream, and even pet foods. Other products such as breads may also be contaminated by ingredients (e.g., eggs) and cause disease if cooking temperatures are not sufficient to kill the *Salmonella* (Lu et al. 2004).

Figure 2-16 illustrates how contamination of foods with *Salmonella* is possible almost anywhere in the food supply chain. This is a topic of discussion in Chapter 4 on prevention principles and in Chapter 8 on safety management of the food supply.

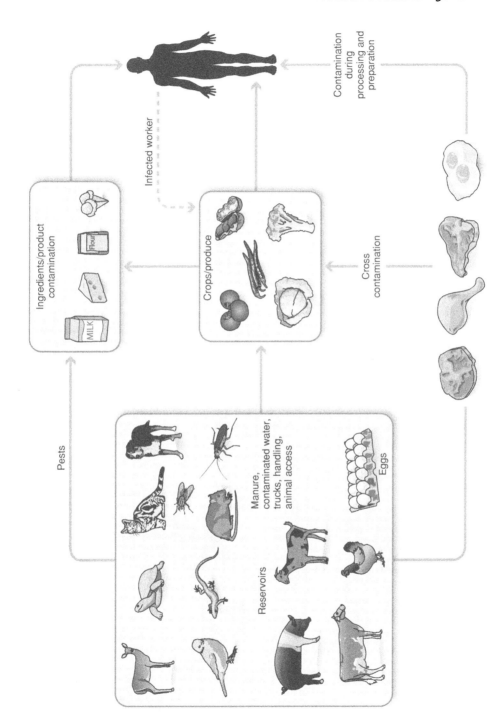

**Figure 2-16** Transmission of Foodborne Salmonellosis

## *Shigella* Species

Dysentery is a disease characterized by frequent, watery diarrhea, often with mucus and/or blood; abdominal cramps; and possibly including fever, nausea, vomiting, and ulceration of the intestinal mucosa. It has been the scourge of humanity since ancient times and traveled with armies around the world, often causing more morbidity and mortality than inflicted by the enemy. One form of the disease is caused by an amoeba (amoebic dysentery) and another is caused by a bacillus (bacillary dysentery). The causative organism of classic bacillary dysentery is *Shigella dysenteriae*. This organism is most often—but not exclusively—encountered in lesser developed countries and is responsible for devastating outbreaks and epidemics. Major complications such as HUS and intestinal perforations are possible, and the fatality rate is as high as 20% among hospitalized cases (Heymann 2008).

Shigellosis refers to all enteric infections caused by *S. dysenteriae* and the other species *S. flexneri*, *S. boydii*, and *S. sonnei*. Approximately 44 serotypes have been established among these four species of *Shigella*. The pathogenicity and geographic distribution of the species and serotypes are quite different. Figure 2-17 shows the most common *Shigella* isolate reported by public health laboratories in the United States is *S. sonnei*, followed by *S. flexneri* (CDC 2006). For a significant number of *Shigella* isolates, the species was not identified. The infective dose for shigellosis is very low compared with other foodborne bacterial pathogens, with infective doses among the species generally ranging from <10 to $10^3$ CFUs (Todd et al. 2008b). The pathogen attaches to the intestinal epithelium and invades the cells, spreading to other adjacent cells of the epithelium. A potent enterotoxin called shiga-toxin is produced by the more virulent strains. Mild cases are very common with some strains, in which case recovery typically happens without medical intervention. Convalescent carriers may continue shedding the pathogen in their feces from days to months, transmitting the pathogen to others via person-to-person contact and vehicles such as food and water. Crowded and unsanitary conditions, such as refugee camps and overloaded day care centers, are breeding sites for the pathogens. Depending on the pathogen strain and host susceptibility, sequelae such as PI-IBS and aseptic or reactive arthritis can occur following recovery from infection (Lindsay 1997; Smith and Bayles 2007).

Humans (and other nonhuman primates) are the primary reservoirs for *Shigella* species. The bacteria do not survive long in the environment, unless they are within a moist and protective medium, such as certain foods. Transmission by person-to-person contact and fomites are important modes for the propagation and continuation of shigellosis epidemics within a community. Drinking water contaminated by feces is probably the most common mode of transmission in lesser developed countries, whereas food is the likely primary mode of transmission in developed countries, thanks in great part to safer water supplies and sewage treatment. Because humans are reservoirs of *Shigella* species, the infected food worker is the likely source of contamination for foodborne outbreaks (Todd et al. 2008b). But food can also become contaminated with *Shigella* species by animals, insects, and water that have come in contact with the feces of infected persons. Foods of greatest concern are those handled and eaten raw, or handled after cooking by an infected preparer. Figure 2-18 illustrates these pathways of contamination and transmission.

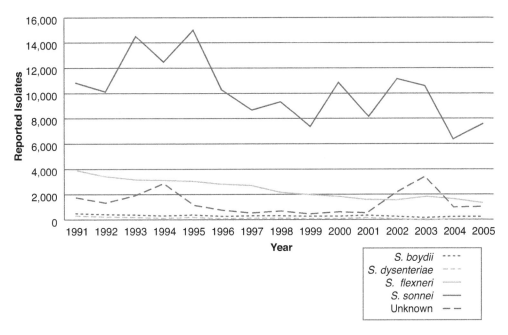

**Figure 2-17** Laboratory-Confirmed Shigella Isolates Reported to CDC by Species and Year for 1991–2005. *Source:* Data from CDC, 2008

Two particularly noteworthy outbreaks demonstrate the importance of food worker hygiene and sanitary conditions in the prevention of foodborne shigellosis. In the summer of 1987, a festival and gathering occurred in western North Carolina. An outbreak of diarrheal disease caused by an antibiotic-resistant strain of *S. sonnei* infected more than half of the estimated 12,700 participants (Wharton et al. 1990). Investigation by public health officials determined multiple modes of transmission were responsible for this massive outbreak: food, water, and person-to-person transmission. The gathering had 47 communal kitchens with questionable or no hand-washing facilities, shallow trench latrines nearby, no refrigeration, and probably infected food handlers. The water supply was also likely contaminated. After disbanding of the gathering, the attendees dispersed and transmitted the infection nationwide, causing at least three outbreaks in other states. Another noteworthy outbreak occurred in 2000 from a commercially produced dip (Kimura et al. 2004). A total of 406 cases of infection by *S. sonnei* were detected nationwide and linked to the contaminated dip. Investigators traced the source of contamination to a sick worker who used his bare hands to help mix the cheese ingredient for the dip. Other settings where outbreaks of shigellosis have occurred include day care centers, airline flights, and cruise ships (CDC 2006; Todd et al. 2007b).

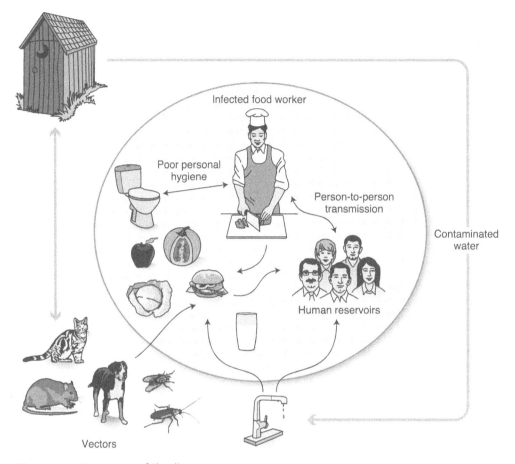

**Figure 2-18** Transmission of Shigellosis

## *Yersinia* **Species**

Yersiniosis is an enigmatic disease compared with other diseases caused by members of the family Enterobacteraciae because several disease states of yersiniosis are possible. After colonization in the small intestine, the *Yersinia* bacteria invade the intestinal mucosa and cause tissue destruction. The most common signs and symptoms are diarrhea, low-grade fever, and abdominal cramps. Vomiting and bloody diarrhea may also be present. Many infected individuals are asymptomatic, while others can develop serious or life-threatening states of disease. In these more serious states, the bacteria invade and colonize the lymphoid tissue and spread to the lymph nodes and beyond, possibly causing septicemia and affecting other organs. Cases of septicemia can have high case-fatality rates (Bottone 1997). The disease may display a variety of manifestations, such as pseudo appendicitis. Reactive arthritis and other sequelae are also risks within a year following acute yersiniosis (Ternhag et al. 2008).

The most deadly species of *Yersinia* is the etiologic agent of plague (*Y. pestis*)—normally transmitted by infected fleas—not food. Another species, *Y. pseudotuberculosis*, is believed to cause epizootic diseases among wild and domestic animals and incidentally infects humans, but knowledge about the transmission of *Y. pseudotuberculosis* is limited. The most important species with regard to foodborne transmission is *Y. enterocolitica*. This bacterium is unique among the Enterobacteriaceae because of its psychrophilic nature, that is, it is capable of reproducing at refrigeration temperatures. Approximately 60 serotypes of *Y. enterocolitica* have been established, though most of them are nonpathogenic (Bottone 1999). The infection is more common in cooler climates such as northern Europe and Japan. In the United States, reported outbreaks and cases are infrequent compared with EHEC and *Salmonella* infections. Prior to 1983, only three well-documented outbreaks of yersiniosis were reported in the United States, and they were linked to contaminated and/or unpasteurized milk, bean sprouts soaked in contaminated water, and tofu (Bottone 1997). More recently, cases of foodborne yersiniosis have been linked to pork products, principally chitterlings, a dish made from the large intestines of pigs (Jones 2003).

Swine are the principal reservoir of *Y. enterocolitica*. Other potential reservoirs include a variety of mammals and birds. However, the majority of pathogenic strains are associated with the pig, and the occurrence of yersiniosis among humans is more prevalent in areas where the pig is a main source of meat (Bottone 1997). Within the United States, the percentage of pig farms with at least one positive test for *Y. enterocolitica* varied by state from 33% to 57% (Wesley, Bhaduri, Bush 2008). Higher rates of positive tests may be found among slaughtered pig carcasses because contamination from the intestines occurs during evisceration procedures. Despite these seemingly high rates of positive tests, the reported human cases of yersiniosis in the United States are comparatively low. Since *Y. enterocolitica* can grow at refrigeration temperatures, the control of foodborne yersiniosis is greatly dependent on good sanitary practices and thorough heating (i.e., milk pasteurization) and/or cooking of foods, particularly pork products.

### *Campylobacter* Species

As one author describes it, *Campylobacter* has gone from complete "obscurity to celebrity" status in 30 years (Butzler 2004). In 1906, British veterinary surgeons isolated these spiral-shaped microorganisms from pregnant sheep, and because of their spiral morphologies (Figure 2-19), the bacteria were considered a member of the genus *Vibrio* until 1963 (Zilbauer et al. 2008). Difficulties in culturing *Campylobacter* over the years delayed its confirmation as a cause of human diarrhea until the 1970s. Since then, *Campylobacter* has been identified as a common cause of diarrheal disease around the world (Petri et al. 2008), and global estimates suggest it may be the leading bacterial cause of outpatient visits for diarrhea in children younger than 5 years (Lanata, Mendoza, Black 2002). In the United States, surveillance programs estimated a decline in the incidence of campylobacteriosis by 32% from 1996 to 2008 (CDC 2009e). Factors attributed to this decline include programs aimed at reducing the rates of infection among chicken flocks. Even with the decline, campylobacteriosis remains a prominent foodborne infection in the United States.

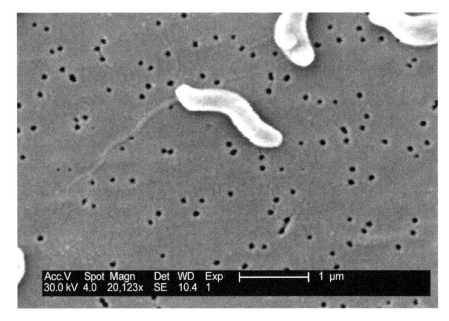

**Figure 2-19** Scanning Electron Micrograph of *Campylobacter jejuni*. *Source:* Courtesy of Dr. Patricia Fields, Dr. Collette Fitzgerald, and Janice Carr/CDC

Among the several species of *Campylobacter* that can cause human disease, *C. jejuni* and *C. coli* are the most important worldwide. About 90% of human campylobacteriosis cases are caused by *C. jejuni*, making it most important in terms of control (Janssen et al. 2008). Serotyping methods for *C. jejuni* are expensive, can be technically difficult to perform, and may yield strains that are difficult to categorize or type. Hence, DNA-based methods and subtyping schemes are often preferable (Altekruse et al. 1999). The infective dose for *Campylobacter* species can be as low as 500 to 800 CFUs (Young, Davis, Dirita 2007). After passage through the stomach, which can greatly reduce the number of viable organisms, the *Campylobacter* colonize the intestine, where they cause diarrhea by either releasing a toxin (secretory or noninflammatory diarrhea) or by invading and damaging the epithelial tissue, resulting in inflammatory diarrhea (Janssen et al. 2008). In most cases, the disease is self-limiting, and the majority of people recover without medical intervention or antibiotic therapy. Some individuals infected with *Campylobacter* become asymptomatic carriers. A small percentage of cases may require antibiotic therapy, and a few cases may have complications arising from septicemia and colonization at extraintestinal sites (Janssen et al. 2008; Zilbauer et al. 2008). Sequelae such as reactive arthritis, PI-IBS, and a neurologic condition known as Guillain-Barré syndrome (GBS) are special concerns with campylobacteriosis. GBS is an autoimmune condition that causes weakness, paralysis, and respiratory insufficiency, possibly requiring artificial ventilation. Among the multiple causes of GBS, *C. jejuni* is the most frequently identified pathogen known to induce it (Zilbauer et al. 2008).

Figure 2-20 illustrates the transmission cycle of foodborne campylobacteriosis.

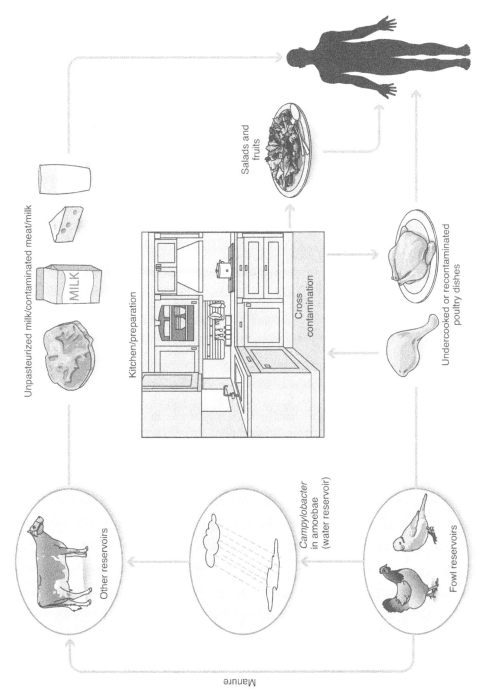

**Figure 2-20** Transmission of Foodborne Campylobacteriosis

Salads and fruits

Unpasteurized milk/contaminated meat/milk

MILK

Kitchen/preparation

Cross contamination

Undercooked or recontaminated poultry dishes

*Campylobacter* in amoebae (water reservoir)

Other reservoirs

Fowl reservoirs

Manure

Reservoirs of *Campylobacter* include a variety of birds and mammals. Chickens are particularly important reservoirs, not only as a source of foodborne infection but also as a source of infection to other farm animals. Normally found in the intestinal tracts, *Campylobacter* are very sensitive to oxygen (microaerophilic) and do not survive long in unfavorable environments. Recent evidence suggests, however, that *Campylobacter* can survive in protozoans such as amoebae living in water and, hence, the waterborne amoebae can be a reservoir of infection for other animals (Young et al. 2007); this same mechanism of survival has been found with other foodborne pathogens (Bleasdale et al. 2009). The formation of biofilms and a state of dormancy known as viable but nonculturable (VBNC) may also contribute to *Campylobacter* survival in the environment, but the relative importance of these factors remains controversial (Murphy, Carroll, Jordan 2006). Whatever the relative importance of the aforementioned survival mechanisms, epidemiologic studies of campylobacteriosis outbreaks have confirmed the prime importance of contaminated, undercooked chicken and the cross-contamination of other foods during preparation and handling (CDC 1998).

A variety of foods has been implicated in epidemiologic studies of campylobacteriosis. The most important categories are poultry, red meats, and raw milk (Altekruse et al. 1999). Figure 2-21 illustrates the types of foods implicated in 145 confirmed and suspected campylobacteriosis outbreaks in the United States from 1990 through 2006. An important observation of these data is that dairy products represent 36% of the total food types, with unpasteurized dairy products—predominantly raw milk—representing the single largest category. The likely *Campylobacter* contamination source for raw milk is infected cows, or the contamination of dairy equipment, and/or the mixing of contaminated milk with uncontaminated milk (CDC 2009a). Of the meats, chicken is implicated most often (17%). This corresponds with surveys indicating retail chicken meats have had historically high rates (up to 98%) of contamination with *C. jejuni* (Altekruse et al. 1999). More recently, efforts by the U.S. poultry industry to reduce chicken infections and carcass contamination have dramatically reduced *Campylobacter* loading on chicken carcasses (Stern and Pretanik 2006). One particularly interesting and important observation in Figure 2-21 is the large percentage of salads, fruits, and mixed-ingredient dishes implicated as vehicles for *Campylobacter* transmission. Because *Campylobacter* species are readily destroyed at cooking temperatures, a likely explanation for this observation is the cross-contamination of cooked food and produce items (most salads and fruits are eaten uncooked) by raw meats and/or contaminated surfaces in the food preparation area.

### Listeria monocytogenes

The bacterium *Listeria monocytogenes* (Figure 2-22) is the etiology of listeriosis—a disease that rightfully frightens pregnant women and immunocompromised individuals. In pregnant women, the disease can result in serious outcomes such as abortion, stillbirth, premature birth, and neonatal infections, along with other serious or life-threatening conditions to newborns. Older adults and others who are immunocompromised are at increased risk of complications such as meningitis and septicemia. Among healthy and intermediate-age individuals, the disease is usually limited to gastroenteritis, diarrhea, vomiting, fatigue, and headache, though some relatively young adults may also experience meningitis and septicemia (Drevets and Bronze 2008).

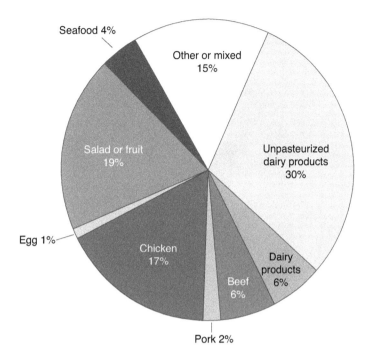

**Figure 2-21** Food Categories Implicated in 145 Campylobacteriosis Outbreaks—U.S. from 1990–2006. *Source:* Data from Center for Science in the Public Interest

Fortunately—compared with other foodborne bacterial infections—the incidence of listeriosis is low in the general population. But certain subpopulations (e.g., those discussed previously) are at increased risk of infection and severe consequences; this risk merits the placement of listeriosis on a priority list of public health problems.

The infective dose of *L. monocytogenes* is relatively high compared with other infectious agents. Outbreaks have been associated with levels approximating $10^4$ to $10^6$ CFUs/g of *L. monocytogenes* (Food and Drug Administration [FDA] et al. 2003). Of course, individuals with impaired immune systems are at increased risk of infection and, hence, have lower infective doses. The subject of infective doses for *L. monocytogenes* has been extensively debated, and new risk assessment approaches advocate using dose-response curves, where the statistical probability of becoming infected increases with the dose of bacteria. (This subject is discussed later under risk assessment.) After access to the body through the consumption of contaminated food, the *L. monocytogenes* bacteria invade the mucosal epithelium and lymphatics of the intestine. The invasive bacteria spread cell to cell in the host using the host cells' membranes as a protective vacuole. Infected lymph nodes disseminate bacteria via blood to other organs. The bacteria are uniquely capable of crossing key protective barriers in the body, for example, the maternofetal barrier and

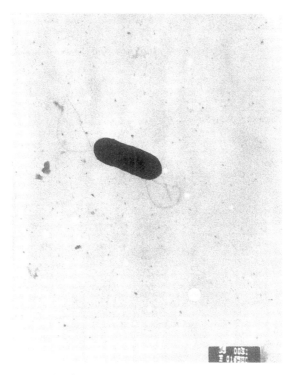

**Figure 2-22** Electron Micrograph of *Listeria monocytogenes*. *Source:* Courtesy of Elizabeth White, Dr. Balasubr Swaminathan, Peggy Hayes/CDC

blood–brain barrier (Drevets and Bronze 2008). This leads to the complications discussed earlier associated with pregnancy and the nervous system.

More than a dozen serotypes of *L. monocytogenes* have been established; nearly all (95%) of human infections are caused by four serotypes, designated as 1/2a, 1/2b, 1/2c, and 4b (Heymann 2008). Because listeriosis is primarily a zoonotic disease, the reservoirs include many species of animals. Yet, the *Listeria* bacteria are found throughout nature in soil, decaying vegetation, water, and other materials and surfaces that come in contact with animals and their feces. This includes food preparation surfaces and processing equipment. The ability of *L. monocytogenes* to produce biofilms contributes to its tenacity and persistence in natural and human environments. Other important survival factors include its ability to grow at a relatively wide range of pH and temperatures—even at refrigeration temperatures—and in relatively high concentrations of salt (Gandhi and Chikindas 2007). Figure 2-23 illustrates the various ways that *L. monocytogenes* contaminates the outdoor/indoor environment and enters the food handling chain. Despite the fact that heat processing (e.g., cooking and pasteurization) of foods usually kills *L. monocytogenes*, it is frequently detected in a wide variety of finished food products, suggesting that postprocessing contamination and cross-contamination are important contributors to foodborne transmission.

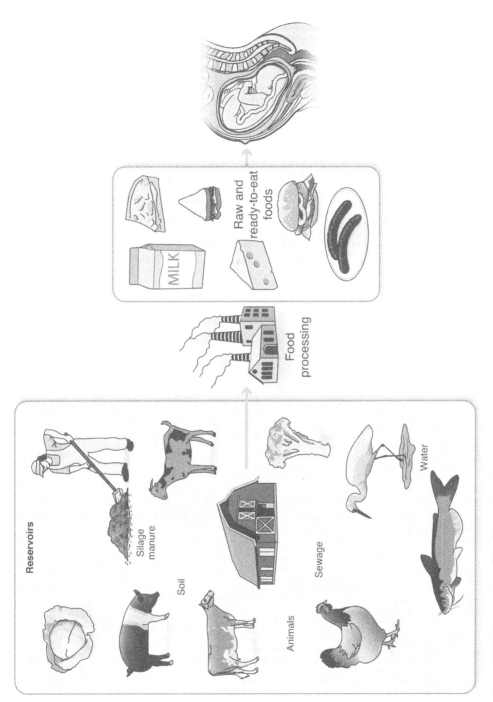

**Figure 2-23** Transmission of Foodborne Listeriosis

Indeed, the establishment of *L. monocytogenes* in the food-processing environment has been clearly established as related to food contamination during production, even over prolonged periods of time (Tompkin 2002).

Outbreaks of listeriosis have been most commonly linked to a variety of meat and dairy products, seafood, and vegetables (Farber and Peterkin 1991; Ramaswamy et al. 2007). In recent years, ready-to-eat (RTE) foods such as deli products have been linked to listeriosis outbreaks. Table 2-5

**Table 2-5** Food Categories Used in the *Listeria monocytogenes* Risk Assessment

*SEAFOOD*

Smoked Seafood (finfish and mollusks)

Raw Seafood (finfish, mollusks, and crustaceans)

Preserved Fish (dried, pickled, and marinated finfish)

Cooked Ready-to-Eat Crustaceans (shrimp and crab)

*PRODUCE*

Vegetables (raw)

Fruits (raw, dried)

*DAIRY*

Fresh Soft Cheese (queso fresco, queso de Crema, Queso de Puna)

Soft Unripened Cheese, >50% moisture (cottage cheese, cream cheese, ricotta)

Soft Ripened Cheese, >50% moisture (brie, camembert, feta, mozzarella)

Semi-soft Cheese, 39–50% moisture (blue, brick, Monterey, Muenster)

Hard Cheese, <39% moisture (cheddar, Colby, parmesan)

Processed Cheese (cheese foods, spreads, slices)

Pasteurized Fluid Milk

Unpasteurized Fluid Milk

Ice Cream and Other Frozen Dairy Products

Cultured Milk Products (yogurt, sour cream, buttermilk)

High Fat and Other Dairy Products (butter, cream, other miscellaneous milk products)

*MEAT*

Frankfurters (reheated)

Frankfurters (not reheated)

Dry/Semi-Dry Fermented Sausages

Deli Meats (cooked, ready-to-eat)

Pâté and Meat Spreads

*COMBINATION FOODS*

Deli-type Salads (fruit, vegetable, meat, pasta, egg, or seafood salads)

*Source:* FDA, 2003.

lists RTE food categories used in assessing the relative risks to the public health from foodborne *L. monocytogenes*. All these foods can be considered risky for susceptible individuals, but the deli meats represent the highest risk on a per annum and per serving basis in the United States (FDA et al. 2003). If control measures involving the processing and retail handling of deli products are not strictly followed, the risks of listeriosis increase greatly (Lianou and Sofos 2007). However, the risks of listeriosis are even greater if deli products are not properly stored (refrigerated at proper temperatures) and handled in the home (Yang et al. 2006).

### *Vibrio* Species

Multiple species of bacteria belonging to the genus *Vibrio* have been implicated and confirmed as an etiology of human infections, but the three most important from a food safety perspective are *V. cholerae*, *V. parahaemolyticus*, and *V. vulnificus* (Figure 2-24). The dreaded disease cholera is caused by different strains of *V. cholerae*, which is categorized by serotypes (predominantly type O1 and O139). Further categorization is done by biotypes on the basis of biochemical testing and the production of cholera toxin (toxigenic), a protein that causes voluminous diarrhea and dehydration. Without oral rehydration solution (ORS) therapy, the mortality from cholera would be greater than the currently reported rate of 0–9% (Heymann 2008). From the nineteenth century to the current date, seven pandemics of cholera have swept across the globe causing great morbidity, particularly in the lesser developed countries. With international laws and mandatory reporting of cholera, the world community has attempted to stem the tide of this communicable disease. But the enforcement of international laws is difficult because environmental conditions within sovereign countries are largely responsible for the persistence of cholera (Jones 1999).

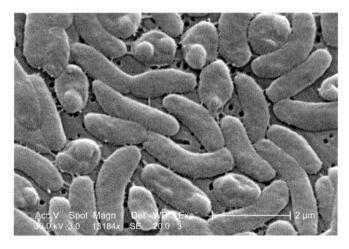

**Figure 2-24**  Scanning Electron Micrograph of *Vibrio vulnificus. Source:* Courtesy of Janice Carr/CDC

Unlike the other *Vibrio* pathogens, the principal reservoir for toxigenic *V. cholerae* is humans. Therefore, eliminating fecal-oral routes of transmission in humans is critical to reducing the incidence of cholera in a community. This involves the assurance of safe drinking water and proper sewage disposal, and excluding the contamination of foods, which frequently occurs from using contaminated water to wash or prepare raw or cooked foods. Beverages and ice prepared from contaminated water are especially risky vehicles of transmission. Another important source of cholera transmission is the consumption of raw seafood (or cross-contamination of cooked seafood) harvested from waters contaminated by inadequately treated sewage or runoff. Although the global leading cause of cholera epidemics is water contamination, food transmission accounted for 32% and 71% of outbreaks in South America and East Asia, respectively (Griffith, Kelly-Hope, Miller 2006). In developed and industrialized countries, where water and wastewater treatment are more common, the consumption of raw seafood and unwashed vegetables is the riskiest transmission vehicle for cholera. Still, increasing international travel and frequent importation of foods make cholera a concern for all countries.

The *Vibrio* species are marine organisms. Being halophilic (salt loving), the habitat of species like *V. parahaemolyticus* and *V. vulnificus* is primarily brackish estuarine waters; they cannot survive in the deep ocean because of the extreme pressures. In terms of ecology, these organisms live in the water column during warmer months and survive winters in the sediments. During the warmer months, *Vibrio* species attach themselves to the surfaces of zooplankton and shellfish, and they become part of the microbiota within shellfish digestive tracts. Their habitat and association with shellfish explain why *Vibrio* infections are seasonal and almost always associated with seafood and, to a lesser degree, contact with seawater.

In January 2007, all cases of *Vibrio* illnesses became nationally notifiable to the CDC, regardless of the species involved. The reports from these cases are compiled, maintained, and periodically analyzed by the CDC. In 2007, a total of 549 *Vibrio* illnesses (excluding toxigenic *V. cholerae* infections) was reported to the CDC. The breakdown of these cases by *Vibrio* species and complications are shown in Table 2-6. A total of 160 *Vibrio* specimens from patients in Table 2-6 were obtained from wound sites. Nearly all *Vibrio* species are capable of causing wound infections, usually following exposure to seawater and/or the handling of seafood; several species also cause septicemia. Among those nonwound infections, 89% reported eating seafood within 7 days prior to illness. The most frequently reported single seafood item eaten was oysters (58%), followed by finfish (13%), and clams (11%); the oysters and clams were eaten raw by 97% and 83%, respectively, of the cases. Other types of shellfish implicated in past outbreaks include mussels, crabs, lobsters, and shrimp. Among the finfish, specialty dishes such as sushi are particularly risky because the fish is eaten raw.

As with many gastrointestinal infections, the symptoms of vibriosis include diarrhea, cramps, nausea, and weakness; some may experience chills, vomiting, and headaches. In the case of *V. vulnificus* infection, the severity of disease is much greater, as indicated by the complication rates in Table 2-6. Acquired primarily by eating seafood, the majority of *V. vulnificus* infection cases develop complications and require hospitalization. More than 50% of septicemic cases may be fatal, and 90% of the hypotensive cases may die (Heymann 2008). Hence, prompt public health action is necessary to minimize the threat of seafood contaminated with *V. vulnificus*.

**Table 2-6** Number of *Vibrio* Illnesses (excluding toxigenic *V. cholerae*) by Species and Complications from the United States, 2007

| Vibrio *Species* | Complications | | | | | |
| --- | --- | --- | --- | --- | --- | --- |
| | Patients | | Hospitalized | | Deaths | |
| | N | % | n/N | % | n/N | % |
| *V. alginolyticus* | 100 | 18 | 15/90 | 17 | 0/88 | 0 |
| *V. cholerae* (nontoxigenic) | 49 | 9 | 21/43 | 49 | 3/37 | 8 |
| *V. damsela* | 2 | <1 | 0/2 | 0 | 0/2 | 0 |
| *V. fluvialis* | 19 | 3 | 3/17 | 18 | 1/17 | 6 |
| *V. hollisae* | 6 | 1 | 4/6 | 67 | 0/6 | 0 |
| *V. mimicus* | 10 | 2 | 4/9 | 44 | 0/9 | 0 |
| *V. parahaemolyticus* | 232 | 42 | 52/221 | 24 | 0/218 | 0 |
| *V. vulnificus* | 95 | 17 | 87/94 | 93 | 30/83 | 36 |
| Species not identified | 23 | 4 | 7/18 | 39 | 1/16 | 6 |
| Other | 4 | 1 | 2/3 | 67 | 0/3 | 0 |
| Multiple species | 9 | 2 | 4/9 | 44 | 1/9 | 11 |
| Total | 549 | 100 | 199/512 | 39 | 36/488 | 7 |

*Source:* Courtesy of CDC, 2008b.

## Spore Formers and Toxicoinfections

An important survival mechanism with certain bacteria is the formation of endospores—highly differentiated cellular structures formed from within the bacterial cells (Figure 2-25). These structures are often simply called spores. They contribute to bacterial survival by switching metabolism into a dormant state and forming barriers that can withstand harsh environmental conditions such as heating, drying, and some chemicals. The formation of spores is called sporulation and occurs when certain key nutrients become absent in the bacteria's environment. The dormant state of spores may last for many years, and when environmental conditions return to a favorable state, germination and outgrowth of the vegetative cells occurs, allowing resumption of multiplication. The genera of spore formers most important to food safety are *Clostridium* and *Bacillus*. These bacteria and/or their spores are very common in soil, dust, plants, and the intestinal tracts of nearly every animal species. Furthermore, the spores can become airborne and dispersed anywhere outside and within building structures. Hence, the complete elimination of spores is difficult to achieve.

## Clostridium perfringens: *Toxicoinfection*

*Clostridium perfringens* (Figure 2-26) is responsible for the most commonly encountered foodborne toxicoinfection. Unlike foodborne infections where attachment and colonization of the

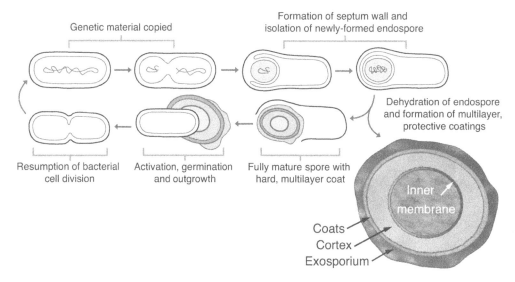

**Figure 2-25** Diagram of a Bacterial Endospore. *Source:* Cross-section of bacterial spore, Courtesy of Lawrence Livermore National Laboratory

intestinal mucosa are necessary, a toxicoinfection occurs when the viable bacteria are present in large numbers within the lumen of the intestinal tract. In the case of *C. perfringens*, the disease results from a toxin released during the sporulation of vegetative cells in the gut lumen. A minimum of $10^5$ CFUs/g or more of *C. perfringens* in food is believed necessary to cause illness (CDC 2009b). The host response to the toxin is typically diarrhea and abdominal cramps. The incubation period ranges from 8 to 24 hours, and symptoms usually subside 1 to 2 days later. In most cases, the disease does not progress to more serious states. However, a severe form of disease called enteritidis necroticans or "pig-bel" can occur with certain populations, usually among refugees or malnourished individuals who lack sufficient proteases to destroy the toxin. Some evidence exists that preformed toxins and/or sporulating bacterial cells in foods may also contribute to illness and to the shortening of incubation periods for some cases (Roach and Sienko 1992).

For a number of reasons, the actual incidence of *C. perfringens* foodborne disease is difficult to determine. One probable reason is that mild cases of the disease and sporadic cases are never reported. Nonetheless, from 1998 to 2002, *C. perfringens* was the third leading bacterial etiology of foodborne disease outbreaks reported in the United States (Lynch et al. 2006). In 2006, it was the second leading bacterial etiology of reported foodborne disease outbreaks (CDC 2009g). Meats and dishes with gravy, casseroles, or stews are frequently associated with *C. perfringens* disease outbreaks (CDC 2009b). The settings for a majority of these outbreaks involve large quantities of food prepared in advance at institutions (e.g., schools and prisons), gatherings (e.g., banquets, catered events), cafeterias, and restaurants. Because *C. perfringens* spores can survive

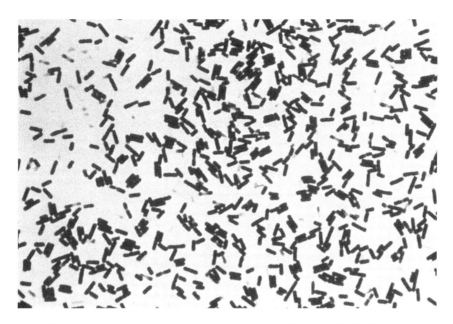

**Figure 2-26** Photomicrograph of Clostridium perfringens. *Source:* Courtesy of CDC/Don Stalons

many cooking processes, the bacteria can germinate and multiply to hazardous levels from inadequate holding temperatures prior to consumption. Thus, attention to time and temperature safety guidelines are critically important to the prevention of this disease.

## Bacillus cereus: *Toxicoinfection and Intoxication*

Two distinct syndromes are attributed to *B. cereus*: a diarrheal syndrome, characterized by abdominal cramps and diarrhea; and an emetic syndrome, characterized by nausea and vomiting. Each syndrome is caused by different types of toxins, though outbreaks with overlapping syndromes have occurred. Table 2-7 highlights key differences in incubation periods and disease characteristics between the two syndromes, along with those from *C. perfringens* toxicoinfection and *C. botulinum* toxicoinfection/intoxication. Note for *B. cereus* that the diarrheal syndrome is believed to be a toxicoinfection, whereas the emetic syndrome is believed to be an intoxication by preformed toxins in the foods prior to consumption. The topic of foodborne intoxication by *B. cereus* is revisited in the section on microbial toxins in Chapter 3. Unlike the toxicoinfection by *C. perfringens*, the toxicoinfection by *B. cereus* does not require sporulation to release toxins.

Like *C. perfringens*, the bacteria and spores of *B. cereus* can be found in soil, dust, and plants, but the bacteria are found less often in the intestinal tracts of animals. The spores of *B. cereus* can also survive most cooking processes and germinate later when conditions become more suitable.

**Table 2-7** Comparison of Spore-Forming Bacteria and Foodborne Diseases

| Disease or Syndrome | Incubation Period | Signs/Symptoms & Recovery Period | Key Differences |
|---|---|---|---|
| C. perfringens Toxicoinfection | 8–16 hours | Watery diarrhea with abdominal cramps and nausea lasting 24–48 hours. | Sporulation in the small intestine is necessary to produce and release toxins. |
| B. cereus Diarrheal Syndrome (Toxicoinfection) | 10–16 hours | Abdominal cramps with watery diarrhea and nausea lasting 24–48 hours. | Sporulation is not necessary; lysis of vegetative cells releases toxins. |
| B. cereus Emetic Syndrome (Intoxication) | 1–6 hours | Sudden and severe nausea and vomiting, possibly diarrhea, typically over in 24 hours. | Toxin is preformed in foods prior to consumption. |
| C. botulinum Infant Botulism or Adult Intestinal Toxemia Botulism | 3–30 days | Lethargy, weakness, poor head control, and other neurological signs in infants. Duration is variable. | The victim or host usually does not possess a fully developed microbiota in the gut. Spores may be ingested from non-food sources. |
| C. botulinum Intoxication (Foodborne Botulism) | 12–72 hours | Vomiting, diarrhea, blurred vision, muscle weakness and other neurological signs, possible respiratory failure and death. Recoveries may take from days to months. | The heat labile toxin is preformed under anaerobic conditions in low-acid foods prior to consumption. |

*Source:* Compiled from Fenicia and Anniballi 2009; Heymann 2008; Stenfors Arnensen et al. 2008.

Therefore, the times and temperatures of cooked foods are critical to inducing the germination and growth of *B. cereus* spores to hazardous levels, usually about $10^5$ to $10^8$ CFUs/g of food (Stenfors Arensen, Fagerlund, Granum 2008). In the United States, the food most often associated with outbreaks from *B. cereus* is fried rice. Other foods include those of plant origin, usually cooked foods and meat dishes with a variety of ingredients.

### Clostridium botulinum: *Infant Botulism and Adult Intestinal Toxemia Botulism*

Although typically not described in the medical literature as a toxicoinfection, the ingestion of *C. botulinum* (and a few other *Clostridia*) spores by susceptible individuals can lead to colonization and release of neurotoxins in the large intestine by these bacteria. The potent neurotoxins are then absorbed by the intestine and transported to neuronal synapses, where the neurotoxic action takes effect. The greatest risk factor for this condition is the absence of a fully developed microbiota; apparently, the microbiota inhibits the colonization of *C. botulinum* in the gut. The most susceptible individuals are infants younger than 1 year who have not yet developed their microbiota (Fenicia and Anniballi 2009). In extremely rare cases, adults with an altered gastrointestinal tract may also develop this type of botulism. The sources of *C. botulinum* spores include household dusts and soil or foods in contact with the soil, such as honey. Classic foodborne botulism is actually an intoxication from preformed neurotoxins and is discussed separately in the section on microbial toxins in Chapter 3.

## FOODBORNE VIRUSES

In terms of food safety, several important points should be remembered about viruses. First, the estimated portion of foodborne illness outbreaks in the United States attributed to one virus alone (*Norovirus*) ranges from 28% to 67% (Mead et al. 1999; Turcios et al. 2006). This is difficult to prove, however, because most foodborne illness outbreaks have an unknown etiology, and diagnostic tests for norovirus infections are lacking. Nevertheless, on the basis of clinical and epidemiologic profiles, norovirus is believed to be the leading cause of foodborne illness (Turcios et al. 2006). Second, viruses do not replicate in food or water. A suitable and living host is necessary for viral replication. Third, infected persons shed large numbers of viruses in their stools, as many as $10^{11}$ particles per gram of stool, and only a few virus particles are necessary to cause infection (Koopmans and Duizer 2002). In the overwhelming majority of cases (with some exceptions), the sources of viruses that cause foodborne illness come from infected people, usually food handlers or workers, or they can come from food contacting water contaminated by feces (Todd et al. 2007a). Finally, viruses transmitted via food are not easily degraded in the environment and may remain infectious for considerable periods of time.

Enteric viruses typically cause gastroenteritis, but some viruses use the enteric route of transmission to access other organs such as the liver (e.g., hepatitis) and the nervous system (e.g., polio). Of the possible foodborne viruses, those of greatest concern in developed countries are noroviruses (formerly Norwalk-like viruses) and hepatitis A virus (Koopmans and Duizer 2002), shown in Figures 2-27 and 2-28, respectively. Other viruses are important to a lesser extent. The difficulty of ranking risks from foodborne viruses is that these viruses are also transmitted by other modes and vehicles (e.g., waterborne, person-to-person), and the proportion of viral infections directly attributable to foodborne transmission cannot be easily ascertained.

### Noroviruses

Noroviruses (Figure 2-27) are considered the most common foodborne viruses. According to the ICTV, the genus *Norovirus* consists of viruses belonging to the family Caliciviridae, which are characterized by single-stranded RNA enclosed in an icosahedral-shaped capsid, without an envelope, and whose natural hosts are vertebrates. Among the different *Norovirus* species, strains, and serotypes is the well-known *Norwalk virus*, named after a 1968 outbreak at an elementary school in Norwalk, Ohio. Since that time, similar viruses were identified in numerous outbreaks, and the genus *Norovirus* was subsequently established (ICTVdB Management 2006). Among noroviruses responsible for epidemics and foodborne outbreaks, humans are the only established reservoirs.

Norovirus infections are relatively mild and self-limiting, except maybe in the very young and old, or those who are immunocompromised. Sometimes referred to as the "stomach flu," typical symptoms include nausea, vomiting, and diarrhea, and possibly abdominal cramps, muscle aches,

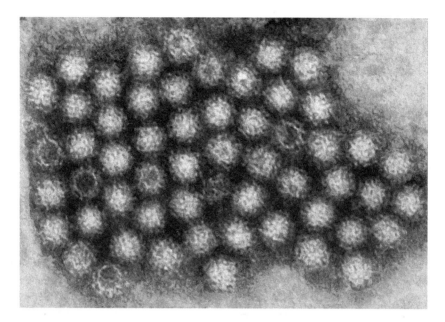

**Figure 2-27** Transmission Electron Micrograph of Norovirus Particles. *Source:* Courtesy of CDC/ Charles D. Humphrey

low-grade fever, and headache. Outbreaks from noroviruses can affect large numbers of people and result in significant suffering and financial expense. Cruise ships were common settings for norovirus infection outbreaks, earning the virus the title of "Cruise Ship Virus" (CDC 2002). Several modes of transmission are involved with norovirus infections, such as person-to-person and contaminated water, but food has a prominent role in outbreaks. Three broad categories of foodborne outbreaks have been recognized (Food and Agriculture Organization [FAO]/World Health Organization [WHO] 2008):

1. Consumption of food contaminated by infected food workers
2. Consumption of contaminated molluscan shellfish
3. Consumption of contaminated produce

Infected food workers are primary sources of norovirus outbreaks. In a review of foodborne illness outbreaks where pathogen contamination was determined to be caused by food workers, norovirus was the etiologic agent most frequently reported (Todd et al. 2007b). In 47.4% of these outbreaks, the food workers had symptoms of infection while at work. Studies have also determined that individuals shed noroviruses in their stools for hours before and many days after becoming symptomatic (Todd et al. 2008a). In addition, the vomit of infected individuals can contain as many norovirus particles as loose stools ($10^5$–$10^{11}$ particles/g), and noroviruses can remain viable on soiled clothing and other surfaces for many hours (Todd et al. 2008a). Because the infective dose of norovirus is estimated between only 10 and 100 particles, secondary and tertiary cross-contamination of foods by objects and surfaces can easily lead to infections (Todd et al. 2009).

Given the great amount of virus shedding by infected food workers, and the transmissibility of norovirus, it is not surprising that foods associated with norovirus outbreaks include salads, sandwiches, and other foods that are handled (Parashar et al. 2001). Contamination of foods with noroviruses can also occur during preharvest, postharvest, and shipping. Molluscan shellfish, particularly oysters, are often associated with norovirus infections. Shellfish harvested from sewage-polluted waters are frequently contaminated with enteric viruses—including noroviruses (FAO/WHO 2008). Other foods that have been implicated in the transmission of noroviruses are produce such as raspberries and green onions. Data and knowledge on the specific sources of produce contamination are incomplete, but pre- and postharvest contact with contaminated water and/or infected workers is considered the most likely sources (FAO/WHO 2008).

## Hepatitis A and E Viruses

Hepatitis is an inflammation of the liver that may have several etiologies. Viruses are common transmissible etiologies of hepatitis among people. Several forms of viral hepatitis have been identified and extensively studied (Figure 2-28). Some are transmitted by percutaneous routes (e.g., needles) or through mucosal contact with infected fluids, while others are transmitted by the fecal-oral route. Those of food safety concern include the latter route. Hepatitis A virus (HAV) is considered more serious in the developed countries because most people in lesser developed countries are infected during childhood and develop immunity by adulthood. Over several decades, HAV has been responsible for large outbreaks frequently traced back to contaminated water and food (Fiore 2004). Humans and other primates are the only reservoirs of HAV, and infected food workers represent the most common sources of food contamination with HAV (CDC 1990). Shellfish harvested from polluted waters are also important sources of HAV infection but considered less common. Yet, one of the largest recorded outbreaks of HAV involved more than 292,000 cases from people consuming clams in China (Halliday et al. 1991). Outbreaks with HAV from produce contaminated during growing, harvesting, and distribution have also occurred, but determining the sources of contamination in these circumstances is difficult at best (Fiore 2004).

Investigating outbreaks from foodborne HAV is difficult for several reasons. Foremost is the long incubation period with HAV infection that averages 28 to 30 days. Most people have difficulty recalling specific meals and food items consumed several weeks prior to the onset of disease. Even if a specific location or meal is implicated, the contaminated food items are probably no longer available for laboratory analysis, and laboratory methods for HAV detection in foods are rife with complications. Another difficulty is the confounding problem arising from sporadic cases in the community at large and other modes of transmission before and after the suspected outbreak. In 2007, only 6.5% of reported HAV cases were suspected to be from food- or waterborne outbreaks, but in 67.7% of cases, the risk factors were unknown (Daniels et al. 2009). People may also have mild cases of HAV infection and fail to seek medical attention, resulting in underreporting of cases. The geographic distribution of cases and extensive travel histories also make it difficult to pinpoint a particular source. All of the aforementioned difficulties suggest

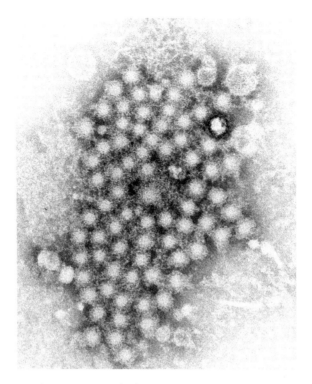

**Figure 2-28** Transmission Electron Micrograph of Hepatitis Virus Particles. *Source:* Courtesy of CDC/ E.H. Cook, Jr.

that the best strategy to prevent foodborne HAV infections is consistent food handler hygiene (at work and home) and safe food practices.

The incidence of HAV infections in the United States has decreased dramatically since it last peaked in 1995 (Daniels et al. 2009). This decrease was attributed primarily to HAV immunizations administered over the following decade. In 1996, the CDC's Advisory Committee on Immunization Practices recommended HAV immunizations for adults at increased risk as a result of lifestyle and to children living in communities with high HAV infection rates. This recommendation was expanded in 1999 to include routine vaccination of children in multiple states with incident rates above certain thresholds. In 2006, the recommendation was expanded further to all children in all 50 states. As a result, the HAV incidence in 2007 was the lowest ever recorded (1.0 case per 100,000 population, see Figure 2-29).

Hepatitis E virus (HEV) infections are endemic in lesser developed countries, where poor sanitation and inadequate water and wastewater treatment are common. The disease is self-limiting but may cause complications during pregnancy, with case-fatality rates reaching 20% among infected women in their third trimester of pregnancy (Heymann 2008). The HEV is distinctly different from other viruses that cause hepatitis and has been taxonomically assigned as the only

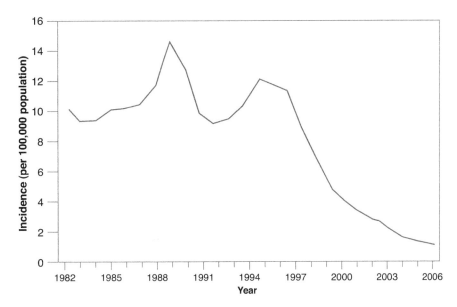

**Figure 2-29** Incidence of Hepatitis A in the United States by Year. *Source:* From Daniels et al. (CDC) 2009

"species" under the genus *Hepevirus*, family Hepeviridae. Only one serotype has been identified, but sequencing of its RNA has identified four major genotypes (Mushahwar 2008). And humans may not be the only reservoirs. Research has identified HEV in domestic swine and several wild animals, suggesting that HEV infections may be zoonotic and potentially foodborne from non-human sources (Aggarwal and Naik 2009). Waterborne outbreaks of HEV infection represent the most documented mode of transmission. Despite the reported low incidence of HEV infection in the United States, the recent detection of HEV in animals used as food merits additional research and enhanced surveillance (FAO/WHO 2008).

## Human Rotavirus

Diarrheal disease is a leading cause of death in the world among children. The human rotavirus (HRV) is a major contributor to this burden by causing severe dehydration. The spread of HRV in lesser developed countries is predominantly person-to-person, with waterborne and foodborne modes contributing to some degree. Within the United States, approximately 80% of infants became infected with HRV by age 5 years, but higher standards of medical care prevented most deaths. A major setting for HRV transmission and outbreaks in the United States has been day care centers. This is changing with the introduction of a HRV vaccination program in 2006 (CDC 2009f). Still, multiple and emerging strains of HRV exist, and the vaccines do not ensure protection against all of them.

### Other Potential Foodborne Viruses

Several other viruses are suspected of being foodborne. Compared with the viruses discussed previously, the incidence of infection is less (or unknown), and supporting evidence for foodborne transmission is usually incomplete or undocumented. Table 2-8 lists the most common and several other possible foodborne viruses, along with the diseases they cause and the likelihood of food/water transmission. This list is not intended to be all inclusive but rather to convey the unexplored and evolving nature of many viruses (Wilhelmi, Roman, Sanchez-Fauquier 2003). Surveillance and research are necessary to identify new strains or emerging foodborne viruses in the near and distant future.

### PROTOZOANS

According to a report by the International Life Sciences Institute (ILSI), the protozoans of greatest concern to food production worldwide belong to the genera *Cryptosporidium, Giardia, Cyclospora,* and *Toxoplasma* (Dawson 2003). Other pathogenic protozoans are transmitted by food and water, but they are not considered to be as important in terms of food processing and distribution.

**Table 2-8** Known Foodborne Viruses

| Virus | Nature of Disease | Food/Water Transmission? |
|---|---|---|
| Noroviruses | Gastroenteritis | Frequently both |
| Hepatitis A Virus | Hepatitis | Frequently both |
| Hepatitis E Virus | Hepatitis | Water, possibly food |
| Human Rotavirus | Gastroenteritis | Sometimes both water and food, usually person-to-person contact and fomites |
| Enteroviruses | Other secondary infections, e.g., neurological; poliomyelitis is the most well known | Sometimes water or food, primarily person-to-person contact |
| Enteric Adenoviruses | Gastroenteritis | Occasional, but fecal-oral route is involved |
| Astroviruses | Gastroenteritis | Occasional, but has been implicated in foodborne transmission |
| Sapovirus | Gastroenteritis | Occasional, possibly foodborne |
| Coronavirus | Gastroenteritis | Uncommon, possibly foodborne |
| Nipah Virus (bat virus) | Neurological | Foodborne; zoonotic disease from pigs |

*Source:* Compiled from FAO/WHO 2008; Heymann 2008; Koopsman and Duzier 2002; and Wilhelmi et al. 2003.

### *Cryptosporidium* Species

The species belonging to the genus *Cryptosporidium* have a wide range of hosts, infecting great numbers of mammals and some birds and reptiles. This parasite (Figure 2-30) belongs to a subclass of protozoans called Coccidia that infect hosts as sporozoites and, following sexual fusion of gametes, produce hardy oocysts. The oocysts are excreted in the feces of infected humans and animals, contaminating the water and food consumed by other hosts and restarting the cycle (Figure 2-31). These cysts are highly resistant to chlorine at levels typically found in treated water supplies. For many years, the majority of human diseases were believed to be caused by a single species, *C. parvum*, but recent molecular techniques have revealed several different genotypes and species, each often associated with specific animal hosts (Yoder, Beach, CDC 2007a). Among the reservoirs of greatest concern are humans, cattle, and other ruminants (hoofed, cud-chewing animals with multiple stomachs); reservoirs of secondary concern include dogs, cats, birds, rodents, and pigs.

The clinical manifestations of cryptosporidiosis caused by the different species are very similar. The infective dose is very low (10–30 oocysts), and infected humans can shed $10^8$–$10^9$ oocysts in a single bowel movement (Chappell et al. 1996; Dupont et al. 1995). In healthy individuals, the disease is relatively mild with signs and symptoms that include watery diarrhea, stomach cramps, nausea and/or vomiting, and low-grade fever. The disease can have serious consequences among those who are immunocompromised, such as HIV-infected persons. The greatest risk factors for cryp-

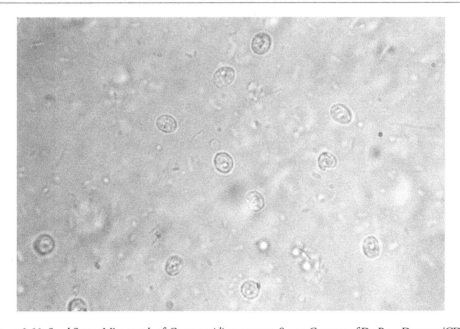

**Figure 2-30** Stool Smear Micrograph of *Cryptosporidium parvum. Source:* Courtesy of Dr. Peter Drotman/CDC

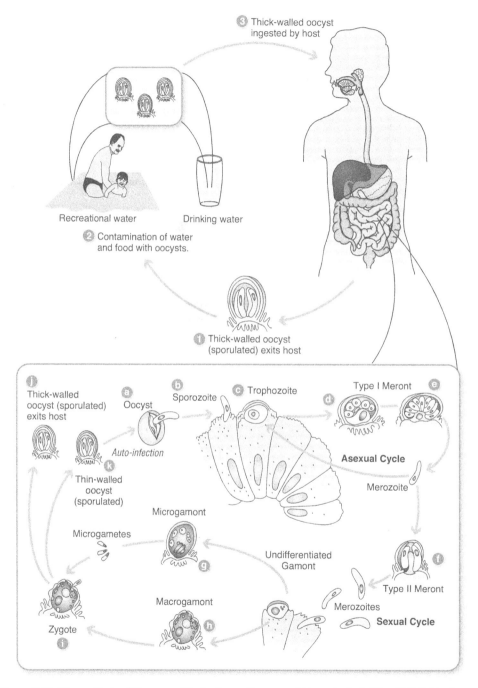

**Figure 2-31** Disease Cycle of Cryptosporidiosis. *Source:* Courtesy of Alexander J. da Silva, PhD/Melanie Moser/CDC

tosporidiosis are contact with infected animals, ingestion of contaminated water, household contact with infected individuals, and international travel (Yoder et al. 2007a). Despite the large numbers of infected farm animals, foodborne cryptosporidiosis is not well documented, partly because methods to detect the oocysts in foods are not well developed (Laberge, Griffiths, Griffiths 1996).

## *Giardia* Species

Several species of *Giardia* are capable of causing disease in humans: *G. lamblia, G. intestinalis,* and *G. duodenalis* (Heymann 2008). Like other protozoans, the infective stage is the trophozoite (Figure 2-32), which rapidly reproduces asexually to colonize the small intestine. They also form cysts that are excreted through defecation into the environment, permitting *Giardia* to survive for long periods of time under damp and cool conditions. The fecal-oral route of transmission is responsible for outbreaks of giardiasis through person-to-person contact, consumption of contaminated water and food, and to a lesser extent animal-to-person contact. Reservoirs of *Giardia* include many domestic and wild mammals. Historically, giardiasis was frequently associated with campers who drank contaminated water, dubbing the disease "Beaver Fever." Although many outbreaks of giardiasis have been documented over the years, including foodborne giardiasis, the relative contribution of different transmission modes to sporadic cases is unknown. To better understand its epidemiology and estimate the burden of disease, giardiasis became a nationally notifiable disease to the CDC in 2002 (Yoder et al. 2007b).

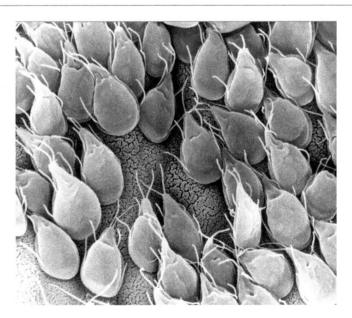

**Figure 2-32** Scanning Electron Micrograph of *Giardia* trophozoites on Intestinal Epithelium of a Gerbil. *Source:* Courtesy of Dr. Stan Erlandsen/CDC

The clinical course of giardiasis is usually self-limiting, and the clinical manifestations are similar to other gastrointestinal infections, namely, diarrhea and abdominal cramps, along with bloating, malabsorption, and weight loss. Although the egg-shaped cysts and pear-shaped trophozoites of *Giardia* are easily discerned in stool specimens, many clinicians do not routinely order laboratory tests for patients with nonbloody diarrhea (Yoder et al. 2007b). Therefore, the true incidence of giardiasis in the United States is unknown.

## Cyclospora cayetanensis

Among the many species of *Cyclospora* that infect animals, only *C. cayetanensis* has been associated with humans as its definitive host. The complete life cycle and biology of *C. cayetanensis* are not well understood, but its development outside of the host makes *C. cayetanensis* different from *Cryptosporidium* and *Giardia*. After the oocysts of *C. cayetanensis* are excreted in the feces of infected hosts, they must sporulate in the environment before becoming infectious to another host. This can take days to weeks (Heymann 2008). Consequently, with a longer time needed outside of the host, the role of person-to-person transmission is less compared with vehicles such as contaminated food and water. The diarrhea and other manifestations of disease can be persistent, often lasting for weeks without treatment, eventually resolving by themselves.

Cyclosporiasis is believed to be endemic in lesser developed countries, where transmission most likely occurs from the consumption of contaminated water and food. In North America, large foodborne outbreaks of cyclosporiasis have been linked to various types of imported produce (snow peas, raspberries, basil, and lettuce) (CDC 2004c). The exact sources of produce contamination were not definitively determined. Without additional research, the sources of produce contamination are speculative but probably involve contact with sewage-contaminated water.

## Toxoplasma gondii

The definitive hosts of *Toxoplasma gondii* are felines, including domestic, feral, and wild cats. Humans and other animals serve as secondary and/or intermediate hosts for the parasite. Approximately 23% of adolescents and adults in the United States may have been infected with *T. gondii* (CDC 2000). For those with normal immune competence, the disease toxoplasmosis is relatively mild and self-limiting, with signs and symptoms similar to the flu, that is, fever, muscle aches, malaise. For immunocompromised individuals, the disease can be serious and even deadly. Three main routes of infection are important:

1. The ingestion of undercooked or raw meats where *T. gondii* has become encysted in the food animal's flesh
2. The accidental ingestion of *T. gondii* oocysts in cat feces (e.g., litterbox changing, gardening in contaminated soil), or by ingesting fruits and vegetables contaminated by cat feces
3. Transplacental infection to a fetus from a mother with toxoplasmosis

Infection of the fetus with *T. gondii* is potentially the most serious form of disease. Mental retardation, epilepsy and blindness are possible outcomes, and 400–4,000 cases of congenital toxoplasmosis are estimated to occur each year in the United States (CDC 2000). Animals used for food, whether wild or domestic, can become infected from ingesting oocysts in the soil. After excystation and further development, the *T. gondii* tachyzoites can invade other tissues in the animal and form tissue cysts that contain bradyzoites. Consumption of these tissue cysts in the meat by humans can cause toxoplasmosis. The most common meat products infected with *T. gondii* are pork.

## Other Protozoans

Other protozoan diseases of foodborne importance include amebiasis and sarcocystosis. Known also as amoebic dysentery, amebiasis is cause by *Entamoeba histolytica* and characterized by the dysentery-type of diarrhea, though many cases may be comparatively mild. *E. histolytica* forms infective cysts that are passed through stools and may remain viable for weeks or months in moist environments. With humans as the only reservoirs of *E. histolytica*, food and water contaminated by human feces are the most common vehicles of transmission, followed by close personal contact in households or institutions.

Many species of the genus *Sarcocystis* that infect and parasitize animal hosts have been identified, but only two species (*S. homonis* and *S. suihominis*) are known to infect humans as their definitive host. Other species of *Sarcocystis* may infect humans accidently, but humans become a "dead-end" host for them, that is, the parasite cannot reproduce in the new host species. The life cycle of *Sarcocystis* species is complex in terms of developmental stages and intermediate and definitive hosts (Fayer 2004). Basically, humans consume undercooked meat, usually beef or pork, containing sarcocysts in the tissue. These sarcocysts release bradyzoites, and they invade the human intestinal epithelium and undergo differentiation into several forms. Ultimately, gametes fuse to form oocysts that sporulate and are shed in the feces. Ingestion of these sporocysts by livestock begins a series of stages that eventually leads to formation of sarcocysts in the muscle tissue, and the cycle repeats itself.

If humans acquire sarcocystosis from ingesting beef with *S. hominis* sarcocysts, the disease is limited to the intestinal tract, and the infections are typically asymptomatic and resolve spontaneously. Ingestion of *S. suihominis* sarcocysts in pork can result in more pronounced illness, such as bloating, diarrhea, nausea, and vomiting. Infections with nonhuman sarcocysts or sporocysts can result in muscular sarcocystosis, a relatively rare occurrence, at least in the developed countries.

## FOODBORNE HELMINTHS

Approximately 300 species of helminths currently infect people around the globe (Cox 2002). Some of them have lineages linked to humans' primate evolution. Other zoonotic helminths have adapted to humans as hosts during the domestication of animals for food or companionship (Sianto et al. 2009). Humans can also become secondary or dead-end hosts for a great number of zoonotic helminths. Most of the 300 or so helminths that infect humans are rare and found only in the tropics. Their life cycles vary in complexity and may involve multiple intermediate and definitive hosts. As part of their life cycles, a few helminths access human hosts by contaminating foods with their eggs or larvae. Many helminths access their hosts primarily through other routes but could incidentally contaminate foods to infect a human host. Because entire textbooks and journals are devoted to helminthology, the following discussion is limited to those helminths considered historically important to the North American food supply.

### *Trichinella* Species

Trichinellosis is a nematode infection caused primarily by *Trichinella spiralis*, though several other *Trichinella* species have been identified in various hosts and different regions of the world. This parasitic roundworm has a grisly life cycle involving larvae encysting themselves in muscles and other tissues (Figure 2-33). Most often associated with the consumption of undercooked or raw pork, trichinellosis was a major concern in the United States during the mid-twentieth century. In 1943, after examining the diaphragm muscles taken from necropsies of human bodies across the country, a report published by the federal government estimated that 16% or more Americans had trichinellosis infections (Wright, Kerr, Jacobs 1943). Since then, federal regulations were developed to ensure safe pork products, dramatically reducing the number of reported trichinellosis cases (Figure 2-34). Over the decades, a link was observed between feeding hogs uncooked garbage and *Trichinella* infections. Consequently, eliminating uncooked or raw garbage from a hog's diet is an important measure in the *Trichinella* control strategy. At the consumer's level, thorough cooking of meats such as pork remains an effective control measure.

The life cycle of *Trichinella* species does not involve a free-living stage outside of the host. The adults live and mate in the mucosa of the duodenum and jejunum of the host. The resulting eggs

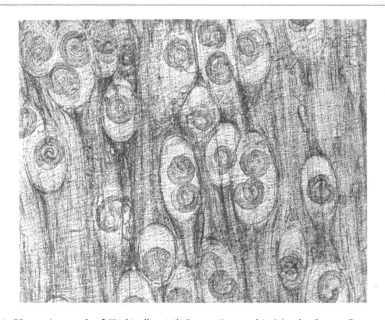

**Figure 2-33** Photomicrograph of *Trichinella spirilis* Larvae Encysted in Muscle. *Source:* Courtesy of CDC

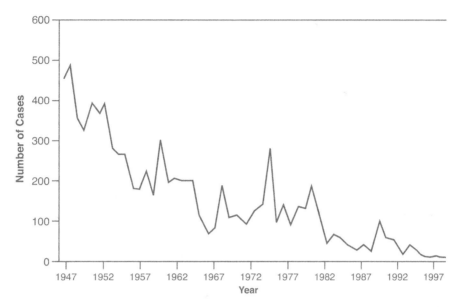

**Figure 2-34** Number of Reported Trichinellosis Cases, by Year—United States, 1947–2001. *Source:* From Roy et al. (CDC) 2003

hatch in the host, and the larvae migrate through the gut wall into other tissues. Several organs, including the heart and eyes, may be affected, but only the larvae that reach the skeletal muscles of the host will ultimately survive, possibly as long as several years. They accomplish this by curling up in the muscle tissue to form a cyst (Figure 2-33). When the host animal's muscle tissue is consumed by another animal or humans, the larvae are liberated by digestive enzymes and mature in the intestines of the new host, starting the cycle over.

Domestic animals that may be hosts to *Trichinella* species include pigs, dogs, cats, rats, and occasionally horses fed items containing animal products. A great variety of wild animals such as bears, foxes, wolves, wild boars, and practically any omnivorous or predatory animal can be a potential host. Although pork was identified as the primary source of human *Trichinella* infections in the past, undercooked wild game has now become the principal source of human cases in the United States (CDC 2004d). This is partly because of the increasing popularity of bear hunting and the consumption of wild game. Furthermore, bears are frequently infected with the *T. nativa*, a species of *Trichinella* that is highly resistant to freezing and may remain viable while frozen for months or years (CDC 2004d). From 1997 to 2001, bear meat was responsible for 40% of reported cases of trichinellosis, whereas pork was responsible for 31% of reported cases; approximately 28% of reported cases were from unknown sources (Roy, Lopez, Schantz 2003).

The signs and symptoms of trichinellosis can vary by the species of *Trichinella*, but generally they coincide with the parasite's development and journey through the host. Depending on the number of larvae ingested, the incubation period can be highly variable. The first indication of infection may be gastroenteritis (e.g., diarrhea, nausea, abdominal pain, and possible vomiting) approximately 2 days after ingestion of the contaminated meat. Invasion of the surrounding tissue by the larvae usually occurs 1 or 2 weeks following initial symptoms. Over the course of larvae migration, several clinical manifestations are possible, such as muscle soreness, fever, ocular signs, and other problems (Heymann 2008). Neurologic and cardiac complications can occur weeks later, and death from myocardial failure is possible. The disease is often misdiagnosed as illnesses such as the flu.

### *Taenia* Species

A great variety of cestodes (tapeworms) infect animals and occasionally humans, but two species of tapeworms parasitize humans as their only definitive hosts: *Taenia saginata* and *Taenia solium*. The intermediate hosts of *T. saginata* and *T. solium* are cattle and swine, respectively. Except for differences in their anatomy and specific intermediate hosts, the life cycles of these *Taenia* species are very similar (Figure 2-35). The cycles begin by humans consuming raw or undercooked meat that contain encysted larval forms called cysticerci in the muscle flesh. The larvae develop into adult tapeworms within the human intestine, where they may live for decades, obtaining all their nourishment from the human host. The adult tapeworm infection is called taeniasis. This form of disease is often mild and variable, consisting possibly of nervousness, weight loss, and abdominal pain. Each segment of the tapeworm, called a proglottid, has reproductive organs that produce tens of thousands of eggs. The gravid proglottids and eggs are shed through human feces each day in great numbers, extensively contaminating the surrounding environment. In the soil, the eggs can survive for months with fully developed embryos. Cattle or swine consume the eggs during grazing or rooting in the soil, and the embryos hatch in the animals' intestine. From there, the embryos migrate to striated muscles and transform into cysterci, starting the cycle over again. The larval form of this infection is called cysticercosis.

The occurrence of cysticercosis is usually limited to the intermediate animal hosts. In the case of *T. solium* infections, however, it is possible for humans to acquire this very serious and sometimes fatal disease. This happens by accidental ingestion of the *T. solium* eggs, either by autoinfection (from one's self) or from contaminated soil. When humans ingest *T. solium* eggs, the cysticerci may become embedded in the muscles, ocular regions, and central nervous system—including the brain. Signs and symptoms of cysticercosis depend on the locations and numbers of the cysticerci in the tissues. With neurocysticercosis, signs and symptoms may range from headaches to seizures and stroke. Cysticercosis is a debilitating disease that merits prevention by strict adherence to sanitation and food safety practices.

From the descriptions provided previously on the life cycle of *Taenia* tapeworms, it makes sense that the disease is more common in regions where sanitation is inadequate and livestock are allowed access to human feces or human feces–contaminated soil. The occurrence of human *Taenia* infections is high in such places as Latin America, perhaps as much as 10–25% incidence in some villages, while the prevalence of cysticercosis in swine may reach 37% in some parts of eastern Tanzania, Africa (Heymann 2008). Infections by *Taenia* have become rare in North America and Europe. However, infections from imported meat are possible in these regions, and the possibility still exists for local transmission of taeniasis or cysticercosis (CDC 1992).

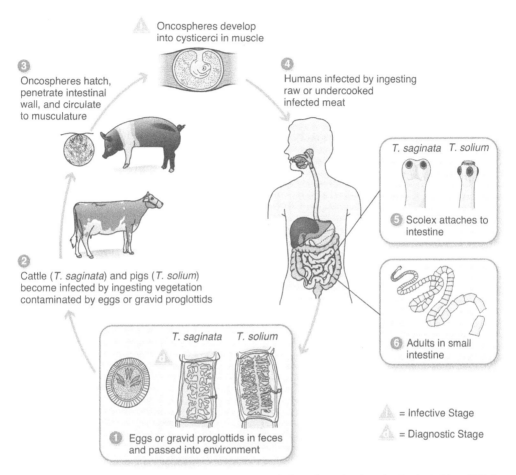

**Figure 2-35** Disease Cycle of Taeniasis. *Source:* Courtesy of Alexander J. da Silva, PhD/Melanie Moser/CDC

## *Diphyllobothrium* Species

Many different species of fish tapeworms belonging to the genus *Diphyllobothrium* have been identified to infect humans and animals (Skeríková et al. 2009). Of the several species known to infect humans, the tapeworm *Diphyllobothrium latum* is considered the most important. Figure 2-36 illustrates the life cycle of *Diphyllobothrium* species and shows at least three intermediate hosts are involved: crustaceans such copepods, freshwater fish, and/or salmon. Humans and other fish-eating mammals and birds are the definitive hosts. These hosts are also responsible for continuation of the *Diphyllobothrium* species life cycle by passing tapeworm eggs (as many as $10^6$ eggs/worm/day) in feces to a body of water. In humans, the disease is called diphyllobothriasis and occurs from eating raw or undercooked fish. Cases of diphyllobothriasis by *D. latum* are usually associated with fish caught in subarctic or temperate regions of the Northern Hemisphere, that is, northern latitudes of North America, Europe, and Asia. For many years, *D. latum* was presumed responsible for diphyllobothriasis from the consumption of raw or undercooked salmon, but in recent years, the species *D. nihonkaiense* has been increasingly identified as the etiologic agent (Arizono et al. 2009). Cases of diphyllobothriasis by *D. pacificum* have been reported in South America and Japan after consuming marine (not freshwater) fish (Scholz et al. 2009; Skeríková et al. 2009).

## Other Helminths of Food Safety Concern

Several other helminths that may be transmitted by foods are included in Table 2-9. The majority of these helminths are usually encountered outside of North America. Nonetheless, with

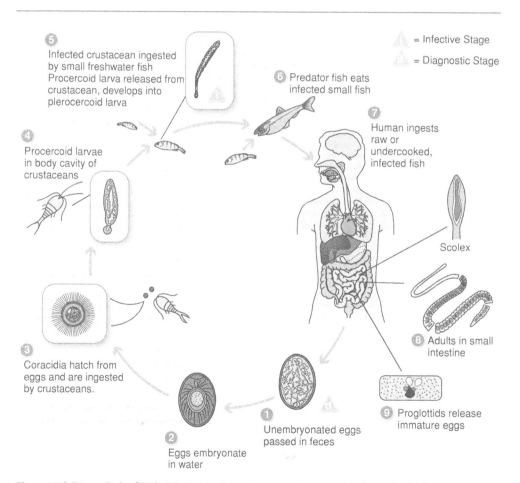

**Figure 2-36** Disease Cycle of Diphyllobothriasis. *Source:* Courtesy of Alexander J. da Silva, PhD/Melanie Moser/CDC

**Table 2-9** Selected Helminths of Food Safety Importance

| Helminth | Occurrence | Foodborne Transmission |
|---|---|---|
| *Trichinella* spp. | Worldwide, with incidence dependent on local cooking and eating habits | Primarily from raw or undercooked pork, and from other meats, frequently from wild game |
| *Taenia* spp. (beef and pork tapeworms) | Worldwide, particularly in regions with poor sanitary conditions and with livestock having access to human feces | Consumption of cystercerci in raw or undercooked beef and pork. Cystircercosis from unintentional consumption of *T. solium* eggs |
| *Diphyllobothrium* spp. (broad or fish tapeworm) | Mostly northern hemisphere and some in the tropics | Consumption of raw or undercooked freshwater fish and salmon. To a lesser degree, marine fish consumed raw |
| *Echinococcus granulosus* | All continents except Antarctica | Contamination of food or water after contact with infected dogs |
| *Fasciola hepatica* and *F. gigantica* (agent of liver rot) | Reported in 61 countries, mostly where sheep and cattle are raised | Consumption of raw aquatic plants (watercress) containing metacercariae |
| *Fasciolopsis buski* | Southeast Asia, particularly in areas with pigs | Consumption of raw aquatic plants (water caltrop nuts, water chestnuts, water bamboo) containing metacercariae |
| *Clonorchis sinensis* (Chinese liver fluke) | Throughout China, occasionally Japan, Korea, and Southeast Asia. Human and multiple animal definitive hosts | Consumption of raw or undercooked freshwater fish containing encysted larvae |
| *Anisakis simplex* (herringworm or whaleworm) and *Pseudoterranova decipiens* (codworm or sealworm) | Throughout the world where individuals eat inadequately cooked fish, squid, and octopus | Consumption of raw or undercooked fish after larvae have migrated from fish's mesentery to muscle flesh, usually after fish die or are killed |
| *Capillaria philipiensis* | Endemic in Philippines and Thailand, but also reported in other countries | Consumption of raw, whole freshwater fish, and autoinfection |
| *Gnathostoma* spp. (agent of a visceral larva migrans) | Anyplace where dogs, cats, and large carnivores may act as definitive hosts | Consumption of undercooked fish, poultry, frogs, or snakes. Common among ethnic dishes such as sashimi, somfak, or ceviche |
| *Ascaris lumbricoides* (agent of intestinal roundworm infection) | Worldwide and common, with incidence exceeding 50% in most tropical countries | Consumption of uncooked produce from soil contaminated with human feces (and infective helminth eggs) |
| *Trichuris trichiura* (human whipworm) | Worldwide but most prominent in warm, moist regions | Consumption of human-feces-contaminated soil or vegetables |

*Source:* Compiled from Heymann 2008; Cox 2002; Scholz et al. 2009; and CDC 1992.

an increasingly global food market and international travel, the possibility of acquiring one of these helminth infections exists, albeit the risk depends on multiple factors and circumstances. Specific measures for controlling foodborne helminths are covered in later chapters.

## PRIONS

For at least 200 years, a neurodegenerative disease known as scrapie has afflicted sheep. In the 1980s, the etiologic agent was tentatively identified as a prion protein (PrP). Several variants of the transmissible PrP have been studied since then, and a collection of diseases called transmissible spongiform encephalopathies (TSE) or prion diseases was identified as afflicting several species—including humans (Chesebro 2003). As a result of additional research, the number of recognized prion diseases continues to grow (Watts, Balachandran, Westaway 2006). The animals identified to be afflicted by TSE include sheep, cattle, mink, elk, deer, and other animals experimentally inoculated.

The public became aware of prion diseases from a highly publicized epidemic of bovine spongiform encephalopathy (BSE), known as "mad cow disease." By 1992, more than 30,000 cattle per year were being identified with the disease in the United Kingdom (Brown et al. 2006). Despite intensive efforts that eventually controlled the epidemic, the disease spread across international borders, and by 2006 it was reported in 24 other countries. The first confirmed case in the United States was a dairy cow from Washington State, reported in December 2003 (CDC 2004a). It was ultimately determined that the BSE epidemic was intensified by the rendering of livestock carcasses to make feed for cattle. The prions apparently survived the ineffective rendering process and were transmitted to healthy cattle through the contaminated feed. The exportation of U.K. feed products to other countries apparently exported the disease as well.

The transmission of TSEs occurs from either consuming materials contaminated with prions or by being inoculated by prion-contaminated materials, for example, by transplanted tissues or contaminated surgical instruments (Chesebro 2003). They do not appear to be transmitted by person-to-person, animal-to-animal, or animal-to-human contact. Prions exert their detrimental effects by causing certain other proteins to misfold into a wrong shape. An accumulation of misfolded proteins in the brain leads to the formation of plaques or spongy voids (spongiform). The associated symptoms become more progressive and may take months or years before becoming clinically recognizable. In cattle with BSE, the symptoms typically include behavioral changes such as nervousness or aggression, unusual posture and incoordination, inability to rise (downer), and unexplained weight loss. Among wild animals such as deer and elk in North America, the TSE is called chronic wasting disease (CWD), a reference to the animals' emaciated appearance. In humans, the primary symptoms are dementia and ataxia. The neurologic pathology ultimately leads to an early death in all species.

Human forms of TSE are called Creutzfeldt-Jakob disease (CJD) or Gerstmann-Straussler-Scheinker syndrome, kuru, and fatal familial insomnia. Several types of CJD are known, and each has been labeled with an adjective that describes the context of its occurrence. Classic CJD (cCJD) includes familial (inherited), iatrogenic, and sporadic forms designated as fCJD, iCJD, sCJD, respectively. As their names suggest, the cCJD forms are either inherited, transmitted by tissue transplantation or surgical instruments (iatrogenic), or occur very infrequently (1 in $10^6$

people) with no identifiable risk factors (sporadic). In 1994, during the BSE epidemic, the United Kingdom identified a new variant of CJD, designated as vCJD. This revelation prompted alarm among public health officials worldwide because epidemiologic and laboratory evidence suggested vCJD was transmitted from BSE-contaminated cattle products (CDC 2004b). The incidence of vCJD dropped off over a period of several years following its initial discovery. Speculation is that a tougher control on beef producers was responsible by limiting BSE in the human food chain.

Even within a species, different strains of prions have been identified, meaning that they differ by their conformational structure and behavior within the animal. Different strains or variants of prions tend to accumulate in different regions of the nervous system, or other tissues may also be involved. Because BSE can have a very long incubation period, BSE-infected cattle could be slaughtered for food before behavioral signs become obvious. Outside of the host, prions are very resistant to degradation from high temperatures, acidity, ultraviolet light, ionizing radiation, common disinfectants, and proteolytic enzymes. In other words, prions are very persistent in the environment. Unfortunately, highly sensitive and accurate methods for detecting prion infectivity in the environment have not been developed (Saunders, Bartelt-Hunt, Bartz 2008). The current food safety strategy focuses on eliminating transmission among livestock by restricting certain rendered feeds, banning certain bovine tissues from entering the human food chain, observational surveillance of cattle for infection, and occasional testing of carcasses for BSE. The risk of prions in the human food chain is difficult to assess but is generally considered to be extremely low. The concern is that complacency may lead to another epidemic similar to the past one in the United Kingdom.

## EMERGING VERSUS CONTEMPORARY FOODBORNE INFECTIONS

According to the Institute of Medicine (IOM), an emerging infectious disease is one where the incidence has increased within the past two decades or poses a threat to increase in the near future (Lederberg, Shope, Oaks 1992). This includes both newly identified diseases and those previously controlled in the past (i.e., reemergence). The majority of foodborne infections discussed in this chapter fit the definition of an emerging infectious disease. But the incidence of foodborne diseases is not static and changes over time. As some diseases become controlled, others may emerge and increase in incidence. The foodborne diseases listed in Table 2-10 were once high-priority concerns in the United States because of their associated morbidity and/or mortality, but their incidences decreased greatly in the latter half of the twentieth century. Several specific control measures are credited for the reduction of these foodborne diseases (Beatty et al. 2003; Tauxe 2002). Although these foodborne diseases have been largely controlled in developed countries, their reservoirs still exist, and under the right conditions, they could reemerge. In fact, most of these diseases still occur in the United States but at very low incidence levels.

A great number of changing conditions and trends contribute to emerging foodborne diseases. Several of these trends were briefly discussed in Chapter 1. In a landmark report, the IOM identified six factors or categories that facilitate the emergence of microbial threats or diseases (Lederberg et al. 1992). Several authors have specifically analyzed the emergence of foodborne diseases in the context of these factors (Altekruse, Cohen, Swerdlow 1997; Buchanan 1997; Skovgaard 2007; Tauxe 2002). Some of their insights are shared in the following subsections on the six factors identified by the IOM.

Table 2-10 Foodborne Diseases of Concern in Early Twentieth Century United States

| Disease | Pathogenic Agent | Key Control Measures |
|---------|------------------|----------------------|
| Typhoid fever | *Salmonella* Typhi | Pasteurization of milk, shellfish sanitation |
| Brucellosis | *Brucella abortus* | Pasteurization of milk |
| Q fever | *Coxiella burnetii* | Pasteurization of milk |
| Bovine tuberculosis | *Mycobacterium bovis* | Pasteurization of milk |
| Scarlet fever | *Streptococcus* spp. | Pasteurization of milk |
| Septic sore throat | *Streptococcus* spp. | Pasteurization of milk |
| Trichinellosis | *Trichinella spirilis* | Ban feeding uncooked garbage to pigs, adequate cooking of pork |
| Tapeworms | *Taenia* spp. | Sanitation, meat inspections |
| Gastrointestinal anthrax | *Bacillus anthracis* | Animal vaccinations and inspections |
| Botulism | *Clostridium botulinum* | Retort food canning |

*Source*: Compiled from Beatty et al. 2003; Tauxe 2002; and Tauxe and Esteban 2007.

## 1. Human Demographics and Behavior

The population in the United States and other developed countries is changing demographically. A greater proportion of the population has a heightened susceptibility to foodborne infections. Individuals such as older adults, people infected with HIV, transplant recipients, and cancer/chemotherapy patients generally have less resistance to foodborne infections. Behavioral and cultural changes are reflected in the eating preferences and habits of people. More health-conscious people are eating raw fruits and vegetables, increasing the demand for fresh produce that may also become contaminated with pathogens during growing, harvesting, processing, and/or distribution. A greater percentage of people are also eating outside of the home. For many reasons related to food safety, the risks of outbreaks are greater (or more easily recognized) at sites where large quantities of food are handled, prepared, and consumed. In addition, with the population growth of developed countries attributed more and more to immigration, ethnic practices by immigrants may put them at increased risk of foodborne diseases. Examples include outbreaks from the consumption of rare pork, resulting in trichinellosis, or cheeses made from raw milk, resulting in listeriosis or brucellosis.

## 2. Technology and Industry

A century ago, the food production industry was not on the same scale as it is today. Technology and industry practices have changed agriculture from a widely dispersed set of company- and family-owned farms to corporate agricultural production, processing, and distribution centers. Although this change has increased food production and helps feed the world, it has also introduced and transmitted zoonotic pathogens across animal stocks and distributed them to human consumers. The emergence of *E. coli* O157:H7 and *Salmonella* species in human populations, sometimes as massive and geographically distributed outbreaks, is reflected in this change. Food processing plants are highly productive and automated, and if adequate food safety practices are not followed, these plants can harbor foodborne pathogens and contaminate multiple lots of foods. Many food products distributed across the country are now made from ingredients provided by multiple companies. If any of these ingredients is contaminated and harbors pathogens, the pathogens are distributed along with the food product. More about this topic is discussed later in the topic of safety management of the food supply.

### 3. International Travel and Commerce

The world has become a smaller place in terms of international travel and commerce. Tourists and businesspeople can eat lunch on the other side of the world and return home before the next day. They can also bring back unwanted souvenirs, such as diarrheal disease and parasites, and unknowingly serve as incubatory carriers of a disease or parasite. But this phenomenon is not limited to international travelers. The exportation and importation of foods around the world are now commonplace. Foodborne diseases considered as emerging or exotic sometimes appear in developed countries from imported foods. This may be the result of poor food safety practices in the country of origin and/or contamination during shipping. International trade has also spread infected breeding stocks of animals across borders. The pandemic of salmonellosis is believed to be the result of chickens being sold for breeding purposes, particularly egg-laying hens.

### 4. Microbial Adaptation and Change

As discussed earlier in this chapter, microorganisms are capable of rapid evolutionary changes that result in adaptation to different environmental conditions. Some of these changes involve acquiring additional pathogenic factors, which in turn increases the virulence of foodborne pathogens. Other changes involve increased pathogen tolerances to temperature extremes, acidic conditions, desiccation, and to some disinfectants. For example, several foodborne pathogens are capable of entering a VBNC state, allowing them to survive unfavorable environmental conditions. Changes can also be very specific, such as the acid tolerance response (ATR) discussed earlier. The greatest change of concern is antibiotic resistance. Multiple strains of foodborne pathogens have been identified as resistant to various antibiotics. The principal selection pressure for antibiotic resistance among foodborne pathogens is the liberal use of antibiotics in farm animals. Patients prescribed antibiotics for foodborne diseases may also contribute to antibiotic resistance, but this selection pressure is more influential in secondary human cases and person-to-person transmission scenarios.

### 5. Economic Development and Land Use

Animals raised for food generate approximately 2 billion tons of manure each year in the United States. Disposal of this manure creates numerous environmental problems, but it also acts as a reservoir of zoonotic pathogens such as *E. coli* O157:H7, *Salmonella* species, *Campylobacter* species, and others. Improper waste management of manure contributes to the spread of zoonotic pathogens among herds of farm animals. Land use and waste management are also influential in the increasing trend of foodborne infections from fresh produce. Poor waste management of manure, and animals in close proximity to field crops, can result in pre- or postharvest contamination of produce with pathogens. A similar problem is the proper treatment and disposal of human wastes. The capacity of sewage treatment plants does not always keep pace with growing human populations, especially in lesser developed countries. Even in developed countries, excessive rains (e.g., hurricanes) or equipment breakdowns can spill raw sewage onto the land and into waterways. Human pathogens in sewage can become foodborne under the right set of circumstances. Shellfish beds in local waters are particularly efficient at concentrating pathogens from raw sewage and farm runoff. Seafood harvested from these contaminated waters can be a source of several pathogens.

## 6. Breakdown of Public Health Measures

Believing that the war on infectious diseases was won in developed countries, the public health priority and research emphasis on infectious diseases began to wane during the mid-twentieth century. Attention and resources were directed from infectious disease control programs to higher priority chronic disease control and other programs. An institutional complacency ensued with infectious diseases, and a false sense of security developed with the public, believing that modern medicine could cure nearly any infection. The recognition of new infectious diseases and old ones reemerging came about in the latter part of the twentieth century, when several epidemics caught the public's attention, most notably the AIDS epidemic. But many public health agencies continued to operate with severely restricted budgets, especially at the state and local levels of government. During the 1990s, several states did not have personnel dedicated to a foodborne disease surveillance program. Federal and state agencies also had limited staffing to effectively conduct food safety inspections and enforcement at commercial food processing plants and restaurants. Events such as natural disasters also lead to the breakdown of public health measures, resulting in inadequate food protection and increased potential for disease transmission.

New and infrequently reported foodborne pathogens have been identified in recent years, albeit knowledge about them is limited for a number of reasons. For example, the bacteria *Aeromonas hydrophila* and *Plesiomonas shigelloides* have been associated with foodborne illnesses from the consumption of fish and shellfish, as well as other modes of transmission. Additional research is needed to characterize their pathogenicity in humans and their significance for foodborne transmission. Other emerging infections of the gastrointestinal tract continue to be identified, but new diagnostic tests and additional epidemiologic studies are needed before specific control measures can be proposed (Schlenker and Surawicz 2009). In the near and far future, humans will likely encounter new foodborne pathogens that will challenge existing food safety programs. Given the scope and magnitude of potential problems, a proactive approach is preferable to a reactive one.

## Intentional Contamination of Foods

Under the auspices of the IOM, a workshop was held to address foodborne threats to health (Institute of Medicine [IOM] 2006). The ease and vulnerability of foods to deliberate adulteration (i.e., terrorism) are frightening to many and a great concern to public officials. Whatever the motivation, the deliberate introduction of a pathogen or toxicant into the food supply could yield catastrophic results, both in terms of morbidity and economic losses. In fact, the IOM now includes a new category, Intent to Harm, for the emergence of infectious diseases (Smolinski, Hamburg, Lederberg 2003). This opens the possibility to a wider array of new or rarely encountered pathogens as agents of foodborne diseases. Even though a determined effort to inflict harm is difficult to thwart, food safety practices and management of the food supply must include reducing vulnerability to the deliberate introduction of harmful agents. This subject is addressed in more depth under safety management of the food supply.

## REFERENCES

Aggarwal R, Naik S. 2009. Epidemiology of hepatitis E: Current status. *J Gastroenterol Hepatol* 24(9):1484–1493.

Altekruse SF, Cohen ML, Swerdlow DL. 1997. Emerging foodborne diseases. *Emerg Infect Dis* 3(3):285–293.

Altekruse SF, Stern NJ, Fields PI, Swerdlow DL. 1999. *Campylobacter jejuni*—an emerging foodborne pathogen. *Emerg Infect Dis* 5(1):28–35.

American Medical Association, American Nurses Association–American Nurses Foundation, Centers for Disease Control and Prevention, Center for Food Safety and Applied Nutrition, Food and Drug Administration, Food Safety and Inspection Service, US Department of Agriculture. 2004. Diagnosis and management of foodborne illnesses: A primer for physicians and other health care professionals. *MMWR Recomm Rep* 53(RR-4):1–33.

Arensen LPS, Fagerlund A, Granum PE. 2008. From soil to gut: *Bacillus cereus* and its food poisoning toxins. *FEMS Microbiol Rev* 32(4):579–606.

Arizono N, Yamada M, Nakamura-Uchiyama F, Ohnishi K. 2009. Diphyllobothriasis associated with eating raw Pacific salmon. *Emerg Infect Dis* 15(6):866–870.

Beatty ME, Ashford DA, Griffin PM, Tauxe RV, Sobel J. 2003. Gastrointestinal anthrax: Review of the literature. *Arch Intern Med* 163(20):2527–2531.

Bell BP, Goldoft M, Griffin PM, Davis MA, Gordon DC, Tarr PI, Bartleson CA, Lewis JH, Barrett TJ, Wells JG. 1994. A multistate outbreak of *Escherichia coli* O157:H7–associated bloody diarrhea and hemolytic uremic syndrome from hamburgers. The Washington experience. *JAMA* 272(17):1349–1353.

Beuchat LR. 2006. Vectors and conditions for preharvest contamination of fruits and vegetables with pathogens capable of causing enteric diseases. *British Food Journal* 108(1):38–53.

Bleasdale B, Lott PJ, Jagannathan A, Stevens MP, Birtles RJ, Wigley P. 2009. The salmonella pathogenicity island 2-encoded type III secretion system is essential for the survival of *Salmonella enterica* serovar Typhimurium in free-living amoebae. *Appl Environ Microbiol* 75(6):1793–1795.

Boirivant M, Strober W. 2007. The mechanism of action of probiotics. *Curr Opin Gastroenterol* 23(6):679–692.

Bottone EJ. 1999. *Yersinia enterocolitica*: Overview and epidemiologic correlates. *Microorganisms Infect* 1(4):323–333.

Bottone EJ. 1997. *Yersinia enterocolitica*: The charisma continues. *Clin Microbiol Rev* 10(2):257–276.

Brenner DJ, Farmer JJ III. 2005. Family I Enterobacteriaceae. In: *Bergey's manual of systematic bacteriology*. Vol. 2. Brenner DJ, Krieg NR, Staley JT, eds. New York, NY: Springer.

Brenner FW, Villar RG, Angulo FJ, Tauxe R, Swaminathan B. 2000. *Salmonella* nomenclature. *J Clin Microbiol* 38(7):2465–2467.

Brown P, McShane LM, Zanusso G, Detwile L. 2006. On the question of sporadic or atypical bovine spongiform encephalopathy and Creutzfeldt-Jakob disease. *Emerg Infect Dis* 12(12):1816–1821.

Buchanan RL. 1997. Identifying and controlling emerging foodborne pathogens: Research needs. *Emerg Infect Dis* 3(4):517–521.

Buck JW, Walcott RR, Beuchat LR. 2003, January 21. Recent trends in microbiological safety of fruits and vegetables. *Plant Health Progress*. doi:10.1094/PHP-2003-0121-01-RV.

Butzler JP. 2004. *Campylobacter*, from obscurity to celebrity. *Clin Microbiol Infect* 10(10):868–876.

Cassin MH, Lammerding AM, Todd FC, Ross W, McColl RS. 1998. Quantitative risk assessment for *Escherichia coli* O157:H7 in ground beef hamburgers. *Int J Food Microbiol* 41(1):21–44.

Centers for Disease Control and Prevention. 2009a. *Campylobacter jejuni* infection associated with unpasteurized milk and cheese—Kansas, 2007. *MMWR* 57(51):1377–1379.

Centers for Disease Control and Prevention. 2009b. *Clostridium perfringens* infection among inmates at a county jail—Wisconsin, August 2008. *MMWR* 58(6):138–141.

Centers for Disease Control and Prevention. 2009c. Multistate outbreak of *Salmonella* infections associated with peanut butter and peanut butter–containing products—United States, 2008–2009. *MMWR* 58(4):85–90.

Centers for Disease Control and Prevention. 2009d. Outbreak of *Salmonella* serotype Saintpaul infections associated with eating alfalfa sprouts—United States, 2009. *MMWR* 58(18):500–503.

Centers for Disease Control and Prevention. 2009e. Preliminary FoodNet data on the incidence of infection with pathogens transmitted commonly through food—10 states, 2008. *MMWR* 58(13):333–337.

Centers for Disease Control and Prevention. 2009f. Prevention of rotavirus gastroenteritis among infants and children: Recommendations of the advisory committee on immunization practices (ACIP). *MMWR Recomm Rep* 58(RR-2):1–25.

Centers for Disease Control and Prevention. 2009g. Surveillance for foodborne disease outbreaks—United States, 2006. *MMWR* 58(22):609–615.

Centers for Disease Control and Prevention. 2008. *Salmonella* surveillance: Annual summary, 2006. *MMWR Surveill Summ* 52(No. SS-6).

Centers for Disease Control and Prevention. 2006, November. *Shigella* surveillance: Annual summary, 2005. Atlanta, GA: U.S. Department of Health and Human Services.

Centers for Disease Control and Prevention. 2004a. Bovine spongiform encephalopathy in a dairy cow—Washington State, 2003. *MMWR* 52(53):1280–1285.

Centers for Disease Control and Prevention. 2004b. Creutzfeldt-Jakob disease not related to a common venue—New Jersey, 1995–2004. *MMWR* 53(18):392–396.

Centers for Disease Control and Prevention. 2004c. Outbreak of cyclosporiasis associated with snow peas—Pennsylvania, 2004. *MMWR* 53(37):876–878.

Centers for Disease Control and Prevention. 2004d. Trichinellosis associated with bear meat—New York and Tennessee, 2003. *MMWR* 53(27):606–610.

Centers for Disease Control and Prevention. 2003. Salmonella *surveillance summary, 2002.* Atlanta, GA: U.S. Department of Health and Human Services.

Centers for Disease Control and Prevention. 2002. Outbreaks of gastroenteritis associated with noroviruses on cruise ships—United States, 2002. *MMWR* 51(49):1112–1115.

Centers for Disease Control and Prevention. 2000. Preventing congenital toxoplasmosis. *MMWR Recomm Rep* 49(RR02):57–75.

Centers for Disease Control and Prevention. 1998. Outbreak of *Campylobacter* enteritis associated with cross-contamination of food—Oklahoma, 1996. *MMWR* 47(7):129–131.

Centers for Disease Control and Prevention. 1992. Locally acquired neurocysticercosis—North Carolina, Massachusetts, and South Carolina, 1989–1991. *MMWR* 41(1):1–4.

Centers for Disease Control and Prevention. 1990. Foodborne hepatitis A—Alaska, Florida, North Carolina, Washington. *MMWR* 39(14):228–232.

Chappell CL, Okhuysen PC, Sterling CR, DuPont HL. 1996. *Cryptosporidium parvum*: Intensity of infection and oocyst excretion patterns in healthy volunteers. *J Infect Dis* 173(1):232–236.

Chesebro B. 2003. Introduction to the transmissible spongiform encephalopathies or prion diseases. *Br Med Bull* 66:1–20.

Cox FE. 2002. History of human parasitology. *Clin Microbiol Rev* 15(4):595–612.

Daniels D, Grytdal S, Wasley A, Centers for Disease Control and Prevention. 2009. Surveillance for acute viral hepatitis—United States, 2007. *MMWR Surveill Summ* 58(3):1–27.

Dawson D. 2003, June. *Foodborne protozoan parasites.* Report prepared under the responsibility of the ILSI Europe Emerging Pathogen Task Force. Brussels: International Life Sciences Institute.

Donlan RM. 2002. Biofilms: Microbial life on surfaces. *Emerg Infect Dis* 8(9):881–890.

Donlan RM. 2001. Biofilm formation: A clinically relevant microbiological process. *Clin Infect Dis* 33(8):1387–1392.

Donlan RM, Costerton JW. 2002. Biofilms: Survival mechanisms of clinically relevant microorganisms. *Clin Microbiol Rev* 15(2):167–193.

Drevets DA, Bronze MS. 2008. *Listeria monocytogenes*: Epidemiology, human disease, and mechanisms of brain invasion. *FEMS Immunol Med Microbiol* 53(2):151–165.

DuPont HL, Chappell CL, Sterling CR, Okhuysen PC, Rose JB, Jakubowski W. 1995. The infectivity of *Cryptosporidium parvum* in healthy volunteers. *N Engl J Med* 332(13):855–859.

Farber JM, Peterkin PI. 1991. *Listeria monocytogenes*, a food-borne pathogen. *Microbiol Rev* 55(3):476–511.

Fayer R. 2004. *Sarcocystis* spp. in human infections. *Clin Microbiol Rev* 17(4):894,902, table of contents.

Fenicia L, Anniballi F. 2009. Infant botulism. *Ann Ist Super Sanita* 45(2):134–146.

Finlay BB, Falkow S. 1997. Common themes in microbial pathogenicity revisited. *Microbiol Mol Biol Rev* 61(2):136–169.

Fiore AE. 2004. Hepatitis A transmitted by food. *Clin Infect Dis* 38(5):705–715.

Food and Agriculture Organization of the United Nations/World Health Organization (FAO/WHO). 2008. Viruses in food: Scientific advice to support risk management activities. Report nr Microbiological Risk Assessment Series No. 13. Rome: Food and Agriculture Organization.

Food and Drug Administration/Center for Food Safety and Applied Nutrition, U.S. Department of Agriculture/Food Safety and Inspection Service, Centers for Disease Control and Prevention. 2003, September. *Quantitative assessment of relative risk to public health from foodborne* Listeria monocytogenes *among selected categories of ready-to-eat foods*. Silver Spring, MD: Food and Drug Administration, U.S. Department of Agriculture, Centers for Disease Control and Prevention.

Gandhi M, Chikindas ML. 2007. *Listeria*: A foodborne pathogen that knows how to survive. *Int J Food Microbiol* 113(1):1–15.

Griffith DC, Kelly-Hope LA, Miller MA. 2006. Review of reported cholera outbreaks worldwide, 1995–2005. *Am J Trop Med Hyg* 75(5):973–977.

Groisman EA, Casadesus J. 2005. The origin and evolution of human pathogens. *Mol Microbiol* 56(1):1–7.

Halliday ML, Kang LY, Zhou TK, Hu MD, Pan QC, Fu TY, Huang YS, Hu SL. 1991. An epidemic of hepatitis A attributable to the ingestion of raw clams in Shanghai, China. *J Infect Dis* 164(5):852–859.

Helman CG. 1981. Disease versus illness in general practice. *J R Coll Gen Pract* 31(230):548–552.

Hennessy TW, Hedberg CW, Slutsker L, White KE, Besser-Wiek JM, Moen ME, Feldman J, Coleman WW, Edmonson LM, MacDonald KL, et al. 1996. A national outbreak of *Salmonella enteritidis* infections from ice cream. The investigation team. *N Engl J Med* 334(20):1281–1286.

Heymann DL, ed. 2008. *Control of communicable diseases manual*. 19th ed. Washington, DC: American Public Health Association.

ICTVdB Management. 2006. 00.012.0.03. norovirus. In: *ICTVdB—the universal virus database*, version 4. Büchen-Osmond C, ed. New York, NY: Columbia University.

Institute of Medicine, Board on Global Health, Forum on Microbial Threats. 2006. *Addressing foodborne threats to health: Policies, practices, and global coordination, workshop summary*. Washington, DC: National Academy Press.

Janssen R, Krogfelt KA, Cawthraw SA, van Pelt W, Wagenaar JA, Owen RJ. 2008. Host-pathogen interactions in *Campylobacter* infections: The host perspective. *Clin Microbiol Rev* 21(3):505–518.

Johnson B. 2003. OSHA infectious dose white paper. *Applied Biosafety* 8(4):160–165.

Jones JA. 1999. International control of cholera: An environmental perspective to infectious disease control. *Indiana Law Journal* 74(3):1035–1088.

Jones TF. 2003. From pig to pacifier: Chitterling-associated yersiniosis outbreak among black infants. *Emerg Infect Dis* 9(8):1007–1009.

Kaper JB, Nataro JP, Mobley HL. 2004. Pathogenic *Escherichia coli*. *Nat Rev Microbiol* 2(2):123–140.

Kimura AC, Johnson K, Palumbo MS, Hopkins J, Boase JC, Reporter R, Goldoft M, Stefonek KR, Farrar JA, Van Gilder TJ, et al. 2004. Multistate shigellosis outbreak and commercially prepared food, United States. *Emerg Infect Dis* 10(6):1147–1149.

Konstantinidis KT, Ramette A, Tiedje JM. 2006, October 11. The bacterial species definition in the genomic era. *Phil Trans R Soc B* (361):1929–1940.

Koopmans M, Duizer E. 2002, September. *Foodborne viruses: An emerging problem*. Report prepared under the responsibility of the ILSI Europe Emerging Pathogen Task Force. Brussels: International Life Sciences Institute.

Laberge I, Griffiths MW, Griffiths MW. 1996. Prevalence, detection and control of *Cryptosporidium parvum* in food. *Int J Food Microbiol* 32(1–2):1–26.

Lamps LW. 2003. Pathology of food-borne infectious diseases of the gastrointestinal tract: An update. *Adv Anat Pathol* 10(6):319–327.

Lanata CF, Mendoza W, Black RF. 2002. *Improving diarrhoea estimates*. Geneva: World Health Organization.

Lederberg L, Shope RE, Oaks JSC, eds. 1992. *Emerging infections: Microbial threats to health in the United States.* Committee on Emerging Microbial Threats to Health, Institute of Medicine. Washington, DC: National Academy Press.

Lianou A, Sofos JN. 2007. A review of the incidence and transmission of *Listeria monocytogenes* in ready-to-eat products in retail and food service environments. *J Food Prot* 70(9):2172–2198.

Lindsay JA. 1997. Chronic sequelae of foodborne disease. *Emerg Infect Dis* 3(4):443–452.

Lu PL, Hwang IJ, Tung YL, Hwang SJ, Lin CL, Siu LK. 2004. Molecular and epidemiologic analysis of a county-wide outbreak caused by *Salmonella enterica* subsp. enterica serovar enteritidis traced to a bakery. *BMC Infect Dis* 4:48.

Lynch M, Painter J, Woodruff R, Braden C, Centers for Disease Control and Prevention. 2006. Surveillance for foodborne-disease outbreaks—United States, 1998–2002. *MMWR Surveill Summ* 55(10):1–42.

Magalhaes JG, Tattoli I, Girardin SE. 2007. The intestinal epithelial barrier: How to distinguish between the microbial flora and pathogens. *Semin Immunol* 19(2):106–115.

Mead PS, Finelli L, Lambert-Fair MA, Champ D, Townes J, Hutwagner L, Barrett T, Spitalny K, Mintz E. 1997. Risk factors for sporadic infection with *Escherichia coli* O157:H7. *Arch Intern Med* 157(2):204–208.

Mead PS, Slutsker L, Dietz V, McCaig LF, Bresee JS, Shapiro C, Griffin PM, Tauxe RV. 1999. Food-related illness and death in the United States. *Emerg Infect Dis* 5(5):607–625.

Molbak K, Olsen JE, Wegener HC. 2005. *Salmonella* infections. In: *Foodborne infections and intoxications.* 3rd ed. Rieman HP, Cliver DO, eds. Amsterdam: Academic Press.

Murphy C, Carroll C, Jordan KN. 2006. Environmental survival mechanisms of the foodborne pathogen *Campylobacter jejuni. J Appl Microbiol* 100(4):623–632.

Mushahwar IK. 2008. Hepatitis E virus: Molecular virology, clinical features, diagnosis, transmission, epidemiology, and prevention. *J Med Virol* 80(4):646–658.

Naimi TS, Wicklund JH, Olsen SJ, Krause G, Wells JG, Bartkus JM, Boxrud DJ, Sullivan M, Kassenborg H, Besser JM, et al. 2003. Concurrent outbreaks of *Shigella sonnei* and enterotoxigenic *Escherichia coli* infections associated with parsley: Implications for surveillance and control of foodborne illness. *J Food Prot* 66(4):535–541.

Navaneethan U, Giannella RA. 2008. Mechanisms of infectious diarrhea. *Nat Clin Pract Gastroenterol Hepatol* 5(11): 637–647.

O'Driscoll B, Gahan CG, Hill C. 1996. Adaptive acid tolerance response in *Listeria monocytogenes*: Isolation of an acid-tolerant mutant which demonstrates increased virulence. *Appl Environ Microbiol* 62(5):1693–1698.

Pace NR. 2008. The molecular tree of life changes how we see, teach microbial diversity. *Microorganism* 3(1):15–20.

Parashar U, Quiroz ES, Mounts AW, Monroe SS, Fankhauser RL, Ando T, Noel JS, Bulens SN, Beard SR, Li JF, et al. 2001. "Norwalk-like viruses". Public health consequences and outbreak management. *MMWR Recomm Rep* 50(RR-9):1–17.

Patrick ME, Adcock PM, Gomez TM, Altekruse SF, Holland BH, Tauxe RV, Swerdlow DL. 2004. *Salmonella enteritidis* infections, United States, 1985–1999. *Emerg Infect Dis* 10(1):1–7.

Petri WA Jr, Miller M, Binder HJ, Levine MM, Dillingham R, Guerrant RL. 2008. Enteric infections, diarrhea, and their impact on function and development. *J Clin Invest* 118(4):1277–1290.

Pizarro-Cerda J, Cossart P. 2006. Bacterial adhesion and entry into host cells. *Cell* 124(4):715–727.

Ramaswamy V, Cresence VM, Rejitha JS, Lekshmi MU, Dharsana KS, Prasad SP, Vijila HM. 2007. Listeria—review of epidemiology and pathogenesis. *J Microbiol Immunol Infect* 40(1):4–13.

Rees JR, Pannier MA, McNees A, Shallow S, Angulo FJ, Vugia DJ. 2004. Persistent diarrhea, arthritis, and other complications of enteric infections: A pilot survey based on California FoodNet surveillance, 1998–1999. *Clin Infect Dis* 38 Suppl 3:S311–317.

Roach RL, Sienko DG. 1992. *Clostridium perfringens* outbreak associated with minestrone soup. *Am J Epidemiol* 136(10):1288–1291.

Roy SL, Lopez AS, Schantz PM. 2003. Trichinellosis surveillance—United States, 1997–2001. *MMWR Surveill Summ* 52(6):1–8.

Ryan CA, Nickels MK, Hargrett-Bean NT, Potter ME, Endo T, Mayer L, Langkop CW, Gibson C, McDonald RC, Kenney RT. 1987. Massive outbreak of antimicrobial-resistant salmonellosis traced to pasteurized milk. *JAMA* 258(22): 3269–3274.

Saunders SE, Bartelt-Hunt SL, Bartz JC. 2008. Prions in the environment: Occurrence, fate and mitigation. *Prion* 2(4):162–169.

Schlenker C, Surawicz CM. 2009. Emerging infections of the gastrointestinal tract. *Best Pract Res Clin Gastroenterol* 23(1): 89–99.

Schmid-Hempel P, Frank SA. 2007. Pathogenesis, virulence, and infective dose. *PLoS Pathog* 3(10):1372–1373.

Scholz T, Garcia HH, Kuchta R, Wicht B. 2009. Update on the human broad tapeworm (genus *Diphyllobothrium*), including clinical relevance. *Clin Microbiol Rev* 22(1):60,146, table of contents.

Schroeder CM, Naugle AL, Schlosser WD, Hogue AT, Angulo FJ, Rose JS, Ebel ED, Disney WT, Holt KG, Goldman DP. 2005. Estimate of illnesses from *Salmonella enteritidis* in eggs, United States, 2000. *Emerg Infect Dis* 11(1):113–115.

Schulz HN, Jorgensen BB. 2001. Big bacteria. *Annu Rev Microbiol* 55:105–137.

Sianto L, Chame M, Silva CS, Goncalves ML, Reinhard K, Fugassa M, Araujo A. 2009. Animal helminths in human archaeological remains: A review of zoonoses in the past. *Rev Inst Med Trop Sao Paulo* 51(3):119–130.

Skerikova A, Brabec J, Kuchta R, Jimenez JA, Garcia HH, Scholz T. 2006. Is the human-infecting *Diphyllobothrium pacificum* a valid species or just a South American population of the holarctic fish broad tapeworm, *D. latum*? *Am J Trop Med Hyg* 75(2):307–310.

Skovgaard N. 2007. New trends in emerging pathogens. *Int J Food Microbiol* 120(3):217–224.

Smith JL, Bayles D. 2007. Postinfectious irritable bowel syndrome: A long-term consequence of bacterial gastroenteritis. *J Food Prot* 70(7):1762–1769.

Smolinski MS, Hamburg MA, Lederberg J, eds. 2003. *Microbial threats to health: Emergence, detection, and response.* Forum on Microbial Threats, Board on Global Health. Washington, DC: National Academy Press.

Stecher B, Hardt WD. 2008. The role of microbiota in infectious disease. *Trends Microbiol* 16(3):107–114.

Stenfors Arnesen LP, Fagerlund A, Granum PE. 2008. From soil to gut: *Bacillus cereus* and its food poisoning toxins. *FEMS Microbiol Rev* 32(4):579–606.

Stern NJ, Pretanik S. 2006. Counts of *Campylobacter* spp. on U.S. broiler carcasses. *J Food Prot* 69(5):1034–1039.

Tauxe RV. 2002. Emerging foodborne pathogens. *Int J Food Microbiol* 78(1–2):31–41.

Ternhag A, Torner A, Svensson A, Ekdahl K, Giesecke J. 2008. Short- and long-term effects of bacterial gastrointestinal infections. *Emerg Infect Dis* 14(1):143–148.

Teunis PF, Nagelkerke NJ, Haas CN. 1999. Dose response models for infectious gastroenteritis. *Risk Anal* 19(6):1251–1260.

Todd EC, Greig JD, Bartleson CA, Michaels BS. 2009. Outbreaks where food workers have been implicated in the spread of foodborne disease. Part 6. Transmission and survival of pathogens in the food processing and preparation environment. *J Food Prot* 72(1):202–219.

Todd EC, Greig JD, Bartleson CA, Michaels BS. 2008a. Outbreaks where food workers have been implicated in the spread of foodborne disease. Part 5. Sources of contamination and pathogen excretion from infected persons. *J Food Prot* 71(12):2582–2595.

Todd EC, Greig JD, Bartleson CA, Michaels BS. 2008b. Outbreaks where food workers have been implicated in the spread of foodborne disease. Part 4. Infective doses and pathogen carriage. *J Food Prot* 71(11):2339–2373.

Todd EC, Greig JD, Bartleson CA, Michaels BS. 2007a. Outbreaks where food workers have been implicated in the spread of foodborne disease. Part 3. Factors contributing to outbreaks and description of outbreak categories. *J Food Prot* 70(9):2199–2217.

Todd EC, Greig JD, Bartleson CA, Michaels BS. 2007b. Outbreaks where food workers have been implicated in the spread of foodborne disease. Part 2. Description of outbreaks by size, severity, and settings. *J Food Prot* 70(8):1975–1993.

Tompkin RB. 2002. Control of *Listeria monocytogenes* in the food-processing environment. *J Food Prot* 65(4):709–725.

Turcios RM, Widdowson MA, Sulka AC, Mead PS, Glass RI. 2006. Reevaluation of epidemiological criteria for identifying outbreaks of acute gastroenteritis due to norovirus: United States, 1998–2000. *Clin Infect Dis* 42(7):964–969.

Viswanathan VK, Hodges K, Hecht G. 2009. Enteric infection meets intestinal function: How bacterial pathogens cause diarrhoea. *Nat Rev Microbiol* 7(2):110–119.

Watts JC, Balachandran A, Westaway D. 2006. The expanding universe of prion diseases. *PLoS Pathog* 2(3):e26.

Wesley IV, Bhaduri S, Bush E. 2008. Prevalence of *Yersinia enterocolitica* in market weight hogs in the United States. *J Food Prot* 71(6):1162–1168.

Wharton M, Spiegel RA, Horan JM, Tauxe RV, Wells JG, Barg N, Herndon J, Meriwether RA, MacCormack JN, Levine RH. 1990. A large outbreak of antibiotic-resistant shigellosis at a mass gathering. *J Infect Dis* 162(6):1324–1328.

Wilhelmi I, Roman E, Sanchez-Fauquier A. 2003. Viruses causing gastroenteritis. *Clin Microbiol Infect* 9(4):247–262.

Wright WH, Kerr KB, Jacobs L. 1943. Studies on trichinosis, Xv. Summary of the findings of *Trichinella spiralis* in a random sampling and other samplings of the population of the United States. *Public Health Reports* 58(35):1293–1327.

Yang H, Mokhtari A, Jaykus LA, Morales RA, Cates SC, Cowen P. 2006. Consumer phase risk assessment for *Listeria monocytogenes* in deli meats. *Risk Anal* 26(1):89–103.

Yoder JS, Beach MJ, Centers for Disease Control and Prevention. 2007a. Cryptosporidiosis surveillance—United States, 2003–2005. *MMWR Surveill Summ* 56(7):1–10.

Yoder JS, Beach MJ, Centers for Disease Control and Prevention. 2007b. Giardiasis surveillance—United States, 2003–2005. *MMWR Surveill Summ* 56(7):11–18.

Young KT, Davis LM, Dirita VJ. 2007. *Campylobacter jejuni*: Molecular biology and pathogenesis. *Nat Rev Microbiol* 5(9):665–679.

Zilbauer M, Dorrell N, Wren BW, Bajaj-Elliott M. 2008. *Campylobacter jejuni*-mediated disease pathogenesis: An update. *Trans R Soc Trop Med Hyg* 102(2):123–129.

## USEFUL RESOURCES

*Bad Bug Book: Introduction Foodborne Pathogenic Microorganisms and Natural Toxins Handbook.* A concise and handy reference to foodborne pathogens and toxins. http://www.fda.gov/Food/FoodSafety/FoodborneIllness/FoodborneIllnessFoodbornePathogensNaturalToxins/BadBugBook/default.htm

Center for Science in the Public Interest, Outbreak Alert! Database. An interesting database of foodborne illness outbreaks compiled from multiple sources dating back to 1990. http://www.cspinet.org/foodsafety/outbreak/pathogen.php

Centers for Disease Control and Prevention sites:

- OutbreakNet Team. Links to Foodborne Illness A–Z, National Outbreak Reporting System (NORS), and Outbreak Surveillance Data, including by year and etiology. http://www.cdc.gov/outbreaknet/
- FoodNet Reports. Annual summaries of nine pathogens that are followed through an active surveillance system (FoodNet) involving participating states. http://www.cdc.gov/foodnet/reports.htm
- Enteric Diseases Epidemiology Branch homepage. http://www.cdc.gov/enterics/index.html
- National Surveillance Team—Enteric Diseases Epidemiology Branch. Links to National Antimicrobial Resistance Monitoring System for selected foodborne pathogens, and National Case Surveillance files for notifiable (and some other) foodborne pathogens. http://www.cdc.gov/nationalsurveillance/index.html
- Public Health Laboratory Information System, Division of Foodborne, Waterborne, and Environmental Diseases. Links to *Salmonella* and *Shigella* annual summaries. http://www.cdc.gov/ncidod/dbmd/phlisdata/d*efault.htm*
- Parasites A–Z Index, food-related parasites. http://www.cdc.gov/ncidod/dpd/food.htm
- Food Safety Office. Links to specific diseases/pathogens, foods and high-risk groups, and other resources. http://www.cdc.gov/foodsafety/
- *Morbidity and Mortality Weekly Report (MMWR).* Important publications on current (and past) disease outbreaks and trends, including foodborne diseases. http://www.cdc.gov/mmwr/
- OutbreakNet: Foodborne Outbreak Online Database. Search OutbreakNet by year, state, location, and etiology. http://wwwn.cdc.gov/foodborneoutbreaks/

Food Safety Network, Canada. Links to food risks and other information. http://www.foodsafetynetwork.ca/aspx/public/default.aspx

Food Safety Research and Response Network. Links to foodborne pathogen research projects and publications. http://www.fsrrn.net/

FoodSafety.org. Gateway to federal food safety information. http://www.foodsafety.gov/

Michigan Department of Agriculture, FPAdvisor (Food Pathogen Advisor). A searchable database used for training exercises that allow the user to enter disease symptoms, incubation periods, foods, and other information to derive a list suspected foodborne pathogens. http://www.mda.state.mi.us/FPAdvisor/FpadvisorHelp.htm

U.S. Department of Agriculture, National Agricultural Library, Food Safety Research Information Office, Pathogens and Contaminants. Pathogen and contaminant fact sheets and links to pathogen biology. http://fsrio.nal.usda.gov/path_contam.php

World Health Organization, Food Safety. Links to microbial risks and foodborne disease. http://www.who.int/foodsafety/en/

CHAPTER **3**

# Foodborne Toxic and Physical Agents

## LEARNING OBJECTIVES

1. Describe and define the major categories and sources of toxicants in foods.
2. Define the terms *toxicants, toxins, poisons, poisoning, toxic effects,* and *intoxication.*
3. Explain the dose-response concept of toxicity and why it is important in food toxicology.
4. List the factors that determine the target organs and the type of effects from toxic agents in foods.
5. Compare and contrast the different scenarios of acute and chronic exposures and effects.
6. List the major types of bacterial toxins in foods, and distinguish the major differences between the toxins.
7. Recognize the most common mycotoxins and whether their major toxic effects are acute and/or chronic.
8. Explain how algal toxins enter the human food chain, and list the major types of syndromes caused by algal toxins and the associated foods.
9. Describe the relevance and significance of plant and animal toxins in terms of the human food chain and health risks.
10. List the major sources, types, and pathways of environmental chemicals that contaminate the human food chain.
11. Discuss the sources and explain the risks of pesticides and veterinary drugs in the human food chain.
12. Explain the difference between food additives and adulterants and give examples of how they may affect human health.
13. Identify the types and sources of toxic substances encountered during food processing, packaging, storage, and preparation.
14. Distinguish the differences between food allergies and food intolerance, and explain their relevance to food safety.
15. Identify the major sources of radionuclides in the environment, and rank their importance in terms of likelihood to contaminate the human food chain.
16. Explain the relevance of foreign objects in foods in terms of safety and aesthetics.

## BASIC FOOD TOXICOLOGY

Chapter 1 introduces *food poisoning* as a colloquial term used to describe foodborne illnesses, whether from infection or intoxication. In the context of chemicals, *poisoning* often implies intentional harm or misuse of a chemical substance that results in harm. Furthermore, a poison or poisonous substance has connotations of causing death or being used in homicide or suicide cases (Hodgson 2004). Various legal documents define poisons more precisely, but most authorities generally consider a poison to be an exceptionally toxic substance. To avoid biases and perceptions associated with the term *poison*, and because most substances have a wide range of possible toxic effects, toxicologists prefer the overarching term toxicant rather than poison. Therefore, this book uses the term *poison* sparingly in this and subsequent chapters, and when used, it shall be in the most commonly accepted context.

Toxicants are often categorized on the basis of different perspectives. These include exposure classes (air, water, food, occupational, etc.), usage classes (solvents, drugs, pesticides, etc.), chemical categories (organic, inorganic, metals, etc.), toxic responses or effects (neurotoxic, hepatotoxic, etc.), and so forth. Within the realm of food safety and toxicology, a convenient categorization of toxicants is by their origin. Figure 3-1 is a Venn diagram that illustrates the categories and sources of toxicants frequently encountered in foods. Toxins are subcategories of toxicants produced naturally from biological sources. And although many food additives and veterinary medications are also derived from biological sources, these substances are refined and used for specific purposes in

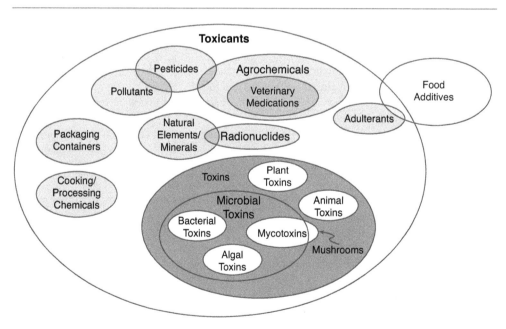

**Figure 3-1** Categories and Sources of Toxicants in Foods

the human food chain. The categories of toxicants presented in Figure 3-1 are the basis for an introduction to food toxicology.

The type and degree of adverse effects from toxicants depend on many factors. In experimental toxicology, the adverse effects are designated as toxic endpoints, whereas epidemiologists who study adverse effects in human populations refer to them as health outcomes. Table 3-1 lists common endpoints and health outcomes used in toxicological experiments and epidemiologic studies. Nearly all toxicants are capable of causing multiple adverse effects, but most toxicants have a predilection to harm specific target organs. Among the factors that influence determination of a target organ are the toxicant's route of exposure, chemical structure, dose, and its distribution throughout the body and metabolic fate. With regard to route of exposure, the most common and greatest concern for food safety is the ingestion route. As for chemical structures of toxicants in foods, they are diverse and range from simple salts to complex, heterocyclic ring structures. The dose of toxicants depends on the concentration of toxicant in the food and the amount of food consumed. Because the concept of dose is very important to understanding the toxicology of foods, it must be explored more fully.

## Dose-Response Relationships

One of the most important premises of toxicology is the dose-response relationship of a toxicant. Essentially, this premise states that the toxicity (i.e., response) of a substance increases with increasing dose. The dose-response relationship of a toxic substance is experimentally measured using responses for a particular endpoint and groups of animals administered different doses of the substance. In quantitative terms, the dose is the amount of substance administered over a specified period of time, while the response for a toxic endpoint is measured as values that are either discrete (i.e., absent or present, such as mortality, or categorical) or continuous (i.e., uninterrupted range of values, such as body weight or enzyme levels). When the response rates or values are plotted against the administered dose, a dose-response curve such as the one shown in Figure 3-2 can be drawn. For different toxicant and endpoint combinations, dose-response curves

**Table 3-1** Common Endpoints and Health Outcomes in Toxicology

| Experimental Endpoints | Health Outcomes |
|---|---|
| Lethality | Death |
| Carcinogenesis and mutagenesis | Cancer and mutations |
| Reproduction and teratogenesis | Birth defects, reproductive health |
| Neurobehavioral effects | Neuropathy, behavior, etc. |
| Organ system dysfunction | Gastro, hepatic, renal, pulmonary, etc. |
| — Gastrointestinal | — Gastroenteritis |
| — Liver, kidney, lungs, etc. | — Organ impairment/failure |
| Immunologic effects | Allergic reactions, immunodeficiency |
| Endocrine disruption | Hormone-related outcomes |

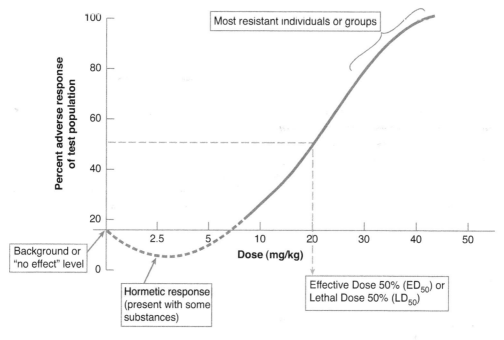

**Figure 3-2**  Idealized Dose-Response Curve

will vary in position and slope along the axes. These variations are related to the type of measured effects and responses, the sensitivity or susceptibility of the animal to the toxicant, the toxicant's potency and specificity, and the rates of toxicant metabolism and elimination. Potent toxicants, for example, have a curve positioned farther to the left, indicating a lesser dose is needed to cause the same level of response. Highly specific toxicants (i.e., those that bind to specific targets) have a steeper slope in the linear portion of the curve, indicating that very little additional dose is needed to increase the level of response.

A historically important indicator of relative lethality for a toxicant is the lethal dose 50 ($LD_{50}$). This is the dose at which an estimated 50% of the test animal population (usually rats) experience fatal effects, indicated by the dotted line in Figure 3-2. This measure of lethality is used less often today because of problematic issues with differences in laboratory methods and interspecies responses. The primary value of the $LD_{50}$ is to compare relative lethality of several toxicants. When nonlethal endpoints are measured, the effective dose 50 ($EF_{50}$) is used as an indicator of relative toxicity. This is the dose at which an estimated 50% of the test animal population experiences a predetermined effect (nonlethal). For both lethal and nonlethal endpoints, the more sensitive individuals experience effects at the lower doses on the dose-response curve, while the most resistant individuals experience the same effects at higher doses.

Virtually any substance can be toxic with too much dose. Many substances confer protection or health benefits at lower doses but become toxic with increasing doses. For example, certain nutrients such as vitamin A are essential to health, and a deficiency of vitamin A can lead to blindness, maternal mortality, and immunodeficiency. On the other hand, excessive amounts of vitamin A are toxic, either acutely or chronically depending on the dose rate, that is, the number and quantity of doses over a period of time. Acute vitamin A toxicity includes signs and symptoms such as nausea, fatigue, headache, and dizziness. Chronic vitamin A toxicity can result in birth defects, liver damage, and/or central nervous system effects. Fortunately, vitamin A toxicity is rare and most likely occurs from using vitamin supplements and/or excessive consumption of animal livers containing high levels of vitamin A (Hathcock et al. 1990). The beneficial response of a toxic substance at low doses is referred to as hormesis, illustrated by the dip in the curve of Figure 3-2.

Besides the toxicant's chemical structure and the dose, other factors also influence determination of the target organ and the types and degree of adverse effects. A useful acronym can be borrowed from the pharmaceutical industry to describe these other factors: ADME (absorption-distribution-metabolism-elimination). Each of these factors is briefly described in the following subsections.

### Absorption

After a toxicant is ingested from contaminated food, it must be absorbed by the mucosal epithelium of the gastrointestinal tract. Otherwise, the toxicant will pass through the gut without significant adverse effects. Most toxicant absorption by the gastrointestinal tract takes place in the small intestine and, to a lesser extent, the stomach. The large intestine is specialized for the absorption of water and does not generally absorb toxicants. The reasons for significant toxicant absorption in the small intestine include a relatively higher pH (~6), a larger surface area with the presence of villi and microvilli, and easy passive diffusion across the cell membranes for most toxicants. With toxicants that are structurally similar to nutrients, the mechanism of transport across cell membranes is active transport. Larger toxicants, particularly carcinogens and some toxins, are transported across the cell membranes through endocytosis or exocytosis. Resident bacteria in the gut (i.e., microbiota) also influence toxicant absorption by metabolizing the toxicants, which changes their chemical structure. The change of a chemical's structure through metabolic processes, whether from a microbe or human, is called biotransformation. Depending on the chemical reactions involved, the biotransformation of toxicants can make them more or less readily absorbed in the small intestine.

A unique phenomenon exists that maintains some toxicants between the small intestine and liver, called enterohepatic circulation. This phenomenon occurs when a toxicant is absorbed by the intestine and transported to the liver by the hepatic vein. Once in the liver, the toxicant can be biotransformed and secreted with bile back into the gastrointestinal tract. The toxicant can then be reabsorbed by the small intestine and again transported back to the liver. This cycle can occur many times, which prolongs the residence time of the toxicant in the intestine, liver, and systemic circulation. The result is continuous or repeated dosing of organs with the toxicant and its metabolites.

### Distribution

For enterotoxic substances, the toxicants only need to be absorbed locally by the gastrointestinal tract. However, toxicants may also be absorbed locally and enter the circulatory system, where they may be distributed to other parts of the body. The ability of a toxicant to be absorbed through the cell membranes and enter the circulatory system is called its bioavailability. The distribution of bioavailable toxicants is influenced by the physiology and anatomy of the organ systems and by the toxicant's physiochemical properties. Organs with significant tissue mass and perfusion of blood (e.g., the liver) can have a high distribution of toxicants in a relatively short period of time. Conversely, fat and bone tissue generally have a lower distribution of toxicants shortly after exposure, but certain toxicants may accumulate in these tissues over extended periods of exposure and time.

Physiochemical properties of a toxicant important to distribution are its molecular weight and structure, lipid solubility, and ionic equilibrium (measured as pKa). These properties influence the toxicant's ability to circulate in the bloodstream and also to cross cell membranes of distant tissues and organs. Highly lipophilic toxicants have a greater tendency to cross cell membranes, and they preferentially accumulate in adipose tissues. Neurotoxicants have properties that permit them to cross highly selective membranes such as the blood–brain barrier. Other toxicants have properties that permit them to bind to specific molecular targets in organs such as the liver and kidneys.

The study and characterization of toxicant distribution in the body is called toxicokinetics. The pharmaceutical industry uses the term pharmacokinetics to describe the distribution of drugs and medications.

## Metabolism

All living organisms can modify substances through their metabolism. Along with metabolic pathways that perform life-sustaining functions such as respiration, organisms also have metabolic pathways adapted to the modification of toxic substances, usually rendering the substances less toxic and more easily eliminated from the organism. The toxic substances that are biochemically modified may be natural by-products of metabolism, or they may be completely foreign to life processes, in which case the toxicants (and medications) are called xenobiotics. The metabolism of xenobiotics is called biotransformation and is traditionally classified into phase I and phase II reactions. Whereas both phases of reactions may occur in tissues throughout the human body, the liver plays the greatest role in using these reactions to detoxify xenobiotics.

The metabolism of xenobiotics involves many enzymes and complex biochemical pathways. In general, phase I reactions add a functional group to the xenobiotic. This typically involves oxidation, reduction, or hydrolysis and makes the xenobiotic compound more amenable to phase II reactions. During phase II reactions, conjugation of the xenobiotic occurs with an endogenous molecule. The resulting conjugate is more water soluble and, thus, more excretable. Several key points should be remembered with regard to xenobiotic metabolism:

- Although most xenobiotics are detoxified during phase I and phase II reactions, these reactions often produce a great number of intermediates and other metabolites, and sometimes the reaction products are more toxic than the original xenobiotic is. This is call bioactivation of a toxicant and is common with many carcinogens.
- A significant difference can exist in the metabolism of xenobiotics between species and among different individuals within the same species. As a consequence of these metabolic

differences, the toxicity may also be different in terms of both type and degree of responses. Within a species, individual responses can vary with different stages of development and life (e.g., embryonic development to senior aging), nutritional status, physiologic stresses, and genetic susceptibility or resistance.

• Many of the enzymes involved in xenobiotic metabolism are inducible. In other words, the toxicant initiates gene induction or increases the rate of induction for genes that encode certain enzymes (i.e., proteins). An increase in the levels of enzymes involved with toxicant metabolism can lead to rapid detoxification and individual tolerance. This is different from population resistance, where the population has genetically changed over generations by selection pressures from toxicants. An example of the former is an individual who requires larger doses of a toxicant (or drug) to get the same effect that was previously experienced. An example of the latter is an insect population that has developed resistance to a commonly used pesticide.

## Elimination

The elimination of toxicants from an organism is essential to homeostasis and survival. The major routes of elimination for animals and humans are through defecation, urination, and exhalation. Minor routes of elimination include the skin, sweat, lactation, and hair. Absorbed toxicants must be transported to the liver, kidneys, and lungs for excretion through the major routes of elimination. The biotransformation of toxicants usually permits them to be more easily transported via the bloodstream and to diffuse or be transported across cell membranes into the excretory organs. Once inside the excretory organs, the toxicants may be further modified to facilitate excretion.

If a toxicant's rate of elimination is less than its rate of absorption, then it is possible for bioaccumulation of the toxicant in the organism. This phenomenon is common with toxicants that are sequestered within the organism. In toxicokinetics, sequestration refers to the storage of toxicants in inert tissues such as fat, bone, nails, and hair in animals, or the bark and leaves of plants. This is different from the bioaccumulation of toxicants across trophic levels of a food chain, referred to as biomagnification. The bioaccumulation and biomagnification of toxicants are very important concepts in food toxicology, particularly with respect to toxicants in seafood.

## Acute vs. Chronic Exposures and Effects

The exposure to toxicants in foods varies from acute to chronic. Similarly, the adverse effects from toxicant exposures can range from acute to chronic. Textbooks and other authoritative sources give several different definitions for acute and chronic exposures. For the purposes of this book, the definitions by the Environmental Protection Agency (EPA) and International Union of Pure and Applied Chemistry (IUPAC) are used (EPA 1997; U.S. National Library of Medicine 2005). Table 3-2 summarizes the types of exposures and effects commonly encountered in toxicology. Note that some exposures may be considered subchronic (or subacute), and other effects may be latent or delayed.

Although it is reasonable to assume that chronic exposures are followed by chronic effects, this is not always the rule. In some cases, a chronic exposure may need to reach a certain absorbed

**Table 3-2** Terms and Definitions for Acute and Chronic Exposures/Effects

| Term | Definition[a] |
|---|---|
| **Acute exposure** | A single exposure to a toxic substance which may result in severe biological harm or death. Acute exposures are usually characterized as lasting no longer than a day, as compared to longer, continuing exposure over a period of time. (EPA) |
| **Acute effect** | An adverse effect on any living organism which results in severe symptoms that develop rapidly; symptoms often subside after the exposure stops. (EPA) |
| **Chronic exposure** | Multiple exposures occurring over an extended period of time or over a significant fraction of an animal's or human's lifetime (usually 7 years to a lifetime). (EPA) |
| **Chronic effect** | An adverse effect on a human or animal in which symptoms recur frequently or develop slowly over a long period of time. (EPA) |
| **Subchronic exposure** | Multiple or continuous exposures lasting for approximately 10% of an experimental species lifetime, usually over a 3-month period. (EPA) |
| **Latent period** | 1. Delay between exposure to a harmful substance and the manifestations of a disease or other adverse effects. <br><br> 2. Period from disease initiation to disease detection. (IUPAC) |
| **Latent/delayed effect** | Consequence occurring after a latent period following the end of exposure to a toxic substance or other harmful environmental factor. (IUPAC) |

[a] Definitions from the Environmental Protection Agency (EPA 1997) and International Union of Pure and Applied Chemistry (IUPAC 2005), as indicated in parentheses.

dose or threshold level before an effect occurs, and then it could be manifested as an acute effect. In other cases, effects can be manifested a period of time after the exposure ceases, that is, they are latent effects. An example of a latent effect is the induction of cancer that may take years to become clinically recognizable. The latency period of toxic agents is analogous to the incubation period of an infectious agent. Figure 3-3 illustrates the different exposure and effect scenarios that are possible (LeBlanc 2004). In epidemiologic studies, the establishment of causation by a particular agent is more easily done in the scenario where the acute effects follow the acute exposure. The establishment of causation is more difficult with the longer timelines depicted in Figure 3-3. The reasons include exposures to other agents over time that may be fully or partly responsible for the health outcome; accountability of all exposures to multiple agents over years of time is very difficult if not impossible. Another reason is related to confounding variables or factors (also called confounders and lurking variables). These are factors that statistically correlate with other exposure and effect factors but that are not causally related to the health outcome.

## MICROBIAL TOXINS

The fact that microorganisms produce toxins is introduced in Chapter 2 in the discussion of foodborne infections. In this chapter, the discussion focuses on the production of microbial toxins in foods rather than those produced *in vivo* during the infection process. Preformed microbial

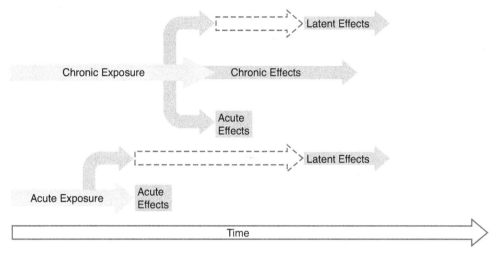

**Figure 3-3** Toxic Exposure and Effects Scenarios. *Source:* Adapted from LeBlanc, 2005.

toxins in foods are toxic agents that conform to the principles of toxicology previously introduced. But unlike synthetic toxicants that may contaminate foods, microbial toxins can increase in quantity (and hence dose) as the responsible microorganisms continue to grow in the foods.

Foodborne intoxications by microbes are caused by the consumption of food with a sufficiently high dose of microbial toxins to produce acute effects. Nearly all reported outbreaks of foodborne illnesses caused by microbial toxins are acute. However, it is well established through experimental research and epidemiologic studies that some microbial toxins, especially certain mycotoxins, can cause chronic diseases such as cancer. Some microbial toxins may also cause both acute and chronic diseases, depending on the dose. By controlling microbial growth in foods, the production of toxins is also limited. This is an important concept in the prevention of foodborne intoxications.

## Bacterial Toxins

### *Staphylococcal Enterotoxins*

Foodborne intoxications from the staphylococcal enterotoxins are common throughout the world. Among the more than 30 species of staphylococci, the one most commonly associated with foodborne outbreaks and intoxications is *Staphylococcus aureus*, though several of the other staphylococci also produce enterotoxins. For historical reasons related to laboratory methods, the other enterotoxin-producing staphylococci have not been adequately studied, and their relative contribution to foodborne intoxications is probably underestimated. Regardless of the species or strain, staphylococcal enterotoxins are recognized as a major cause of foodborne disease. During the 1960s and 1970s, they were a leading cause of foodborne illness in the United States, but the reported number of cases and outbreaks decreased by the late 1980s (Bergdoll and Wong 2006). Several reasons were believed responsible for this trend; among them was better attention to sanitation and temperature controls by the food industry, thereby reducing the incidence of large outbreaks that were associated with commercial sources. Smaller outbreaks and sporadic cases are still very common in noncommercial settings, such as picnics and family meals, but because the intoxication can be relatively mild with a short duration (1–2 days), most cases likely are not reported.

Although intoxication by staphylococcal enterotoxins is considered relatively mild by clinical standards, anyone who has experienced the disease will not forget it. The severity of symptoms varies with the dose of enterotoxins, but the onset of vomiting is generally abrupt and violent, with retching, cramps, and prostration. Diarrhea is also common along with lowered blood pressure. In many cases, the dizziness and vertigo are temporarily disabling. Although death is rare, severe cases may last several days, often leading to hospitalization in an attempt to make a diagnosis (Heymann 2008). During the disease, the individual is essentially incapacitated, which is dangerous if operating machinery or piloting an aircraft. For this reason, some staphylococcal enterotoxins are regarded as potential biological warfare or bioterrorist agents (Ecker et al. 2005).

As a result of research interests and scientific publications, the number of staphylococcal enterotoxins identified has continued to grow over the years. At least 19 different staphylococcal enterotoxins have been identified to date (Thomas et al. 2007). As they were discovered, the enterotoxins were designated with successive letters of the alphabet. For many years, staphylococcal enterotoxins A (SEA) and D (SED) were the ones most frequently associated with foodborne illness outbreaks (Balaban and Rasooly 2000; Jay, Loessner, Golden 2005). It has been suggested, however, that newly identified staphylococcal enterotoxins may be overlooked in outbreaks because of poor quantitative assessments of incriminated foods (Le Loir, Baron, Gautier 2003). The clinical severity of disease and effective dose can also vary with different staphylococcal enterotoxins. An effective dose of some staphylococcal enterotoxins can be as low as 200 nanograms (Balaban and Rasooly 2000).

Staphylococcal enteroxotins are considered to be superantigens: They interact with T cells and antigen-presenting cells (APC) in a manner that causes excessive proliferation of T cells and massive secretion of cytokines, the signaling molecules of the immune system. The result is a hyperimmune response that can lead to severe inflammation, organ failure, and/or toxic shock syndrome. Whereas the superantigenic activity of ingested staphylococcal enterotoxins contributes to gastroenteritis, the greatest clinical concern with superantigenic activity is from wound infections by *S. aureus*—not foodborne intoxications. The primary symptom of emesis (vomiting) is believed to be a distinctly separate activity of the staphylococcal enterotoxins (Le Loir et al. 2003). In fact, the emetic activity may limit biological damage from superantigen activity by rapidly eliminating the staphylococcal enterotoxins from the gastrointestinal tract.

Staphylococcal enterotoxins are small proteins that are soluble in water. They are resistant to proteolytic enzymes and can withstand boiling temperatures for as long as 30 minutes (Le Loir 2003). These characteristics are challenging to food safety because killing the staphylococci after the production of enterotoxins does not eliminate the hazard. Therefore, a two-pronged prevention strategy is necessary: (1) minimize the contamination of food with staphylococci, and/or destroy them before enterotoxin production; and (2) inhibit the growth of staphylococci and/or toxin production. Because animals and humans are primary reservoirs of *Staphylococcal* species, they are virtually everywhere. An estimated one-third of Americans have *S. aureus* colonized in their nasal passages (Kuehnert et al. 2006), suggesting human contact is an important source of food contamination. Compared with other bacteria, *S. aureus* also has a relatively high tolerance to salt and pH ranges. Fortunately, *S. aureus* is easily destroyed with heat treatment processes, and with regard to growth parameters, the optimum production of enterotoxins has a more restricted range.

Foodborne illness outbreaks from staphylococcal enterotoxins involve a wide variety of protein-based foods that provide a good growth medium for staphylococci. Foods such as meats, fish, casseroles, sandwiches, and dishes with eggs or other protein ingredients are common sources of intoxication. Food contamination with *S. aureus* is frequently from food workers that carry the bacterium in their nasal passages or who have acne, infected cuts, or sores (Todd et al. 2007). Secondary or cross-contamination in food preparation areas is also common. Initial food contamination with *S. aureus* is usually followed by poor temperature controls that permit the bacteria to grow and produce enterotoxins. Generally, sufficient production of enterotoxins is suspected with a population of *S. aureus* around $10^5$ CFUs/gram of food (Heymann 2008).

### Botulinum Toxins

Chapter 2 briefly introduces the various clinical syndromes of botulism. This chapter emphasizes the ingestion of preformed botulinum toxins in foods—not toxicoinfections. Botulinum toxins are the most potent neurotoxins known to humans. From historical accounts, botulism outbreaks have occurred in human civilizations for centuries, most notably as "sausage poisoning" in Europe during the seventeenth and eighteenth centuries (*botulus* is Latin for sausage). During the twentieth century, a total of seven botulinum toxins were discovered (designated A to G), each produced by different strains of *Clostridium botulinum*. Fortunately, this knowledge about botulinum toxins led to tougher food safety standards to control them, decreasing the incidence of botulism cases and outbreaks greatly over the twentieth century. Nevertheless, considering the potent and often lethal effects of botulinum toxins, they rightly remain high on the list of food safety priorities.

Not all botulinum toxins affect humans. Only four types (A, B, E, and F) are associated with toxicity in humans, with type A being the most lethal. After absorption of the botulinum toxins, the initial signs and symptoms typically include nausea, vomiting, and diarrhea. These usually occur 12–36 hours after consuming the contaminated food. The toxins are also transported via the bloodstream to the motor neurons of the peripheral nervous system (PNS), where they enter the neurons and interfere with the release of neurotransmitters. The clinical result is the development of neurological symptoms such as muscle weakness, blurred vision, difficulty speaking, and other symptoms. Progression of toxicity can lead to flaccid paralysis and paralysis of the diaphragm and respiratory muscles, causing respiratory failure. Even with advanced medical care, the case-fatality rate of foodborne botulism can reach 5–10% in the United States, and the recovery of those affected can take months (Heymann 2008). The case-fatality rate among untreated cases can reach 60–70% (Sobel 2005).

The bacteria that produce botulinum toxins, principally *C. botulinum*, are spore-formers found in the soil and marine sediments. As such, the spores are virtually unavoidable in all agricultural products (including plants and animals) and fish or anywhere dirt or dust can be deposited. Like other bacterial endospores, they are hardy and can withstand high temperatures and harsh environmental conditions. However, to produce botulinum toxins, the spores must germinate and grow under specific, suitable conditions. In the case of *C. botulinum*, these conditions include the appropriate anaerobic environment, activating temperature, incubation temperature, moisture and nutrient content, and pH. More specific details about these conditions are discussed later in Chapter 4. From epidemiologic investigations, however, the foods most often involved are either canned, wrapped, or stored in a manner that creates anaerobic conditions; they are held at moderate or unrefrigerated (shelf) temperatures; and they have a pH above 4.6. Nearly all (92%) of botulism events (single cases or outbreaks) in modern U.S. history have been associated with home-processed foods, mostly home canning, while only a small portion (8%) were associated with commercially processed foods (Centers for Disease Control and Prevention [CDC] 2001). Among the commercial products responsible for botulism outbreaks are salted or fermented white fish; jars of garlic packed in oil; potato-based and eggplant-based dips; canned tuna, liver paste, vichyssoise, beef stew, and hotdog chili; and carrot juice (Angulo et al. 1998; CDC 2007a, 2007b, 2006a).

The single most important preventive measure for botulism is the proper canning of foods. During the canning process of low-acid foods, the temperature must be sufficiently raised (110°–121°C) to destroy any Clostridia spores, and the canned product must maintain its integrity to prevent recontamination with spores. Most commercial canning operations follow strict guidelines and quality control measures to ensure that canned products are free of viable spores that could germinate and produce botulinum toxins. Although voluntary food recalls are issued whenever certain lots of cans were not properly processed, the retort canning process has rarely resulted in botulism outbreaks. In the United States between 1950 and 2007, only five botulism outbreaks were attributed to deficiencies in the commercial canning process (CDC 2007a). Considering the disease severity of botulism and number of cases possible from an outbreak with commercially canned products, any deficiency in the retort canning process must be promptly identified and immediately corrected.

As stated previously, most foodborne botulism outbreaks are associated with home-processed foods. Improper home canning of foods is the greatest culprit, but any food processing technique that creates ideal conditions for the survival, germination, and growth of *C. botulinum* is a potential source of botulinum toxins. Sometimes, the combination of modern and traditional food processing techniques proves to be hazardous. For example, Alaskan Natives have a long tradition of fermenting foods for weeks or months using grass-lined holes or barrels in the ground. The introduction of modern conveniences such as jars and plastic wraps spurred innovation by sealing the foods and allowing them to ferment above ground. This modification of food processing created an anaerobic environment at warmer temperatures, a condition conducive to the germination and growth of *C. botulinum*, and hence the production of toxins. As a consequence of these practices, Alaska had the highest incidence of foodborne botulism in the United States, and among the highest in regions of the world (CDC 2001).

The potency and lethality of botulinum toxins make them potential weapons for biological warfare and terrorism (Madsen 2001). The neurotoxin can cause botulism through the inhalation of aerosols, injection, or ingestion. The intentional contamination of foods with botulinum toxins is a threat that warrants safeguarding against (Wein and Liu 2005). Fortunately, in contrast to staphylococcal enterotoxins, and unlike the spores of *C. botulinum*, the botulinum toxins can be destroyed by cooking temperatures (80°C/176°F for 10 minutes, or boiling for a few minutes). Thus, as a last line of defense, the thorough heating of food products prior to consumption can reduce the risk of botulism.

## Other Preformed Bacterial Toxins

### *Bacillus cereus* Enterotoxin

The foodborne illnesses caused by *Bacillus cereus* were introduced in Chapter 2. Two types of illness syndromes have been identified: (1) diarrheal syndrome, caused by a toxicoinfection; and (2) emetic syndrome, caused by preformed toxin in food. The epidemiology of *B. cereus* illnesses and the diarrheal syndrome are sufficiently covered in the previous chapter. This section briefly discusses the toxin responsible for the emetic syndrome.

The emetic syndrome is caused by a preformed toxin recently discovered and named cereulide (Agata et al. 1995). Recognition that cereulide causes intoxication is most evident by the short incubation/latency period, usually within 0.5 to 6 hours following consumption. The mechanisms of emesis by cereulide have not been conclusively determined and need further study (Stenfors Arneson, Fagerlund, Granum 2008). Different strains of *B. cereus* may produce different levels of cereulide. The production of cereulide in foods by *B. cereus* strains takes place from 12°C/53.6°F to 37°C/98.6°F, but the level of production also varies with the type of food. A variety of foods has been associated with the emetic syndrome caused by cereulide, but the most commonly reported foods are rice dishes (Schoeni and Wong 2005). Cereulide is heat stable and usually is not destroyed by reheating foods that have been stored at room temperatures.

### Bacterial-Produced Histamines (Scombroid Fish Poisoning)

A very common type of seafood-related illness is called scombroid fish poisoning. This foodborne intoxication is caused by histamine and other amines that are produced when marine bacteria metabolize histidine (an amino acid) in the muscle of fish. The term *scombroid* originated from the *Scombridae* family of fish because these fish have high levels of histidine in their muscles and are historically associated with the intoxication. Scombroid fish are deep-seas species such as tuna, bonita, and mackerel. These fish are most commonly implicated in scombroid fish poisoning, but other nonscombroid fish such as mahi mahi, bluefish, amberjack, abalone, and sardines have also been responsible for outbreaks (CDC 2007c). From 1998 to 2002, there were 168 outbreaks of scombroid intoxication reported to the CDC (Sobel and Painter 2005).

The onset of symptoms from scombroid intoxication is very rapid (almost instantaneous) and somewhat similar to an allergic-type response, though it is actually a toxic response to the histamine-like compounds. The cluster of symptoms may include rashes, flushing, sweating, dizziness, nausea, diarrhea, swelling and burning of the mouth, and a metallic taste (Brett 2003). The intoxication usually resolves itself within 24 hours, but severe cases may need antihistamine treatment at emergency rooms. Misdiagnosis of the intoxication is not uncommon, and sometimes concurrent allergies can complicate the condition and diagnosis.

The marine bacteria responsible for producing the histamine-like compounds proliferate after the fish is caught and allowed to remain at temperatures greater than 45°F/7.2°C for several hours (CDC 2007c). The toxic compounds cannot be sensed (i.e., by taste or smell), and cooking or freezing the fish does not destroy them. Prompt refrigeration at 40°F/4.4°C or lower temperatures from the time of catch until consumption is the best method of prevention. This limits the growth of bacteria and the conversion of histidine to histamine.

## Mycotoxins

### *Mycotoxins from Molds*

The term mycotoxin is used primarily to describe various toxins produced by molds (filamentous fungi), though it can also be used for toxins produced by yeasts and mushrooms. Mycotoxins are considered to be secondary metabolites, which are metabolic by-products that have no apparent purpose in the growth and development of fungi. Between 300 and 400 compounds are identified as mycotoxins, but only about a dozen groups of them receive regular attention for their toxicity to humans and animals (Bennett and Klich 2003). They are diverse in chemical structure and may originate from a variety of fungal species and biosynthetic pathways. The biological responses to mycotoxins include a myriad of toxic endpoints or health outcomes. All of the aforementioned characteristics make the classification of mycotoxins extremely difficult. Often, mycotoxins are classified by different perspectives of the professionals involved (clinicians, toxicologists, biochemists, organic chemists, etc.). Table 3-3 lists some major mycotoxins along with their sources and toxic effects.

The latency period of adverse effects from mycotoxins may range from acute to chronic. The diseases caused by exposure to mycotoxins are collectively called mycotoxicoses and include afflictions to both humans and animals, particularly farm animals. As with other toxicants, the symptoms and severity of mycotoxicoses depend on the type of mycotoxin, the dose, susceptibility of the species exposed, and individual susceptibility within a species. Along with genetic predisposition, individual susceptibility to mycotoxicosis is compounded with malnutrition, concurrent exposures to other toxicants, and preexisting disease or infection. Conversely, exposure to mycotoxins can increase susceptibility to infection and worsen conditions such as malnutrition and existing diseases, or mycotoxins may act with other chemicals synergistically to enhance toxicity. Historical accounts of acute mycotoxicoses outbreaks are the best-known examples of mycotoxin hazards, but an abundance of scientific literature suggests that chronic hazards (e.g., cancer) may be much more prevalent. The link between mycotoxin consumption and chronic diseases is more difficult to prove with existing scientific methods and techniques.

Mycotoxins can contaminate foods at virtually any point in the food chain, from crops in the field to storage containers in the home. Most mycotoxin contamination is associated with the colonization of fungi on crops, and because mycotoxins are resistant to decomposition and temperature treatments (e.g., cooking and freezing), they can remain in the food chain until consumed. If farm animals consume mycotoxin-contaminated feeds, some toxic metabolites may remain in the tissues or milk, eventually reaching the consumer. In many lesser developed countries, and sometimes in developed countries, improper storage of postharvest foods promotes the

**Table 3-3** Examples of Selected Mycotoxins in Foods and Toxicity Concerns

| *Selected Mycotoxins (examples of types)* | *Fungal Producers (foods with fungi often present)* | *Toxicity/Health Concerns* |
|---|---|---|
| Aflatoxins<br>≥16 types, most studied: B1, B2, G1, G2 | *Aspergillus flavus, A. parasiticus* (corn, peanuts, tree nuts, dried fruits, rice, other foods) | Acutely toxic (aflatoxicosis) and confirmed as carcinogenic (liver) |
| Ochratoxins<br>≥7 types or metabolites | Produced by many storage-related fungi, particularly of the genera *Aspergillus* and *Penicillium* (corn, peanuts, coffee, dried beans, soybeans, oats, dried and citrus fruits, cured hams, cheeses, others) | Nephrotoxic, hepatotoxic, teratogenic, immunosuppressive, carcinogenic |
| Ergot alkaloids | *Claviceps purpurea* (infected rye and other grains) | "Ergotism" |
| Fumonisins<br>≥15 types; FB1, FB2, FB3, etc. | *Fusarium verticilliodes* and other *Fusarium* spp. (corn, sorghum, rice, other grains) | Human carcinogenicity (esophagus), hepatotoxic, serious organ diseases in animals |
| Trichothecenes<br>Many structurally related toxins (>80)<br>T-2 toxin<br>vomitoxin<br>(deoxynivalenol, DON) | *Fusarium* spp., *Trichoderma* spp., *Myrothecium* spp., and others (corn, wheat, barley, oats, rye, hay, feeds) | Hepatotoxic, nephrotoxic, multi-organ toxic, immunosuppressive, hemorrhagic syndrome, alimentary toxic aleukia (ATA), "scabby wheat" disease |
| Patulin | *Penicillium claviforme, P. griseofulvum, P. expansum,* other *Penicillium* spp. and genera (apples, other fruits, juices and ciders, beans, wheat, sausage, moldy foods) | Genotoxic, possibly carcinogenic. |
| Yellow rice toxins<br>Citrinin<br>Citreoviridin<br>Luteoskyrin<br>Related compounds | *Penicillium citrinum, Penicillium viridicatum* (rice, moldy bread, cured hams, wheat, rye, oats) | Nephrotoxic, hepatotoxic, paralytic effects, respiratory disorders, carcinogenic |
| Other mycotoxins<br>(300–400 known) | *Alternaria* spp., *Aspergillus* spp., *Fusarium* spp., *Penicillium* spp., many others | Potentially genotoxic, carcinogenic, toxic to specific organs, endocrine disrupting |

growth of fungi and the production of mycotoxins. In general, the storage of foods under high relative humidity and warm temperatures promotes the growth of fungi and the production of mycotoxins. Additional details on this topic, along with measures for controlling fungal growth, are discussed in Chapters 4 and 8.

Since the late twentieth century, the most studied mycotoxins are a class of structurally related compounds called **aflatoxins**. These mycotoxins are produced primarily by two fungal species, *Aspergillus flavus* and *A. parasiticus*, though other fungi are also known to produce aflatoxins. Of the dozen or more known aflatoxins, the most important ones are designated as B1, B2, G1, and G2 on the basis of blue (B) or green (G) fluorescence under ultraviolet light. Aflatoxins are frequently detected in human foods such as corn, peanuts, spices, dried fruits, tree nuts, and numerous other agricultural products. In addition, farm animals that are fed aflatoxin-contaminated feeds produce toxic metabolites (e.g., M1) in their urine and/or milk. For dairy cows, the presence of M1 is a human health concern, and the concentration of aflatoxins in the feed of cows and M1 in their milk are regulated within the United States.

The mycotoxicoses caused by alfatoxins are sometimes referred to as aflatoxicosis. Acute forms of the disease may occur among both animals and humans from relatively high doses of aflatoxins. The latency period and severity of disease is dose-dependent. For humans, consumption of 2–6 mg per day of aflatoxins for a month can cause acute liver injury (e.g., hepatitis) and death (Patten 1981). Other possible health outcomes from acute disease include hemorrhage, edema, and alterations in nutrient absorption and metabolism. Recent outbreaks of aflatoxicosis occurred in Kenya in 2004 (CDC 2004b). In this outbreak, a total of 317 cases were reported with 125 deaths. The source of aflatoxin was traced to locally grown maize that had been stored under damp conditions, allowing the growth of mold and the production of aflatoxins.

An equal or greater concern is the chronic effects of low or moderate levels of aflatoxins in the human diet. Laboratory evidence has demonstrated that aflatoxins, in particular B1, are potent carcinogens in many species of animals, with the liver being a primary target organ. And epidemiologic studies of humans around the world have found a strong association of alflatoxins in the diet and liver cancer. The risk of liver cancer is greatly compounded with infections by hepatitis B virus (Hussein and Brasel 2001). Although a direct cause-and-effect relationship between liver cancer and aflatoxin consumption is difficult to establish, animal experiments and epidemiologic studies on the subject strongly suggest that aflatoxins are a major source of carcinogens in the human diet. Consequently, the regulation of aflatoxin levels in pre- and postharvest foods has become critical to limiting population exposure to them.

Ochratoxins are produced by common fungi of the genera *Aspergillus* and *Penicillium*. They are usually produced during the storage of foodstuffs, including a diverse range of commodities. These mycotoxins are very common during the storage of grains in temperate climates. When consumed by farm animals, ochratoxins have a long biological half-life in the animal tissues and fluids. This makes them a concern in meat and milk products. Ochratoxin "A" is a potent nephrotoxin (toxic to the kidney), and with sufficient dose, it will also damage the liver (Richard 2007). Ochratoxin A is believed to be responsible for the occurrence of human renal diseases in certain regions of the world such as the Balkans. In animals, ochratoxin A has also been determined to be immunosuppressive, teratogenic, and carcinogenic. The increasing detection of ochratoxins in food products of animal and plant origin has prompted some countries to regulate the level of them in certain foods.

Ergot alkaloids include a large group of compounds produced primarily by *Claviceps purpurea*. These mycotoxins are produced when *C. purpurea* parasitizes grasses and food grains such as rye. Several ergot alkaloids are often produced together to yield a mix of biologically active compounds with a range of adverse effects. The diseases caused by these mycotoxins are called ergotisms and have a long recorded history dating back many centuries. Two distinct syndromes have been observed: convulsive and gangrenous. As the name implies, the convulsive syndrome results in spasms and/or convulsions, accompanied with tingling sensations in muscles. Some ergot alkaloids include lysergic acid and related compounds that cause hallucinations; several historians have suggested this may explain frequent accounts of witchcraft and demonic possession over the centuries. The gangrenous syndrome is characterized by swollen and inflamed body parts with a burning sensation, often resulting in shrunken or loss of limbs. Other signs and symptoms of ergotism include gastrointestinal and central nervous system effects. Ergotism occurs much less often in modern times as a result of better quality control of managing grain crops.

Fumonisins are produced by *Fusarium* species that grow on corn and other grains. Most of the toxic effects of fumonisins have been observed in animals, but these effects have been extrapolated to humans. Liver and kidney tumors in rats administered fumonisins are among the experimental observations. Serious diseases that affect the brains of horses have been caused by fumonisins, and lung edema in swine has been caused by fumonisins (Richard 2007). In epidemiologic studies in several countries, the consumption of fumonisins has been associated with a high rate of human esophageal cancer (Bennett and Klich 2003). These observations highlight the multiple organ toxicity possible with fumonisins.

Trichothocenes include a large number (>80) compounds produced by *Fusarium* species and other genera. The mechanisms of toxicity differ with structural variations of the individual toxins but seem to be related to their ability to inhibit protein synthesis. Tragically, disease outbreaks from these mycotoxins have occurred during times of war and food shortages when grain crops were left in the fields too long under wet conditions. In 1913 and during World War II, Russians were afflicted by epidemics of alimentary toxic aleukia (ATA), a disease attributed to the consumption of grains contaminated with trichothocenes (Bennett and Klich 2003). The disease ATA begins with an acute phase of gastroenteritis, necrosis of the oral cavity, bleeding from several orifices, and central nervous system effects. Later stages of ATA include massive necrosis of the gastrointestinal tract, accompanied with hemorrhagic spots and ulcers on the skin. The immunosuppressive effects of trichothocenes can also lead to severe infections and septicemia.

Patulin is produced by *Penicillium* species and other genera. It is most often associated with apples and apple juice, and to some degree with other fruits, vegetables, cereals, and other foods (Kabak, Dobson, Var 2006). Compared with the other mycotoxins, patulin is considered less toxic. At one time, patulin was used as an antibiotic, but its toxicity was too great for clinical use (Bennett and Klich 2003). In laboratory experiments using high concentrations, patulin is genotoxic and can induce tumors in rats. Because the molds that produce patulin are associated with the spoilage of fruits, patulin is useful to apple growers and juice producers as a quality control indicator. High levels of patulin in juices and cider are indicative of moldy fruits used for production.

The yellow rice toxins get their name from a series of historical episodes in Asia, principally Japan, where the affected moldy rice had a yellowish appearance. Certain species of the genus *Penicillium* primarily produce yellow rice toxins, and other genera of molds have also been determined to produce these mycotoxins. The name "yellow rice toxins" is a misnomer because rice is not the only foodstuff to be contaminated with these mycotoxins. The most well-known mycotoxin in this group is citrinin. This mycotoxin is an established nephrotoxin in animals and is strongly suspected of causing nephrotoxicity in humans (Peraica et al. 2008).

### Toxic or Poisonous Mushrooms

Mushrooms are fungi that have differentiated into multicellular and macroscopic structures called *fruiting bodies*. In many parts of the world, edible mushrooms are used to supplement diets or add flavor and texture to foods. Over the centuries, human populations have learned to distinguish between "poisonous" and edible mushrooms, often by unfortunate trial and error, while the cultivation and marketing of edible mushrooms has become commonplace. Despite centuries of accumulated knowledge, mushroom poisoning still occurs all too frequently in modern times—occasionally reported as foodborne illness outbreaks (CDC 2009). Globally, since the 1950s, the reported number of severe and fatal cases of mushroom poisoning has increased (Diaz 2005a). In a review of mushroom exposures reported to Texas Poison Control Centers during the years 2005–2006, a total of 742 exposures occurred (Barbee et al. 2009). In all these cases, the exposures were acute and intentional. Among those admitted to the hospital, and for whom the mushroom exposure was known, the most common toxin was psilocybin, a hallucinogen in certain mushrooms frequently used for substance abuse purposes.

Approximately 5,000 species of mushrooms are known, but the number confirmed as poisonous or toxic is much less, only about 100 species (Barceloux 2008). Still, only 200–300 mushrooms are clearly established as safely edible (Berger and Guss 2005b). The most dangerous groups of mushrooms (many—but not all—called toadstools) have the common names of amanitas, false morels, and a group called little brown mushrooms. It is beyond the scope of this text to review all the possible species of toxic mushrooms. Furthermore, the toxins produced by these mushrooms are structurally diverse and have a variety of adverse effects on different target organs. Therefore, the purpose of the following discussion is to emphasize the potential harm from mushroom toxins and to convey the importance of ensuring that only safe mushrooms are consumed.

Medical syndromes or health outcomes from consuming mushroom toxins are often used as a scheme for classification. This is a practical approach to deal with the fact that many times the offending mushroom and its toxins may not be identified during and after the illness. There are two dimensions helpful in describing mushroom poisonings. The first dimension is based on the latency period: rapid onset (<6 hours) and delayed onset (≥6 hours) (Barceloux 2008). The second dimension is based on either the target organ(s) or the set of signs and symptoms that constitute a syndrome (Diaz 2005b). Often, the syndromes seem to overlap. The classification scheme is limited by the following: (1) variability associated with the types and mix of mushroom toxins consumed; (2) the toxin concentration in the mushroom, as well as the amount of mushroom consumed (i.e., dose); and (3) individual differences in response to the toxins. Despite these limitations, the classification scheme does provide a framework for discussion.

The types of syndromes in the rapid onset time scale (<6 hours) include neurotoxicity, severe allergic reactions, and gastrointestinal symptoms. The neurotoxic symptoms are related to the specific biological activity of the toxins. Some neurotoxins affect key neurotransmitters such as acetylcholine or glutamine, which may determine whether they are psychoactive or affect the peripheral nervous system. Depending on the toxins, the symptoms of neurotoxicity can range from dizziness and weakness to hallucinations, seizures, and coma. The allergic reactions are rare and include the *Paxillus involutus* immunohemolytic syndrome, characterized initially by symptoms of gastroenteritis within 30 minutes to 3 hours and progressing to hemolytic anemia and acute renal failure (Diaz 2005b). The gastrointestinal symptoms or syndrome can range from mild to severe. The symptoms often include nausea, projectile vomiting, diarrhea, and may include tachycardia (rapid heart beat) with chest pains, mimicking a heart attack.

The delayed onset syndromes are more likely to be severe and potentially fatal. Depending on the toxins involved, the target organs include the liver, kidney, hematopoietic system, central and peripheral nervous systems, and cardiopulmonary system. The potential hepatotoxic and nephrotoxic complications may require liver and kidney transplants, respectively, for survival of the patient. The most commonly encountered mushroom toxins, and those responsible for the majority of reported deaths, are a group of toxins called cyclopeptides (Berger and Guss 2005a). The most toxic variety of mushroom that contains cyclopeptides is *Amanita phalloides*, one of many toxic species characterized by their parasol shape and white gills (the thin flaps under the mushroom cap). The toxins within *A. phalloides* are so potent that reportedly a capful ingested by an adult can cause liver failure and death (Scheurlyn et al. 1994). Among the cyclopeptide-containing toxins, the most well known is amanitin. Other groups of mushroom toxins are listed in Table 3-4.

Knowledge is the key to determining whether a mushroom is edible and safe. A growing trend to collect wild mushrooms has contributed to cases of accidental poisonings. Many folk sayings and myths purport to have methods for determining the safety of a mushroom, but most of these methods are unproven scientifically, and field guides are inadequate for identifying mushrooms for human consumption. Furthermore, cooking and drying do not destroy most toxins. The best way to determine the safety of a mushroom is through identification by a competent mycologist (CDC 1997). For commercial food establishments, extra care is necessary to ensure mushrooms are procured only from sources regulated by food regulatory authorities.

## Algal Toxins

Algae encompass a wide variety of eukaryotic organisms that range in size from unicellular microbes to macroscopic, multicellular structures. They are photosynthetic but differ significantly from plants in structure. Algae are most prominent in aquatic environments, where microscopic forms are found in the water column and form a food base for marine ecosystems. Approximately 5,000 species of algae are known, from which about 40 species, mostly the dinoflagellates, produce secondary metabolites that also act as potent toxins (Sobel and Painter 2005).

The secondary metabolites produced by dinoflagellates are biologically active compounds that elicit diverse responses in many organisms. Marine scientists theorize that these metabolites are involved with broader ecological functions, but the study of them has been limited mostly to their toxicity in animals and humans (Paul et al. 2007). The dinoflagellate toxins are notorious for causing serious human illnesses following the consumption of certain seafood. Like many toxins, the classification of dinoflagellate toxins is often based on the perspective of the classifier. Recently, the World Health Organization (WHO) decided to classify these toxins on the basis of

**Table 3-4** Mushroom Poisoning Syndromes, Principal Toxins, and Target Organs

| Syndromes | Principal Toxins | Mushroom Genera | Target Organs | | | |
|---|---|---|---|---|---|---|
| | | | Liver | Kidney | CNS[a] | GI[b] Tract |
| Amatoxin-containing mushrooms | Cyclopeptides: Amatoxins, phallotoxins, virotoxins | Amanita Galerina Lepiota | Delayed-onset | Delayed-onset | Likely from hepatorenal effects | Early-onset |
| False morel and gyromitrin poisoning | Gyromitrin, MFH, MMH | Gyromitra | Possible complication | Possible complication | Mild (early) to seizures and coma (delayed) | Early and/or delayed onset |
| Gastroenteritis-producing mushrooms | Most are unidentified | Great variety | | | | Early-onset |
| Inky cap and coprine toxicity | Coprine (disulfiram-like) | Coprinus | | | Early and/or delayed onset | Early and/or delayed onset |
| Isoxazole-containing mushrooms and pantherina syndrome | Muscimol, ibotenic acid | Amanita | | | Early-onset | |
| Muscarine-containing mushrooms and muscarine toxicity | Muscarine | Inocybe Clitocybe Mycena | | | Early-onset | Early-onset |
| Orellanine-containing Mushrooms and nephrotoxicity | Orellanine | Cortinarius | | Delayed-onset | | Early and/or delayed onset (mild) |
| Hullucinogenic | Hullucinogenic Indoles: psilocybin | Psilocybe Panaeolus Inocybe Others | | | Early-onset | |
| Paxillus and other mushroom syndromes | Not well defined | Paxillus Tricholoma Amanita | | Delayed-onset | | Early-onset |

[a] Central Nervous System.
[b] Gastrointestinal.

Source: Compiled from Barceloux 2008.

their chemical structure (Toyofuku 2006), but many health authorities still classify the toxins on the basis of disease syndromes. Although these toxins have very diverse chemical structures, most of them are clinically recognized as neurotoxic and/or hepatotoxic, depending on the predominant signs and symptoms of the patients (Wang 2008). Several structurally similar toxins are also produced by dinoflagellates that act exclusively as enterotoxins, causing severe but self-limiting diarrhea. Table 3-5 lists the best-known toxins produced by dinoflagellates, along with their associated diseases/syndromes and occurrence.

Dinoflagellates and other toxigenic algae are common in the seas throughout many parts of the world. In most ecosystems, their population sizes are limited by natural constraints, and their toxins are not overtly harmful to wildlife and humans. This changes when population levels of the algae increase and they are consumed by various forms of marine life. The toxins then bioaccumulate within various species of the food web. The filter feeders, including the molluscan shellfish (oysters, mussels, clams, etc.), are particularly efficient at concentrating the algae and their toxins. Sometimes the toxins can magnify in concentration with animals in the upper trophic levels, a process called biomagnification. The population levels of algae can increase to the point of becoming obvious, as evidenced by decreased water quality, eutrophication, and/or the death of marine life. These conditions are known as "harmful algal blooms" and have been increasing in frequency and type worldwide, mostly as a result of human activities (Glibert et al. 2005). The phenomenon of "red tide" is an example of a harmful algal bloom, though not all algal blooms have a red color. Harmful algal blooms usually increase the risks from algal toxins, but they are not reliable predictors of seafood safety: High concentrations of algal toxins can be detected in seafood harvested from waters without algal blooms. More recently, concerns have been expressed about the presence of algal toxins in freshwater and the possible bioaccumulation of these toxins in aquatic and terrestrial food animals (Deeds et al. 2008).

The first five groups of toxins and syndromes in Table 3-5 (ciguatera, DSP, NSP, PSP, ASP) are historically important to food safety (Food Code 2009). The other toxins (azaspiracids, palytoxin, yessotoxins, pectenotoxins, cyclic imines) have been identified and characterized more recently, and additional toxins will likely be identified in the future (Toyofuku 2006; Wang 2008). The dinoflagellate toxins are generally heat stable and are not affected greatly by cooking (Sobel and Painter 2005). Diagnostic tests for algal toxins are not available, so diagnosis is based on clinical presentation and a recent history of seafood consumption. The consequences of intoxication can be severe and debilitating, particularly for the neurotoxic effects, and antidotes to the toxins are unavailable. Therefore, treatment is mostly limited to supportive care.

Ciguatera is caused by the ingestion of carnivorous reef fish that contain ciguatoxins in their flesh. The toxins originate as maitotoxins produced by a dinoflagellate (*Gambierdiscus toxicus*) and are biotransformed to ciguatoxins by herbivorous fish and invertebrates that feed upon the dinoflagellates (Wang 2008). The ciguatoxins are then biomagnified when carnivorous fish prey on herbivorous fish and concentrate the ciguatoxins. Humans then consume the carnivorous fish and suffer ciguatera. The clinical presentation of ciguatera may include "gastrointestinal, cardiovascular, neurological and neuropsychiatric symptoms and signs" (Friedman et al. 2008). Death can occur in severe cases, but most cases usually resolve themselves in 1–4 days. Chronic symptoms may persist in some patients anywhere from days to months following the acute illness.

**Table 3 5** Important Algal (Dinoflagellate) Toxins Associated with Seafood

| Algal (Dinoflagellate) Toxins | Foodborne Diseases/Syndromes | Associated Foods/Occurrence |
|---|---|---|
| Ciguatoxins (Maitotoxins are precursors produced by dinoflagellates.) | Ciguatera | Coral reef fish from extreme southeastern United States, Hawaii, and subtropical/tropical regions worldwide. Recently reported in fish from the northern Gulf of Mexico |
| Okadaic Acid Group Dinophysis Toxins | Diarrheic shellfish poisoning (DSP) | Molluscan shellfish. Reported in Japan, Southeast Asia, New Zealand, western Europe and Scandinavia, and eastern Canada |
| Brevetoxin Group | Neurotoxic shellfish poisoning (NSP) | Molluscan shellfish harvested from coastal Gulf of Mexico and southern Atlantic. Similar toxins in New Zealand and suggested occurrences elsewhere |
| Saxitoxin Group | Paralytic shellfish poisoning (PSP) | Molluscan shellfish harvested from U.S. northwest and northeast coasts. Reports from temperate to tropical regions elsewhere in the world. Toxins found in the viscera of mackerel and several species of crustaceans (lobster and crabs) in the United States |
| Domoic Acid Group | Amnesic shellfish poisoning (ASP) | Molluscan shellfish harvested from U.S. northwest and northeast coasts. Toxin-producing algae are found in Gulf of Mexico. Toxins found in viscera of several crab species and anchovies from United States |
| Azaspiracid Group | Azaspriacid poisoning (diarrheic, systemic and neurotoxic) | Molluscan shellfish in Europe |
| Palytoxins | Palytoxin poisoning (neurotoxic and systemic effects) | Crabs, sea urchins, and fish. Reported in Southeast Asia, Japan, and Brazil |
| Yessotoxin Group | No confirmed human cases but potent toxin in animal studies. Once suspected of causing DSP but now confirmed as neurotoxic | Detected in molluscan shellfish from Europe, Asia, and North America |
| Pectenotoxins Group | No confirmed human cases but potent toxin in animal studies | Detected in molluscan shellfish from Europe, Asia, and Australia |
| Cyclic Imines Group | No confirmed human cases but highly toxic in animal studies | Detected in molluscan shellfish and microalgae from several parts of the world |

*Source:* Compiled from Food Code 2009; Toyofuku 2006; and Wang 2008.

Okadaic acid and related *Dinophysis* toxins are responsible for diarrheic shellfish poisoning (DSP), recognized to cause human illnesses since the late 1970s. These toxins are produced by the dinoflagellate genera of *Dinophysis* and *Prorocentrum* that accumulate in the digestive tracts of molluscan shellfish. As the name DSP implies, the predominant symptoms are severe diarrhea and abdominal cramps, which appear approximately 30 minutes after consuming the shellfish (Sobel and Painter 2005). The illness usually resolves itself within 3–4 days following onset. These algal toxins are among the few that seem to exclusively affect the gastrointestinal system.

The brevetoxins are produced by several genera of dinoflagellates and cause neurotoxic shellfish poisoning (NSP). Following the consumption of shellfish with the accumulated toxins, gastrointestinal and neurological symptoms appear within 3–6 hours. The neurological symptoms include paresthesias around the mouth and of the extremities, affected gait, and dizziness (Heymann 2008). Neurological and gastrointestinal symptoms usually resolve completely and rapidly, typically within 48 hours. One of the dinoflagellates responsible for producing brevetoxins (*Gymnodinium breve*) causes "red tides" in Florida, resulting in massive fish kills and sometimes inhalation hazards to humans from aerosolized toxins.

The saxitoxins are potent neurotoxins produced by several genera of dinoflagellates that usually affect shellfish beds in colder waters (e.g., northern latitudes of North America) but may also affect tropical waters. Exposure to saxitoxins usually occurs from consumption of molluscan shellfish but occasionally from consumption of fin fish, crustaceans, and gastropods (Sobel and Painter 2005). In stark contrast to NSP, the disease syndrome caused by saxitoxins, called paralytic shellfish poisoning (PSP), is severe with a rapid onset ranging from minutes to hours after consumption. Death from respiratory distress is possible within 12 hours. The initial symptoms include gastrointestinal disturbances accompanied by paresthesias of the mouth and extremities. These symptoms may resolve within a few days among the milder cases, while the more severe cases progress to muscle paralysis and respiratory distress.

Amnesiac shellfish poisoning (ASP) was first reported in Canada in 1987. Along with gastrointestinal symptoms of diarrhea and vomiting, patients also experienced headaches and short-term memory losses (Heymann 2008). Several months after acute intoxication, patients still showed memory deficits along with evidence of motor neuropathy and sensorineural effects. The causative agent was determined to be domoic acid, found in the blue mussels consumed by the victims. The neurotoxin is produced by a dinoflagellate recently renamed as *Pseudonitzschia multiseries* (Toyofuku 2006). Monitoring studies of this dinoflagellate and domoic acid determined that the toxin can move up the food chain, but human illnesses have not been reported with seafood from higher trophic levels. The implementation of monitoring programs and the closing of shellfish beds when domoic acid levels reach 20 parts per million (ppm) in the water have been effective in preventing outbreaks of ASP. The chronic effects of low-level exposures (i.e., <20 ppm) to domoic acid have not been fully determined.

## PLANTS AND ANIMAL TOXINS

### Plant Toxins

Secondary metabolites were introduced earlier as compounds derived from metabolism that are not involved in the primary physiology of an organism, that is, they play no apparent role in respiration, digestion, reproduction, structure, and so forth. Indirect functions of these secondary metabolites may exist, but their specific roles are often unknown. One likely role of secondary metabolites is to influence interactions among various species, possibly leading to an advantage in the competition for survival. Some secondary metabolites are employed in "chemical defense" against other species and may be considered "poisons" or toxins by humans. Plants are probably the greatest producers of toxins because they lie stationary at the bottom of the food chain, unable to flee from being consumed by herbivores (Berenbaum 1995). Within parts of a plant (stem, leaves, seeds, fruits, roots, flowers, etc.), the quantity of toxins can differ greatly. The presence of toxins can also change during particular life stages of the plant, and temporal variations in toxin concentration may occur over a plant's lifetime. The production of some toxins is induced by environmental factors, parasitic diseases, and injuries to the plant, such as inflicted by insects or animals.

Like most natural substances of biological origin, plant toxins have chemical structures that are diverse and variable. Furthermore, many plant toxins have not been identified, and plants often produce multiple toxins that complicate individual toxin isolation and characterization. This makes the classification of poisonous plants and their toxins into discrete categories very difficult. In general, the major toxins in plants are organic compounds, and their biochemical derivations are associated with the metabolic pathways of plants. Selected categories of plant toxins are listed in Table 3-6. Certain organic compounds in plants are considered antivitamins rather than toxins. These compounds interfere with either the absorption or utilization of important vitamins. In addition to organic compounds and toxins, elements and inorganic compounds from the soil can accumulate in some plants to the level of causing toxicity in animals and humans.

Throughout human history, plants were deemed safe for consumption after years of uneventful experience, usually as a staple food over multiple human generations. Some toxins in staple foods were unavoidable, but human cultures learned to remove or render harmless these toxins by food preparation methods. With the beginning of agriculture, some 10,000 years ago, plants were selectively bred and domesticated to enhance their nutritional content and diminish their toxic characteristics (Diamond 2002). Nowadays and worldwide, about 30 plants account for 95% of the plant-derived calories in the human daily diet, and about 300 plants account for nearly 5% of the remaining plant caloric intake (Kundsen et al. 2008). Yet, nearly 7,000 plant species are cultivated or collected in the wild and used to supplement human diets, and more than 20,000 plant species throughout the world are thought to be edible (Plants for a Future 2008). Foods that are used exclusively in some regions of the world and introduced into developed countries are considered "novel," and although most novel food plants appear safe in terms of acute toxicity, the potential long-term health effects (adverse or beneficial) of most novel plant foods are unknown (Kundsen et al. 2008).

Approximately 100,000 exposures to toxic plants are reported each year to poison control centers in the United States (Froberg, Ibrahim, Furbee 2007). The majority of these exposures involve children eating or tasting nonfood plants, usually ornamental or wild plants. However, the most serious reported poisonings are among adults who mistakenly identified a plant as edible or who deliberately ingested a plant for medicinal or other purposes. Those who gather wild plants for intentional consumption have the greatest risk for intoxication or poisoning. Considering that approximately 250,000 flowering plants exist, the total number of toxic/poisonous plants in nature is virtually impossible to determine.

**Table 3-6** Selected Categories of Plant Toxins

| Plant Toxin Categories | Foods and Other Plants |
| --- | --- |
| Alkaloids | |
|   Glycoalkaloids | Potatoes, tomatoes, eggplants |
|   Pyrrolizidine alkaloids | Cereals contaminated with weeds, herbal teas, medicinal preps |
|   Pyridine alkaloids | |
|     Nicotine | Tobacco |
| Glycosides | |
|   Cyanogenic glycosides | Cassava root, bitter almonds, lima beans, apple and apricot seeds |
|   Cardiac glycosides | Christmas rose, foxglove, certain lilies |
|   Coumarins | Celery, parsnips, sweet clover |
| Oxalates and Oxalic Acids | Rhubarb leaves, tomatoes, spinach |
| Proteins and Amino Acids | |
|   Allergens | Variety of foods and plants |
|   Lathyrogens | Chick peas, vetch |
|   Lectins | Red kidney beans, soybeans, cereals, potatoes |
|     Ricin | Castor beans |
| Antivitamins | Mung beans, berries, Brussels sprouts, beets |
| Phenolic Compounds | |
|   Tannins | Coffee, tea, cocoa |
| Toxins in Honey | |
|   Grayanotoxin | Honey made with nectar from rhododendron plants |

Intoxication from domesticated food plants is rare but can occur under the right circumstances. For example, food plants of the genus *Solanum* (e.g., potatoes, tomatoes, eggplants) produce a class of compounds known as glycoalkaloids, characterized by steroidal and ring structures with a carbohydrate side chain. Reports of foodborne illness outbreaks from plant toxins in foods such as potatoes are extremely rare, especially considering that millions are consumed everyday in the world. But such outbreaks have been documented during the twentieth century, when outbreaks were reported among both animals and humans fed potatoes, including fatal cases (Hopkins 1995; Lee 2006). Apparently, two glycoalkloids ($\alpha$-solanine, $\alpha$-chaconine) increase to toxic levels in potatoes that are turning green and sprouting. The toxin levels are highest just underneath the skin and in areas of high metabolic activity (e.g., the "eyes"). The glycoalkloid concentration in potatoes can also increase under certain growth and storage conditions, and genetic varieties of potatoes may contain higher levels of glycoalkloids (Korpan et al. 2004). Cooking does not effectively destroy these glycoalkaloids. Fortunately, most potatoes on the market shelves have glycoalkaloid concentrations well below the acutely toxic level, but some health scientists are concerned about low levels of gylcoalkaloids in foods, particularly for sensitive individuals (Korpan et al. 2004).

Some common food plants have toxins that can be avoided or removed with proper preparation. The toxin phytohaemagglutinin, belonging to the lectin group of toxins, is reduced in red kidney beans by boiling for 10 minutes or more. Raw or undercooked (under 80°C/176°F) kidney beans can result in foodborne intoxications. Ironically, cooking kidney beans at lower temperatures can make the toxins even more potent, an important point to remember when cooking raw kidney beans in a crockpot (Food and Drug Administration [FDA] 2009). Toxins in some plant foods are avoided by not eating certain parts (e.g., seeds from apples) and by discarding damaged or poorly stored fruits and vegetables. In the tropical and lesser developed countries, an important food crop is cassava root, a hardy and reliable source of carbohydrates. The bitter variety of cassava contains high levels of cyanogenic glycosides (linamarin and lotaustralin) that are converted to hydrocyanic acid (HCN) by the natural enzymes in cassava. These toxins must be removed by soaking, boiling, fermenting, and/or other processing methods before the cassava can be safely consumed.

An interesting and unusual source of plant toxins is honey made from the nectar of rhododendrons and a few other plants. Theses toxins, called grayanotoxins, have been associated with illnesses known as "mad honey poisoning" since ancient times (Gunduz et al. 2008). Bees ingest the toxins in nectar while foraging, and when the honey is made at the hive, the grayanotoxins become concentrated. The clinical presentation of grayanotoxicosis is similar to pesticide poisoning in that it affects the nervous system. Patients experience dizziness, weakness, nausea and/or vomiting, hypotension (low blood pressure), bradycardia (slow heart beat), and often other symptoms such as blurred vision and impaired consciousness. Recovery is usually within 24 hours, though serious complications can occur. Commercial honey operations are actually safer than independent bee keepers because large quantities of honey are pooled from many hives, diluting the concentration of any grayanotoxins in honey from contaminated hives (FDA 2009).

The risks from plant toxins in everyday foods are minimal or rare—unless the preparer uses exotic or novel foods or prepares traditional foods in an unconventional manner. The best prevention strategy is obtaining foods from reputable and approved sources and ensuring that foods not usually eaten raw are thoroughly cooked. As stated previously, some toxins are not easily destroyed by cooking, so using poorly stored or spoiled fruits and vegetables increases the risks of consuming toxins—both from plants and fungi on the plants. In a rarely documented event, one foodborne illness outbreak was traced to toxins called raphides, belonging to the oxalates group of plant toxins (Watson et al. 2005). The entrée dish implicated in the outbreak was Chinese braised vegetables. The toxins were detected in the dish by a forensic laboratory and appeared to be from plant debris that had contaminated edible mushrooms, an ingredient in the dish. An attempted trace back to the source of ingredients was unsuccessful because the mushrooms and vegetables were obtained from an Asian market that no longer had packages of the products, and the executive chef was uncertain of the products' origins. A second hypothesis for the outbreak was deliberate contamination of the entrée with poisonous plants (i.e., bioterrorism), but the evidence for criminal activity was insufficient to make such allegations.

## Animal Toxins

Approximately 120,000 species of animals in the world are considered either venomous or poisonous. The distinction between a venomous and poisonous animal is based on several characteristics. Venomous animals have specialized cells and glands that produce and store mixtures of toxins that make up venom, and most venomous animals have a "venom apparatus" (e.g., stingers, fangs) that delivers the venom to the animal's prey or enemy (Mebs 2002). In contrast, poisonous animals lack a venom apparatus to deliver the toxins. Some poisonous animals may produce toxins from specialized glands, but they may also acquire the toxins from other animals, microbes, or the environment and store them somewhere in their bodies, often compartmentalized in certain organs and tissues. In this sense, shellfish and fin fish that accumulate algal toxins could be considered poisonous animals. This is debatable, but the distinction may be that poisonous animals acquire toxins for "chemical defense" against predators, whereas other animals may store toxins through sequestration to prevent toxicity from exposures. Certain organs of some animal species are toxic because of high concentrations of seemingly innocuous substances such as retinol (vitamin A) (Lips 2003).

If ingested, most venoms are destroyed by digestive enzymes. The potency of venom is usually greatest when it enters the bloodstream of an organism through the parenteral route. Despite this generalization, care is necessary to avoid venom glands if a venomous animal is used for food, as may be done in some cultures. In contrast, toxic substances in poisonous animals may be distributed across many tissues, or they may be associated with offal, a culinary term for the internal organs of food animals. Some species of animals may have high concentrations of toxins in their internal organs. In cultures that traditionally consume offal, the specific organs that can be safely consumed are well established, and their proper preparation is knowledge passed down through several generations. When foodborne intoxication occurs from eating internal organs, it usually happens when the culinary habits of a culture are brought by immigrants to a region where different animal species or environmental conditions exist (CDC 1995).

Besides the issues discussed earlier with the accumulation of algal toxins in marine animals, the most frequently reported problem with consuming animal toxins is the puffer fish (known as fugu). The substance responsible for this intoxication is a powerful neurotoxin called tetrodotoxin, named after the biological order of fish Tetraodontoidae (CDC 1996). Tetrodotoxin is found in many species of marine animals and some species of amphibians (Noguchi and Arakawa 2008). The fugu is most often associated with intoxications because of its popularity as a delicacy in Japan and occasionally in the United States (CDC 1996). The death rate of those who become ill from tetrodotoxin is approximately 60% (CDC 1996). Certified chefs carefully prepare the fugu to minimize its toxicity, producing only a mild tingling sensation. Despite careful preparation, fugu is a common source of fatal foodborne intoxication in Japan; outbreaks from tetrodotoxin are also associated with the consumption of certain gastropods and shellfish, but much less frequently compared with the fugu (Noguchi and Arakawa 2008).

## ENVIRONMENTAL AND AGRICULTURAL CHEMICALS

The discussion of toxic substances thus far has dealt with toxins, that is, biologically produced substances by different organisms. Although toxins represent a prominent and pervasive hazard in foods, other environmental chemicals associated with anthropogenic (human) activity and geologic processes are important to recognize and eliminate. Unlike food additives, which are intentionally put into foods, these chemicals are unintentional contaminants. Some chemicals are pollutants discharged from industrial sources and may contaminate foods via the pathways of soil, air, and/or water. Other chemicals are used to increase agricultural productivity but are undesirable—possibly hazardous—in the final food product. Still other chemicals are naturally present as a result of geologic processes and may contaminate preharvest foods.

## Environmental Chemicals

The industrialization of nations brought unprecedented prosperity and quality of life to millions of people around the world, but whether from ignorance or indifference, it also resulted in widespread environmental pollution. Factories produce uncontrolled emissions and effluents that pollute the air, water, and soil. Power plants and transportation sources produce pollution from burning fossil fuels, yielding a complex mixture of hydrocarbons, gases, and heavy metals. In turn, these pollutants often find their way into the human food chain. At the same time, the introduction of pesticides destroys pests that damage crops and transmit diseases to farm animals and humans. But an unanticipated consequence of pesticide usage is the accumulation of chemical residues in wildlife and in the human food chain. Most of the concerns with chemical residues in food from pollution are chronic exposures, such as cancer and organ system dysfunction, but several episodes in modern history highlight that sometimes the hazards can be acute or subchronic.

As Japan began its postwar reconstruction in the 1950s, several epidemics of disease were linked to industrial processes and emissions. As part of mining operations in the mountains of Japan, cadmium found its way into the Jinzu River and surrounding tributaries, where it accumulated in the water column and sediments. These sources of water were used for fishing, drinking, and irrigation of the rice crops. Throughout the history of mining in the region, local residents had experienced an affliction called itai-itai disease, translated into English as "ouch-ouch" disease. The disease was characterized by a painful spine and legs, brittle bones that easily fractured, and complications that included renal dysfunction/failure and death. For many years, health experts speculated the etiology was either genetic or infectious, but in a series of studies spanning several decades, the link between cadmium exposure and itai-itai disease was clearly established (Nogawa and Kido 1993). The highest and most persistent concentrations of cadmium were measured in the soils of irrigated rice fields, and the rice harvested from these fields contained significantly higher levels of cadmium compared with other rice (Aoshima 1987). Despite pollution limits imposed on mining operations in Japan, some soils still have high levels of cadmium and have been banned from use for commercial farming.

Another tragedy that involved industrial pollution and contamination of the food chain was dubbed Minimata disease. Named after the Japanese fishing city of Minimata, the disease was the result of methylmercury that had bioaccumulated in the local seafood. The source of pollution was a nearby factory that produced methylmercury as a by product. The factory's wastewater contained methylmercury and was released into Minimata Bay from 1938 until 1968. Methylmercury is very soluble and a potent neurotoxin that is capable of causing birth defects (teratogenic). This form of mercury bioaccumulates in organisms, particularly in shellfish and fin fish. Inhabitants of the Minimata area caught and consumed the local seafood as a main source of protein. In 1965, a similar epidemic of Minimata disease occurred in another region of Japan and was linked to methylmercury. Over the years, exposure to methylmercury caused thousands of birth defects, at least 1,784 deaths, and permanently affected more than 10,000 people (Imamura, Ide, Yasunaga 2007).

For decades, environmental scientists have studied the transport and fate of toxicants in the environment, and many thousands of publications and databases exist on the subject. The pathways from an environmental source of pollution to the human food chain are frequently indirect, as illustrated in Figure 3-4 (Vaughan 1984). The health risks of chemicals in the human food chain depend on many factors, chief among them is a chemical's persistence in the environment and ability to bioaccumulate in organisms. Chemicals with a long history of persistence and bioaccumulation include metals (Cd, Pb, Hg, Cr, As), polycyclic aromatic hydrocarbons (PAHs), and chlorinated hydrocarbons (PCBs, DDT, etc.). In recent years, a more inclusive grouping of

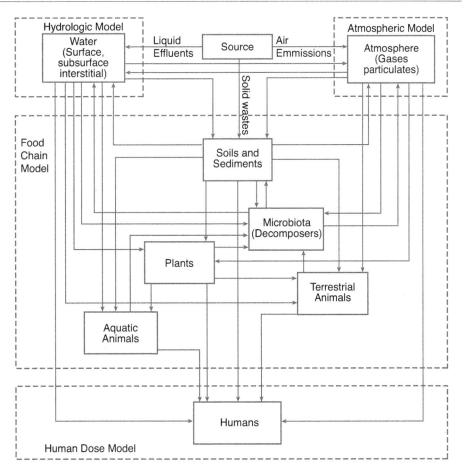

**Figure 3-4** Conceptual Framework for Modeling Contamination of the Food Chain. *Source*: Modified from Vaughn, 1984. Reproduced with permission from *Environmental Health Perspectives*.

organic chemicals with environmental persistence has been made, called persistent organic pollutants (POPs). This category of chemicals includes a variety of pesticides, solvents, flame retardants, oils, pharmaceuticals, and other types of synthetic chemicals. Studies of chemical residues in U.S. foods demonstrate that POPs are detected in nearly all food categories (Schafer and Kegley 2002). Many of these chemicals have been determined to cause adverse effects ranging from cancer to endocrine disruption in animal experiments, though at much higher dose levels than usually detected in foods. The chronic risks of POPs in the food supply are the subject of constant debate and scientific inquiry. Discussions of these risks are centered around a methodology called risk assessment, which is discussed in greater detail later.

Some sources of chemicals in the environment are naturally occurring from geologic processes. Mercury (Hg) and arsenic (As) are classic examples. Natural sources of mercury include volcanoes, geologic deposits, and the ocean. Mercury naturally cycles through the environment, often transforming between inorganic and organic forms, but the amount of mercury in the environment has been greatly augmented by human activity, predominantly from the burning of fossil fuels. The methylation of inorganic or elemental mercury is the primary means of bioaccumulation in the food chain. The aquatic food web is particularly efficient in the bioaccumulation and biomagnification of methylmercury. Similarly, arsenic is abundant in the earth's crust and exists in a variety of chemical forms, each with different toxic potential. The greatest exposure to arsenic is from drinking well water or using it to prepare foods, particularly in certain regions where the underlying geologic strata contain high levels of arsenic. Human activities and pollution also augment arsenic levels in the environment. Unlike mercury, the inorganic forms of arsenic are more toxic because most organic forms of arsenic are readily excreted from the body.

Nearly all environmentally persistent chemicals contaminate bodies of water and accumulate in the sediments. This means the aquatic food web is especially vulnerable to the bioaccumulation of chemicals. Fish and seafood are potentially major sources of environmental chemicals in the human diet. State and local jurisdictions in the United States monitor local waters and the fish for certain chemical contaminants and issue advisories regarding the safe consumption of fish. These advisories may be very specific or broad, ranging from consumption advisories for particular fish species and sensitive human subpopulations to complete commercial fishing bans in designated waters. For many years, the EPA has maintained and analyzed trends in the fish consumption advisories (EPA 2007). At the end of the calendar year 2006, the total number of active fish consumption advisories in the United States was 3,852 for 44 different chemical contaminants. Of the 44 contaminants, 88% of the advisories involved only five chemicals, those with a high potential for bioaccumulation: mercury, polychlorinated biphenyls (PCBs), chlordane, dioxins, and DDT. The issuance of fish consumption advisories for all five chemicals increased over previous years, but the primary reason is believed to be an increase in monitoring activities rather than an increase in environmental contamination. One presumed reason for the increased monitoring was a joint FDA-EPA advisory issued in 2004 on the hazards of eating certain seafood containing mercury (FDA and EPA 2004). The advisory was intended primarily for women who were anticipating pregnancy, already pregnant, or nursing children. Among the recommendations were the following (paraphrased): (1) Do not eat top predator marine fish (sharks, swordfish, king mackerel, etc.); (2) eat 12 ounces per week of selected fish and shellfish that are low in mercury content; and (3) for locally caught fish, check fish consumption advisories, or limit consumption to 6 ounces per week.

## Agricultural Chemicals (Agrochemicals or Agrichemicals)

The "Green Revolution" of the twentieth century dramatically increased food production and saved billions of people—in great part because of the use of agricultural chemicals, or agrochemicals. The bulk of agrochemicals are pesticides and fertilizers, but they also include veterinary medications such as antibiotics and growth regulators or hormones. Agrochemicals are intended to minimize losses caused by pests, enhance production through rapid growth and shorter time to market, and/or increase yield in a limited amount of space. Very few agrochemicals are intended to remain as residues in the final food product. Nonetheless, residues from agrochemicals are practically unavoidable in raw and finished food products. Food safety measures are necessary throughout the food chain to limit agrochemical residues to acceptable levels in the final food product.

### *Pesticides*

Pesticides are legally and broadly defined under the U.S. Federal Insecticide, Fungicide, and Rodenticide Act (FIFRA). In practice, pesticides are categorized by their target pest and further subdivided into chemical classes and structure. Pesticide categories include insecticides (insects), herbicides (weeds), rodenticides (rodents), fungicides (fungi), nematicides (nematodes), and so forth. The United States produces approximately 1.6 billion pounds of active ingredients used in conventional pesticides each year; this excludes nonconventional pesticides used as industrial wood preservatives, specialty biocides, and chlorine and hypochlorites (Kiely, Donaldson, Grube 2004). Agricultural applications account for 78% of all conventional pesticide use (herbicides, pesticides, fungicides, nematicides, other). Among insecticides, the most commonly used chemical classes are organophosphates, carbamates, and pyrethroids. The chlorinated hydrocarbon insecticides, known for their environmental persistence and bioaccumulation potential (e.g., DDT), have largely been replaced by the organophosphates and carbamates.

Pesticides are semantically referred to as either pollutants or agrochemicals, depending on their transport and fate in the environment. Obviously, pesticides applied directly on crops to control insects, weeds, fungi, or other pests and that remain as residues on the food product are defined straightforwardly as agrochemicals. However, pesticides often travel from application sites by overspray, drift, runoff, and spills to contaminate foodstuffs, in which case the pesticide is a pollutant. Regardless of the viewpoint, pesticide residues in foods represent a major concern to consumers, regulators, and public health officials. After all, pesticides are designed to kill or repel an organism, and they are applied in many places where exposure to nontarget organisms can occur—including wildlife, farm animals, and humans. Consequently, regulatory controls on pesticide application and the monitoring of residues have become an important part of their use, at least in the developed countries.

In general, after many years of monitoring and scientific study, the levels of pesticide residues in the U.S. food supply are very low compared with other types of chemical exposures. The majority of health scientists conclude that the health risks posed by pesticide residues in foods are much less than those posed by microbial contaminants, naturally produced toxins, and environmental pollutants (Winter 2001). Yet, it is also important to remember that pesticide safety is dependent on their proper application and handling. Pesticides are extremely toxic, and several documented foodborne illness outbreaks attest to the misuse of pesticides. For example, in 1971, an outbreak of methylmercury intoxication occurred in Iraq after people consumed breads made from fungicide-treated grains intended to be used as seeds (Clarkson 1995). The largest recorded outbreak of foodborne intoxication by pesticides in North America occurred in 1985 (CDC 1986). Thousands of probable cases were reported among several states and Canada after the consumption of watermelons and cantaloupes contaminated with aldicarb, a carbamate insecticide. Aldicarb is easily transported from a plant's roots to the stems, leaves, and fruits; it is not EPA-registered for use on melons. Another concern is the misuse of pesticides in foreign countries that export foods to the United States. Compliance with pesticide application regulations is dependent on the foreign government's diligence and enforcement. Finally, of all the possible hazards associated with pesticide residues in foods, the most immediate risk is the use of pesticides in food storage and preparation areas (CDC 1999). Special precautions are always necessary whenever pesticides are applied in food storage and preparation areas.

### Veterinary Drugs

Modern agriculture is very dependent on the use of veterinary drugs to raise livestock for human food. Veterinary drugs are used to prevent or fight infections, treat injuries, promote rapid growth, and/or increase milk production. Domesticated animals are raised in greater density than in previous centuries, increasing the risk of infectious disease transmission among a herd or flock and causing stress on the animals. Veterinary drugs such as antibiotics and topical antiseptics reduce the risk of disease transmission and ensure good health among the animals. In turn, this reduces the risk of transmitting zoonotic pathogens to humans via the food chain. Antibiotics and hormone-like steroidal compounds also promote the rapid and efficient growth of animals, lowering overall costs and increasing productivity. With all these obvious benefits, the risks of veterinary drugs in food animals are less clear.

The overwhelming majority of scientific literature on the use of veterinary drugs in food animals is focused on the use of antibiotics and the risk of developing antibiotic-resistant strains of pathogens, some of which may infect humans via the food chain. The risks of other veterinary drugs appear to be of lesser concern by public health experts. If the drugs are used responsibly and according to labeling instructions, there should be little or no drug residues in the animal tissues consumed by humans. The problem is that veterinary drugs may be used "extra label" and bypass rigorous drug approval processes, usually without adequate enforcement of extra-label policies (Government Accountability Office [GAO] 1992). Furthermore, not all veterinary drugs are procured and administered by appropriately trained individuals, allowing the opportunity for misuse of the drugs in animals raised for food purposes. Although rarely reported, acute foodborne illnesses have been linked to drug residues in animal tissues. In Europe, the drug clenbuterol was approved for therapeutic use in farm animals, but the drug also has anabolic effects on muscle mass and body fat. These properties have been improperly and illegally exploited, resulting in serious foodborne intoxications (Salleras et al. 1995). To minimize the risks from drug residues in the food supply, a system of veterinary drug approval/use and enforcement is necessary, along with a robust monitoring program of drug residues in foods.

The issues associated with the use of antibiotics in food animals are complicated and controversial (Mathew, Cissell, Liamthong 2007). Evidence exists that pathogens in animals have acquired antibiotic resistance genes, possibly from nontherapeutic uses of antibiotics, and some of these pathogens have infected humans. On the other hand, restricting nontherapeutic use of antibiotics in food animals has led to increased infections in animals and the heavy use of other, more potent antibiotics for treatment. The antibiotics used for treating animal infections are usually more clinically important to human populations. In the United States, a mixed strategy is being advocated: (1) impose restrictions on selected antibiotics, and (2) provide education, surveillance, and research to identify and solve problems (Mathew et al. 2007).

## FOOD ADDITIVES, ADULTERANTS, AND CHEMICALS ASSOCIATED WITH PROCESSING AND PACKAGING

Throughout human history, foods have been subjected to treatment processes (e.g., smoking, drying, salting, grinding). The main purpose of food treatment in early human communities was to preserve foods for later use, usually during times of seasonal changes and famine, or to remove toxic or inedible parts. Over time, besides serving essential purposes, food treatment also improved the palatability of food and enhanced the pleasure of eating. As civilizations and empires flourished, the spice trade became established, and explorers and merchants traveled the world in search of exotic flavors. Thus, the processing of foods by treatments and additives is not a recent innovation, but modern times have introduced sophisticated technology and a greater complexity to the science of food processing.

Previous discussions in this chapter highlight the unwanted or unavoidable chemical substances that may contaminate foods. In this section, the discussion focuses on chemical substances that are deliberately added to foods and chemical substances that become incorporated into foods as part of processing, distribution, cooking, and serving of foods. Most of these chemicals are beneficial at the proper concentrations and safe at certain ingested doses, but they can become toxic at higher concentrations and doses. Some chemicals are undesirable in foods at any concentration but also may be unavoidable, and methods to reduce their concentration to an acceptable level may be necessary. Finally, chemical substances may be added or incorporated into foods without consumers' knowledge for malicious reasons, from ignorance, or as a result of incompetent food safety management.

### Food Additives and Adulterants

The key difference between a food additive and adulterant is consent and approval. Both food additives and adulterants are *avoidable* substances, but a food additive is legally allowed to be a part of foods *if* the proper conditions of its use are followed. In the United States, the FDA is responsible for regulating and monitoring food additives. A program called the Priority Based Assessment of Food Additives (PAFA) accomplishes this aim (Rangan and Barceloux 2009a). An essential tool of PAFA is a database maintained by the FDA that contains oral toxicology information on more than 2,100 substances added directly to foods and minimal information on more than 3,200 indirect additives in foods. Selected fields from this database are made available to the public as the Everything Added to Food in the United States (EAFUS) database. The legal definition of a food additive is contained in Section 201(s) of the Food, Drug, and Cosmetic Act. In short, according to this definition, a food additive includes any substance that can become directly or indirectly incorporated into a food during the entire production, distribution, and holding processes. Compared with a layperson's definition, the legal definition of a food additive is far-reaching and wide. The FDA even regulates the use of radiation to sterilize food like a food additive (21 CFR 179).

Food additives are used for a variety of purposes, everything from flavor enhancement and coloring to preservation and nutritional fortification. Table 3-7 lists examples of common food additives. To legally use a substance as a food additive, the substance must meet at least one of two conditions: (1) The substance must receive approval from the FDA for an intended use, or (2) the substance must be exempt from regulation as a food additive by being generally recognized as safe (GRAS). Most GRAS substances have a history of safe use dating back before 1958, the date that legislation established the initial GRAS list. Procedures are available to add substances to the GRAS list on the basis of an established history of safe use, but most new food additives must receive premarket approval by FDA following an extensive review of the scientific data on safety.

Even if a substance is approved for use as a food additive, it can still be illegally or improperly used and may cause foodborne illnesses. Improper use of food additives has been suspected in many reported foodborne intoxication outbreaks. Between May 2003 and February 2004, 10 outbreaks of foodborne intoxications occurred among children at nine different schools in Massachusetts (CDC 2006b). An investigation of the outbreaks linked the illnesses to tortillas, which were traced back to a flour tortilla manufacturer in Chicago. At the manufacturing plant, investigators found several deficiencies such as unlabeled food additives and ingredients; improper storage, use, and labeling of chemicals; and food contact surfaces that were not protected from chemical contamination. Laboratory analysis of leftover tortillas from the outbreaks found unusually high concentrations of two food additives, calcium propionate and potassium bromate used as a mold inhibitor and dough strengthener, respectively. These two food additives were strongly suspected of causing the outbreaks. Similar outbreaks had been reported years earlier in other parts of the United States.

The most serious foodborne illness outbreaks have involved the use of unapproved or illegal food additives—that is, adulterants. Foods have been adulterated for centuries, often in an effort to increase sales through false presentation (color, texture, weight, etc.) or to increase profits by substitution with cheaper ingredients (Jackson 2009). Some of the older techniques involved adding sawdust to bread, chalk to flour, and various pigments to give color. Most of the time, these adulterations to foods were economically damaging but not serious in terms of causing diseases. However, when a toxic adulterant is introduced into a food supply, the result can be catastrophic. One of the worst incidents of poisoning by food adulteration in modern history was the Spanish toxic oil syndrome. This occurred in the early 1980s when vendors diverted refined rapeseed oil intended for industrial purposes and sold it as olive oil to unsuspecting customers (Rangan and Barceloux 2009b). The incident resulted in an epidemic that killed more than 600 people and affected some 25,000 people, many of whom suffered permanent damage to their health.

**Table 3-7** Examples of Food Ingredients and Additives

| Category of Ingredient/Additive | Purposes of Additives | Common Examples |
| --- | --- | --- |
| **Preservatives** (antimicrobials and antioxidants) | Prevent food spoilage from microbes; prevent undesirable changes in flavor, color, or texture; preserve freshness | Ascorbic acid, citric acid, sodium benzoate, calcium propionate, sodium erythorbate, sodium nitrite, calcium sorbate, potassium sorbate, BHA, BHT, EDTA, tocopherols (vitamin E) |
| **Sweeteners** | Sweeten the food product, with or without the extra calories | Sucrose (sugar), glucose, fructose, sorbitol, mannitol, corn syrup, high fructose corn syrup, saccharin, aspartame, sucralose, acesulfame potassium (acesulfame-K), neotame |
| **Color additives** | Replace or offset color loss from environmental conditions and processing; enhance or add colors to food products for appeal | FD&C Blue Nos. 1 and 2, FD&C Green No. 3, FD&C Red Nos. 3 and 40, FD&C Yellow Nos. 5 and 6, Orange B, Citrus Red No. 2, annatto extract, betacarotene, grape skin extract, cochineal extract or carmine, paprika oleoresin, caramel color, fruit and vegetable juices, saffron |
| **Flavors, spices, and flavor enhancers** | Add or enhance specific flavors in food products | Natural flavoring, artificial flavor, and spices, monosodium glutamate (MSG), hydrolyzed soy protein, autolyzed yeast extract, disodium guanylate or inosinate |
| **Nutrients** (enrichment and fortification) | Replace vitamins and minerals lost in processing, or add nutrients that may be lacking in the diet | Thiamine hydrochloride, riboflavin (vitamin $B_2$), niacin, niacinamide, folate or folic acid, betacarotene, potassium iodide, iron or ferrous sulfate, alpha tocopherols, ascorbic acid, vitamin D, amino acids (L-tryptophan, L-lysine, L-leucine, L-methionine) |
| **Texturizers/stabilizers/thickners/binders/emulsifiers** | Used in foods to allow smooth mixing, prevent separation, help maintain uniform texture or consistency, and thicken | Soy lecithin, mono- and diglycerides, egg yolks, polysorbates, sorbitan monostearate, gelatin, pectin, carrageenan, xanthan gum, whey |
| **pH control agents and acidulants** | Control acidity and alkalinity, prevent spoilage | Lactic acid, citric acid, ammonium hydroxide, sodium carbonate |

Modified from FDA.

In developed countries, the legal and law enforcement infrastructure is usually sufficient to minimize the risk of economically motivated adulteration of foods. With the global economy, however, foods are exported and imported around the world, increasing the public's risk of encountering adulterated foods. The rapid economic growth of the People's Republic of China has brought attention to the challenges of controlling food adulteration (Zamiska 2007). Dozens of incidents have been identified over the last decade where foods were contaminated with substances either deliberately or incidentally. The most notable incidents involved the use of melamine, an industrial chemical used to make plastics, cleaners, glue, ink, and other products. Melamine was added to wheat gluten, used as thickener or binder, to give the false appearance of higher protein content. The melamine-tainted wheat gluten was sold and used in several products, including pet foods distributed in the United States. Tragically, in 2008, melamine also contaminated baby formula in China and caused the death of 6 infants and sickened 294,000 babies. In late 2009, China executed 2 individuals, and another 19 were convicted with lesser sentences, for their roles in the tainted baby formula.

Intentional adulteration of food for malicious purposes is an event that must be guarded against. Throughout history, the poisoning of food and drink has been used to assassinate leaders and to terrorize citizens. In these times, the possibility of terrorists deliberately contaminating the food supply with a toxic substance is a concern for everyone. Several incidents of deliberate adulteration with toxic materials have occurred in the United States but on a relatively small scale. In one incident, the pesticide endrin was found in suspected poisonings using tortillas as the vehicle (CDC 1989). In another incident, hamburger meat was poisoned with nicotine, causing approximately 100 intoxications and prompting the recall of 1,700 pounds of ground beef (CDC 2003). Whatever the motivations of a criminal to poison people or animals, food safety programs must include vulnerability assessments and security measures to minimize the risk of malicious adulteration.

## Chemicals Associated with Processing, Packaging, Storage, and Preparation

The processing, distribution, and preparation of foods expose them to a variety of potential chemical contaminants. During processing, chemical changes can occur in the food itself that generate toxic by-products. Modern machinery used in food processing plants may be a source of inadvertent contamination from oils, solvents, cleaners, insecticides, or other materials used for maintenance and normal operations. The packaging and containers used to ship and store food products may contain substances that can migrate into foodstuff. Improperly stored foods in warehouses, supermarkets, and at home can result in contamination from a nearby source of chemicals, such as pesticides, fertilizers, and commercial or household cleaners. Finally, the careless preparation of food and the use of some containers may result in chemical contamination.

Most food products undergo a series of steps in processing to prepare them for the marketplace. Depending on the final product, these steps may involve mechanical manipulation (slicing, dicing, crushing, mixing, etc), incorporation of additives for seasoning and/or to assist in processing, thermal treatment, gas treatment, packaging, and other steps or processes. In the modern food industry, these steps are highly automated whenever possible using machines, conveyors, massive cookers, sterilizers, blast freezers, and so forth. Chemicals are associated with modern machinery and technology, and when a malfunction occurs, the food products can become contaminated. Two notable epidemics occurred in Yusho, Japan, in 1968 and Yu-Cheng, Taiwan, in 1979 when rice oil became contaminated with fluids from a leaking heat exchanger, part of the food processing equipment (Rangan and Barceloux 2009a). The heat exchanger fluids contained polychlorinated biphenyls (PCBs) and polychlorinated dibenzofurans (PCDFs), and high temperatures further degraded the fluids into a mix of other chlorinated compounds. A total of approximately 4,000 people from the two epidemics suffered acute effects ranging from chloracne to neurobehavioral disorders. PCBs are also suspected human carcinogens and have a strong bioaccumulation potential.

Food processing operations frequently use heat to treat foods and ingredients, usually to kill pathogens, sterilize the product, precook the food, and/or make it ready-to-eat (RTE). Significant changes can occur to the food's chemical makeup based on the temperature, duration of heating, and other conditions. Most of these changes are beneficial, such as improving flavor, destroying certain toxins, or making nutrients more available for digestion. Other changes are undesirable, for example, causing a loss of nutrients or producing potentially toxic substances. In recent years, the compound acrylamide was detected in certain foods, among them a favorite of Americans, french fries (Stadler 2005). Acrylamide is a neurotoxicant and potential human carcinogen that is also used in industry to make polyacrylamide. It is produced under high heat ($>120°C/248°F$) in foods with abundant amounts of carbohydrates and the amino acid asparagine. The longer such foods are cooked at high temperatures, the more acrylamide is formed. The health risks of acrylamide in the human diet are still being assessed, but WHO and other organizations have expressed concerns about dietary exposure to acrylamide. In 2004, FDA issued an action plan for acrylamide in foods (FDA 2004). The action plan's goals include the development of methods to detect acrylamide in foods, research to determine the chemical mechanisms involved with acrylamide formation, determination of the U.S. consumer's dietary intake of acrylamide, and completion of a health risk assessment.

Heat treatment processes also produce other potential carcinogens. Foods that are heated sometimes produce classes of chemicals called heterocyclic aromatic amines (HAAs) and polycyclic aromatic hydrocarbons (PAHs), several known as mutagens and carcinogens. The best-known carcinogenic PAH, benzo(α)pyrene, is produced during the combustion and pyrolysis of organic compounds. Flame-grilled and smoked meats often contain significant amounts of benzo(α)pyrene, and the charred parts of foods usually have the highest levels (Kazerouni et al. 2001). Fried foods such as bacon contain detectable levels of carcinogens called N-nitrosamines. Other heating processes such as cooking, bottling, and canning may produce a class of carcinogens known as furans. The number and types of chemical reactions that occur during various heating processes, along with the different compositions of foods, make it impossible to predict all the potentially toxic compounds produced. The main concerns with these compounds are chronic, low-dose exposures in the human diet and possible long-term health effects. Additional research is necessary in the future to identify new potential toxicants from thermal processes, and risk assessment methods are needed to prioritize risks to public health.

Foods come in contact with many surfaces throughout processing, packaging, distribution, storage, preparation, and serving. Food contact surfaces are found in cookers, holding vessels, wrappers, packaging materials, cans, bottles, cutting boards and countertops, and dishes. The materials used for food contact surfaces have changed significantly over the last half century. Technological advances have introduced materials with functional properties such as reduced weight, protection against microbial contamination, easily cleanable surfaces, disposability, preservation of freshness, and other properties. These new materials appeal to consumers because of their convenience, but the discovery that some chemical components in materials migrate into foods also raises concerns.

Conventional food contact materials are divided into the following categories:

- Plastics
- Metals
- Glass and ceramics
- Paper and board
- RCF (regenerated cellulose film)
- Elastomers (natural and synthetic rubbers) (Katan 1996)

Several metal alloys are used for food processing equipment and containers. Canned foods were once a source of lead exposure from soldered seams prior to substitution with nonlead solder. In cans with unlacquered interior surfaces, significant dissolution of tin into the food could cause acute gastroenteritis, but this type of foodborne intoxication is relatively rare when canning regulations are followed (Boogaard et al. 2003). The most likely reason for metals migrating or leaching into foods is using the wrong alloy for a particular application. Innovation can be a hazardous and sometimes illegal undertaking. For example, certain metal alloys used in the food industry are not intended to be subjected to heat or acidic conditions. In the past, cadmium intoxications have occurred from using refrigerator shelves (intended for cold-holding applications) as barbeque grills and using cadmium-plated containers to store or prepare foods (Baker and Hafner 1961). Other metals such as zinc and copper have caused gastroenteritis after leaching from containers into acidic beverages (CDC 1983; Witherell, Watson, Giguere 1977). Galvanized containers contain zinc and should never be used for food preparation and storage. Care is necessary to ensure that appropriate metals (e.g., high-quality stainless steel) are used for food contact surfaces and containers (Morgan 1999).

Glass and ceramic containers are generally considered very safe for holding foods and beverages, but sometimes these materials can leach metals. High levels of lead can leach from lead crystal glassware into alcoholic beverages, citrus juices, and baby formula. Ceramic materials can also be a significant source of lead and cadmium (CDC 2004a). The greatest risks of metal contamination from ceramic dishes and cups come from lead glazing; improperly formulated or fired glazes; broken, worn, or cracked surfaces; and highly decorated surfaces, indicating pigments such as lead and cadmium. Enamelware is another source of metals when used with acidic drinks or foods; intoxications from the metal antimony have been reported in the past from storing citrus drinks in gray enamelware. Glass and ceramic materials that meet regulatory requirements for food contact surfaces are generally considered safe, but homemade or imported products may not meet regulatory standards, especially older and antique dishes and utensils.

Paper has been used as food packaging since the seventeenth century. Over the years, the number of paper and cellulose products has grown to encompass a diverse group of papers, paperboards, and laminates (Marsh and Bugusu 2007). The specific applications for food contact surfaces include cartons, wrappers, sacks, tissues, and plates and cups. Paper and cellulose products are made from chemical processes and additives that can be a source of metals (Zn, Sn, Al, Mn, Ba), dioxins, furans, and other organic compounds (Arvanitoyannis and Bosnea 2004). The propensity of chemicals to migrate into foodstuff from paper products depends greatly on the aqueous and fat content of the food. The properties of paper and cellulose products are carefully designed for specific food applications and to minimize the migration of chemical contaminants. From a food safety perspective, the greatest risk of exposure to chemicals probably results from using nonfood paper products for food contact surfaces.

Polymeric materials like plastics and elastomers contain residual monomers and additives (plasticizers, pigments, stabilizers, etc.) that migrate into foods to some degree. Polymers are chemically different from one another and are employed in many food contact applications. Various types of plastics are used to package, store, and even cook foods. Special polymeric materials are used as nonstick coatings in pots and pans or as lacquers to coat the inside of food cans. With a steadily increasing use of polymeric materials, the migration of chemicals to food and drink has been a growing concern among health scientists and consumers. Highly publicized issues in the past include carcinogenic chemicals migrating from plastics during microwaving and the migration of PFOA (perfluorooctanoic acid, or C-8, a possible human carcinogen) from Teflon and other nonstick coatings. More recently, revelations about the migration of phthalates from soft plastics and bisphenol A (BPA) from hard plastics and lacquer coatings have caused alarm among consumers. The health concerns with phthalates and BPA are possible developmental effects in children and endocrine disruption, though the health significance of low concentrations found in foods is hotly debated.

From a legal perspective, the chemical components that migrate from food contact surfaces are considered "indirect" food additives. As such, these chemicals are considered "avoidable" and are regulated by the FDA. Therefore, any material intended for use as a food contact surface with potential chemical migrants must meet one of the following conditions: (1) The chemical is not expected to become a "component" of a food with the material's intended use; (2) the chemical is on the GRAS listing; (3) the chemical has been prior-sanctioned (under the PAFA program); or (4) a "no migration" determination of the material has been made (Heckman 2005). The "no migration" determination is controversial and the subject of many court cases. The problem stems from whether "no migration" literally means absolutely no migration or minimal migration.

## Allergens and Food Intolerance

Certain individuals experience adverse reactions to particular foods without exposure to known toxicants or toxins. Such nontoxic reactions are classified as either food allergies or food intolerance (Atkins 2008). The primary difference between these two categories is involvement of the immune system. Food allergies are abnormal immunologic responses to proteins in foods, whereas food intolerance is a nonimmunologic response to a substance in the food and/or a specific physiologic abnormality in the individual (Hare and Fasono 2008). Food allergies are further classified on the basis of involvement by a particular antibody protein, called immunoglobulin E (IgE). Allergies that are IgE-mediated produce immediate hypersensitivity reactions to food proteins, typically within minutes to one hour, and may involve the gastrointestinal tract, skin, and/or respiratory tract (Nowak-Wegrzyn and Sampson 2006). If the IgE-mediated reaction is broadly systemic, then a potentially deadly condition known as anaphylactic shock is possible. Anaphylactic reactions occur among sensitized individuals most often after consuming peanuts, tree nuts, fish, and shellfish.

A second type of food allergy is a combination of IgE- and cell-mediated mechanisms. In this type of allergy, both IgE antibodies and T-lymphocyte cells are involved. The typical types of responses with the mixed mechanisms of allergy are eosinophilic esophagitis and eosinophilic gastroenteritis, with possible atopic dermatitis or asthma (Atkins 2008). In this type of allergy, white blood cells called eosinophils infiltrate the mucosa of the gastrointestinal tract. The third type of allergy is cell-mediated (non-IgE) and principally involves the gastrointestinal tract with a clinical presentation of vomiting, abdominal pain and cramps, and occasionally bloody stool. This type of allergy is also known by syndromes called food-protein-induced enterocolitis, celiac disease, and infantile colic (Nowak-Wegrzyn and Sampson 2006). Celiac disease, often confused with gluten intolerance, is an autoimmune disorder that is triggered by the alcohol-soluble portion of gluten called gliadin.

The incidence of food allergies has been increasing over the past 20 years, but the exact percentage of the population affected is difficult to estimate because of erroneous self-reporting and misunderstandings about true food allergies. Some estimates of food allergies are 8% in infants and children and 4% in adults, and recent studies report a doubling in peanut-associated allergies (Nowak-Wegrzyn and Sampson 2006). The most common food allergies among children involve cow's milk, eggs, peanuts, soy, wheat, tree nuts, and fish; among adults, the most common food allergies involve shellfish, peanuts, tree nuts, and fish (Hare and Fasano 2008). Prevention of allergic food reactions is best accomplished by complete avoidance of the offending foods. This is difficult for a number of reasons. First, the individual must identify beforehand the allergens or foods involved, either through specific medical testing and/or the process of elimination. Second, foods are often mixtures of poorly defined ingredients and may contain the specific allergens, or other proteins may have cross-reactive properties with the antigens. Third, labels on food ingredients are helpful in avoidance diets but not always fool-proof sources of information. For severe food allergies, a complete elimination diet may be necessary. In this approach, a great variety of foods are removed from the individual's diet at one time, but drawbacks of this approach include unknown allergens in other foods, poor nutritional intake, and unpalatable diets (Atkins 2008). If all avoidance and elimination diets do not work, pharmacological interventions and prophylactic treatments are clinical options for some individuals.

Food intolerance is a nonallergic sensitivity to certain foods or ingredients. The underlying biological mechanisms can be specific, multicausal, or not clearly understood in some cases. The majority of food intolerances are the result of genetic or acquired deficiencies in metabolism. Lactose and fructose intolerance are examples of genetic deficiencies that result from low production levels of enzymes (i.e., lactase and fructase) necessary to digest these sugars. Favism is a genetic condition in which an enzyme (G6PD) deficiency causes an increased sensitivity to hemolytic toxins in fava beans (Taylor, Helfe, Gauger 2001). Other food intolerances are considered idiosyncratic reactions, meaning they are unusual and exaggerated responses to a substance. For some idiosyncratic reactions, the exact mechanisms are either unknown, involve several possible mechanisms, and/or are difficult to prove scientifically. Idiosyncratic reactions to sulfites added to foods can result in asthmatic responses, sometimes quite severe. Monosodium glutamate (MSG) is a common food additive that has been blamed for foodborne illness outbreaks dubbed the "Chinese restaurant syndrome," but despite decades of scientific research, the relationship between MSG ingestion and various idiosyncratic reactions has not been clearly established (Williams and Woessner 2009). Individual sensitivities to MSG may certainly exist, but they are considered extremely rare. Other substances and food additives have been implicated in idiosyncratic reactions, but most remain unproven scientifically. The options for prevention of food intolerance are essentially the same as for food allergies.

From a food safety perspective, food allergies and food intolerance represent special challenges for food manufacturers, supermarkets, and food service establishments. Careful accountability and listing of ingredients on food labels are important to warn consumers with allergies or intolerance. Precautions during food processing and preparation are necessary to prevent cross-contamination of foods with potential allergenic or intolerant substances. Failure to minimize the risks to sensitive consumers could result in serious and possibly life-threatening reactions.

## RADIATION AND RADIOISOTOPES

The words *radiation* and *nuclear* evoke a range of emotional responses among different people. Fear and apprehension are common responses that hinder the rational discussion of risks and benefits of technology such as food irradiation. The reasons for such emotional responses are based on perceptions stemming from cultural differences, personal experiences, distrust of authority, limited technical knowledge, or other factors. The inability to "sense" ionizing radiation exposures is particularly frightening for most people. Events in modern history related to threats of nuclear war and nuclear power plant accidents have justified some fears and concerns. Residual fallout from nuclear weapons testing in the twentieth century still accounts for the most widespread source of artificial radionuclides in the terrestrial environment. The Chernobyl nuclear power plant accident in 1986 resulted in the widespread contamination of ecosystems and the human food chain with radionuclides (Alexakhin et al. 2007). Despite these tragic events, the vast majority of exposure to ionizing radiation in the United States is from natural background sources (i.e., cosmic radiation and radionuclides) and medical X-rays and procedures (National Council on Radiation Protection and Measurements 2009).

Radiation is generally divided into ionizing and nonionizing types within the electromagnetic spectrum. Common and familiar sources of nonionizing radiation include microwaves and radio waves. Ionizing radiation can be produced and emitted from devices (e.g., X-ray machines), or it can be emitted from isotopes undergoing radioactive decay, also called radionuclides. Several different types of ionizing radiation occur ($\alpha$ and $\beta$ particles, $\gamma$-rays and X-ray, neutrons) with different levels of energy. An important property of ionizing radiation is that it removes electrons from the orbits of atoms, producing chemically active ions and free radicals. In biological cells, ionizing radiation causes damage by either directly breaking DNA or producing ions and free radicals that react with DNA and other biologically important molecules. Fortunately, because organisms are exposed to natural radiation, they have evolved mechanisms to repair damaged

DNA and scavenge free radicals. The hazard occurs when the ionizing radiation dose, a function of energy deposition over time, exceeds the repair capacity of the cells.

Highly energetic radiation produced by some radionuclides can directly penetrate the skin, but the greatest hazards from radionuclides are from their internalization by inhalation or consumption. About 60 radionuclides are common sources of natural radiation in the environment. Radon and its decay products are radionuclides that constitute the most common source of internalized radiation, nearly all it from inhalation, with possible contributions from drinking water. Radionuclides such as carbon-14 (C-14) and potassium-40 (K-40) are ubiquitous and are incorporated into every plant and animal. Radioactive isotopes of the elements uranium, thorium, and radium are radionuclides that produce intense radiation, but they exist naturally at relatively low abundances. Some parts of the world have unusually high background levels of radiation from naturally occurring radionuclides. Interestingly, people living in the high radiation background areas (HRBAs) do not appear to suffer adverse health effects and may actually live longer compared with people in non-HRBAs (Dissanayake 2005).

The greatest risks of food contamination with radionuclides are from uncontrolled releases by artificial (human) sources and from technologically enhanced, naturally occurring radioactive materials (Technologically-Enhanced Naturally Occurring Radioactive Material, TENORM). Table 3-8 lists artificial sources of potential radionuclides that could enter the human food chain under the right circumstances. The first few entries in Table 3-8 are sources related to nuclear technologies (power, weapons) and are highly regulated. The TENORM sources are less well known and have a variety of physical forms such as soils, sludge, pipe scale, and ore wastes (Schultheisz, Czyscinski, Klinger 2006). These sources of radionuclides are essentially wastes produced by extracting materials from the earth's crust or water, leaving behind a concentrated level of naturally occurring radioactivity. Even so, TENORM wastes are considered "low-level" radioactive waste in terms of regulatory controls. Human exposure to TENORM can occur from using wastes to make products (e.g., concrete aggregate) or from improper disposal, which may contaminate the air, groundwater, and soil—including food crops. The last category of Table 3-8, radiological terrorism, is a threat that has received greater attention in recent years (Kuna, Hon, Patočka 2009).

After the Chernobyl nuclear power plant accident in 1986, countries scrambled to put together guidelines to limit radionuclides in foodstuffs. However, regulators and toxicologists were ill prepared to tackle the complications of calculating acceptable dose levels of radionuclides in foods, partly because the radionuclides also have chemical properties that influence their internal distribution (toxicokinetics) to different target organs (Rubery 1989). Years later in the United States, the FDA established limits, called Derived Intervention Levels (DILs), for radionuclide activity in foods. If the DILs are exceeded, FDA can take several actions to protect public health. Minimal monitoring is performed by FDA for radionuclides in imported foods and foods sold through interstate commerce. Most states are responsible for radiological monitoring of agricultural and food products produced and sold within their states.

## CONTAMINATION WITH FOREIGN OBJECTS (FILTH, TOO)

All of the previous agents discussed cause foodborne illnesses by somehow interacting with the host or victim, producing either an infection, intoxication, irradiation exposure, or disruption of

**Table 3-8** Possible Artificial Sources of Radionuclides in Foods

| *Sources of Radionuclides* | *Radionuclides of Primary Concern* |
|---|---|
| Nuclear reactors | I-131; Cs-134 + Cs-137; Ru-103 + Ru-106 |
| Nuclear fuel processing plants | St-90; Cs-137; Pu-238 + Pu-239 + Am-241 |
| Nuclear waste storage facilities | Sr-90; Cs-137; Pu-238 + Pu-239 + Am-241 |
| Nuclear weapons, (i.e., dispersal of nuclear weapon material without nuclear detonation) | Pu-239 |
| Radioisotope thermoelectric generators and radioisotope heater units used in space vehicles | Pu-238 |
| Technologically enhanced, naturally occurring radiation materials (TENORM): <br><br> Geothermal energy production wastes, oil and gas production wastes, drinking water treatment wastes, waste water treatment wastes, aluminum production wastes, coal ash, copper mining and production wastes, fertilizer and fertilizer production wastes, gold and silver mining wastes, rare earths mining wastes, titanium production wastes, uranium mining wastes, zircon mining wastes | U-238/235/234 + decay products; Ra-238/226 + decay products; Th-232 + decay products; Pb-210 |
| Radiological terrorism | Commercially available radionuclides/ radioisotopes |

*Source:* Compiled from the FDA and the EPA.

homeostasis. Another form of harm is simply physical injury caused by foreign objects in food. The number and types of injuries caused by foreign objects in foods are not tracked very well, and the true extent of harm from such contamination is difficult to assess. Nevertheless, a few studies from decades ago have been conducted on foreign objects in foods (Hyman, Klontz, Tollefson 1993; Olsen 1998b). From the limited data analyzed, the following objects, in order of reported frequency, were most responsible for injury:

1. Glass
2. Metal
3. Plastic
4. Stone or rock
5. Capsules or crystals
6. Pits or shells
7. Wood
8. Other miscellaneous objects

The frequency of injury from encountering a foreign object in food is rare, anywhere from 1–14% (Hyman et al. 1993; Olsen 1998b). Furthermore, a small percentage of those who were injured sought medical attention. The most common types of injuries involved cuts to the mouth and throat, and chipped or broken teeth. Occasionally, swallowed objects may need surgical removal, or lacerations may become infected. Deaths are extremely rare and usually result from choking. One of the most disconcerting findings was the relative frequency of injuries to infants and children from glass fragments. Decades ago, manufacturers had quality control problems with glass fragments in jarred baby food. Glass "slivers" posed the greatest risk of perforating an infant's intestines. Another possible source of glass particles and slivers were broken light bulbs in food processing and preparation areas. The types of metals encountered included bolts, nails, blades, shavings, and wire. These items were most likely contaminants from food processing operations, but food preparation or kitchen activities can also be a source of metal contaminants like paper clips, staples, lids, broken utensils, etc. Plastics are virtually ubiquitous in the food industry, so a piece of hard plastic can come from practically anywhere.

Hard foreign objects may also originate in the preharvest portion of the food handling chain. Stones, rocks, burrs, pieces of wood, and other objects may be caught in combines or swept into storage bins. Other hard objects are not considered "foreign" in foods but could nonetheless cause injuries. Examples include fish bones, a common source of injury, and fractured or splintered animal bones in meat products. Vegetable and fruit products may contain unwanted pits, seeds, and hard/sharp stems. With raw or unprocessed foods, it is reasonable to anticipate and avoid naturally hard items such as bones and pits. On the other hand, food products marketed to the consumer as deboned or pitted imply a reasonable expectation of safety from naturally hard objects.

Finally, some foreign objects in foods are not necessarily hazardous but are objectionable and distasteful. Commonly known as filth, objects such as dirt, insect parts, animal and human hairs, slime, and severely damaged or fragmented food parts are considered undesirable and aesthetically unpleasing. But do they represent a food safety hazard? In most cases, the answer is no. However, the determination of safety is not always straightforward. Although most insect parts are not toxigenic if consumed, evidence exists that mite infestations can cause allergic and anaphylactic reactions; several species of insects are known transmitters of enteric diseases, or they are indicators of unsanitary conditions (Olsen 1998a, 1998c). In other words, filth may be considered either hazardous or nonhazardous. Under the Food, Drug, and Cosmetic Act, contaminants such as filth and foreign objects are regulated by the FDA as adulterants. Some of these adulterants are avoidable, whereas others are unavoidable and must be limited as much as practical. To determine the proper enforcement options under the law, FDA uses three categories for objects in foods: Category 1 represents health hazards; category 2 represents indicators of insanitation; and category 3 represents natural or unavoidable defects (Olsen et al. 2001). To withstand a possible court challenge, detailed scientific criteria have been developed to assign the appropriate category for filth and foreign objects in foods.

---

## REFERENCES

Agata N, Ohta M, Mori M, Isobe M. 1995. A novel dodecadepsipeptide, cereulide, is an emetic toxin of *Bacillus cereus*. *FEMS Microbiol Lett* 129(1):17–20.

Alexakhin RM, Sanzharova NI, Fesenko SV, Spiridonov SI, Panov AV. 2007. Chernobyl radionuclide distribution, migration, and environmental and agricultural impacts. *Health Phys* 93(5):418–426.

Angulo FJ, Getz J, Taylor JP, Hendricks KA, Hatheway CL, Barth SS, Solomon HM, Larson AE, Johnson EA, Nickey LN, et al. 1998. A large outbreak of botulism: The hazardous baked potato. *J Infect Dis* 178(1):172–177.

Aoshima K. 1987. Epidemiology of renal tubular dysfunction in the inhabitants of a cadmium-polluted area in the Jinzu river basin in Toyama prefecture. *Tohoku J Exp Med* 152(2):151–172.

Arvanitoyannis IS, Bosnea L. 2004. Migration of substances from food packaging materials to foods. *Crit Rev Food Sci Nutr* 44(2):63–76.

Atkins D. 2008. Food allergy: Diagnosis and management. *Prim Care* 35(1):vii,40,119.

Baker TD, Hafner WG. 1961. Cadmium poisoning from a refrigerator shelf used as an improvised barbecue grill. *Public Health Rep* 76:543–544.

Balaban N, Rasooly A. 2000. Staphylococcal enterotoxins. *Int J Food Microbiol* 61(1):1–10.

Barbee G, Berry-Caban C, Barry J, Borys D, Ward J, Salyer S. 2009. Analysis of mushroom exposures in Texas requiring hospitalization, 2005–2006. *J Med Toxicol* 5(2):59–62.

Barceloux DG. 2008. *Medical toxicology of natural substances: Foods, fungi, medicinal herbs, plants, and venomous animals.* Hoboken, NJ: John Wiley.

Bennett JW, Klich M. 2003. Mycotoxins. *Clin Microbiol Rev* 16(3):497–516.

Berenbaum MR. 1995. The chemistry of defense: Theory and practice. In: *The chemistry of biotic interaction.* Eisner T, Meinwald J, eds. Washington, DC: National Academy Press.

Berger KJ, Guss DA. 2005a. Mycotoxins revisited: Part II. *J Emerg Med* 28(2):175–183.

Berger KJ, Guss DA. 2005b. Mycotoxins revisited: Part I. *J Emerg Med* 28(1):53–62.

Bergdoll MS, Wong AC. 2006. Staphylococcal intoxications. In: *Foodborne infections and intoxications.* 3rd ed. (pp. 523–562). Reimann HP, Cliver DO, eds. Amsterdam: Elsevier.

Boogaard PJ, Boisset M, Blunden S, Davies S, Ong TJ, Taverne JP. 2003. Comparative assessment of gastrointestinal irritant potency in man of tin(II) chloride and tin migrated from packaging. *Food Chem Toxicol* 41(12):1663–1670.

Brett MM. 2003. Food poisoning associated with biotoxins in fish and shellfish. *Curr Opin Infect Dis* 16(5):461–465.

Centers for Disease Control and Prevention. 2009. Surveillance for foodborne disease outbreaks—United States, 2006. *MMWR* 58(22):609–615.

Centers for Disease Control and Prevention. 2007a. Botulism associated with commercially canned chili sauce—Texas and Indiana, July 2007. *MMWR* 56(30):767–769.

Centers for Disease Control and Prevention. 2007b. Foodborne botulism from home-prepared fermented tofu—California, 2006. *MMWR* 56(5):96–97.

Centers for Disease Control and Prevention. 2007c. Scombroid fish poisoning associated with tuna steaks—Louisiana and Tennessee, 2006. *MMWR* 56(32):817–819.

Centers for Disease Control and Prevention. 2006a. Botulism associated with commercial carrot juice—Georgia and Florida, September 2006. *MMWR* 55(40):1098–1099.

Centers for Disease Control and Prevention. 2006b. Multiple outbreaks of gastrointestinal illness among school children associated with consumption of flour tortillas—Massachusetts, 2003–2004. *MMWR* 55(1):8–11.

Centers for Disease Control and Prevention. 2004a. Childhood lead poisoning from commercially manufactured French ceramic dinnerware—New York City, 2003. *MMWR* 53(26):584–586.

Centers for Disease Control and Prevention. 2004b. Outbreak of aflatoxin poisoning—eastern and central provinces, Kenya, January–July 2004. *MMWR* 53(34):790–793.

Centers for Disease Control and Prevention. 2003. Nicotine poisoning after ingestion of contaminated ground beef—Michigan, 2003. *MMWR* 52(18):413–416.

Centers for Disease Control and Prevention. 2001. Botulism outbreak associated with eating fermented food—Alaska, 2001. *MMWR* 50(32):680–682.

Centers for Disease Control and Prevention. 1999. Aldicarb as a cause of food poisoning—Louisiana, 1998. *MMWR* 48(13):269–271.

Centers for Disease Control and Prevention. 1997. *Amanita phalloides* mushroom poisoning—northern California, January 1997. *MMWR* 46(22):489–492.

Centers for Disease Control and Prevention. 1996. Tetrodotoxin poisoning associated with eating puffer fish transported from Japan—California, 1996. *MMWR* 45(19):389–391.

Centers for Disease Control and Prevention. 1995. Acute hepatitis and renal failure following ingestion of raw carp gallbladders—Maryland and Pennsylvania, 1991 and 1994. *MMWR* 44(30):565–566.

Centers for Disease Control and Prevention. 1989. Endrin poisoning associated with taquito ingestion—California. *MMWR* 38(19):345–347.

Centers for Disease Control and Prevention. 1986. Aldicarb food poisoning from contaminated melons—California. *MMWR* 35(16):254–258.

Centers for Disease Control and Prevention. 1983. Illness associated with elevated levels of zinc in fruit punch—New Mexico. *MMWR* 32(19):257–258.

Clarkson TW. 1995. Environmental contaminants in the food chain. *Am J Clin Nutr* 61(3 Suppl):682S–686S.

Deeds JR, Landsberg JH, Etheridge SM, Pitcher GC, Longan SW. 2008. Non-traditional vectors for paralytic shellfish poisoning. *Mar Drugs* 6(2):308–348.

Diamond J. 2002. Evolution, consequences and future of plant and animal domestication. *Nature* 418(6898):700–707.

Diaz JH. 2005a. Evolving global epidemiology, syndromic classification, general management, and prevention of unknown mushroom poisonings. *Crit Care Med* 33(2):419–426.

Diaz JH. 2005b. Syndromic diagnosis and management of confirmed mushroom poisonings. *Crit Care Med* 33(2):427–436.

Dissanayake C. 2005. Global voices of science. Of stones and health: Medical geology in Sri Lanka. *Science* 309(5736): 883–885.

Ecker DJ, Sampath R, Willett P, Wyatt JR, Samant V, Massire C, Hall TA, Hari K, McNeil JA, Buchen-Osmond C, et al. 2005. The microbial Rosetta Stone database: A compilation of global and emerging infectious microorganisms and bioterrorist threat agents. *BMC Microbiol* 5:19.

Environmental Protection Agency. 2007. *2005/2006 national listing of fish advisories.* Report nr EPA-823-F-07-003. Washington, DC: Environmental Protection Agency. Available from: http://www.epa.gov/fishadvisories.

Environmental Protection Agency. 1997. *Terms of environment: Glossary, abbreviations, and acronyms.* Report nr 175-B-97-001. Washington, DC: Environmental Protection Agency. Available from: http://www.epa.gov/glossary/.

Food and Drug Administration. 2009. *Foodborne pathogenic microorganisms and natural toxins handbook: The "bad bug book."* Washington, DC: U.S. Food and Drug Administration.

Food and Drug Administration. 2004. *FDA action plan for acrylamide in food.* Washington, DC: Food and Drug Administration. Available from: http://www.fda.gov/Food/FoodSafety/FoodContaminantsAdulteration/ChemicalContaminants/Acrylamide/ucm053519.htm.

Food and Drug Administration and Environmental Protection Agency. 2004. *2004 EPA and FDA advice for: Women who might become pregnant; women who are pregnant, nursing mothers; young children.* Report nr EPA-823-R-04-005. Washington, DC: Food and Drug Administration, Environmental Protection Agency.

Food Code. 2009. *Recommendations of the United States Public Health Service, Food and Drug Administration.* Report nr PB2009112613. Alexandria, VA: National Technical Information Service Publication.

Friedman MA, Fleming LE, Fernandez M, Bienfang P, Schrank K, Dickey R, Bottein MY, Backer L, Ayyar R, Weisman R, et al. 2008. Ciguatera fish poisoning: Treatment, prevention and management. *Mar Drugs* 6(3):456–479.

Froberg B, Ibrahim D, Furbee RB. 2007. Plant poisoning. *Emerg Med Clin North Am* 25(2):375,433, abstract ix.

Glibert PM, Anderson DM, Gentien P, Graneli E, Sellner KG. 2005. The global, complex phenomena of harmful algal blooms. *Oceanography* 18(2):136–147.

Government Accountability Office. 1992. *Food safety and quality: FDA strategy needed to address animal drug residues in milk.* Report nr GAO/RCED-92-209. Washington, DC: General Accounting Office.

Gunduz A, Turedi S, Russell RM, Ayaz FA. 2008. Clinical review of grayanotoxin/mad honey poisoning past and present. *Clin Toxicol (Phila)* 46(5):437–442.

Hare ND, Fasano MB. 2008. Clinical manifestations of food allergy: Differentiating true allergy from food intolerance. *Postgrad Med* 120(2):E01–05.

Hathcock JN, Hattan DG, Jenkins MY, McDonald JT, Sundaresan PR, Wilkening VL. 1990. Evaluation of vitamin A toxicity. *Am J Clin Nutr* 52(2):183–202.

Heckman JH. 2005. Food packaging regulation in the United States and the European Union. *Regul Toxicol Pharmacol* 42(1):96–122.

Heymann DL, ed. 2008. *Control of communicable diseases manual.* 19th ed. Washington, DC: American Public Health Association.

Hodgson E. 2004. *A textbook of modern toxicology.* 3rd ed. Hoboken, NJ: John Wiley.

Hopkins J. 1995. The glycoalkaloids: Naturally of interest (but a hot potato?). *Food Chem Toxicol* 33(4):323–328.

Hussein HS, Brasel JM. 2001. Toxicity, metabolism, and impact of mycotoxins on humans and animals. *Toxicology* 167(2):101–134.

Hyman FN, Klontz KC, Tollefson L. 1993. Food and drug administration surveillance of the role of foreign objects in foodborne injuries. *Public Health Rep* 108(1):54–59.

Imamura T, Ide H, Yasunaga H. 2007. History of public health crises in Japan. *J Public Health Policy* 28(2):221–237.

Jackson LS. 2009. Chemical Food Safety Issues in the United States: Past, Present, and Future. *J Agric Food Chem* 57(18):1861–1870.

Jay JM, Loessner MJ, Golden DA. 2005. *Modern food microbiology.* 7th ed. New York, NY: Springer Science+Business Media.

Kabak B, Dobson AD, Var I. 2006. Strategies to prevent mycotoxin contamination of food and animal feed: A review. *Crit Rev Food Sci Nutr* 46(8):593–619.

Katan LL. 1996. *Migration from food contact materials.* London: Blackie Academic and Professional.

Kazerouni N, Sinha R, Hsu CH, Greenberg A, Rothman N. 2001. Analysis of 200 food items for benzo[α]pyrene and estimation of its intake in an epidemiologic study. *Food Chem Toxicol* 39(5):423–436.

Kiely T, Donaldson D, Grube A. 2004. *Pesticides industry sales and usage: 2000 and 2001 market estimates.* Report nr EPA-733-R-04-001. Washington, DC: Environmental Protection Agency. Available from: http://www.epa.gov/opp00001/pestsales/01pestsales/market_estimates2001.pdf.

Knudsen I, Soborg I, Eriksen F, Pilegaard K, Pedersen J. 2008. Risk management and risk assessment of novel plant foods: Concepts and principles. *Food Chem Toxicol* 46(5):1681–1705.

Korpan YI, Nazarenko EA, Skryshevskaya IV, Martelet C, Jaffrezic-Renault N, El'skaya AV. 2004. Potato glycoalkaloids: True safety or false sense of security? *Trends Biotechnol* 22(3):147–151.

Kuehnert MJ, Kruszon-Moran D, Hill HA, McQuillan G, McAllister SK, Fosheim G, McDougal LK, Chaitram J, Jensen B, Fridkin SK, et al. 2006. Prevalence of *Staphylococcus aureus* nasal colonization in the United States, 2001–2002. *J Infect Dis* 193(2):172–179.

Kuna P, Hon Z, Patočka J. 2009. How serious is threat of radiological terrorism? *Acta Medica* 52(3):85–89.

LeBlanc GA. 2004. Acute toxicity. In: *A textbook of modern toxicology.* 3rd ed. Hodgson E, ed. Hoboken, NJ: John Wiley.

Le Loir Y, Baron F, Gautier M. 2003. *Staphylococcus aureus* and food poisoning. *Genet Mol Res* 2(1):63–76.

Lee MR. 2006. The Solanaceae: Foods and poisons. *J R Coll Physicians Edinb* 36(2):162–169.

Lips P. 2003. Hypervitaminosis A and fractures. *N Engl J Med* 348(4):347–349.

Madsen JM. 2001. Toxins as weapons of mass destruction. A comparison and contrast with biological-warfare and chemical-warfare agents. *Clin Lab Med* 21(3):593–605.

Marsh K, Bugusu B. 2007. Food packaging—roles, materials, and environmental issues. *J Food Sci* 72(3):R39–55.

Mathew AG, Cissell R, Liamthong S. 2007. Antibiotic resistance in bacteria associated with food animals: A United States perspective of livestock production. *Foodborne Pathog Dis* 4(2):115–133.

Mebs D. 2002. *Venomous and poisonous animals: A handbook for biologists, toxicologists and toxinologists, physicians and pharmacists.* New York, NY: CRC Press.

Mebs D. 2001. Toxicity in animals. Trends in evolution? *Toxicon* 39(1):87–96.

Morgan JN. 1999. Effects of processing of heavy metal content of foods. *Adv Exp Med Biol* 459:195–211.

National Council on Radiation Protection and Measurements. 2009. *Ionizing radiation exposure of the population of the United States (2009).* Report nr No. 160. Bethesda, MD: National Council on Radiation Protection and Measurements.

Nogawa K, Kido T. 1993. Biological monitoring of cadmium exposure in itai-itai disease epidemiology. *Int Arch Occup Environ Health* 65(1 Suppl):S43–46.

Noguchi T, Arakawa O. 2008. Tetrodotoxin—distribution and accumulation in aquatic organisms, and cases of human intoxication. *Mar Drugs* 6(2):220–242.

Nowak-Wegrzyn A, Sampson HA. 2006. Adverse reactions to foods. *Med Clin North Am* 90(1):97–127.

Olsen AR. 1998a. Regulatory action criteria for filth and other extraneous materials. III. Review of flies and foodborne enteric disease. *Regul Toxicol Pharmacol* 28(3):199–211.

Olsen AR. 1998b. Regulatory action criteria for filth and other extraneous materials. II. Allergenic mites: An emerging food safety issue. *Regul Toxicol Pharmacol* 28(3):190–198.

Olsen AR. 1998c. Regulatory action criteria for filth and other extraneous materials. I. Review of hard or sharp foreign objects as physical hazards in food. *Regul Toxicol Pharmacol* 28(3):181–189.

Olsen AR, Gecan JS, Ziobro GC, Bryce JR. 2001. Regulatory action criteria for filth and other extraneous materials v. strategy for evaluating hazardous and nonhazardous filth. *Regul Toxicol Pharmacol* 33(3):363–392.

Patten RC. 1981. Aflatoxins and disease. *Am J Trop Med Hyg* 30(2):422–425.

Paul VJ, Arthur KE, Ritson-Williams R, Ross C, Sharp K. 2007. Chemical defenses: From compounds to communities. *Biol Bull* 213(3):226–251.

Peraica M, Domijan AM, Miletic-Medved M, Fuchs R. 2008. The involvement of mycotoxins in the development of endemic nephropathy. *Wien Klin Wochenschr* 120(13–14):402–427.

Plants for a Future. 2008. Edible plants. Cornwall, England: Plants for a Future. Available from: http://www.pfaf.org/leaflets/edible_uses.php.

Rangan C, Barceloux DG. 2009a. Food additives and sensitivities. *Dis Mon* 55(5):292–311.

Rangan C, Barceloux DG. 2009b. Food contamination. *Dis Mon* 55(5):263–291.

Richard JL. 2007. Some major mycotoxins and their mycotoxicoses—an overview. *Int J Food Microbiol* 119(1–2):3–10.

Rubery ED. 1989. Radionuclides in food: A neglected branch of toxicology? *Hum Toxicol* 8(2):79–86.

Salleras L, Dominguez A, Mata E, Taberner JL, Moro I, Salva P. 1995. Epidemiologic study of an outbreak of clenbuterol poisoning in Catalonia, Spain. *Public Health Rep* 110(3):338–342.

Schafer KS, Kegley SE. 2002. Persistent toxic chemicals in the US food supply. *J Epidemiol Community Health* 56(11):813–817.

Scheurlen C, Spannbrucker N, Spengler U, Zachoval R, Schulte-Witte H, Brensing KA, Sauerbruch T. 1994. *Amanita phalloides* intoxications in a family of Russian immigrants. Case reports and review of the literature with a focus on orthotopic liver transplantation. *Z Gastroenterol* 32(7):399–404.

Schoeni JL, Wong AC. 2005. *Bacillus cereus* food poisoning and its toxins. *J Food Prot* 68(3):636–648.

Schultheisz DJ, Czyscinski KS, Klinger AD. 2006. Improving radioactive waste management: An overview of the environmental protection agency's low-activity waste effort. *Health Phys* 91(5):518–522.

Sobel J. 2005. Botulism. *Clin Infect Dis* 41(8):1167–1173.

Sobel J, Painter J. 2005. Illnesses caused by marine toxins. *Clin Infect Dis* 41(9):1290–1296.

Stadler RH. 2005. Acrylamide formation in different foods and potential strategies for reduction. *Adv Exp Med Biol* 561:157–169.

Stenfors Arnesen LP, Fagerlund A, Granum PE. 2008. From soil to gut: *Bacillus cereus* and its food poisoning toxins. *FEMS Microbiol Rev* 32(4):579–606.

Taylor SL, Helfe SL, Gauger BJ. 2001. Food allergies and sensitivities. In: *Food toxicology*. Helferich W, Winter CK, eds. (pp. 1–36). Boca Raton, FL: CRC Press.

Thomas D, Chou S, Dauwalder O, Lina G. 2007. Diversity in *Staphylococcus aureus* enterotoxins. *Chem Immunol Allergy* 93:24–41.

Todd EC, Greig JD, Bartleson CA, Michaels BS. 2007. Outbreaks where food workers have been implicated in the spread of foodborne disease. Part 3. Factors contributing to outbreaks and description of outbreak categories. *J Food Prot* 70(9):2199–2217.

Toyofuku H. 2006. Joint FAO/WHO/IOC activities to provide scientific advice on marine biotoxins (research report). *Mar Pollut Bull* 52(12):1735–1745.

U.S. National Library of Medicine. 2005. IUPAC glossary of terms used in toxicology. Bethesda, MD: National Library of Medicine. Available from: http://sis.nlm.nih.gov/enviro/iupacglossary/references.html.

Vaughan BE. 1984. State of research: Environmental pathways and food chain transfer. *Environ Health Perspect* 54:353–371.

Wang DZ. 2008. Neurotoxins from marine dinoflagellates: A brief review. *Mar Drugs* 6(2):349–371.

Watson JT, Jones RC, Siston AM, Diaz PS, Gerber SI, Crowe JB, Satzger RD. 2005. Outbreak of food-borne illness associated with plant material containing raphides. *Clin Toxicol (Phila)* 43(1):17–21.

Wein LM, Liu Y. 2005. Analyzing a bioterror attack on the food supply: The case of botulinum toxin in milk. *Proc Natl Acad Sci U S A* 102(28):9984–9989.

Williams AN, Woessner KM. 2009. Monosodium glutamate "allergy": Menace or myth? *Clin Exp Allergy* 39(5):640–646.

Winter CK. 2001. Pesticide residues in the food supply. In: *Food toxicology*. Helferich W, Winter CK, eds. (pp. 163–186). Boca Rotan, FL: CRC Press.

Witherell LE, Watson WN, Giguere GC. 1980. Outbreak of acute copper poisoning due to soft drink dispenser. *Am J Public Health* 70(10):1115.

Zamiska M. 2007, April 13. Who's monitoring Chinese food exports? *YaleGlobal Online Magazine*.

## USEFUL RESOURCES

Environmental Protection Agency. Fish Advisories. http://water.epa.gov/scitech/swguidance/fishshellfish/fishadvisories/advisories_index.cfm

ExToxNet FAQs. Natural Toxins in Food Topics. http://extoxnet.orst.edu/faqs/natural/page1.htm

FAO Corporate Document Repository. *Marine Biotoxins.* http://www.fao.org/docrep/007/y5486e/y5486e00.htm#Contents

Food Allergy and Anaphylaxis Network (FAAN). www.foodallergy.org

Food and Drug Administration. CPG Sec. 560.750 Radionuclides in Imported Foods—Levels of Concern. http://www.fda.gov/ICECI/ComplianceManuals/CompliancePolicyGuidanceManual/ucm074576.htm

Food and Drug Administration. FDA Poisonous Plant Database. http://www.accessdata.fda.gov/scripts/Plantox/

Food and Drug Administration. Food Ingredients & Packaging. http://www.fda.gov/Food/FoodIngredientsPackaging/default.htm

FoodContactMaterials.com. The Internet resource for materials that come into contact with food. http://www.foodcontactmaterials.com/

Harmful Algae. Distribution of HABs in the U.S. http://www.whoi.edu/redtide/page.do?pid=14898

International Programme on Chemical Safety. Joint FAO/WHO Expert Committee on Food Additives (JECFA). http://www.who.int/ipcs/food/jecfa/en/

Linus Pauling Institute at Oregon State University. Mission statement. http://lpi.oregonstate.edu/ *Mycotoxicology Newsletter.* http://www.mycotoxicology.org/

National Council on Radiation Protection and Measurements. http://www.ncrponline.org/

National Institutes of Health, Office of Dietary Supplements. http://ods.od.nih.gov/index.aspx

Society for Mycotoxin Research. http://www.mycotoxin.de/docs/public/home.asp

U.S. National Library of Medicine. Environmental Health and Toxicology resources page. Diseases and the Environment. http://sis.nlm.nih.gov/enviro.html

U.S. National Library of Medicine. IUPAC Glossary of Terms Used In Toxicology—Introduction. http://sis.nlm.nih.gov/enviro/iupacglossary/frontmatter.html

# CHAPTER 4

# Food Safety: Principles of Prevention

## LEARNING OBJECTIVES

1. Explain the differences between primary habitats/reservoirs and secondary sources of microbial contamination.
2. For important pathogenic and toxigenic microorganisms, identify the primary habitats/reservoirs and secondary sources of food contamination.
3. Define the terms *intrinsic* and *extrinsic parameters* with respect to microbial growth in foods.
4. List and describe the intrinsic and extrinsic parameters of foods, and describe the importance of each parameter in terms of microbial survival and growth.
5. Recognize the range of values for intrinsic and extrinsic parameters that support the growth of pathogenic and toxigenic microorganisms.
6. Explain why pathogens are of more concern in certain food types compared with other food types.
7. Define the term *predictive microbiology* with respect to food science and protection.
8. Describe the benefits and limitations of modeling microbial survival and growth in foods.
9. Define the terms *potentially hazardous food* (PHF) and *temperature controlled for safety* (TCS).
10. Given the necessary information, determine whether a food is considered PHF/TCS.
11. Explain how chemicals and toxins can be eliminated or excluded from foods.
12. Describe the importance of sanitary principles and practices with respect to food safety.
13. Recognize inadequate practices in cleaning and sanitizing surfaces/equipment, waste disposal, and pest control.
14. Identify and describe the relative importance of risk factors that contribute to foodborne illnesses in retail food facilities.
15. Explain how the source of foods is important in preventing foodborne illnesses.
16. Recognize inadequate cooking temperatures for common food types.

17. Differentiate between acceptable and unacceptable scenarios in the time/temperature holding requirements of foods.
18. List and describe factors that contribute to inadequate cleaning of food equipment and contact surfaces.
19. Describe several scenarios of how cross-contamination occurs.
20. Explain the importance of food worker hygiene in foodborne illness prevention.
21. Identify the causes of and solutions to poor worker hygiene.
22. Describe the need for and challenges of food worker education and training.

## INTRODUCTION

According to the Codex Alimentarius Commission, a food hazard is a "biological, chemical or physical agent in, or condition of, food with the potential to cause an adverse health effect" (Codex Alimentarius Commission 2010). From the material presented earlier in Chapters 2 and 3, it should be apparent that the etiologic agents of foodborne diseases are numerous and originate from many sources. To test all foods for the presence of every etiologic agent is impractical and unrealistic. Therefore, standards are used to guide the food industry in controlling food hazards and preventing foodborne illnesses; these standards also assist food safety professionals in determining whether or not food products are deemed "safe." Food safety standards vary in degree of complexity and enforceability, from federal regulations that mandate specific standards for a particular food product to general advice for the consumer on safe food handling practices at home. Over the past several decades, greater emphasis has been placed on the use of scientific and factual information in the prioritization and setting of food safety standards. The preferred approach to incorporating scientific information into setting food safety standards is called risk analysis, which is discussed in greater detail in Chapter 6. Because of the growing complexity of food operations, greater emphasis is also being placed on the systematic control of food hazards by using food safety management tools, such as the Hazard Analysis and Critical Control Point (HACCP) process. This food safety management tool and others are discussed in Chapters 6 and 8.

The purpose of this chapter is to familiarize the student with the basic principles of prevention in food safety. Furthermore, this chapter provides a background in the scientific underpinnings and public health rationale of the prevention principles, which are the basis of most food safety standards. This chapter makes frequent references to the retail food establishment model standards known as the Food Code (Food and Drug Administration and Public Health Service [FDA and PHS] 2009). This document is periodically updated and provides public health rationale for retail food safety standards. Most food safety standards for the nonretail portion of the food industry are contained in federal and/or state regulations; this chapter and the rest of the book make occasional referrals to these regulations. The Food Code provides an excellent point of reference for principles of prevention that are relevant for most food handling operations.

This chapter begins with a section on the most common and important type of food hazards, microbial contamination and growth. Unlike Chapters 2 and 3, this section emphasizes the sources of microbial contamination and the relevance of microbial growth in the causation of foodborne diseases. Parameters for controlling microbial growth are introduced; the importance of this topic is a recurring theme in other chapters. The next section discusses the prevention of contamination with chemical pollutants and toxins. Next, the principles and purposes of sanitation are examined. Sanitation is the cornerstone of food safety, and the student must become very familiar with sanitary practices, sanitization of surfaces and equipment, waste disposal, and pest/disease vector control. The next section is on foodborne illness risk factors, which brings the other topics together into a comprehensive perspective of prevention. Finally, given the great importance of food workers in the prevention and causation of foodborne illnesses, the topic of food worker education and training is covered.

## REDUCE MICROBIAL CONTAMINATION AND CONTROL GROWTH

A simplistic viewpoint is that germs are everywhere; care is necessary to keep food clean; and cooking is needed to kill the germs. Whereas food safety guidance must be simple enough for most people to understand, the food safety professional needs a greater depth and breadth of knowledge to prioritize and solve problems. This begins with understanding the relative importance of different microbial sources—specifically for the pathogenic and toxigenic microorganisms relevant to food safety. The control of microbial hazards in foods has become increasingly sophisticated over the decades. Basic food sanitation has been augmented with volumes of regulations, engineering controls, veterinary medicine, applied microbiological sciences, and disease surveillance programs. All of these contributions are essential to controlling microbial hazards in the modern food industry. Yet, despite the sophistication and multidisciplinary involvement, the control of microbial hazards in foods is rooted in two basic principles: (1) exclude and/or reduce microbial contamination of foods, and (2) limit or control microbial growth in foods.

### Sources of Contamination

Microorganisms have adapted to specific niches, and in the process, new species and strains have evolved. The main sources of microorganisms in foods are typically associated with their primary habitats. For example, most species within the bacterial family Enterobacteriaceae live in the intestinal tracts of animals, and the primary source of Enterobacteriaceae in foods is the feces of animals. Similarly, microorganisms that normally live in the soil contaminate foods through contact with dirt and objects in contact with soil. The spore-forming bacteria of the genera *Bacillus* and *Clostridium* are normally found in the soil and water runoff/sediments. The bacterium *Listeria monocytogenes* has adapted to living in both the environment and animal hosts. For pathogenic microorganisms that require living hosts, the degree of host specificity is very important in determining the main source of food contamination. With a few exotic exceptions, enteric viruses that infect humans are very host-specific, and the human gastrointestinal tract is the primary habitat and source of these viruses. Table 4-1 lists the primary habitats and reservoirs for important pathogenic and toxigenic microorganisms. Details on the reservoirs for each infectious agent were previously provided, and the student is referred to Chapter 2 for review.

Under ideal conditions, the exclusion of microbial contamination starts with the primary habitats and reservoirs of foodborne pathogenic and toxigenic microorganisms. In the case of zoonotic pathogens, infected animals should be excluded from slaughter and treated with antimicrobials to prevent the spread of infection throughout a herd or flock. The intestines of slaughtered animals

**Table 4-1** Primary Habitats/Reservoirs and Secondary Sources of Important Pathogens and Toxigenic Microorganisms

| Pathogens or Toxigenic Microorganisms | Primary Habitats and Reservoirs | Secondary Contamination Sources |
|---|---|---|
| **Bacteria** | | |
| Family Enterobacteriaceae *Escherichia Salmonella Yersinia Shigella* | Intestinal tracts of infected animals and/or humans | Cross contamination of meats, other foods, contact surfaces, and food handlers. Feces-contaminated water. Runoff/manure contamination in produce fields. Shellfish from sewage-contaminated waters |
| *Campylobacter* | Intestinal tracts of infected animals, possibly humans. Protozoa in waters/puddles | Cross contamination of meats, other foods, contact surfaces, and food handlers |
| Spore-Forming Bacteria *Bacillus Clostridium* | Soil and water | Plants, animals, airborne dust, food handlers, utensils, contact surfaces |
| *Listeria* | Soil, water, plants, silage, and GI tracts of infected animals and humans | Cross contamination of foods and contact surfaces in food processing plants and preparation areas |
| *Staphylococcus* | Nasal passages, GI tracts, skin/hides, and infected tissues of humans and/or animals | Cross contamination of foods and contact surfaces in food processing plants and preparation areas |
| Marine/Aquatic Bacteria *Vibrio Aeromonas* Histamine-toxin producers | Marine or estuarine waters, sediments. Shellfish | GI tracts for *Cholera*-infected humans. Water/food contact surfaces |
| **Enteric Viruses** Hepatitis viruses, Noroviruses, Rotavirus | Human gastrointestinal tracts | Contamination and cross contamination of food contact surfaces, utensils, clothing, etc. Shellfish from sewage-contaminated waters |
| **Protozoans** *Cryptosporidium, Giardia, Cyclospora, Toxoplasma* | Intestinal tracts of mostly animals and sometimes humans | Contaminated water and plants, including crops. Cross contamination of foods and contact surfaces |
| **Helminths** *Trichinella, Taenia, Diphyllobothrium* | Intestinal tracts and muscle/organ tissues of animals and/or fish | Possibly food contact surfaces. Crops contaminated with feces for certain helminths (e.g., *Ascaris*) |
| **Toxigenic Molds (Fungi)** | Soil, water, plants, animals, humans | Plants, animals, airborne dust, food handlers, utensils, contact surfaces |

should be carefully removed to prevent contaminating the meat with feces. Harvested foods should be thoroughly washed and/or disinfected to eliminate soil-dwelling and aquatic microorganisms responsible for infections or intoxications. Sanitation and cleanliness throughout the food handling chain should prevent microbial contamination from other sources. Finally, human carriers of disease should be excluded from food handling jobs. All of the aforementioned preventive measures are desirable goals, but they cannot be accomplished with practicality and 100% effectiveness. Thus, the reduction of microbial contamination in foods must include controlling the secondary contamination sources listed in Table 4-1.

The sources of microbial contamination in the food chain begin with preharvest on the farm and extend to the point of consumption. This encompasses a wide range of activities under vastly different environmental conditions. Livestock raised for food become infected with pathogens from other animals or from reservoirs in the environment. The incidence rate of infection among farm animals is influenced by herd immunity, crowding or density of animals, prophylactic treatments, and management of manure wastes. Animals infected with zoonotic pathogens often do not exhibit signs of disease and enter the human food chain. During slaughter and meat processing, an infected animal may contaminate the production lines, and subsequent carcasses and meats will become contaminated from the production lines. Additional contamination in the food chain occurs when meats directly or indirectly contact other foods during transport, sale, and preparation. The most important microbial contaminants associated with meat and poultry products include certain Enterobacteriaceae, *Campylobacter* species, *Listeria monocytogenes*, protozoans, and helminths.

The microorganisms with primary habitats in the ambient environment often cycle back and forth between soil and water with the help of wind, rain, and runoff. These microorganisms are generally adapted to surviving austere environmental conditions and flourishing when the conditions become more favorable for growth. The spore-forming bacteria and fungi are typical examples of microorganisms adapted to surviving in the environment. Because crops in the field are in constant contact with soil and water, they are expected to be contaminated with soil-dwelling microorganisms, and dirt from fresh produce can contaminate other foods during handling, transport, and preparation. These environmental microorganisms may also survive in the guts of animals, but the toxigenic microorganisms of food safety importance usually do not proliferate in the gastrointestinal tract. The soil and water become contaminated with enteric pathogens excreted by infected animals, but most of these organisms cannot persist in the environment for extended periods of time. They typically have a transient existence in the environment until a new host is accessed. An exception to this generalization is *Listeria monocytogenes*, which can survive and multiply in intestinal tracts, soils, water, sewage, feces, and decaying vegetation. Despite an increasing number of infections by enteric pathogens (e.g., *Salmonella* spp. and *E. coli* O157: H7) from fresh produce, vegetables and fruits typically are not the primary source of enteric pathogens. The ultimate source of enteric pathogens in fresh produce is contact with infected animals or workers, or from soil, water, and/or equipment contaminated with feces.

Humans and food workers are very important primary and secondary sources of contamination. Infected humans can shed pathogens, and poor hygienic habits increase the likelihood of directly or indirectly contaminating food. In the case of enteric viruses and certain bacteria, humans are the primary reservoir. Thus, by ensuring the food worker is healthy and has good hygienic habits, the risk of contaminating food with human pathogens is greatly reduced. Even with good health and hygienic practices, the food worker may be responsible for contamination problems by improperly handling meats and other potential sources of contamination. All raw meats are presumed contaminated with zoonotic pathogens, and all produce is presumed contaminated with soil-dwelling microorganisms. The prevention of cross-contamination between foods, utensils, equipment, and food contact surfaces is the primary responsibility of food workers and the facility management. Additional food safety responsibilities include preventing the growth of microorganisms that may already be present.

## Extrinsic and Intrinsic Growth Parameters of Foods

All biological processes are influenced or limited by physiochemical parameters. The biochemical reactions that constitute metabolism are dependent on parameters such as temperature, pH, nutrients, water, and oxygen. Microorganisms are particularly vulnerable to changing parameters in the environment because of their small size and lack of specialized, multicellular structures. Nevertheless, morphological and biochemical adaptations have allowed microbial species to survive in different environments under various conditions. The important parameters with regard to microbial growth in foods have been divided into intrinsic and extrinsic parameters by Jay, Loessner, and Golden (2005).

The intrinsic parameters are considered inherent properties of foods. They include the following:

- Acidity or pH
- Moisture and water activity
- Oxidation-reduction potential
- Nutrient content
- Antimicrobial constituents
- Biological structures

The extrinsic parameters are not considered inherent properties of foods. Rather, they are properties of the environment where the foods are stored or prepared. The most important extrinsic parameters are the following:

- Storage and holding temperatures
- Relative humidity
- Types and concentrations of gases present
- Presence of competitive microbiota

Under conditions with ideal intrinsic and extrinsic parameters, the growth curve of bacteria is characterized by four distinct phases and resembles Figure 4-1. During the lag phase (A), bacterial cells must adapt to new environmental conditions, usually because the intrinsic and extrinsic parameters are somewhat different from the original source of bacteria. Although not undergoing reproduction, the bacteria are actively growing in size, storing nutrients, and synthesizing enzymes during the lag phase. Rapid reproduction of bacteria then occurs in the logarithmic or exponential growth phase (B). From binary fission, the number of bacteria doubles with each generation. The time required for a new generation differs by species and with the intrinsic and extrinsic growth parameters. At some point, the bacterial population begins altering the microenvironment by depleting nutrients, creating toxic by-products, or changing other intrinsic and extrinsic parameters. This affects the reproductive and death rates, and when the rates equalize, a plateau or stationary phase (C) is reached. Further depletion of nutrients and alteration of the microenvironment leads to a decline phase (D), where the death rate exceeds the reproductive rate. Usually, some bacterial cells remain viable and capable of starting a new population if transferred to another environment.

An important point to remember about intrinsic and extrinsic parameters is that they sometimes interact. Changes in one parameter may alter the optimum and/or limiting ranges of growth for another parameter. Therefore, whenever an intrinsic or extrinsic parameter is changed and used to control microbial growth, the other parameters should be evaluated with respect to their influence on microbial growth.

## Intrinsic Parameters

### Acidity (pH)

The pH is relevant from the standpoint of proper enzyme functioning and nutrient transport into the microbial cell. Enzyme functioning is dependent on protein shape and structure. Outside of certain pH ranges, the structure of enzymes and their active sites are modified and may not function properly. Changes in pH at the microbial cell's exterior also change the residual electrical charge of the cell's surface. This is important to nutrient trans-

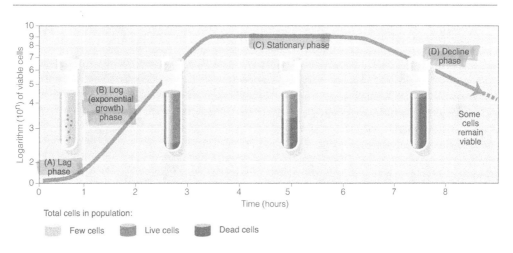

**Figure 4-1** The Growth Curve for a Bacterial Population

port because the electrical charge at the cell's surface determines the ease of nutrient transport into the cell. Extremes of pH may also affect the microorganism's ability to tolerate toxic substances in the local environment. Microbial species have an optimum pH range that is characteristic of their natural habitats. Outside of this optimum range, an increase in the lag phase of the growth curve can be observed. This increased lag phase usually corresponds with the microorganism changing the pH of its surroundings to an optimum level for growth. Figure 4-2 illustrates the pH ranges for the growth of common pathogenic and toxigenic bacteria.

From Figure 4-2, it is apparent that most foodborne pathogens have a relatively narrow pH range for growth. The optimum pH growth range is even narrower. This partly explains why foods such as milk and meats are excellent growth media for foodborne pathogens compared with fruits and vegetables. Milk and meats have a pH range of around 5.5 to 6.8, whereas fruits have a pH range around 3.9 to 4.5, and vegetables generally have a pH range from 3.8 to 6.0. In general, pathogens grow very slowly with a pH of less than 4.6, and the growth of most pathogens can be minimized with a pH of 4.2. Increasing the acidity of foods (i.e., lowering the pH) has been used for centuries to preserve foods and is still used today to destroy or retard the growth of pathogens.

## Moisture and Water Activity

Water is the universal solvent. The availability of water is why organisms flourish on earth, while other planets appear devoid of life. Without water, the biochemical reactions necessary for

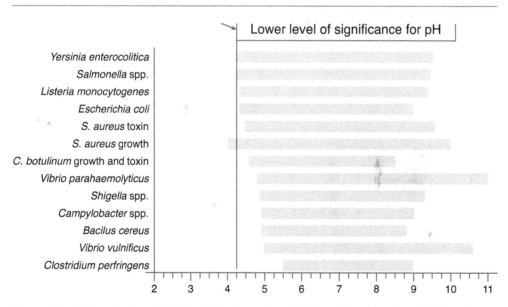

**Figure 4-2** pH Growth Ranges for Selected Foodborne Bacteria. *Source:* Data taken from IFT (2001) report

life cannot take place. The small dimensions of microorganisms make them susceptible to desiccation, and drying foods is one of the oldest treatment processes used for preservation, even though ancient people did not understand the underlying reasons. The biological effects of limiting water to microorganisms include the unavailability of nutrients, improper functioning of the cell membrane, and reduced metabolic activity. Water is necessary to facilitate the transfer of nutrients, maintain a fluid state in the cell membrane, and provide an aqueous environment for the biochemical reactions of metabolism.

The total amount of water in foods is the moisture content, but not all of this water is available to microorganisms. Water molecules are physically and chemically bound to the food matrix in a number of ways. Some water is unavailable because of osmotic pressures and capillary effects. Water is also chemically bonded to solutes and other molecules in the foods. Some of these bonds can be strong and may involve hydroxyl groups of polysaccharides, functional groups of proteins, hydrogen bonding, ion-dipole bonding, and other strong interactions. Microorganisms must compete with the various physical and chemical forces within the food matrix for water. The availability of water in foods is measured as the water activity ($a_w$). Mathematically, $a_w$ is expressed as the ratio of the partial pressure of water measured above the food to the partial pressure of pure water under the same conditions:

$$a_w = p \,/\, p_0$$

where $a_w$ = water pressure, p = partial pressure of water above food, and $p_0$ = partial pressure of pure water.

The $a_w$ is related to another measure of water availability called the equilibrium relative humidity (ERH). The relationship is simply the multiplication of $a_w$ by 100:

$$ERH = a_w \times 100$$

Because water vapor pressure changes with temperature, the food must be measured at the same temperature as the pure water used for reference. The $a_w$ is expressed as a ratio from 0.0 to 1.0, whereas the ERH is expressed as a percentage.

Water activity has a great influence on the capability of pathogenic and toxigenic microorganisms to survive and reproduce in foods. The $a_w$ is altered by various parameters such as osmotic pressure, temperature, pH, and oxidation-reduction potential. Osmotic pressure frequently determines the $a_w$ of food substrates. Increasing the concentration of solutes in a substrate increases osmotic pressure, and in turn, the $a_w$ decreases. The addition of salt is sometimes used to lower the $a_w$ of foods. The molar concentration of salt is inversely related to the $a_w$, and salty foods prevent water from diffusing into microbial cells. Similarly, solutes such as sugars also create osmotic pressures that reduce the $a_w$. Table 4-2 lists some common foods and their typical $a_w$ values.

In general, moist foods with high $a_w$ values permit the survival and growth of pathogens and toxigenic microorganisms. Table 4-3 lists the minimum water activities for the growth of microorganisms important to food safety. Notice that most pathogenic bacteria do not grow below an $a_w$ of 0.92, whereas most molds can grow at relatively lower $a_w$ values (0.61–0.92). An exception to the bacteria is *Staphylococcus aureus*, which is capable of growing at a 0.83 $a_w$ value. This adaptation to lower $a_w$ values provides *S. aureus* with a competitive advantage over other bacteria in certain foods (e.g., salted hams). Because foods often consist of heterogeneous parts or unblended

**Table 4-2**  Estimated Intrinsic Parameters and Other Factors Affecting Microbial Growth in Common Food Types

| Food Type | pH | $a_w$ | Eh | Other Parameters and Factors |
|---|---|---|---|---|
| **Fresh meat and poultry products** | 5.1–6.4 | 0.99–1.0 | −200 to > +300 | High protein content supports rapid microbial growth—unless processing controls are used. Cooked foods destroy microbial competitors |
| **Fresh fish and seafood products** | 4.8–7.0 | 0.99–1.0 | −400 to > +300 | High protein and soluble nitrogen content support rapid microbial growth—unless processing controls are used. Microbial activity leads to rapid spoilage but is not a reliable indicator of pathogens |
| **Fruits and vegetables** | 1.8–6.7 | 0.97–1.0 | +74 to > +400 | Intact (e.g., uncut/unpeeled) raw produce does not generally support rapid microbial growth; yeasts and molds may be more prevalent. |
| **Cereal grains and related products** | > 6.0 | 0.1–0.8 | −470 to +360 | Uncooked/dried grains and milled products do not support rapid microbial growth. Cooked products and those with other ingredients require product assessment. |
| **Fats, oils, and salad dressings** | 3.2–4.0 | ~0.92 | NR[a] | Low pH and water-in-oil emulsion are important in limiting microbial growth. Changes in these parameters/factors could favor microbial growth. |
| **Butter and margarine** | 6.1–6.4 | 0.88–0.96 | +290 to +350 | The composition and manufacturing process are critical to $a_w$ and microbial growth potential. Blended products may require product assessment. |
| **Sugars and syrups** | 5.0–7.0 | 0.1–0.8 | NR[a] | High sugar content results in low $a_w$ and limited microbial growth. Low-sugar products may require product assessment. |
| **Eggs and egg products** | 6.0–9.5 | 0.97 | +500 | Intact shell eggs are often sterile except possible salmonellae. High protein content of egg products supports rapid microbial growth— unless processing controls are used. |
| **Milk and milk products (except cheeses)** | 3.8–6.5 | 0.83–1.0 | +300 to +340 | High protein content and $a_w$ supports rapid microbial growth— unless processing controls are used. Pasteurization eliminates most pathogens from initial sources. |
| **Cheeses** | 4.7–6.1 | 0.68–1.0 | −200 to +300 | More than 500 types of cheeses are known. Pathogen survival and growth depend on many factors in the cheese-making process. |

[a]Not Reported.

*Source:* Compiled from Jay et al. 2005, IFT 2001, and other sources

**Table 4-3** Water Activity and Influence on Microbial Growth

| Water Activity ($a_w$) | Significance of $a_w$ in Terms of Microbial Growth |
| --- | --- |
| 0.92–0.99 | Minimum and optimum $a_w$ range for most pathogenic and toxigenic bacteria. Optimum conditions for toxigenic fungi. |
| 0.83–0.87 | Critical point. Minimum $a_w$ for growth of *Staphylococcus aureus*. Higher $a_w$ results in toxin formation by *S. aureus* and growth of other pathogenic and spoilage bacteria. Most spoilage yeasts are capable of growing at and above this $a_w$. Minimum $a_w$ for aflatoxin formation by toxigenic fungi is 0.82. |
| 0.80 | Most spoilage molds grow at and above this $a_w$. |
| 0.75 | Halophilic bacteria grow at this $a_w$. |
| 0.61 | Xerophilic molds and osmophilic yeasts are can grow at this $a_w$. |
| 0.5–0.3 | No microbial growth or proliferation. |

*Source*: Compiled from FT 2001; Jay et al. 2005; and Kabak et al. 2006.

ingredients, the $a_w$ can be different in microenvironments or component interfaces of foods. Caution is necessary whenever the $a_w$ is measured or used to control pathogens in foods because the $a_w$ may be higher within the microenvironments and at component interfaces.

## Oxidation-Reduction Potential

Microbial species are adapted to growing under different environmental concentrations of oxygen. As such, they are categorized as aerobic, anaerobic, facultative aerobic, and microaerophilic. Along with dissolved molecular oxygen, foods may contain other chemical substances that act as electron acceptors or, conversely, electron donors. When electrons are transferable between elements or compounds, an electrical potential exists that can be measured in millivolts (mV) as either positive or negative values. The relative ease of a substrate losing or gaining electrons is called its oxidation-reduction or redox potential (Eh). As an intrinsic parameter, the Eh of foods determines whether conditions of growth are favorable or inhibiting for different microorganisms. The Eh measured in foods is highly variable and can change with pH, partial pressure of oxygen, composition of the food, added ingredients, and alterations from microbial growth. Foods that continue to respire (e.g., muscle meats, fruits, and vegetables) change the Eh to lower values.

Aerobic microorganisms require more positive Eh values for growth, and the anaerobic microorganisms require more negative Eh values for growth. Strict anaerobes such as *C. botulinum* can grow only at relatively low Eh values (< +60 mV). Other anaerobes such as *C. perfringens* are capable of growing at relatively higher Eh values (< +200 mV), while aerobes only grow at much higher Eh values (+300 to +500 mV). The measurement of Eh in foods is rather easy, but the Eh values may not be consistent throughout the food matrix, and changes in other growth parameters may also change Eh values. The measurement of Eh is useful for determining microbial growth potential in foods, but manipulating Eh values to control microbial growth is rarely done without also manipulating other growth parameters.

### Nutrient Content

Along with water, microorganisms have metabolic and growth requirements that rely on the nutrient content of foods. The specific nutrients needed for metabolic functions and growth vary greatly with different microbial species, but all species require sources of energy and nitrogen, as well as key vitamins and minerals. Energy sources for most microorganisms include sugars, alcohols, and amino acids. With enzymatic breakdown and degradation, some microorganisms are capable of utilizing more complex sources of energy such as starches, cellulose, and fats (Jay et al. 2005). The primary sources of nitrogen are amino acids, and to a lesser extent, compounds such as proteins, peptides, ammonia, urea, creatinine, and other sources. The essential vitamins are acquired from foods, or they can be synthesized by certain microbial species. Mineral requirements (P, Fe, Mg, S, Mn, Ca, K, etc.) are generally needed in smaller amounts compared with other nutrients.

The nutritional makeup of foods greatly determines the types and numbers of microorganisms that can survive and grow. The predominant microbial population in a particular food may change as the complexity and presence of nutrients also change, either from microbial activity or by treatment processes. The simplest forms of nutrients such as sugars and amino acids are generally utilized first, followed by the more complex forms of nutrients. Microorganisms capable of utilizing more complex forms of nutrients may predominate after the simpler forms of nutrients are depleted. In most food matrices, the types and complexity of nutrients are varied, and several types of microorganisms may be growing at the same time. The effect of limited nutrients on a microbial population is the reduction of growth and reproduction.

### Antimicrobial Constituents

Plants contain a number of natural compounds that act as antimicrobial constituents, acting to either inhibit or limit the growth of microorganisms. Some compounds, such as the lectins, are associated with human toxicity, while other compounds are not apparently toxic to humans but still possess antimicrobial properties. Animal-based foods can also contain antimicrobial constituents. Fresh eggs have a combination of lysozyme and conalbumin that provide an efficient antimicrobial system (Jay et al. 2005). Lysozyme is also present in cow's milk along with lactoferrin, conglutinin, and a combination of components called the lactoperoxidase system. The components associated with the lactoperoxidase system are lactoperoxidase, thiocyanate, and hydrogen peroxide (Institute of Food Technologists [IFT] 2001). These three components work together to inhibit several important bacterial pathogens, and they somehow work together to reduce the amount of heat needed to kill pathogens when milk is heated. The lactoperoxidase system is so effective that enhancement of the system by adding more thiocyanate and/or hydrogen peroxide has been proposed for regions where refrigeration of milk is unavailable or inadequate (Jay et al. 2005).

Food treatment or processing may also produce antimicrobial constituents. Certain substances are deposited during the smoking of meats and fish that have antimicrobial properties. Condensation reactions similar to the type that produce acrylamide during the heating of foods, called the Maillard reaction or pathway, can yield products with antimicrobial properties. Along with changing the pH, the fermentation of foods may also produce antimicrobial constituents such as bacteriocins, antibiotics, and other related compounds (IFT 2001). The best characterized bacteriocin is the antibiotic nisin produced by lactic acid bacteria. Nisin can be introduced into foods by starter cultures of bacteria or added directly as a standardized preparation. A number of other food additives are also incorporated into the food matrix for the purpose of preservation and/or to inhibit the growth of pathogens.

### Biological Structures

In the raw state, foods of plant and animal origin have natural structures that exclude the entry and growth of microorganisms. Biological structures such as the skin of fruits and vegetables, hides of animals, coats of seeds, and the shells of eggs are primary barriers to the entry of microorganisms into the organism. These primary barriers are not easily penetrated because most microorganisms lack the enzymes necessary to digest the tough biological structures. However, the internalization of microorganisms is possible from physical damage to these structures during the handling and preparation of foods. Unintentional damage such as bruising, puncturing, abrasion, and so forth permits the entry of microorganisms into other tissues where the intrinsic parameters are more suitable for survival and growth. Similarly, the intentional alteration of biological structures by husking, skinning, chopping, cutting, slicing, grinding, and other processes can contaminate the internal portions of foods. Furthermore, the aforementioned processes can further spread contamination throughout the foodstuff. Heating and other processes can also break down biological structures. Besides spreading microbial contamination, disruption of biological structures frequently changes the pH and $a_w$ characteristics of foods, providing more favorable microbial growth conditions.

## Extrinsic Parameters

### Storage and Holding Temperatures

Microbial species have a minimum and maximum temperature range of growth, and within this range are optimum growth temperatures characterized on the growth curve as a short lag time and a rapid rise in microbial reproduction. Microorganisms are traditionally categorized by their temperature growth ranges and optima as either psychrophiles, psychotrophs, mesophiles, or thermophiles (IFT 2001). In reality, many microorganisms overlap these traditional categories and are difficult to classify solely by temperature. Figure 4-3 illustrates the temperature growth ranges for important foodborne pathogenic and toxigenic bacteria. All of these bacteria are considered mesophiles. None of the bacteria in Figure 4-3 are true psychrophiles, but *L. monocytogenes* and *C. botulinum* type E could be considered as psychrotrophs, though their maximum temperature ranges exceed those typical for most psychrotrophs. The pathogen *Y. enterocolitica* is considered to be mesophilic, but it has a psychrophilic nature compared with the other members of the family Enterobacteriaceae. Most psychrophilic/psychrotrophic microorganisms relevant to food microbiology are spoilage bacteria, yeasts, and molds.

Temperature is important to the growth of microorganisms from the standpoint of metabolic activity and structural integrity. Low temperatures slow the reaction times by enzymes in the microorganism, and low temperatures interfere with nutrient transport by reducing fluidity of

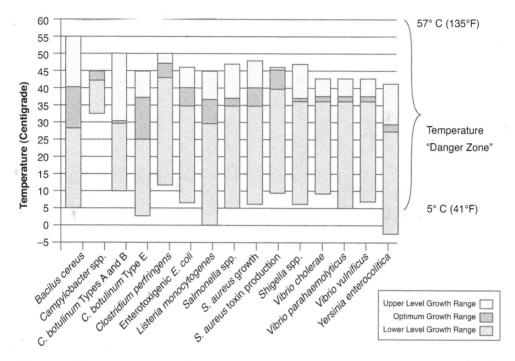

**Figure 4-3** Minimum, Maximum, and Optimum Temperature Growth Ranges for Selected Pathogenic and Toxigenic Bacteria. *Source:* Data from IFT (2001)

the cytoplasmic membrane. With increasing temperatures, the growth rate of microorganisms increases until the optimum temperatures are reached. Thereafter, the growth rate rapidly declines and stops at the maximum temperature. Above optimum temperatures, heat inactivates the heat-sensitive enzymes, and structural components of the cell become denatured (IFT 2001). Some bacteria form endospores when temperatures exceed the optimum. Spores can survive temperatures that destroy most vegetative cells.

Of all the intrinsic and extrinsic parameters, temperature is the most easily manipulated (or abused) in the control of pathogenic and toxigenic microorganisms. Cold temperatures using refrigeration and freezing are commonly employed to preserve foods and their freshness, and cold holding temperatures are used to control the growth of pathogenic or toxigenic microorganisms. Cooking and other heat treatments are essential for destroying pathogens, toxigenic microorganisms, and some toxins. Holding hot foods above the maximum growth ranges of pathogens and toxigenic microorganisms is an important control measure, but it must be carefully practiced because the optimum growth temperatures of most foodborne pathogens lie somewhere between 25°C (77°F) and 47°C (116.6°F). Whenever temperature is used to control microbial growth or destroy microorganisms, the time at the temperature must be considered an integral component.

Given the importance of the time/temperature combination in food safety, it is discussed additionally throughout the book.

## Relative Humidity

Relative humidity (RH) directly influences the $a_w$ of foods. With sufficient time, the $a_w$ of foods equilibrates with the RH of the surrounding environment. This means that foods stored under humid conditions acquire water content until equilibrium is reached. Conversely, foods with high $a_w$ stored under dry conditions lose water content to the surrounding environment. The surface of foods is most affected by the difference in $a_w$ and RH, but the interior portion of foods also changes $a_w$ over time. Much of the concern with RH comes from spoilage problems and food quality, but RH also influences the growth of pathogens and toxigenic microorganisms. The RH of storage areas should be appropriate to ensure the desired $a_w$ is maintained in foods. Covering and wrapping foods can minimize the effects of RH from the surrounding environment.

## Types and Concentrations of Gases Present

The presence of gases, primarily within packages and storage containers of foods, has an important effect on microbial survival and growth. Anaerobes are very sensitive to molecular oxygen ($O_2$) and ozone ($O_3$), mostly from the free radicals produced that exert toxic effects. Most of the food spoilage microorganisms and several pathogens are aerobes, but sufficiently high concentrations of $O_2$ and $O_3$ can even inhibit or destroy aerobic microorganisms. Carbon dioxide ($CO_2$) is very inhibitive to the growth of strict aerobes, and high concentrations of $CO_2$ can deter the growth of anaerobes as well. Carbon dioxide is widely used to control microbial growth in foods with technologies such as modified atmosphere packaging (MAP). Nitrogen is sometimes used in combination with other gases to control microbial growth. Gas composition and concentration also indirectly influence microbial growth by changing the microbial ecology, allowing some microbial populations to outcompete others in the foods (IFT 2001).

## Presence of Competitive Microbiota

Competing microorganisms that are either indigenous or added to the foods can interfere with the survival and growth of spoilage, pathogenic, and/or toxigenic bacteria and fungi. Microbial interference often results from faster growing microorganisms that utilize certain nutrients in the foods, and by the production of substances that change the intrinsic characteristics of the foods. For example, some microbial species produce antimicrobial constituents and/or alter the pH, $a_w$, and Eh of the foods. Deliberate modification of intrinsic or extrinsic parameters by food processing and preparation can also provide a competitive advantage for certain microbial populations. Changes in the microbial ecology of foods can be detrimental when innocuous microorganisms are destroyed during cooking, and subsequent contamination of the foods allows the growth of pathogens without any microbial interference.

## Predictive Microbiology and Potentially Hazardous Foods

Since the early days of microbiology, scientists have described the growth and destruction of microorganisms in qualitative and quantitative terms. A practical application of this science has been the control of pathogens through environmental manipulation and engineering design. Over the past three decades, advances in computational science and computer technology have enabled the modeling of microbial growth and destruction with unprecedented speed and predictive ability. Consequently, within the specialty of food microbiology, a discipline called predictive microbiology has emerged based on the modeling of microbial survival and growth. The primary goal of predictive microbiology is to improve food safety and quality by modeling microbial growth, survival, and inactivation for different values of intrinsic and extrinsic parameters.

Computer modeling and simulation have become commonplace in applications ranging from weather forecasting to the social sciences. All models have limitations and require an appropriate level of validation before they can be used to assist in decision making. Whenever a model is used for an application, the user must understand its limitations. The models developed for predictive microbiology are based on carefully designed experiments with regard to the species and strains of microorganism, food test matrix, inoculums preparation, and selected values of intrinsic and extrinsic parameters. From the experimental data, a primary model is developed that describes the relationship between microbial numbers and the values of intrinsic and/or extrinsic parameters over time. A secondary model is then developed that predicts the results for many different values of the parameters. The tertiary model converts the primary and secondary models into computer software routines that can be easily used. Validation of the model is performed by comparing model predictions to new experimental data. The model's performance is judged by both bias and accuracy factors. The least biased and most accurate models are developed for very specific applications (e.g., a particular food produced by a particular process). Model performance degrades outside of its intended application, and caution is necessary when interpreting the results of model predictions.

Most food microbiologists generally agree that temperature, pH, and $a_w$ are the most important parameters for controlling microbial growth, followed by antimicrobial constituents and the concentration of certain gases. Whereas temperature can be consistently maintained through the application of heat and cold, the other parameters may change over time from microbial growth and/or chemical reactions. Furthermore, interactions between parameters do occur and are not easily determined. Models are helpful in this regard because many "what if" scenarios can be tested without the expense and time associated with laboratory experiments. Another application of models is the training of food safety professionals about how the rates of microbial growth, survival, and inactivation change with different values of intrinsic and extrinsic parameters. Figure 4-4 illustrates the relationship between time–temperature and microbial growth for *Salmonella* species in broth culture. Although the temperature range of growth for salmonellae is estimated to be 5°–47°C, the curves in Figure 4-4 illustrate that the rates of growth and reproduction increase dramatically as temperatures approach the optimum level. The modeled growth curves of other bacteria may have similar overall shapes, but the scales on the axes will be different based on the minimum, maximum, and optimum growth temperatures of individual species and strains.

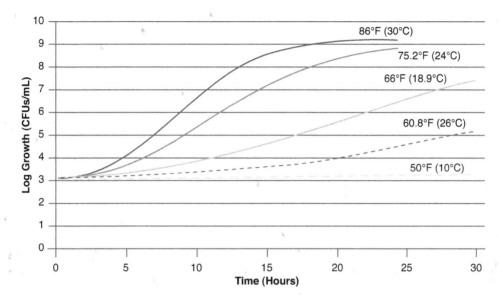

**Figure 4-4** Growth Curve Modeling of *Salmonella* at Different Temperatures. *Source*: Based on data generated by the Pathogen Modeling Program Version 7.0, USDA

As part of an overall prevention strategy, the intrinsic and extrinsic parameters of foods are modified or controlled to limit microbial growth. The rationale or theory is based on the minimum infective dose for pathogens and the effective dose for toxin formation. If the microbial population size is restricted below a critical level, insufficient numbers of pathogenic or toxigenic microorganisms are present to cause foodborne illness. The most widely practiced method of limiting microbial growth in food involves time/temperature controls. For foods that support bacterial growth, the "danger zone" of temperatures is considered between 5°C and 57°C (41°F and 135°F) by the U.S. Public Health Service's Food Code (FDA and PHS 2009). Holding food temperatures above or below the danger zone (i.e., at or below 41°F and at or above 135°F) limits the growth rate of pathogenic and toxigenic microorganisms. In practice, the temperature danger zone is crossed during the preparation, display, and holding of foods. For these situations, the total amount of time in the danger zone becomes important to limiting the cumulative microbial population growth.

Foods with intrinsic parameters that support rapid microbial growth were historically designated as "potentially hazardous foods" (PHF) and were subjected to time/temperature controls. In recognition of new food preservation technologies and to avoid confusion, an expert panel assembled by the Institute of Food Technologists (IFT 2001) recommended using the term "temperature controlled for safety" (TCS) foods instead of PHF. Furthermore, the expert panel recommended using a science-based framework for defining TCS foods. The recommended framework includes the following: (1) evaluation of the food product to determine whether treatment processes destroy pathogens and prevent recontamination (e.g., commercial sterility), (2) the evaluation of microbial growth potential using validated modeling programs (i.e., predictive microbiology), and (3) microbial challenge testing in the laboratory when necessary. To accommodate both points of view and provide a transition period, the latest version of the Food Code (FDA and PHS 2009) incorporates both terms as PHF/TCS foods.

The IFT expert panel emphasized that modifying multiple intrinsic and extrinsic parameters was more effective in limiting microbial growth than simply modifying one parameter. In other words, microbial growth is best controlled with a combination of proper storage temperatures, modification of the pH and $a_w$, addition of preservatives, and other parameter modifications. For some foods, modifying a single parameter is ineffective in controlling microorganisms, whereas modifying two or more parameters inhibits microbial growth. The use of multiple controls for microbial growth is called the "hurdle concept" because a pathogenic or toxigenic microorganism must overcome several barriers to growth (IFT 2001). Hurdles also provide an added margin of safety. Modern food processing technologies use the hurdle concept to extend the shelf life of foods and prevent the growth of pathogens.

Protein-based foods of animal origin (meats, poultry, fish, eggs, milk, etc.) are nearly always considered PHF/TCS foods unless processed and packaged in a manner to destroy potential pathogens, inhibit microbial growth, and prevent recontamination. Foods such as fresh produce generally have a low potential for supporting microbial growth. However, a few fruits and vegetables have a history of supporting the growth of pathogens. Bean and alfalfa sprouts, for example, have been associated with outbreaks of salmonellosis and *E. coli* O157:H7; initial contamination of the seeds with pathogens can lead to rapid microbial growth during the sprouting process. Cutting and other preparation methods may change the intrinsic parameters of fruits and vegetables in a manner that supports microbial growth. Raw foods such as cantaloupes, tomatoes, and leafy greens that have been cut are considered PHF/TCS foods. Most uncooked grains and milled products are not considered PHF/TCS foods. This is not the case when the $a_w$ changes, such as happens during cooking. Raw rice is not considered a PHF/TCS food, but cooked rice can support the growth of *Bacillus cereus* in the temperature danger zone. Combination food products can be problematic because the intrinsic parameters are difficult to predict for mixtures of different foods. Assessments are required for foods whenever the microbial growth potential is unknown or uncertain.

Compared with the early days of food safety, the designation of foods as PHF/TCS food is more involved. The Food Code (FDA and PHS 2009) offers decision guidelines to help determine whether a food product is considered a PHF/TCS food. Figure 4-5 is the decision tree for determining if a food requires time/temperature control for safety. The first question deals with the issue of whether a food will be held without time or temperature controls. Obviously, if the food is handled as PHF/TCS food anyway, the point is moot, and no further action is required. The next step deals with heat treatment of the food product. Adequate cooking temperatures are capable of destroying vegetative forms of microbial cells, but spores are not destroyed by most cooking processes. Thus, the primary concern with heat-treated foods is the spores—unless the food product is not adequately packaged to prevent recontamination with vegetative cells. Spores have different requirements for germination in terms of $a_w$ and pH compared with the growth of vegetative cells. Knowledge of the food product's heat treatment, packaging, $a_w$, and pH allows

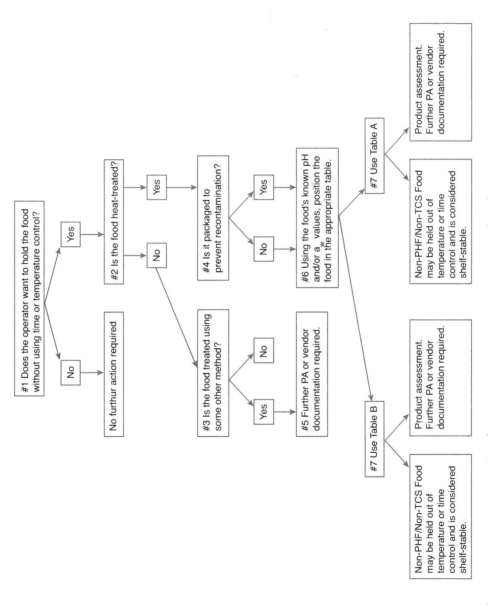

**Figure 4-5** Decision Tree Using $a_w$ and pH for Determining Time/Temperature Control for Safety. *Source:* The Food Code 2009

the selection of Table 4-4A or 4-4B for the final determination. Notice that Table 4-4A allows more neutral pH and higher $a_w$ combinations to control spores, whereas Table 4-4B is more restrictive in the combinations of pH and $a_w$ for controlling vegetative cells. In the absence of formal product assessments that state otherwise, all food products that fall within the "PA" category are considered as PHF/TCS foods. Product assessments are based on appropriately designed laboratory studies of the food product.

**Table 4-4** Interaction of pH and $a_w$ for Controlling Microbial Growth

**1-201, 10(B)—Table A and Table B**

**Table A.** Interaction of pH and $a_w$ for control of spores in food heat-treated to destroy vegetative cells and subsequently packaged

| $a_w$ values | pH values | | |
|---|---|---|---|
| | 4.6 or less | > 4.5–5.6 | > 5.6 |
| ≤ 0.92 | non-PHF[a]/non-TCS FOOD[b] | non PHF/non TCS FOOD | non PHF/nonTCS FOOD |
| > 0.92–.95 | non-PHF/non-TCS FOOD | non-PHF/non-TCS FOOD | PA[c] |
| > 0.95 | non-PHF/non-TCS FOOD | PA | PA |

[a]PHF means Potentially Hazardous Food
[b]TCS food means TIme/Temperature Control for Safety food
[c]PA means Product Assessment required

**Table B.** Interacation of pH and $a_w$ for control of vegetative cells and spores in food not heat-treated or heat-treated but not packaged

| $a_w$ values | pH values | | | |
|---|---|---|---|---|
| | < 4.2 | 4.2–4.6 | > 4.6–5.0 | > 5.0 |
| < 0.88 | non-PHF[a]/non-TCS food[b] | non-PHF/non-TCS food | non-PHF/non-TCS food | non-PHF/non-TCS food |
| 0.88–0.90 | non-PHF/non-TCS food | non-PHF/non-TCS food | non-PHF/non-TCS food | PA[c] |
| > 0.90–0.92 | non-PHF/non-TCS food | non-PHF/non-TCS food | PA | PA |
| > 0.92 | non-PHF/non-TCS food | PA | PA | PA |

[a]PHF means Potentially Hazardous Food
[b]TCS food means TIme/Temperature Control for Safety food
[c]PA means Product Assessment required

*Source:* The Food Code 2009

## ELIMINATE SOURCES OF CONTAMINATION FROM CHEMICAL POLLUTANTS AND TOXINS

For the majority of situations, microbial toxins represent the greatest risk of foodborne intoxications and chronic exposure to carcinogens or other toxic substances. The formation of enterotoxins by the bacteria *S. aureus* and *B. cereus* is widely recognized and best prevented by reducing food contamination with these bacteria and inhibiting their growth. The measures previously discussed for reducing microbial contamination and growth are applicable for preventing formation of these enterotoxins. Similarly, the formation of mycotoxins is also best prevented by minimizing contamination with fungal spores and controlling the growth of molds. However, fungi are comparatively more pervasive compared with toxigenic bacteria, and fungi have different growth requirements in terms of intrinsic and extrinsic parameters compared with bacteria.

Fungi have a competitive advantage over bacteria in produce, grain products, and spices and herbs, primarily because these products have intrinsic parameters that are relatively unfavorable for the majority of bacteria (Moss 2008). For fruits and vegetables, spoilage by mold is primarily a food quality issue, but the presence of mycotoxins such as patulin may be a problem, particularly for fruit juice producers. The foods contaminated most often with a variety of mycotoxins are grains, cereal products, nuts, spices, and herbs. Animals fed with mycotoxin-contaminated grain or feeds can be a source of mycotoxins and/or toxic metabolites in meats and dairy products. Some fermented foods may also be a source of mycotoxins, if the growth of toxigenic fungi occurs during or after the fermentation process.

The Codex Alimentarius Commission, established by the Food and Agriculture Organization (FAO) and WHO, has developed several codes for the prevention and reduction of mycotoxins in food products. Prevention of mycotoxin contamination involves preharvest, harvest, and postharvest control strategies (Kabak, Dobson, Var 2006). The preharvest control strategies differ among various crops, but generally the strategies include using fungal-resistant strains of plants, field management practices, and biological or chemical agents. Harvest control strategies involve choosing the optimum time for harvest, avoidance of mixing different quality crops, and moisture management practices. Postharvest control strategies involve minimizing contamination with toxigenic fungi during transportation and storage, and controlling the storage conditions of raw and finished products. The improper storage of crops and processed products represents the dominant place where fungal growth and mycotoxin production occur. Moisture control is critical. Improper drying and rewetting of grains or nuts after harvest provides ample $a_w$ for the growth of toxigenic fungi, and high relative humidity contributes directly to the $a_w$ of stored raw and finished products. Postharvest control strategies also involve the use of fungicides and other chemical agents, some that involve modifying the atmosphere of stored grains with $CO_2$ and other gases (Magan and Aldred 2007). Fungicides and other chemical agents that inhibit fungal growth must be used properly to minimize residual contamination of the food product with the control agents.

The presence of mold on foods is not always an indication of mycotoxin contamination. Although most foods with signs of mold growth should not be consumed, the only way of determining the presence of mycotoxins is with analytical testing methods. Furthermore, the absence of mold does not mean the absence of mycotoxins because fungal growth is not always visible and mycotoxin generation and contamination can occur throughout the food handling chain. Complete elimination of mycotoxins in foods is practically unachievable. Many countries and international organizations have established permissible limits for mycotoxins in foods, but monitoring programs are required to ensure mycotoxin levels do not exceed these limits. In the United States, FDA and state agencies provide various degrees of sampling and monitoring to estimate levels of certain mycotoxins in domestic and imported foods. Action levels are established by FDA for selected mycotoxins in foods and animal feeds. Residues detected at or above the action levels trigger legal action by FDA to remove the contaminated products from market.

From the perspective of a food safety professional, the elimination of algal toxins associated with seafood is difficult because the ultimate source of the toxins resides in marine waters. Some local public health authorities monitor fish and shellfish, or the waters from whence they came, for levels of toxins produced by dinoflagellates. The banning of fishing and shellfish harvesting when algal toxins exceed a tolerable level, or when harmful algal blooms occur, is successful in many cases. However, analytical methods for most algal toxins are not field-portable or easily performed, and contamination of seafood without associated algal blooms is always a possibility. At the retail food facility, the best prevention method is ensuring all seafood is from an approved source and shellfish shipments are properly tagged and labeled. An important distinction between algal toxins and scombrotoxin is the latter comes from bacterial decomposition of certain fin fish, and prompt refrigeration and cold holding are necessary to prevent scombrotoxin formation.

The elimination of anthropogenic toxicants (i.e., xenobiotics) in foods is dependent on the regulation of environmental pollution, farming practices and agrochemical use, the food processing industry, food contact materials, food ingredients, and the storage and use of chemicals in the vicinity of foodstuff. A maze of regulations covering environmental protection, agricultural practices, and public health is promulgated by multiple federal and state agencies. It is incumbent upon the producers, processors, distributors, and retailers to comply with these regulations for a safe food supply. For food safety programs at the retail level, the source of foodstuff is important to know and check. In other words, the vetting of food suppliers is necessary to ensure a safe source. This becomes increasingly complex in the era of global trade, when foods and ingredients are imported from various countries that may have lax regulation of food safety standards.

Cleaning compounds, sanitizers, pesticides, air fresheners, polishing compounds, and other potentials sources of chemicals are usually found in food production, processing, and preparation facilities. Without care and due diligence, food can become contaminated with toxic chemicals and cause serious illnesses or death. Only authorized chemicals should be located in a food facility, and all chemicals must be stored separately from food items and areas where food is processed or prepared. Chemicals must never be stored in food containers or packaging, and all chemicals must be in their original containers and clearly labeled. Furthermore, the chemicals should be used according to label instructions, and the food or cleaning staff must be trained in the safe use of chemicals.

## SANITATION: PRINCIPLES AND PURPOSES

"Sanitation" was derived from the word *sanitary* and did not appear in print until the nineteenth century. The origin of *sanitary* is from the Latin words *sanitas* (health) and *sanus* (healthy, sane). During the golden age of microbiology and the early years of modern public health, the term *sanitary* became associated with hygienic disposal of wastes, particularly human and animal wastes, and the prevention of water contamination. Over the last century, the term *sanitation* came to encompass a wide variety of environmental control measures to protect and promote human health. In most usages, *food sanitation* refers to the hygienic and healthful handling of foods in a manner that eliminates or reduces the levels of disease-causing microorganisms. Some health scientists consider food sanitation as encompassing all aspects of ensuring a safe food supply. In this book, the term *sanitation* shall refer to specific measures intended to reduce the presence of pathogenic and toxigenic microorganisms through sanitary practices, sanitization of surfaces and equipment, waste disposal, and pest/disease vector control.

## Sanitary Practices and Cleaning

Basic sanitary practices begin with cleanliness and proper waste disposal. The removal of filth and the cleaning of surfaces are fundamental, but not all filth and surfaces are equally important with regard to disease transmission. Most enteric diseases have a fecal-oral route of transmission, thereby making sources of fecal matter paramount with regard to food safety. The isolation and removal of fecal wastes from food operations are essential to reduce the risks of transmitting enteric pathogens. Properly located and functioning toilet facilities accomplish this purpose for human feces, while the exclusion of animals and their intestinal contents from food operations is necessary to eliminate sources of zoonotic pathogens. Animate and inanimate objects that directly or indirectly contact feces must be treated to reduce the number and type of potential pathogens transferrable to foods. Food contact surfaces are particularly important, and treatment of these surfaces involve cleaning and sanitization.

The removal of nonfecal wastes from food premises, equipment, and contact surfaces is necessary for other reasons. First, organic matter provides a growth medium for bacteria and fungi that may be pathogenic or toxigenic. The growth and reproduction of these microorganisms increases their numbers and the risk of contaminating foods. Second, the accumulation of organic matter makes cleaning and sanitizing surfaces difficult and less effective. Surfaces coated with organic matter are not being cleaned or sanitized, and organic matter may react with chemical sanitizers, making them less effective against microorganisms. Third, pests and disease vectors such as cockroaches, flies, and rodents are nearly impossible to control without the elimination of organic matter and food debris. Food particles and the accumulation of garbage are attractants to pests and sustain their population growth, increasing the likelihood of these organisms contacting and contaminating food products.

Prioritization of sanitary practices is necessary to minimize disease risks within the constraints of time and resources. The most relevant sanitary and insanitary practices may not always be obvious to the untrained observer. Unattractive walls in a retail food facility may be aesthetically unpleasing and require periodic cleaning to remove splatters and buildup of materials, but they are less important to food safety compared with surfaces that contact foods. The procedures and processes involved with food operations must be examined from start to finish to identify and evaluate where diligent sanitary practices are most needed. For example, the contact of cooked food with surfaces that were used with raw meat, a potential source of zoonotic pathogens, is not always discovered during brief inspections. Using the same surfaces for another type of food can result in the transfer of contamination. This indirect contact between contaminated and uncontaminated foods is known as "cross contamination." A particularly risky scenario is the cross contamination between raw meats and cooked foods or salad ingredients. Sanitary practices that minimize the risk of cross contamination involve separating food items and cleaning/sanitizing the contact surfaces between uses.

The term *soil* is used to describe undesirable materials such as dirt, dust, food debris and scraps, lubricants, mineral deposits, and other residues on surfaces (Marriott 1997). Soils can be visible to the naked eye, or they can be microscopic deposits on a surface. The type and mix of materials determine soil properties and the cleaning practices needed to remove the soil. Organic soils include food deposits (sugars, fats, proteins, etc.) and petroleum- or oil-based residues. The importance of removing organic soils was discussed earlier as a high priority for sanitary practices. Inorganic soils include "hard water" mineral deposits, oxidation/rust of metals, and deposits or films from cleaners or other chemicals. Inorganic soils are important from the standpoint of interfering with the cleaning and sanitizing of surfaces, forming crevices or pores that harbor microorganisms, and preventing heat transfer to foods. Soil is attached to surfaces by different chemical and physical forces, and disruption of these forces is needed before soil can be separated from a surface.

A particularly persistent form of soil is the formation of biofilms. The phenomenon of biofilms was introduced in Chapter 2 as it pertains to the establishment of an infection. Biofilm formation on inanimate objects in the food handling chain is important with respect to sanitary practices. Several species of pathogenic and spoilage bacteria are known to form biofilms on certain foodstuff and food contact surfaces. Among the pathogens known to form biofilms are *Listeria monocytogenes*, *Shigella* species, *Salmonella enterica*, and *Escherichia coli*. The material type and topographic features of food contact surfaces are important in the formation of biofilms (Chmielewski and Frank 2003). Surfaces that are rough, porous, abraded, or that possess other defects tend to accumulate minute amounts of organic soil and bacteria that are not removed during cleaning and sanitizing. This allows bacteria to regrow and to form biofilms, which can build up as matrix layers. These layers are teeming with bacteria and capable of breaking off as microscopic particles. Within biofilms, the bacteria are protected from sanitizers and other antimicrobials. Foods in contact with the biofilm matrix become contaminated with viable pathogens. The removal of established biofilms from a food contact surface is difficult and usually requires scraping along with heat and a strong combination of cleaners and sanitizers.

The basic sequence for cleaning and sanitizing food contact surfaces is the following:

Rinse → Clean → Rinse → Sanitize → Air Dry → Protect from contamination and moisture

Effective cleaning of surfaces involves mechanical action and cleaning compounds. Mechanical action can come from high pressure water and/or physical scrubbing by workers or machinery. The selection of cleaning methods is based on the primary composition of the soil, type of surface to be cleaned, and chemical safety precautions for food workers and consumers. In all cases, good quality water is necessary to wet the soil and food contact surface, allowing the cleaner to penetrate and separate the soil attached to the surface, and to rinse away the dispersed soil. The water must be potable and free of pathogens, and the pH and mineral content of the water must be considered when selecting cleaners and sanitizers. The use of nonpotable water in food operations has been linked to outbreaks of foodborne illnesses throughout history and in modern times. Excessively low or high pH ($< 5$ or $> 8.5$) of water can alter the properties of cleaning and sanitizing compounds, and buffering agents may be needed to minimize the effects of pH on these compounds. Water "hardness" or mineral content is most important with regard to the effectiveness of cleaners and sanitizers. In particular, calcium and magnesium salts associated with hardness can neutralize some compounds (i.e., quaternary ammonium), and they can form films or cause corrosion on some surfaces. Minor water hardness can be overcome by adding sequestering agents to the cleaning compounds, but very hard water may require "softening" treatment prior to use.

The chemical composition and formulation of individual cleaning compounds vary and are proprietary among companies that provide them. The company representative should be consulted prior to selecting a cleaning compound. Generally, cleaning compounds can be grouped into the following types (Marriott 1997):

- Alkaline cleaning compounds, formulated as either mild, strong, or heavy-duty cleaners
- Acid cleaning compounds with either mildly or strongly acidic properties
- Solvent cleaners based on ether or alcohol
- Soaps and detergents that contain chemical "builders," compounds added to make them clean more effectively

Different types of additives are used in cleaning compounds by manufacturers to improve cleaning properties and/or protect surfaces. Sequestrants, also called chelating agents, are added to soften or condition the water used with cleaning compounds. Emulsifiers are added to break down fats and oils into very small droplets that can be suspended and rinsed away. Complex molecules known as surfactants are added to cleaning and sanitizing compounds to enhance the wetting and penetration of soil, allowing closer contact with the cleaning/sanitizing agent and disrupting the soil–surface binding forces. Some cleaners have abrasive materials called scouring compounds added to assist with the mechanical loosening of soil. Other types of additives may include oxidizers to remove protein residues, fillers to add bulk or mass, and enzyme-based detergents to degrade soils composed of specific biomolecules (carbohydrates, proteins, fats).

Safety evaluations and precautions are paramount in the selection of chemicals used as cleaners and sanitizers. Corrosiveness and toxicity are potential hazards to workers that must be evaluated, and protective measures are necessary to minimize risks. Mixing different chemical products is potentially dangerous because chemical reactions can produce extremely toxic gases or violent reactions that can cause injury or chemical burns. Additionally, cleaners and sanitizers used on food contact surfaces must not leave chemical residues that could become part of the foodstuff. Chemicals used as cleaners, sanitizers, and antimicrobial agents in the food industry must be registered with EPA, which reviews efficacy data, safety data, and labeling requirements prior to approval. Since FDA regulates acceptable levels of chemical residues/additives in foods, chemical and antimicrobial agents used on foods and food contact surfaces must be approved by FDA. Furthermore, sanitizers used as no-rinse products for food contact surfaces must be listed in the

*Code of Federal Regulations* (21 CFR 178.1010). These sanitizers are regulated as indirect food additives. A list of nonfood chemical compounds used in meat, poultry, and related food industries was once maintained by USDA, but the list has been discontinued. The NSF International (formerly National Sanitation Foundation) has taken over the USDA registration process as a voluntary effort on behalf of the food industry.

## Sanitizing Methods and Chemicals

"Sanitize means to adequately treat food-contact surfaces by a process that is effective in destroying vegetative cells of microorganisms of public health significance, and in substantially reducing numbers of other undesirable microorganisms, but without adversely affecting the product or its safety for the consumer" (21 CFR 110.3).

The preceding definition of *sanitize* succinctly captures the purpose of sanitizing food contact surfaces. By reducing the numbers of pathogenic and toxigenic microorganisms, the likelihood of these organisms contaminating foods in sufficient numbers to cause harm is also reduced. Several methods are available to sanitize food contact surfaces. One method involves the use of heat from conduction, convection, steam, or hot water. Another method is applying chemical sanitizers to a cleaned surface. An increasingly accepted method is the use of radiation, including both ionizing and nonionizing radiation. The irradiation of foods is sometimes controversial and is discussed separately in a Chapter 5.

Using heat to sanitize a food contact surface has the advantage of destroying many different types of pathogenic and toxigenic microorganisms without leaving a chemical residue. The major disadvantages include energy costs and possible safety hazards to workers. Heating elements in equipment such as cookers is one way of utilizing heat to sanitize food contact surfaces. Steam can also be used to sanitize food contact surfaces, but the energy costs are high, and maintaining sufficient time and temperature on food contact surfaces can be difficult to ensure while manually applying steam. Hot water can be used to sanitize food contact surfaces provided sufficient contact time is maintained at the correct time–temperature relationship for biocidal activity. When hot water immersion is used for sanitizing food contact surfaces, the Food Code (FDA and PHS 2009) stipulates that a temperature of 77°C (171°F) or above must be maintained for at least 30 seconds. Some food equipment can be sanitized by pumping hot water through it. Most restaurants, institutional kitchens, and retail food facilities use hot water in warewashing (i.e., dishwashing) machines to sanitize dishware, cooking ware, utensils, and other food contact surfaces that can be placed in the machine. The temperature of the food contact surfaces passing through a warewashing machine must reach a minimum of 71°C (160°F) for proper sanitizing (FDA and PHS 2009). Many warewashing machines use a combination of hot water and chemical sanitizers.

Chemical sanitizers used on permanent or semipermanent food contact surfaces are considered as antimicrobial pesticides under the Federal Insecticide, Fungicide, and Rodenticide Act (FIFRA). As such, all sanitizers marketed in the United States must be registered with EPA and demonstrate efficacy and safety for its intended application. The EPA protocols for testing efficacy of a sanitizer follow the guidelines by the Association of Official Analytical Chemists (AOAC). For sanitizing rinses on food contact surfaces, the performance standards stipulate that a sanitizer must meet one of the following, depending on the type of chemicals used (Environmental Protection Agency [EPA] 2010):

- The sanitizer demonstrates a 99.999% (5 logs) reduction in the number of specified test microorganisms within 30 seconds of contact.
- The sanitizer's concentration effectiveness is equivalent to available chlorine concentrations (from sodium hypochlorite) of 50, 100, and 200 ppm.

Several points should be remembered with regard to the efficacy and use of chemical sanitizers. First, sanitizers used on food contact surfaces must be designated for such use; food contact sanitizers are considered "sanitizing rinses," that is, the sanitizer is applied without rinsing off the surface. Sanitizers designated for cleaning floors, walls, toilets, and so forth may have hazardous characteristics for food contact surfaces, possibly leaving behind a toxic residue. In fact, some nonfood antimicrobial chemicals are actually disinfectants, a stronger antimicrobial with greater potential toxicity. Second, the minimum efficacy of EPA-registered sanitizers is based on clean food contact surfaces. Some products combine a detergent and sanitizer, but the surface must still be clean for effective sanitizing. Third, the performance standard for sanitizer efficacy is based on 99.999% reduction of a clearly established microbial population in a laboratory setting. A clean surface with few microorganisms may not achieve an additional 99.999% reduction because such efficacy would be approaching sterility, a condition that sanitizers are not intended to achieve. Fourth, several chemical factors affect the efficacy of sanitizers. The pH of a solution can dramatically change the sanitizer's efficacy, particularly chlorine solutions. Other chemical properties of water and the presence of inactivating compounds (such as found in some detergents) can alter the sanitizer's efficacy. Finally, several physical factors influence the efficacy of sanitizers:

1. Surfaces with characteristics such as cracks and crevices or that are porous reduce sanitizer efficacy.
2. The presence of soil and/or biofilms on the surface reduces sanitizer efficacy.
3. A short contact or exposure time reduces efficacy.
4. Lower temperatures are less efficacious.
5. Low concentrations of sanitizers are less efficacious; efficacy increases with greater sanitizer concentrations. Above certain concentrations, the efficacy of a sanitizer plateaus.

Chemical sanitizers permitted for use on food contact surfaces associated with public eating facilities, dairy processing equipment, and food processing equipment and utensils are listed in federal regulations (40 CFR 180.940). The exact composition and formulation of sanitizers may vary by manufacturer. General types of chemical sanitizers used on food contact surfaces are chlorine-bearing compounds, quaternary ammonium compounds, iodophors or iodine compounds, bromine compounds, ozone, acid sanitizers, and peroxides. Table 4-5 lists these chemical sanitizers along with important characteristics. Labeling requirements for sanitizers are regulated by EPA, and users should follow the manufacturer's instructions on the label for safe and effective application of the sanitizer.

**Table 4-5** Chemicals Commonly Used to Sanitize Food Contact Surfaces

| Chemical Groups | Specific Examples | Notable Characteristics |
|---|---|---|
| Chlorine-releasing compounds | Calcium hypochlorite, sodium hypochlorite, chlorine dioxide, inorganic and organic chloramines, dichloroisocyanuric acid, trichloroisocyanuric acid | Broad spectrum antimicrobial action. Activity varies with pH. Corrosive to many metals. Potential safety and health hazards during use |
| Quaternary ammonium compounds | Cetyltrimethyl ammonium bromide, lauryldimethylbenzyl ammonium chloride, n-alkyl dimethyl ethylbenzyl ammonium chloride, many other substitutions for hydrogens in $[NH_4]^+$ cation | Effective against most but not all bacteria. Effective against molds. Stable with some detergent properties and not greatly affected by light soil. Activity good at high pH. Noncorrosive to metals. Reacts with anionic-type detergents. Forms film on surfaces |
| Iodophors or iodine solutions | Alcohol-iodine solutions (iodophors), aqueous iodine solutions from gas or other compounds | Broad-spectrum antimicrobial action. Activity much less at high pH and high temperatures. Less corrosive to skin than chlorine. Staining possible on some surfaces |
| Bromine compounds | Potassium bromide, calcium bromide | Bromine added to chloramines make sanitizer more effective at high pH ($\geq$ 7.5). Used more often for water disinfection treatment |
| Ozone | Ozone gas introduced into water solution by various methods. Use of ozone gas for some surfaces is being explored | Broad spectrum antimicrobial action. Unstable. Created on-site for immediate use. Leaves no residue. Approved as a food additive under 21 CFR 173.368 |
| Acid sanitizers | Organic acids: acetic acid, lactic acid, formic acid, proprionic acid, etc. Acid-anionic formulations consisting of inorganic acids and a surfactant | Antimicrobial action against a variety of microbes. Not easily degraded by heat or minor soil. Shorter contact times for effectiveness. Effective low pH ($<$ 4) but ineffective at neutral and high pH. Slightly corrosive to metals |
| Peroxides | Hydrogen peroxide and related compounds, peroxyacetic acid and related compounds | Limited applications in the food industry. Slightly corrosive to metals. Not irritating to skin. Less effective at high pH |

*Source*: Compiled from 40 CFR 180.940 and multiple other sources.

## Food Contact Surfaces and Equipment

A great many different materials are used for food contact surfaces. These include various metals and alloys, plastics, rubber and other polymers, glass and ceramics, wood and paper, concrete or earthenware, laminates, and combinations of materials. The surfaces of materials are often coated with finishes to facilitate cleaning, provide nonstick functions, and/or for aesthetic appeal. The importance of preventing the migration of chemical constituents from food contact surfaces to foods is discussed in Chapter 3. Chemicals that migrate from food contact surfaces are regulated as food additives by FDA. Materials used for food contact surfaces should be inert, and they should neither absorb from nor impart chemicals, odors, tastes, or colors to foods. Other characteristics of materials are important in terms of cleaning and sanitizing food contact surfaces.

The principles of sanitary practice dictate that all food contact surfaces are smooth and nonporous, and incapable of harboring food, microorganisms, and other unwanted residues or filth. Smooth surfaces are also more easily cleaned and effectively sanitized. All food contact surfaces encountered in food processing and preparation should be readily visible and accessible for inspection, cleaning, and sanitizing. Materials that are reusable (i.e., nondisposable) as food contact surfaces should be durable and capable of withstanding frequent cleaning and sanitizing without degrading their integrity. This means that the surfaces should not crack, splinter, scratch, distort, form crevices or pits, or otherwise modify the surface in a manner that provides harborage of microorganisms and/or prevents proper cleaning and sanitizing. Furthermore, the materials that comprise food contact surfaces should be compatible with the choice of detergents and sanitizers. For example, glass can be etched by strong alkaline cleaning solutions; rubber is depolymerized by organic solvents and strong acids; and some metals are easily corroded by acid and chlorine solutions. Another important consideration of materials is they should be used only in applications where they are unlikely to break and contaminate foods with hard or sharp objects.

The preferred material for food contact surfaces is stainless steel because it is strong, easily cleaned, and resistant to rust and many cleaning/sanitizing compounds. Stainless steel comes in a variety of grades and finishes. Depending on the particular application, the correct grade and finish should be used for food operations. Another popular material in the food industry is plastic. Applications of plastic involving food contact range from cutting boards to margarine containers, but not all plastics are alike. Plastics are broadly categorized as either thermoplastics or thermosets. The thermoplastics include a variety of materials composed from ethylene-based monomers, and sometimes nylons. Each thermoplastic product has physical properties that determine its utility and limitations in the food industry. Some thermoplastics are fairly durable and provide smooth, easily cleanable surfaces, such as polyethylene cutting boards, while other thermoplastics are used only for cold-holding applications and wraps. Thermoset plastics, such as polyesters and polyurethanes, generally have greater tolerance for a wider range of temperatures.

From a sanitary perspective, plastics have contributed greatly to cleanliness and minimizing cross contamination in food handling operations. The disadvantage of plastics is that some retain colors from certain substances (e.g., iodine, certain oils) and are vulnerable to degradation by certain cleaners and sanitizers. Over time, plastics can also become scored and degraded, leaving behind crevices and other imperfections on the surface. The right plastic must be chosen for the right application. Regulatory oversight of plastics in the food industry by FDA involves the potential migration of chemical substances to foods (i.e., indirect food additives). The condition of the plastic's surface that contacts food is generally regulated as a sanitary inspection item.

Cleaning and sanitizing food processing/preparation equipment is important but can present major challenges. The equipment must be constructed with acceptable materials from the perspectives of sanitary practice and chemical migration to foods. The food contact parts of equipment must be easily accessible so that they can be properly cleaned and sanitized. The equipment construction must be in a manner that does not allow accumulation of food soils and also separates toxic machinery lubricants and materials from food contact. The major types of cleaning systems for equipment are mechanical cleaning or clean-in-place (CIP), clean-out-of-place (COP), and manual cleaning. For applications where food equipment is difficult or impractical to disassemble for routine cleaning, CIP equipment has become popular. CIP equipment typically employs a circulating system that provides mechanical action with washes and rinses using detergents and sanitizers (FDA and PHS 2009). The design and operation of CIP equipment must ensure that circulating detergents and sanitizers reach all food contact surfaces and that no accumulation of food debris and microbial growth is possible. COP equipment requires various degrees of disassembly by workers and cleaning in a separate production area. The parts from COP equipment may be cleaned in specialized washer tanks or compartmented sinks equipped with mechanical brushes, heating elements, and pumps. Manual cleaning of equipment requires complete disassembly before the parts can be inspected, cleaned, sanitized, and reassembled.

Although some equipment and food contact materials are not allowed in commercial food operations, most food safety regulations and local ordinances covering the construction of food processing and service equipment are performance based. In other words, laws and ordinances may specify criteria such as acceptable temperatures and use words such as "durable, corrosion-resistant, easily cleanable," and so forth, but they do not mandate a particular piece of equipment. In many cases, the acceptability of materials or food equipment requires the judgment of a qualified inspector. This can sometimes be contentious. To assist all concerned with acceptable materials and the construction of food equipment, several so-called third-party organizations have developed "consensus standards" and certify materials and equipment used in the food industry. Two notable organizations in the United States are 3-A Sanitary Standards, Inc., and NSF International. These organizations have steering committees and procedures for food industry suppliers who want third-party certification of their products. Food industry products that meet the standards specified by these organizations may display the organizations' logo or symbol, indicating the products meet minimum requirements of the consensus standards.

## Waste Disposal

Proper waste disposal is the original basis of sanitation. Large volumes of solid, semisolid, and liquid wastes are produced by food processing and preparation facilities. These wastes typically include trimmings and leftover portions of foods, packaging materials, contaminated wash and rinse water, and human excrement from staff and patrons. Wastes are often sources of pathogenic and toxigenic microorganisms, and organic wastes provide an excellent growth medium for microorganisms. Poorly managed wastes are also an attractant and food source for a variety of pests capable of vectoring diseases and contaminating foodstuff. From an aesthetic viewpoint, the accumulation of wastes produces unpleasant odors and sights, discouraging customers from consuming food from the facility. Outside of the food facility, improper waste disposal can create public health hazards in the surrounding community and cause environmental damage.

Toilet and hand washing facilities are essential for people who work in or visit a food facility. The proper number and types of toilets are necessary to ensure people can access and use toilets when needed, without excessive waiting times. Local ordinances and codes usually specify requirements for the number, type, location, and installation of plumbing fixtures such as toilets and hand washing sinks. In general, toilets should not be located in or open into food handling, storage, or dining areas. They should be enclosed in a manner to exclude access by flies or other pests, and the toilet area should be kept clean with plenty of toilet paper, soap for hand washing, and a means of drying hands in a hygienic and sanitary manner. Of course, any food or objects that contact foods should not be permitted in toilet rooms or facilities. The sewage system for removing wastes must conform to local sanitary ordinances or laws for the type of system (either a public sewer system or an individual sewage disposal system).

Garbage and other food wastes must be disposed in a manner that does not provide a medium for microbial growth, source of food for insects or other pests, or public health nuisance for customers and the community. Because 70% of food composition is water, garbage disposal units are effective and sanitary means of eliminating food scraps from the facility. Unfortunately, garbage disposal units have several disadvantages that include high energy costs and extensive water use, and not all food wastes can be ground for wastewater disposal. Furthermore, a garbage disposal unit must be attached to a sewage line leading to a wastewater treatment plant capable of handing the organic loading from food wastes. In some jurisdictions, garbage disposal units for commercial food facilities are not allowed, in which case the food facility must treat its own wastewater or handle food waste as solid wastes. A hierarchical approach to managing food wastes is preferable. The hierarchy begins by source reduction. This involves minimizing food wastes by purchasing and using foods before they expire or perish and carefully planning the amount of food prepared to reduce leftovers and waste. When food is disposed as solid waste, sanitary practices should be employed in its handling and disposal. Containers with food wastes should be lined with plastic bags whenever possible and cleaned and sanitized regularly. For large volumes of food wastes and high capacity containers, a professional cleaning and sanitizing system is necessary. All waste receptacles and containers should be covered and have sufficient integrity to exclude pests when not in use. Local laws and ordinances regarding solid waste disposal must also be followed.

Single-use and disposable items have become a modern convenience and help reduce cleanup activities, particularly for temporary or mobile food service operations. After becoming soiled, single-use dishes and utensils are simply discarded, eliminating the need to bring soiled items back into the facility for washing. The disadvantage of single-use items is the volume of solid waste that must be managed and disposed, and the soiled items must be handled in a sanitary manner to prevent contact with clean surfaces and exclude access by pests. In recent years, environmental concerns about littering and conservation have prompted some communities to require single-use items be recycled or composted. If not properly managed, the storage of soiled recyclable materials can cause sanitation problems in food facilities.

## Pest Control

Pests usually refer to rodents and arthropods, but pests may include any domesticated and wild animals. The arthropods of greatest public health significance in food facilities are the insects commonly known as cockroaches, flies, and ants. These insects are most frequently associated with (contaminative) mechanical transmission of vertebrate pathogens—frequently from contact with food (Foil and Gorham 2004). Within the taxonomic orders of Blattaria (cockroaches) and Diptera (flies, mosquitoes, etc.), dozens of species are associated with human habitation; the most important species with regard to food sanitation number around two dozen. In the United States, the most frequently encountered cockroaches in dwellings and food facilities are German cockroaches (*Blattella germanica*), brown banded cockroaches (*Supella longipalpa*), American cockroaches (*Periplaneta americana*), Oriental cockroaches (*Blatta orientalis*), smokybrown cockroaches (*Periplaneta fuliginosa*), and the less widely distributed Asian cockroaches (*Blattella asahinai*). Cockroaches are prolific breeders, and once established in a food facility, controlling them becomes more difficult and costly. By foraging and feeding, cockroaches pick up pathogens and disperse them to other areas, resulting in direct or indirect contact with foods.

Approximately 21 species of flies are hazards to human health from contact with food (Olsen 1998). These hazards include foodborne myiasis and mechanical transmission of pathogens. Foodborne myiasis is a condition where fly larvae invade the gastrointestinal tract. This condition is relatively rare in the United States, and only certain flies are associated with the disease. The greatest hazard from flies is their role as mechanical vectors of enteric disease. Several species of domestic flies are known transmitters of enteric diseases, and they amplify the risk of disease transmission by contaminating foods. Mechanical transmission occurs by flies transporting pathogens from contaminated sources (e.g., feces, sewage, offal) to foods. Once the food is contaminated, the pathogens may multiply to greater numbers and increase the risk of an infection. Flies belonging to the families Muscidae (house flies), Calliphoridae (blow flies), and Sarcophagidae (flesh flies) are most important in the mechanical transmission of pathogens to foods.

Rodents cause the greatest problems among the vertebrate pests. Known throughout history as carriers of disease, rodents such as rats and mice have become unwanted co-inhabitants with people. They are attracted to wherever food, shelter, and water can be found. Food facilities make ideal habitats for rodents because all their biological needs are met. Rodents are carriers of zoonotic pathogens, and they can mechanically transmit pathogens from contaminated sources to foodstuff. While foraging and feeding, rodents constantly urinate and defecate, leaving contamination throughout a food facility. Excrement from rodents can be deposited directly on food contact surfaces or be transferred by air movement and food worker activities. The two most common rats in the United States are the Norway or brown rat (*Rattus norvegicus*) and the roof or black rat (*Rattus rattus*). Mice are much smaller than rats and can enter a food facility through very small openings or be brought in with crates and boxes.

Birds and other pests are less frequently encountered in food facilities, but when present, they pose a significant threat of food contamination from pathogen-laden droppings. Wild and feral animals should be prevented from breeding around and having access to food facilities. Pets and other domestic animals should not be allowed to enter food facilities because they may be carriers of zoonotic pathogens, and they often carry toxigenic bacteria such as *Staphylococcus aureus.*

Waiting until a pest problem becomes apparent increases the risk of food contamination and makes control of the pests more difficult and expensive. With adequate food and harborage, the population growth of most pests is rapid. The female housefly (*Musca domestica*) lays batches of 100 to 150 eggs every 3 or 4 days. From eggs to adult flies takes about 8 to 12 days in warm weather. The female German cockroach (*Blatella germanica*) carries an egg case with her during the incubation period, around 16 to 28 days, and deposits the egg case just before hatching time. About 40 nymphs will emerge from the egg case and begin foraging for food. The nymphs become adults after several growth stages and molting. From eggs to adult cockroaches takes about 3 to 4 months, during which time the adult female cockroach has deposited additional egg cases. Norway rats (Rattus *norvegicus*) produce litter sizes of 6 to 12 young about 21–23 days following conception. At 3 or 4 weeks old, the rat pups are sufficiently independent to forage for food, and they reach reproductive maturity between 2 and 3 months old. Female Norway rats can produce four to six litters per year.

Surveys and monitoring are necessary to detect the presence of pests before the population grows to significant numbers. Monitoring for pests requires inspections under, above, around, and sometimes within equipment and supplies. Ideally, storage shelves and attached equipment should be visible for inspection from all angles and without clutter. Floor space should also be completely visible throughout the facility. This usually requires that equipment and storage units be elevated 6 inches off the floor or sealed completely to the floor and/or wall to eliminate cracks or openings. Cockroaches and rodents are nocturnal pests, rarely leaving their hiding spaces during daylight hours. A large population of these pests forces some individuals to forage and seek shelter during atypical times. Thus, seeing cockroaches or rodents during daylight hours is an indication of a serious pest problem. Indirect signs of rodents include the presence of droppings, gnawing marks on foodstuff and nonfood materials, and rub marks or streaks along floors or walls from frequent contact with their fur. Indirect signs of cockroaches include much smaller fecal particles and sometimes the presence of an oily odor. Turning on a light in a dark room may also reveal the presence of cockroaches as they scurry to hide.

Along with inspections, other monitoring techniques are effective for detecting the presence of pests. Rodents can be detected by spreading talc on the floor to capture track marks, and rat urine stains on certain surfaces fluoresce when illuminated with a UV light. Cockroach populations can be monitored using several trapping techniques. Companies produce commercial cockroach traps that consist of a chemical attractant and sticky surfaces. By placing traps at strategic locations in a facility, the type of cockroach species and problem areas can be identified. If carefully and knowledgably performed, surveys using chemical flushing agents can also detect the presence and hiding spots of cockroaches.

The control of pests in food facilities is best accomplished by using an approach called integrated pest management (IPM). This approach exploits knowledge about the biology of pests to limit their population density and uses pesticides sparingly and only when necessary to maintain control. An important part of IPM is excluding access by pests to the food facility. The facility's construction and condition are important in excluding access. Closed or screened windows/doors and air curtains at entrances are effective means of excluding flies. Rat proofing a facility involves systematically surveying access points into the facility and eliminating them through repairs and modifications. Inspecting incoming crates, boxes, and packages can spot cockroaches and mice that may be hitching a ride into the facility. Another means of reducing access is by eliminating breeding sites around the facility. This includes the sanitary management of solid and liquid wastes outside of the food facility.

While the exclusion of pests from a facility is important, it is not foolproof, especially with larger facilities and older buildings. Therefore, pest control efforts must include measures inside of the facility. The IPM approach requires implementing good sanitary principles. By eliminating wastes and food residues, the pests are not attracted to the facility, and the population density is limited by the availability of food, water, and shelter. Wastes must be removed and surfaces cleaned to eliminate food sources for insects and rodents. The design and construction of equipment, walls, floors, counters, and other structures must allow easy inspection, access, and cleaning. Attached and free-standing equipment should not have hidden areas that can accumulate food debris and harbor pests. All foodstuffs must be stored in containers that are inaccessible by pests. For rodents, this requires sealed metal containers. Leaking and standing water sources should not be permitted.

When needed, pesticides are carefully selected and used in food facilities. The improper use of pesticides in a food facility can result in contamination of foodstuff and human poisonings. Poison baits are often used to eliminate rodents, but poisons are dangerous to nontarget organisms, including humans. Furthermore, rodents frequently die in inaccessible areas, resulting in smells and maggot problems. Trapping is the preferred method for eliminating rodents in a structure, and a variety of safe and effective traps have been developed in recent years. With regard to cockroaches, the application of selected insecticides and bait stations are the most effective means of pesticide use. The spraying of insecticides must be carefully performed to minimize risks to applicators, staff, and customers. Insecticide application is performed during times when the food facility is not in operation (e.g., nights or weekends), and application techniques such as "crack and crevice" spraying are safer and most effective for cockroaches. When using pesticides, the level of required training is commensurate with the risks of the pesticide type and application method. In most cases, a licensed or certified pesticide applicator under the supervision of a professional pest controller is recommended and/or legally required.

## FOODBORNE ILLNESS RISK FACTORS

An epidemiologic analysis of foodborne disease outbreaks in the United States from 1988–1992 by the Centers for Disease Control and Prevention (Bean et al. 1996) identified five broad categories of factors that contributed to the outbreaks. The Retail Food Team of FDA slightly modified these contributing factors and designated them as foodborne illness risk factors (FDA 2004):

- Food from unsafe sources
- Inadequate cooking
- Improper holding time and temperatures
- Poor personal hygiene
- Contaminated equipment/prevention of contamination

Foodborne illness risk factors represent critical items for nearly all food safety programs. Periodically, FDA uses these risk factors to survey retail food establishments and determine the prevalence of unsafe food handling practices (FDA 2004). The food safety student must commit to memory the foodborne illness risk factors, given their importance.

## Food from Unsafe Sources

The majority of biological and toxic agents that cause foodborne illnesses originate from sources early in the food handling chain, before the foods enter the kitchen. In the United States and other developed countries, the responsibility for food safety starts on the farm and extends to the consumer. Regulations govern farm land use, animal feed, agrochemical use, sanitary practices in abattoirs and processing facilities, food additives and packaging, and other aspects of food safety. At the retail food facility and consumer levels, trust is implicit that agricultural producers and food processors comply with the maze of regulations. When noncompliance occurs, it is often identified early by regulators or epidemiologists, and food recalls are initiated and/or other interventions are implemented. Foods from unregulated sources pose the greatest risk of contamination with biological, chemical, and physical agents.

Retail food facility managers are responsible for ensuring that wholesale and raw foods are purchased from regulated sources. Reputable wholesalers can provide documentation to show their approval as food suppliers. Retail food facilities should maintain purchase receipts from all food suppliers. Furthermore, retail food facilities should inspect incoming food supplies for expiration dates, proper temperature control, pests, protection from contamination, and obvious signs of adulteration, contaminants, or damage. Foods that are received processed as ready-to-eat (RTE) should be so labeled and properly packaged to prevent contamination. The risk of contaminated foods is greatest with home processed or canned foods, where the food processes may be unsafe and not subject to inspection.

Other possible unsafe sources of foods include wild game and mushrooms or plants gathered from nature. Only under specially regulated circumstances should foods collected in the wild be used by retail food facilities. Wild game animals pose unique risks, and knowledge about the local area and species, as well as any special handling, is important prior to preparation and consumption (Friend 2006). Laws governing the sale and consumption of live-caught or field-dressed wild game animals are much more restrictive and vary by state. Game animal species raised on farms may be sold for food under a voluntary USDA inspection program. Imported game animal species are regulated under the jurisdiction of FDA.

Fish and shellfish are examples of foods collected in the wild that are specifically regulated. Commercial fishermen and seafood dealers are regulated by federal and state agencies to ensure safe and sanitary practices are followed. Nevertheless, even with regulatory oversight, the risks are not completely eliminated. Contamination of fish and shellfish with chemicals, algal toxins, parasitic worms, bacteria, protozoans, and viruses can still occur from the fishing waters and shellfish beds. The monitoring and restriction of fishing waters help reduce these risks, but the fishermen must heed these restrictions when issued by regulatory authorities. Molluscan shellfish represent an exceptional risk because they are often eaten raw or undercooked. Shellfish harvested from waters that contain hepatitis A, *Vibrio* species, and other pathogens are known to transmit enteric diseases. Under the National Shellfish Sanitation Program (NSSP), waters are monitored, and shellfish harvesting is regulated on the basis of water quality. Listings of approved shellfish harvesters, dealers, and processors are available from FDA. Each container of shellfish must have an identity tag affixed to it that identifies relevant information about the harvester, dealer, and location and date of harvest. For raw shellfish that are sold or served, these tags must be retained by the retail food facility for 90 days to allow traceback investigation in the event of a foodborne illness outbreak.

The consumption of raw fish in dishes such as sushi and ceviche has become popular in recent years. Fish caught or harvested from natural bodies of water may carry parasitic worms that can either infect or injure consumers. Some worms are deeply embedded in the muscle tissue of fish, the part most often consumed raw. Parasitic worms can be killed if the fish are thoroughly frozen for a sufficient amount of time. Following are the prescribed combinations of freezing temperatures and times (FDA and PHS 2009):

- The fish must be frozen and stored frozen at a temperature of –20°C (–4°F) or below for at least 168 hours.
- The fish must be frozen solid and stored frozen at –35°C (–31°F) or below for at least 15 hours.
- The fish must be frozen until solid at –35°C (–31°F) or below and then stored at –20°C (–4°F) or below for at least 24 hours.

Retail food facilities that receive fish intended to be eaten raw must ensure that they have been properly frozen to kill parasitic worms. If the freezing process has been done off-premises by the supplier, purchase specifications should be provided that states the fish have been adequately treated with proper freezing techniques; the raw fish should also be labeled to advise food handlers whether it has been properly frozen.

## Inadequate Cooking

Done properly with regard to time and temperature, cooking can destroy human pathogens, zoonotic pathogens, and vegetative forms of toxigenic microorganisms. Cooking guidelines and requirements are based on the microbial population density (i.e., loading) and heat resistance of those pathogens associated with certain foods. Dishes containing meats and eggs warrant particular attention because the raw animal products may be contaminated with zoonotic pathogens. In the past, guidance was provided for cooking meat and poultry based on the interior color of the meat, but subsequent studies revealed that color was not always a good indicator of pathogen destruction. Nowadays, cooking temperatures are measured with a thermometer, and minimum holding times are provided as guidance. Table 4-6 summarizes minimum food cooking temperatures recommended by the U.S. Public Health Service's Food Code (FDA and PHS 2009). These minimum cooking temperatures are based on thorough heating of the entire food product. Some deviations from these cooking temperatures may be encountered in food safety references, but these deviations are usually higher temperatures—not lower.

**Table 4-6** Summary of Minimum Internal Cooking Temperatures and Holding Times

| Foods | Minimum Internal Temperatures | Minimum Holding Times at Specified Temperatures |
|---|---|---|
| Raw eggs prepared for immediate service | | |
| Commercially raised game animals | 63°C (145°F) | 15 seconds |
| Fish, pork, or other meats not specified below or in section ¶3-401.11(B)[a] | | |
| Raw eggs not prepared for immediate service | 68°C (155°F) or one of the following combinations: | 15 seconds |
| Comminuted meats, fish, or commercially raised game animals | 70°C (158°F) | < 1 second |
| Mechanically tenderized meats | 66°C (150°F) | 1 minute |
| Ratites (ostrich, rhea, and emu) | 63°C (145°F) | 3 minutes |
| Poultry (e.g., chicken, turkey) | | |
| Baluts (fertilized eggs) | | |
| Stuffed fish, meats, pasta, poultry, and ratites | 74°C (165°F) | 15 seconds |
| Stuffing containing fish, meat, poultry, or ratites | | |
| Wild game animals | | |
| Food cooked in a microwave | 74°C (165°F) | Hold covered for 2 minutes after removal from microwave oven. |
| Whole meat roasts | Refer to cooking charts in ¶3-401.11(B)[a] | |

[a]Refers to a section in the Food Code.

*Source*: Modified from the Food Code (2009).

Federal officials strengthened regulations on egg production and transport following reported outbreaks and the estimated incidence of *Salmonella enteritidis* infections in the United States during the 1980s and 1990s. A public education campaign was also launched to discourage eating raw or undercooked eggs. The current guidance is to cook fresh eggs at 63°C (145°F) or higher for 15 seconds. Many people prefer their eggs to be soft or runny, increasing the risk of acquiring salmonellosis. For consumers without thermometers, CDC recommends cooking eggs until the white and yolk are both firm (Centers for Disease Control and Prevention [CDC] 2003). Young children, older adults, and people with weakened immune systems or debilitating illness have an increased risk of complications from salmonellosis, possibly resulting in hospitalization or death. People at high risk of complications should always avoid raw or undercooked eggs or egg products.

Beef steak is one of the few meat products in the United States that consumers prefer to eat rare. The risks of eating rare steak are minimal if the meat is taken from a healthy animal and handled in a manner to prevent contamination with pathogens. Steaks cut from meats that are USDA-inspected and butchered under sanitary conditions are more likely to be safe for consumption. But visual inspections of carcasses and meats do not ensure the surface of steak is free of contamination with pathogenic microorganisms. Therefore, steak surfaces should be heated sufficiently to kill any pathogenic microorganisms. The Food Code (FDA and PHS 2009) permits raw or undercooked beef (steak) to be served if the following are applicable:

- The population served is not considered highly susceptible to infections.
- The steak is cut from whole-muscle, intact beef.
- The steak is labeled by the food processing plant to indicate that the steak meets the definition of whole-muscle, intact beef.
- The steak is prepared in a manner to remain intact.
- The steak is cooked on the top and bottom to a surface temperature of 63°C (145°F) or higher.
- The steak has a cooked color change on all external surfaces.

Ground or comminuted meat, particularly hamburger, should be cooked at higher temperatures. The Food Code specifies an internal temperature of 68°C (155°F) or higher for 15 seconds or longer. The USDA recommends cooking ground beef, veal, lamb, and pork to an internal temperature of 71.1°C (160°F), and it recommends ground turkey and chicken be cooked to an internal temperature of 73.9°C (165°F). The higher cooking temperatures for ground meat are deemed necessary for several reasons. One reason is the established history of *E. coli* O157:H7 outbreaks from hamburger meat, along with numerous food recalls over the past few decades. A second reason is that ground meat consists of raw ingredients mixed together from different animals and even from different ranches or companies. One infected animal can contaminate tons of ground meat, and the likelihood of encountering contaminated ground meat at the consumer level is increased. In addition, the grinding process distributes pathogens throughout the meat product—both externally and internally—requiring heating throughout the entire product. Higher heat is also needed because the bactericidal effect of heat is less efficient in fatty foods such as hamburger. Finally, microbial challenge testing has demonstrated that higher temperatures are necessary to ensure complete pathogen destruction in ground meats.

Unlike beef steak, pork products should never be eaten rare or undercooked. The long history of trichinellosis and the consequences of taeniasis or cysticercosis from pork warrant caution. These parasites embed themselves within the swine muscle and other tissues, and cooking only the surfaces of chops and other cuts of pork is not adequate to destroy the parasites. The Food Code requires cooking all parts of pork to an internal temperature of 63°C (145°F) or higher for 15 seconds or longer. The USDA recommends an internal cooking temperature of 145°F and a three-minute rest period for whole cuts of pork, steaks, and chops. Parasitic worms in pork can also be destroyed by proper freezing techniques, but the correct combination of freezing temperatures and duration are dependent on the thickness of meat cuts and packaging. Thorough cooking of pork is the preferred method to ensure destruction of parasitic worms, as well as other pathogens.

Raw poultry is potentially contaminated with a number of zoonotic pathogens, and thorough cooking is necessary to ensure complete pathogen destruction. Chickens and turkeys are often cooked as whole birds or cut-up pieces. Sometimes the pieces are deboned and comminuted or minced and used as ingredients in a variety of dishes. Regardless of the form, raw poultry should be cooked so that all parts reach an internal temperature of 74°C (165°F) or higher for 15 seconds or longer. The baking of whole birds requires care to ensure the minimum cooking temperature and time are reached in areas where heat transfer is not efficient, for example, the innermost parts of thighs and wings and the thickest part of the breast. If the bird is stuffed, the interior of the stuffing must reach the minimum cooking temperature and time. Because stuffing may not reach the required temperature and time before the bird is done, USDA recommends cooking stuffing in a separate container rather than in the bird's cavity.

Game animals that are procured from approved sources must be cooked thoroughly or otherwise treated to ensure destruction of parasites and microbial pathogens. This is challenging for low-fat game meats because excessive cooking can result in drying and unpalatable tastes. A variety of cooking and preservation methods are used for wild game, and if not done properly, the risks of consuming game meat can be serious (Friend 2006). The health of the game animal is important when choosing to consume its meat. The Food Code recommends cooking wild game animals to an internal temperature of 74°C (165°F) or higher for 15 seconds or longer. For game animals raised commercially for food and subjected to the voluntary inspection program, the Food Code (FDA and PHS 2009) recommends cooking the meat thoroughly to an internal temperature of 63°C (145°F) or higher for 15 seconds or longer. If the commercially raised game meat is comminuted, the recommended internal cooking temperature is 68°C (155°F) or higher for 15 seconds or longer or one of the temperature–time combinations of the chart shown in Table 4-6.

Some fruits and vegetables are intended to be eaten raw or partially cooked, in which case they should be peeled or washed in a sanitary and hygienic manner before being served to consumers. An exception to this general rule is when the food has been received in RTE form from the supplier. Fruits and vegetables intended for cooking should be washed to remove soil and other debris. Plant-based foods such as certain raw beans must be cooked at prescribed temperatures and times to ensure doneness and the destruction of natural plant toxins. The prescribed temperatures and times vary with the type of plant and plant part, but the Food Code (FDA and PHS 2009) stipulates that foods made from plants be cooked to a temperature of 57°C (135°F) and transferred to hot holding prior to serving. Many dishes contain a combination of vegetables, fruits, and meats. For combination dishes, the cooking temperatures and times must meet the requirements specified for the type of raw meat ingredient. Sometimes the meat ingredient is precooked prior to combining with the other ingredients. For these dishes, the recommended cooking procedure is to heat all parts of the food to a temperature of 74°C (165°F) or higher for 15 seconds or longer. Additionally, whenever PHF/TCS foods are cooked in a noncontinuous manner, the requirements for time/temperature control must be carefully followed between cooking sessions.

Microwave cooking has become commonplace in retail food establishments and home kitchens. The heat generated in food by microwaves is not uniform and must transfer throughout the food product or dish. To ensure adequate heating, raw meats and dishes containing raw meats or eggs must either rotate on a carousel or be stirred halfway through the cooking period. The food should also be covered to retain surface moisture and prevent the spattering of debris. Raw meat foods heated with a microwave should reach a temperature of 74°C (165°F) or higher throughout the food product or dish, and the food should stand covered for 2 minutes after cooking. Heat equilibrium is usually attained during this time period, ensuring that all parts of the dish are adequately cooked.

While cooking is an effective method of destroying most pathogens, it is often not effective in destroying spores and certain preformed toxins. The vegetative forms of bacteria such as *Clostridium* species and *Bacillus cereus* are destroyed at normal cooking temperatures, but their spores can survive cooking and germinate later when the temperatures become favorable. Misconceptions that all cooked food is sterile have led to unsafe food holding temperatures that allowed the germination and multiplication of spore-forming microorganisms. Reheating or recooking foods may once again destroy the vegetative forms, but the number of surviving spores will be greater with each successive heating and cooling period. And although *Staphylococcus aureus* is readily destroyed by cooking temperatures, staphylococcal enterotoxins are not. Measures such as time/temperature control are important to preventing the germination of spore-forming bacteria and the growth of staphylococci. Other heat-stabile toxins can be controlled by eliminating the source.

## Improper Holding/ Time and Temperatures

The risk factor observed most often in foodborne illness outbreaks and surveys of unsafe food practices is the improper holding temperatures of PHF/TCS foods (Bean et al. 1996; FDA 2004). The significance of time–temperature combinations on the population growth of pathogenic and toxigenic microorganisms was examined at length earlier in this chapter. Some important temperatures for the control of microorganisms in food are shown in Figure 4-6. Foods with intrinsic and extrinsic parameters that are favorable to microbial growth (i.e., PHF/TCS foods) need very little contamination with bacteria before rapid growth to hazardous population levels. Therefore, foods that meet the definition of PHF/TCS foods must be time/temperature controlled to limit pathogen growth and toxin formation. This applies principally to bacteria but includes all rapidly or slowly growing pathogenic or toxigenic microorganisms (except for viruses because they require a living host). A temperature difference of a few degrees can result in exponential differences in microbial population levels. The time–temperature combinations for safe holding of foods are proposed on the basis of laboratory studies and the modeling of microbial population growth. When available, timelines from epidemiologic studies of outbreaks also contribute. The cold holding temperature/time guidelines for most foods are based primarily on the growth of *Listeria monocytogenes*, a commonly detected pathogen capable of reproducing at colder temperatures (FDA and PHS 2009). For shell eggs, the growth of salmonellae is the primary basis for cold holding. In developing time/temperature holding guidelines or regulations, the risks are balanced against the feasibility of achieving and maintaining various temperatures.

The Food Code (FDA and PHS 2009) stipulates that all PHF/TCS food held for consumption must be maintained at either 5°C (41°F) and lower or 57°C (135°F) and higher. This represents the outer boundaries of the temperature "danger zone." *An important point to remember is that these temperatures refer to the measured temperature of the* food *itself—not the air temperature.*

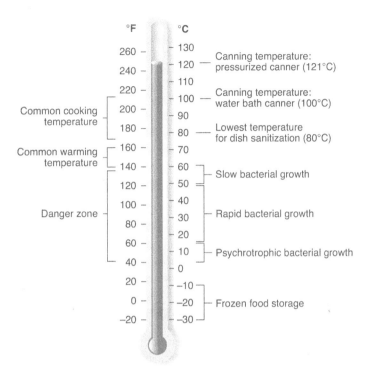

**Figure 4-6** Important Temperature Considerations in Food Microbiology

Exemptions to the time/temperature rule are permitted for roasts being cooked to specific temperatures, eggs stored under 7°C (45°F) conditions, and homogenous liquid foods stored in specially designed equipment. Under certain situations and within very specific time limits, PHF/TCS food may be allowed within the temperature "danger zone." These situations are referred to as using "time as a public health control" by the Food Code (FDA and PHS 2009). After PHF/TCS food is removed from initial holding temperatures of 5°C (41°F) and lower or 57°C (135°F) and higher, it can be held prior to serving at any temperature for a total maximum time of 4 hours. The total maximum time can be 6 hours if the food is removed from an initial holding temperature of 5°C (41°F) and lower—not warmer—and the PHF/TCS food does not exceed a temperature 21°C (70°F) during the entire 6 hours. Because microbial growth has likely occurred during the 4 or 6 hour times in the temperature danger zone, the food must be discarded at the end of these time limits. To ensure the time limits are not exceeded, the PHF/TCS food must be marked or otherwise identified with the time it was removed from safe holding temperatures and when it must be discarded.

In large facilities or complex food operations, many foods are prepared and/or cooked in advance of consumption. Commercial food processors also prepare foods in advance for the convenience of consumers. Any prepared food, whether done in advance or prior to serving, is considered ready-to-eat (RTE) food. Preparing foods in advance frequently leads to time/temperature abuse, microbial growth, and foodborne illness outbreaks. Therefore, foods prepared in advance must be specially processed and/or subjected to strict time/temperature controls to prevent microbial growth. When prepared on the premises of a retail food facility, RTE foods may be maintained under refrigeration with a temperature of 5°C (41°F) and lower for a maximum of 7 days, provided the product is clearly marked with the date when it must be consumed on the premises, sold, or discarded (FDA and PHS 2009). Supermarkets, delis, and restaurants may also receive RTE foods from commercial food processors. These RTE foods may be processed and packaged in a manner to safely extend the shelf life, but the safety of the processed food can be compromised once opened by the retail food facility. In general, the RTE food from a commercial processor cannot be used (consumed) past the "use-by" date marked on the unopened package, and once the package is opened, the RTE food must be date-marked for consumption, sale, or discarding within 7 days of opening. Exemptions are provided in the Food Code for commercially processed RTE foods that are specially regulated to ensure product safety.

Cold holding/storage of foods require refrigeration and freezing temperatures of 0°–5°C (32°–41°F) and –10°C (14°F) and lower, respectively. Properly frozen foods should remain safe indefinitely, but the quality of the food product diminishes over time. The potential for microbial growth with frozen foods is greatest during the freezing and thawing periods. For foods stored under refrigeration, the pathogens *L. monocytogenes* and *Y. enterocolitica* are primary safety concerns. These bacteria may continue to grow very slowly under proper refrigeration. The retention times of food held under refrigeration are often derived from various spoilage bacteria and molds. Nonetheless, the growth of pathogens and toxin formation can occur from temperature changes during the opening of refrigerator doors, loss of electrical power, failure of the refrigeration unit, improper cooling of cooked food, and improper reheating of refrigerated foods. Leftover foods can be problematic because tracking the total time the food was in the temperature danger zone is difficult to ascertain. For consumers in the home, USDA recommends discarding foods left out at room temperature for more than 2 hours, or 1 hour if the ambient temperature is above 32.2°C (90°F). Rapidly cooled leftovers stored under proper refrigeration should be eaten within 3 or 4 days. Retail food establishments must adhere to federal and state regulations concerning RTE foods, including leftovers.

Prior to freezing or refrigerating cooked foods, a rapid cool-down or chill period is required to minimize pathogen growth and toxin production. Large food items or big batches of foods can take unacceptably long to chill, and placing hot items in conventional refrigerators and freezers results in heat transfer to other foods. In industrial and food processing facilities, the chilling and freezing operation may be done rapidly in one step with specially designed blast freezers. Some food processors and retail food facilities use special equipment to shorten the chilling period. In retail food facilities without specialized equipment, a rapid chilling period may be accomplished with alternative methods. Foods separated into smaller containers or batches have better heat transfer and chill faster. Shallow dishes or pans (≤ 2 inches deep) chill faster compared with deeper pots and pans. Removing the lid from a hot container accelerates the loss of heat, and placing pots in ice water baths and stirring the food shorten the chilling period. Whatever methods are used for chilling, two critical time/temperature limits must be met. First, hot PHF/TCS food must be chilled from 57°C (135°F) to 21°C (70°F) within 2 hours, and second, the total amount of time to reach 5°C (41°F) or lower from 57°C (135°F) must not exceed 6 hours (FDA and PHS 2009). The reason for a more rapid cool-down between 57°C (135°F) and 21°C (70°F) is related to the optimum growth temperatures of most foodborne pathogens (see Figure 4-3). For PHF/TCS foods that were prepared at ambient temperatures (e.g., canned meat used in a dish), the chilling period to reach 5°C (41°F) or lower is within 4 hours.

Thawing frozen foods is another temperature transition period that requires careful attention. Because of inefficient heat transfer, the outer portions of frozen foods thaw more quickly compared with the internal portions. Within the temperature danger zone, the outer portions of a PHF/TCS food can support rapid microbial growth for several hours, while the inner portions remain frozen. Furthermore, when the internal portions of a raw food are frozen, pathogen destruction may be incomplete during the cooking process. A safe method of thawing frozen foods is by maintaining them under refrigeration temperatures of 5°C (41°F) or lower. This requires advance meal planning to allow sufficient time for complete thawing. Other acceptable thawing methods involve submergence of the food in a running water bath with a temperature of 21°C (70°F) or lower and with sufficient agitation to remove any food debris. For raw animal foods that will be thoroughly cooked, the water bath must not allow any portion of the food to be above 5°C (41°F) for longer than 4 hours. Some processed foods are intended to go from freezer to cooking without thawing, in which case the preparation instructions must be carefully followed. If properly operated and/or programmed, microwave ovens can effectively thaw frozen foods in short periods of time, but the Food Code (FDA and PHS 2009) requires transfer of PHF/TCS food to conventional cooking processes immediately after microwave thawing.

The reheating of prepared foods represents yet another temperature transition period that could result in a potential hazard. Proper reheating of foods can ensure certain pathogens are destroyed and limit the growth of spore-formers such *C. perfringens*. Conversely, improper reheating of PHS/TCS foods can allow the rapid growth of pathogens and/or toxin formation. Cooked foods are more likely to support the growth of pathogenic or toxigenic microorganisms because competing spoilage microorganisms have been destroyed by previous cooking, and intrinsic parameters such as $a_w$ may become more favorable after cooking. To ensure destruction of vegetative bacteria and minimize time in the temperature danger zone, cooked foods should be reheated to 74°C (165°F) or higher for at least 15 seconds within a 2-hour time frame. Foods reheated using a microwave should reach the same temperature of 74°C (165°F) or higher and be held for at least 2 minutes to ensure complete heat equilibrium is attained. Foods from hermetically sealed containers are considered commercially sterile, and the reheating temperature needs to reach only 57°C (135°F) or higher for any length of time.

## Poor Worker Hygiene

Food workers are frequently the primary and secondary sources of pathogenic or toxigenic microorganisms. As carriers of enteric diseases, people transmit pathogens by direct or indirect contact with foods. They also transfer microbial contamination to foods from touching raw meats and other contaminated items. In a pivotal report, CDC (Bean et al. 1996) identified poor personal hygiene as the second most important contributing factor to foodborne illness outbreaks between 1988 and 1992. Poor personal hygiene of food workers was also the second most observed risk factor during surveys of retail food facilities by FDA (2004). Good personal hygiene by food workers is critically important to preventing microbial contamination of food, regardless of the source within the food facility. Despite a great amount of time and money spent by the food industry on educating workers, the problem of poor worker hygiene is a recurring one.

The role of food workers in the transmission of foodborne disease was evaluated in a series of publications by the Committee on Control of Foodborne Illnesses of the International Association for Food Protection (IAFP) (Todd et al. 2009, 2008a, 2008b, 2007a, 2007b and Greig et al. 2007). The study looked at 816 reports of worker-associated foodborne illnesses dating from 1927 to early 2006. Among the outbreaks, 14 biological agents were identified as responsible. The reported agents were viruses (60.2%), bacteria (34.3%), protozoans (2.8%), and unknown etiology (2.7%). The largest outbreaks involved thousands of cases and usually had a continuous source of infection that extended over several days. These large outbreaks also tended to be associated with special events, resorts, or food products distributed to large numbers of customers. The most frequently reported settings for worker-related outbreaks were foodservice facilities (46.1%), catered events (15.4%), homes (10.2%), schools and day care centers (6.0%), and health care facilities (5.3%).

The insights provided by the IAFP study support existing knowledge about the importance of food workers in disease outbreaks. Certainly, food workers are vitally important to sanitary practices and time/temperature controls, but as primary and secondary sources of microbial contamination, their hygienic practices can have a direct impact on food safety. An infected food worker is the reservoir of pathogens such as noroviruses, hepatitis virus, rotavirus, *Shigella* species, and *Vibrio cholerae*. Food workers are also reservoirs and secondary sources of salmonellae, pathogenic *E. coli*, staphylococci, streptococci, and other pathogenic or toxigenic microorganisms. During the incubatory, symptomatic, and convalescent phases of infection, food workers shed enteric pathogens in their vomitus, feces, and urine. A norovirus-infected individual can shed $10^6$ virus particles per milliliter in vomitus and $10^{11}$ virus particles per gram in feces, and only a few viruses are necessary to cause infection (Koopmans and Duizer 2002; Todd et al. 2008b). Chronic and asymptomatic carriers of disease may shed pathogens indefinitely with little or no indication of illness. Approximately one-third of Americans are chronic carriers of *S. aureus* in their nasal passages (Kuehnert et al. 2006), and staphylococci are common with skin infections, boils, or acne.

Direct contact with foods by infected workers is the primary food safety concern, but other items in contact with infected food workers become secondary sources of contamination. For virulent bacterial pathogens and enteric viruses, only a small infective dose is necessary to cause illness. The risk is multiplied when bacterial pathogens contaminate PHF/TCS foods because the bacteria rapidly multiply to infectious dose levels and spread contamination throughout the facility. Foods that are extensively handled by workers pose the greatest risks. This is particularly true for foods that do not have a pathogen destruction step (e.g., eaten raw) and foods that are handled by workers after cooking. Salads, hors d'oeuvres, and similar foods are usually made with raw ingredients, prepared by hand, and/or served at room temperature. These foods are excellent vehicles for the transmission of enteric pathogens. And because these foods often contain PHF/TCS ingredients, the growth of pathogenic and/or toxigenic bacteria is also likely to occur. Except in preapproved and carefully supervised situations, RTE foods should never be handled with bare hands. The use of disposable gloves, spatulas, tongs, or other hand-free methods are alternatives to handling RTE foods. The entire food handling process from procurement to serving must be examined to identify possible contamination from workers or customers, and measures should be implemented to minimize the risks.

The exclusion of infected workers from food facilities has mixed results in prevention efforts. As previously indicated, asymptomatic carriers may unwittingly shed pathogens. Policies such as stool testing to identify carriers have not been effective in the risk reduction of enteric diseases in food facilities (Todd et al. 2008a). Because a food worker with an illness or skin infection should be restricted from food-related jobs, many food workers conceal their illness for fear of losing their jobs or income. Some guidance documents recommend food workers with diarrhea or vomiting—the peak period of pathogen shedding—not work until after 24 hours have passed without symptoms. Even when an acutely ill food worker is removed from food operations, the risk of disease transmission from residual contamination remains great without meticulous cleaning and sanitization. Of course, a suspected outbreak or disease transmission by an infected food worker warrants prompt action to interrupt the chain of infection and prevent further cases. This may involve screening food workers for disease/carrier status and excluding them from the job for specific periods of time. Unfortunately, knowledge about the infection status of food workers will always be incomplete, and the best prevention strategies emphasize good worker hygiene.

For good personal hygiene to be practiced, the food facility must have properly located and sufficient numbers of lavatories and toilets. The Food Code (FDA and PHS 2009) and public health regulations by individual states delineate requirements for these essential utilities. Generally, separate hand washing sinks should be located in toilet rooms and the kitchen or other food handling areas. Along with soap dispensers and single-use towels or hand dryers, the sinks should have faucets that mix running hot and cold water to provide a hot ($\geq 38°C$ or $100°F$) but not scalding temperature. Whenever possible or required by law, food workers should have separate toilet facilities from the customers. Some states require the posting of a sign in the food workers' restroom stating they must wash their hands after using the toilet. Because food workers can bring pathogens to work from ill family members, a separate changing room with clean work clothes and lockers is desirable, and sometimes required by law. Food workers should also be provided hats or hair nets and should not wear jewelry at work.

Food workers should be instructed in how, when, and where to wash their hands. The hand washing technique should begin with a warm water rinse followed by a lathering scrub of hands, fingers, under fingernails, and exposed parts of arms for at least 10 to 15 seconds; a complete and thorough drying with single-use towels or hand dryer. The hand soap type should provide adequate cleaning but not be too harsh to cause skin irritation. Workers will not wash their hands frequently if the soap causes excessive drying or irritation. Hand antiseptics (formerly known as hand sanitizers) *cannot* be used as a substitute for hand washing. In addition to restroom visits, food workers should wash their hands in the following situations: after handling raw meats or other potentially contaminated items, at the beginning of shifts and after breaks, between changes of disposable gloves, or anytime good hygienic practices dictate (e.g., sneezing, nose blowing/wiping). Disposable gloves can actually be worse than bare hands if the gloves are not changed often and after handling potentially contaminated items.

### Contaminated Equipment/Prevention of Contamination

The importance of cleaning equipment and the prevention of contamination were covered in previous sections of this chapter. During surveys of retail food facilities, FDA found that full-service restaurants were "out-of-compliance" for this risk category in more than 37% of observations (FDA 2004). The most commonly observed deficiency was improper cleaning and sanitizing of utensils, equipment, and work surfaces. The second most commonly observed deficiency was inadequate separation of RTE foods from raw animal foods or from surfaces that were in contact with raw animal foods. These deficiencies pose a significant risk of contaminating foods with pathogenic or toxigenic microorganisms. Other deficiencies observed were inadequate protection of foods from environmental contamination (dusts, condensate, etc.) and faulty packaging. Some common reasons for failing to meet standards for this risk factor are poorly trained staff, inadequately designed or accessible equipment, and insufficient allocation of time for cleaning/sanitizing activities. Good management and supervision within the food facility play an important role in meeting the standards for this risk category.

## FOOD WORKER EDUCATION AND TRAINING

Given the central role that food managers and workers play in food safety, their training is a critical part of any food safety program. Training employees in food sanitation and safety is challenging for a number of reasons. The educational and literacy levels of employees in the food industry vary widely. Many employees in the food industry speak English as a second language, and communication can become a hindrance to training. The number of different jobs in the food industry also makes training challenging because training should emphasize aspects of food safety related to the employee's primary duties and responsibilities. And knowledge attained through training does not necessarily translate into the desired practices and behavior in the food workplace. A major concern for many businesses is the time taken away from job duties while employees undergo training. Finally, the effectiveness of different training techniques is difficult to evaluate. When the costs of training employees are factored in, the cost-effectiveness of training programs is an important consideration.

Regulations generally require some level of training for employees engaged in most food-related operations, but the specific requirements vary greatly. The Food Code (FDA and PHS 2009) recommends certification of a food safety manager in foodservice establishments. Mandatory requirements for certification and/or permitting of food workers are common in many—but not all—states. Among the states with certification or permitting requirements, proof of training in food sanitation or safety is necessary. However, in some cases, only one certified food safety manager is required per facility, and the food safety manager is not required to be onsite at all times (Almanza and Nesmith 2004). Certain food operations are required by federal regulations to have personnel trained in the Hazard Analysis and Critical Control Point (HACCP) procedures of food safety, but this requirement does not extend to most foodservice facilities. In the majority of cases, the adequacy of food safety training is judged by the results of sanitation inspections conducted by local health departments. Although the training of food workers has corresponded with higher sanitation inspection scores, such findings are not always consistent among studies (Mitchell, Fraser, Bearon 2007). Perhaps, the inspection scores are not sufficiently sensitive to indicate food worker knowledge and behavior. The effectiveness of food safety training is also influenced by reinforcement practices in the workplace, usually through a combination of incentives and other good management practices.

Food workers are part of an overall "system" of food safety that includes the facility, equipment, and procedures. Unlike other parts of the food safety system, workers need training and appropriate levels of supervision to ensure that procedures are properly followed. This is accomplished by classroom teaching and on-the-job training. The responsibility for providing training of food workers usually falls upon the food establishment, or the corporation if it belongs to a chain. Several commercial companies, industry associations, and nonprofit organizations provide services for the food industry to train food safety managers and employees. The National Restaurant Association established the ServSafe Food Safety Program to deliver consistent food safety training to managers and employees. The Conference for Food Protection (CFP) partnered with the American National Standards Institute (ANSI) to create the ANSI-CFP Accreditation Committee to accredit food safety manager certification programs provided by other organizations. Along with responsibilities of day-to-day food safety management, a Certified Food Safety Manager is qualified to coordinate the training of employees and to oversee and ensure safe food preparation practices.

## REFERENCES

Almanza BA, Nesmith MS. 2004. Food safety certification regulations in the United States. *J Environ Health* 66(9): 10,4, 20.

Bean NH, Goulding JS, Lao C, Angulo FJ. 1996. Surveillance for foodborne-disease outbreaks—United States, 1988–1992. *MMWR CDC Surveill Summ* 45(5):1–66.

Centers for Disease Control and Prevention. 2003. Outbreaks of *Salmonella* serotype enteritidis infection associated with eating shell eggs—United States, 1999–2001. *MMWR* 51(51–52):1149–1152.

Chmielewski RAN, Frank JF. 2003. Biofilm formation and control in food processing industries. *Comprehensive Reviews in Food Science and Food Safety* 2:22–32.

Codex Alimentarius Commission. 2010. *Codex Alimentarius Commission procedural manual.* 19th ed. Rome, Italy: Joint Food and Agricultural Organization/World Health Organization Food Standards Programme.

Environmental Protection Agency. 2010. Confirmatory efficacy data requirements. Available from: http://www.epa.gov/oppad001/dis_tss_docs/dis-05.htm.

Foil LD, Gorham JR. 2004. Mechanical transmission of disease agents by arthropods. In: *Medical entomology.* 2nd ed. (pp. 461–514). Eldridge BF, Edman JD, eds. Dordrecht, NL: Kluwer Academic Publishers.

Food and Drug Administration. 2004. *2004 report on the occurrence of foodborne illness risk factors in selected institutional foodservice, restaurant, and retail food store facility types.* Washington, DC: U.S. Department of Health and Human Services. Available from: http://www.fda.gov/Food/FoodSafety/RetailFoodProtection/FoodborneIllnessandRiskFactor Reduction/RetailFoodRiskFactorStudies/ucm089696.htm.

Food and Drug Administration and Public Health Service. 2009. *Food code 2009.* Washington, DC: U.S. Department of Health and Human Services. Available from: http://www.fda.gov/Food/FoodSafety/RetailFoodProtection/FoodCode/FoodCode2009/default.htm.

Friend M. 2006. *Disease emergence and resurgence: The wildlife–human connection.* Report nr Circular 1285.Reston, VA: U.S. Geological Survey.

Greig JD, Todd EC, Bartleson CA, Michaels BS. 2007. Outbreaks where food workers have been implicated in the spread of foodborne disease. Part 1. Description of the problem, methods, and agents involved. *J Food Prot* 70(7): 1752–1761.

Institute of Food Technologists. 2001. *Evaluation and definition of potentially hazardous foods: A report of the Institute of Food Technologists for the Food and Drug Administration of the U.S. Department of Health and Human Services.* IFT/FDA Contract No. 223-98-2333, Task Order No. 4. Washington, DC: Food and Drug Administration. Available from: http://www.fda.gov/Food/ScienceResearch/ResearchAreas/SafePracticesforFoodProcesses/ucm094141.htm.

Jay JM, Loessner MJ, Golden DA. 2005. *Modern food microbiology.* 7th ed. New York, NY: Springer Science+Business Media.

Kabak B, Dobson AD, Var I. 2006. Strategies to prevent mycotoxin contamination of food and animal feed: A review. *Crit Rev Food Sci Nutr* 46(8): 593–619.

Koopmans M, Erwin Duizer E. 2002, September. *Foodborne viruses: An emerging problem.* Prepared under the responsibility of the ILSI Europe Emerging Pathogen Task Force. Brussels: International Life Sciences Institute.

Kuehnert MJ, Kruszon-Moran D, Hill HA, McQuillan G, McAllister SK, Fosheim G, McDougal LK, Chaitram J, Jensen B, Fridkin SK, et al. 2006. Prevalence of *Staphylococcus aureus* nasal colonization in the United States, 2001–2002. *J Infect Dis* 193(2):172–179.

Magan N, Aldred D. 2007. Post-harvest control strategies: Minimizing mycotoxins in the food chain. *Int J Food Microbiol* 119:131–139.

Marriott NR. 1997. *Essentials of food sanitation.* New York, NY: Chapman & Hall.

Mitchell RE, Fraser AM, Bearon LB. 2007. Preventing food-borne illness in food service establishments: Broadening the framework for intervention and research on safe food handling behaviors. *Int J Environ Health Res* 17(1):9–24.

Moss MO. 2008. Fungi, quality and safety issues in fresh fruits and vegetables. *J Appl Microbiol* 104(5):1239–1243.

Olsen AR. 1998. Regulatory action criteria for filth and other extraneous materials. III. Review of flies and foodborne enteric disease. *Regul Toxicol Pharmacol* 28(3):199–211.

Todd EC, Greig JD, Bartleson CA, Michaels BS. 2009. Outbreaks where food workers have been implicated in the spread of foodborne disease. Part 6. Transmission and survival of pathogens in the food processing and preparation environment. *J Food Prot* 72(1):202–219.

Todd EC, Greig JD, Bartleson CA, Michaels BS. 2008a. Outbreaks where food workers have been implicated in the spread of foodborne disease. Part 5. Sources of contamination and pathogen excretion from infected persons. *J Food Prot* 71(12):2582–2595.

Todd EC, Greig JD, Bartleson CA, Michaels BS. 2008b. Outbreaks where food workers have been implicated in the spread of foodborne disease. Part 4. Infective doses and pathogen carriage. *J Food Prot* 71(11):2339–2373.

Todd EC, Greig JD, Bartleson CA, Michaels BS. 2007a. Outbreaks where food workers have been implicated in the spread of foodborne disease. Part 3. Factors contributing to outbreaks and description of outbreak categories. *J Food Prot* 70(9):2199–2217.

Todd EC, Greig JD, Bartleson CA, Michaels BS. 2007b. Outbreaks where food workers have been implicated in the spread of foodborne disease. Part 2. Description of outbreaks by size, severity, and settings. *J Food Prot* 70(8):1975–1993.

U.S. Government Printing Office. Title 21 *Code of Federal Regulations,* Part 110 Section 3. Available from: http://www.gpoaccess.gov/cfr/retrieve.html.

U.S. Government Printing Office. Title 21 *Code of Federal Regulations,* Part 178 Section 1010. Available from: http://www.gpoaccess.gov/cfr/retrieve.html.

U.S. Government Printing Office. Title 40 *Code of Federal Regulations,* Part 180 Section 940. Available from: http://www.gpoaccess.gov/cfr/retrieve.html.

## USEFUL RESOURCES

AIB International. https://www.aibonline.org/

Agricultural Research Service. Pathogen Modeling Program (PMP) Online. http://pmp.arserrc.gov/PMPOnline.aspx?ModelID=10

BACANOVA, Understanding the Microbiology of Safe, Minimally Processed Food. http://www.ifr.ac.uk/bacanova/project_backg.html

ComBase. Data and predictive tools for food microbiology. http://www.combase.cc/

Conference for Food Protection. Food Protection Manager Certification. http://www.foodprotect.org/manager-certification/
EPA Resources for Pest Management. http://www.epa.gov/pesticides/controlling/resources.htm

Food and Drug Administration. *Retail Food Protection: Employee Health and Personal Hygiene Handbook.* http://www.fda.gov/Food/FoodSafety/RetailFoodProtection/IndustryandRegulatoryAssistanceandTrainingResources/ucm113827.htm

Food Safety and Inspection Service. Freezing and Food Safety Fact Sheets. http://origin-www.fsis.usda.gov/Fact_Sheets/Focus_On_Freezing/index.asp

Food Safety and Inspection Service. Refrigeration and Food Safety Fact Sheets. http://origin-www.fsis.usda.gov/Fact_Sheets/Refrigeration_&_Food_Safety/index.asp

FoodSafety.gov. Gateway to Federal Food Safety Information. http://www.foodsafety.gov/

International Commission on Microbiological Specification for Foods. http://www.icmsf.iit.edu/main/home.html

Michigan State University Pesticide Safety Education. http://www.pested.msu.edu/index.html

National Restaurant Association. http://www.restaurant.org/

NSF International. http://www.nsf.org/

NSF International. White Book—Nonfood Compounds Listing Directory. http://www.nsf.org/usda/psnclistings.asp

Predictive Microbiology Information Portal (PMIP). http://portal.arserrc.gov/ or http://portal.arserrc.gov/GettingStarted.aspx

ServSafe. http://www.servsafe.com/

3-A Sanitary Standards, Incorporated. http://www.3-a.org/

Washington State Pest Management Resource Service. http://wsprs.wsu.edu/index.html

# CHAPTER 5

# Food Safety:
# Engineering Controls and Technology

## LEARNING OBJECTIVES

1. Explain the hurdle concept of food protection and how it affects food safety.
2. List and explain important factors that affect the resistance of microorganisms to temperature extremes.
3. Define the D-value, z-value, thermal death time, and F-value, and explain how these values are helpful in thermal treatments.
4. Describe the purpose of pasteurization, and recognize the different time–temperature combinations of pasteurization.
5. Distinguish between complete sterilization and commercial sterilization.
6. Describe the process of retorting and contrast it with aseptic packaging.
7. Recognize the purpose and different types of cooking processes.
8. Explain the effects of freezing on pathogens and parasites.
9. Identify the key parameters in controlling the freezing process.
10. Recognize the major chemical methods of food protection and their effectiveness in the control of pathogenic/toxigenic microorganisms.
11. Describe the purpose and uses of food contact sanitizers/antimicrobials and fumigation.
12. Define and discuss the methods of reducing water activity and pH in foods.
13. Describe the principles and food safety concerns of vacuum and modified atmosphere packaging.
14. Explain how fermentation is used to preserve foods and protect them from pathogens.
15. Discuss the concepts of microbial inference/antagonism and biocontrol using bacteriophages.
16. Explain the microbicidal effectiveness of ionizing radiation and identify its legal applications.
17. Address the safety and food quality concerns of food irradiation.
18. Describe new and emerging physical processes of food protection.
19. Provide an overview of the potential food safety issues linked to the technology of creating genetically modified organisms (GMOs).

## FOOD PROTECTION AND THE HURDLE CONCEPT

### Food Preservation, Spoilage, and Protection

The preservation of food was an early innovation by humans. By drying, smoking, and salting foods, they were saved for later consumption and as a safeguard against famine. Preservation methods also permitted the trade of foodstuffs by allowing them to be transported greater distances without spoilage. As food production, processing, and distribution became more sophisticated, so did the methods of food preservation, thanks to scientific discoveries and engineering development. Today, the methods of food preservation are technologically advanced and have become essential to feeding populations around the world.

Spoilage of food is considered any change that makes it unacceptable for human consumption (Forsythe and Hayes 2000). The "acceptability" of food for human consumption depends on the type of change and the preferences of consumers. Many ethnic cultures age or ferment certain foods to produce a desired flavor, aroma, color, and/or texture. The changes in foods one culture considers preferable may be considered unacceptable in another culture and, hence, deemed spoiled food. The causes of food spoilage can be traced to several sources. Insects may damage foods to an unacceptable level, and even the infestation of food with insects is considered objectionable to most consumers. Activities related to food handling and processing may cause unacceptable physical changes to the foodstuff, such as bruising, freezer "burns," excessive drying, and other changes in color, texture, taste, or consistency. Food spoilage also occurs as a result of nonmicrobial chemical reactions with local atmospheres, solutions, and contact surfaces. An objectionable form of this type of spoilage is the oxidative rancidity of oils and fats. The most well known source of food spoilage is microbial activity. A great variety of microorganisms, particularly bacteria and fungi (yeasts and molds), causes food spoilage through biochemical (enzyme-mediated) reactions.

Most technologies used for food preservation are designed to destroy or inhibit spoilage microorganisms, in particular certain species of bacteria and fungi. From a food safety perspective, the use of preservation technology does not guarantee food is free from pathogenic or toxigenic microorganisms. Although many food preservation technologies also destroy or inhibit pathogenic or toxigenic microorganisms, this is not always the case. If not properly utilized, some food preservation technologies may actually increase the risks from pathogens or toxins. In other words, food preservation is not synonymous with food safety. A broader term known as *food protection* is often used to encompass both food safety and preservation. It is important for food safety professionals to understand the basic scientific principles that underlie technologies for food protection.

### Hurdle Concept of Food Protection Technology

The intrinsic and extrinsic parameters (introduced in Chapter 4) that govern microbial growth form the basis of the hurdle concept. *Hurdles* are technological barriers to the growth and reproduction of microbial agents. A single-target approach to hurdles is using only one technological barrier to control microbial growth. The use of multiple technological barriers to control microbial growth is a multitargeted approach, particularly when each hurdle is aimed at a specific target of the microbial cell structure and/or physiology (Gorris 2000). The multitargeted approach is desirable for several reasons. First, a single treatment or hurdle to microbial growth (e.g., heat treatment) is often too severe in terms of food palatability and nutritional value. Consumers have recently expressed a preference for minimally processed foods, but minimal processing can increase the risk of foodborne disease and food spoilage, reducing the product shelf life. Multiple hurdles can offer food protection without overly severe treatments. Second, the effectiveness of multiple hurdles may be synergistic when it comes to inhibiting microbial growth. In other words, the effectiveness of modifying multiple parameters is usually multifold rather than additive. Third, the use of multiple hurdles may reduce the likelihood of developing microbial resistance and protective stress responses. Fourth, multiple hurdles provide an added margin of safety because the microbial agent must overcome more than one hurdle to survive and reproduce.

Food science professionals must carefully design, test, and scientifically verify as effective the food protection technologies used in the hurdle approach. Because minimally processed foods imply the use of less severe preservation treatments, microbial agents are often inactivated—not destroyed, as happens with complete sterilization. Food protection engineers and technologists must characterize the degree of uncertainty and understand the limits of the multiple hurdles used. This is especially important for the control of foodborne pathogens and toxigenic microorganisms. Minimally processed foods must not allow for increased risk of foodborne illnesses.

## THERMAL TRANSFER METHODS

Technologies that use hot or cold temperatures to destroy microorganisms and/or control microbial growth have existed for centuries. Food protection technologies that use heat are most commonly categorized as either pasteurization or sterilization temperatures. Pasteurization by heat is used primarily to destroy disease-causing microorganisms, though it is also used to destroy or reduce populations of spoilage microorganisms. If done correctly, pasteurization destroys most non–spore-forming pathogenic or toxigenic microorganisms, but it does not destroy spore-forming bacteria such as those belonging to the genera *Clostridium* and *Bacillus*. Sterilization temperatures are necessary to destroy spore-forming bacteria.

Strictly speaking, sterilization is a method of destroying all viable organisms as measured by a specific plating technique or other enumeration test. In contrast with absolute sterility, the condition known as "commercial sterility" is allowed for certain food treatment processes (known as shelf stability under federal regulations 9 CFR 318.300 and 9 CFR 381.300). Commercially sterile products are not guaranteed to be free of all viable organisms. Instead, commercially sterile products are sufficiently treated with heat and/or combined with other treatments or ingredients to destroy or inactivate microorganisms that grow at nonrefrigeration temperatures—including any pathogens of concern. This permits food processors to distribute and store foods without refrigeration. In recent years, food processors have used ultrahigh temperature (UHT) technology, which applies very high temperatures for short periods of time, to achieve commercial sterility to make shelf-stable products.

Food protection technologies that use cold are commonly categorized into three temperature ranges (Jay, Loessner, Golden 2005): chilling temperatures (usually between 7° and 15°C), refrigeration temperatures (0° and 7°C but ideally not above 4.4°C or 40°F), and freezer temperatures (≤ –18°C). Chilling temperatures are used primarily for the storage of certain fruits and vegetables, that is, non–potentially hazardous foods (PHF)/temperature controlled for safety (TCS) foods, whereas the refrigeration temperatures are used for transport and storage of perishable and PHF/TCS foods. Freezing temperatures are used primarily for food preservation by halting microbial growth and preventing autolysis; freezing may also be used to ensure the destruction of some multicellular parasites, such as certain helminths associated with fish, pork, and beef. The growth of most microorganisms is halted under freezer temperatures, albeit some species may continue to grow at an extremely slow rate.

## Factors Affecting the Resistance of Microorganisms to Heat and Cold

The section titled "Extrinsic and Intrinsic Growth Parameters of Foods" in Chapter 4 briefly discusses the effects of temperature changes on microbial physiology. In terms of microbicidal effectiveness, certain factors determine the relative resistance of microorganisms to temperature extremes. Table 5-1 lists important factors related to microbial resistance to extreme heat and cold. Most of these factors indirectly change the resistance of microorganisms by altering the transfer of heat throughout the food matrix, while some factors are inherently genetic with the particular species or strain or genetically induced through environmental changes or manipulation. Some of the most important factors are discussed in the following paragraphs.

The water content of foods is very influential in the resistance of microorganisms to heat and cold. With respect to heat resistance, microbial populations become less resistant with increasing amounts of water, whether measured as humidity, water activity, or moisture content. The most often cited reasons for decreasing heat resistance with increasing water is the denaturation of proteins at a faster rate and the easier breakage of peptide bonds (Jay et al. 2005). The water content

---

**Table 5-1** Important Factors Affecting Microbial Survival During Hot and Cold Treatments

Species and strain of the microorganism

Induced resistance (adaptive response) environmental stresses or sensitivity from injury

Nutritional status of the microbial population

Microbial age and population growth phase

Microbial population numbers and density

Water composition and availability in the food matrix

Intrinsic parameters and other extrinsic parameters ("hurdles")

Inhibitory compounds in the food matrix (natural or additives)

Nutrient composition of the food matrix (carbohydrates, proteins, oils, fats, etc.)

Rate of heating or cooling (including thawing or cooldown periods)

Holding temperatures of the food (prior to and after thermal treatment)

Resident time at highest or lowest temperatures

Density, thickness, and thermal transfer properties of the food matrix

Laboratory methods used for resuscitation and enumeration of microbial populations

of foods and its effects on cold resistance of microorganisms is more complex. During freezing, only "free" water becomes frozen, while "bound" water does not freeze. Water that is either frozen or otherwise bound in the food matrix is unavailable and can cause the dehydration of microorganisms. Although some microbial populations may die off over time in a frozen state, freezing should not be considered a method of microbial destruction (with the exception of certain nematodes discussed previously).

The fat, oil, carbohydrate, and protein composition of foods also influence microbial resistance to heat and cold. In general, an increase in any of these constituents also increases resistance of a microbial population to heat. In large part, the reason for increased resistance is related to slower heat transfer and penetration within the food. Another possible contributing factor is lower moisture content within the microbial cell from osmotic pressure, which protects the intracellular proteins to some degree. Certain foods with a high content of fat, sugar, or protein are also known to maintain cell viability of pathogenic and toxigenic bacteria during freezing. This protective effect varies considerably with the particular type of macromolecules involved.

The pH of foods is yet another factor affecting the resistance of microorganisms to temperature extremes. The heat resistance of microorganisms is greatest around their optimum pH of growth. Microbial resistance to heat decreases as pH deviates further from the optimum pH, whether acidic or basic. This relationship is important to the heat processing of foods, allowing acidic or basic foods to be treated with less heat compared with more neutral pH foods. This permits the pasteurization or sterilization of certain foods without degradation in quality or nutritional content. The pH of foods also influences microbial resistance to cold; highly acidic or low pH food decreases cell viability during freezing.

Salts and inhibitory or protective compounds often contribute to the thermal resistance of microorganisms. These substances may be added during food processing, naturally produced by tissues of the food, or produced by microbiota in the food. Some substances act as thermoprotectants or cryoprotectants to microbial populations that are subjected to temperature extremes. Other substances may actually increase the microbicidal effects of heat or cold. The overall effects of different substances and combinations of substances are difficult to generalize or predict without microbial challenge testing. This requires testing of specific products and formulations to determine how microbial resistance and survival are affected.

The age, number, and population density of microorganisms directly influence their resistance to heat and cold. Some evidence exists that large microbial populations excrete substances that confer protection from heat (Jay et al. 2005). Because proteins increase resistance to heat and cold, the totality of proteins produced by a microbial population may contribute to a protective effect. The age and physiologic status of microorganisms, along with the population growth phase, also affect resistance to heat and cold. Spores are very resistant to heat, and they are unaffected by freezing temperatures. Microbial cells in the stationary phase of growth are older and most resistant to heat and cold. Conversely, microbial cells most vulnerable to temperature extremes are those in the beginning of the logarithmic phase, that is, the very youngest cells.

With regard to the species and strains of microorganisms, resistance to heat and cold is an adaptation that has evolved as a survival mechanism. Thermophiles are obviously more resistant to heat, whereas psychrotrophs and psychrophiles are more resistant to cold. Differences in resistance are even recognized between various strains within a species. Some types of resistance arc adaptive responses induced by certain environmental stresses, which may confer cross-protection against other stresses (Wesche et al. 2009). The best-known examples are the production of compounds known as heat shock proteins, genetically induced by stress, that provide protection against heat and possibly other stresses. Extreme stress, however, may injure a microbial cell beyond the point of adaptation and cellular repair, and subsequent stress (e.g., heat or cold) may produce a greater microbicidal effect. An example of this phenomenon is the increased thermal sensitivity of several *E. coli* O157:H7 strains in hamburger meat after first being subjected freezing, but this observation is not universal to all *E. coli* O157:H7 strains (Zhao et al. 2004).

Of all the factors that affect resistance and survival of microorganisms in temperature extremes, the most important are the rate of temperature change and the time–temperature relationship. These factors must be carefully controlled during food processing to ensure the safety and quality of foods.

## Heat Treatments

The thermal properties of foods and materials are critical to using heat treatment technology. The most important properties are described as specific heat, thermal conductivity, and thermal diffusivity (Fellows 2009). The specific heat of a food is the amount of thermal energy (expressed as kilojoules) necessary to raise 1 kilogram of the food by 1° Centigrade (kJ kg$^{-1}$ °C$^{-1}$). The composition of the food greatly determines its specific heat, with the moisture content being particularly important. Thermal conductivity is another property that characterizes the heat transfer of materials during food processing; with foods, it is influenced by a number of factors such as air spaces, moisture content, and structure of the tissues and cells of the foodstuff. Along with thermal conductivity, materials and foods also have different capacities to store and dissipate heat. The ability of a material to conduct heat relative to its ability to store heat is measured as thermal diffusivity. It is used in calculations to determine the temperature distribution over time in materials and foods.

Figure 5-1 illustrates several basic formulae for the important thermal properties. Additional formulae are derived and available from those in Figure 5-1, and the student is referred to Fellows (2009) and other sources for more detailed explanations.

## *Predicting Microbial Survival and Death from Heat*

The destruction of microorganisms is the primary objective of most heat treatments. Mathematical models help predict the amount of heat and time necessary for microbicidal heat treatments. The prediction of conditions necessary to destroy microorganisms is important because excessive heat reduces the nutritional value and quality of foods. The most frequently used model is based on the D-values of microorganisms. The D-value, also known as the decimal reduction time, is the time interval required at a particular temperature to reduce the microbial population by 10-fold. This is derived from plotting the survival rate of a particular microorganism against time (in minutes) at a specified temperature. The resulting death rate curve typically displays an exponential reduction and can be converted to a straight line by graphing logarithmic values or by using a logarithmic scale. Figure 5-2 illustrates a death rate curve used to derive a D-value.

$$c_p = \frac{Q}{m(\theta_1 - \theta_2)}$$

$c_p$ = **specific heat** of food at constant pressure; this is the amount of heat needed to raise the temperature of 1 kg of food by 1°C. Expressed in the units J kg$^{-1}$ °C$^{-1}$.

$Q$ = total amount of heat gained or lost in J.

$m$ = mass in kg.

$\theta_1 - \theta_2$ = temperature difference in °C.

$$k = \frac{Q}{t\theta}$$

$k$ = **thermal conductivity** of the food, that is, how well the food conducts heat. Expressed in the units J s$^{-1}$ m$^{-1}$ °C$^{-1}$ or W m$^{-1}$ °C$^{-1}$.

$t$ = time in s.

$$\alpha = \frac{k}{\rho c_p}$$

$\alpha$ = **thermal diffusivity** of food, that is, the ability of food to conduct heat relative to its ability to store heat. Expressed in the units m$^2$ s$^{-1}$.

$\rho$ = density of food in kg m$^{-3}$.

**Figure 5-1** Basic Formulae of Important Thermal Properties of Foods. *Source:* Adapted from Fellows 2009

The D-values are different for various microorganisms (known as their heat resistance) and vary with different foods and ingredients. Higher D-values indicate greater heat resistance of a particular microbial species and strain. But other factors listed in Table 5-1 also contribute to the differences and variability associated with D-values. Thus, the D-value is applicable under the following conditions: (1) for particular microorganism at a specific, constant temperature; (2) a

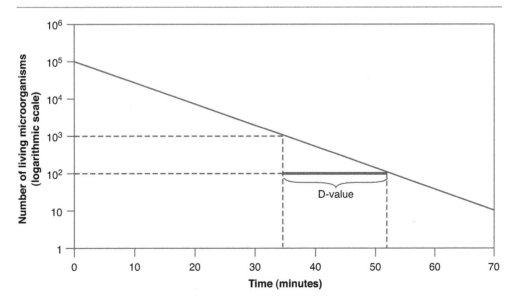

**Figure 5-2** Death Rate Curve

particular medium or food type; and (3) defined and consistent factors identified in Table 5-1. Because many factors influence the death rates of microorganisms, it is not uncommon to find a range of D-values for a microbial species in the published literature.

To predict the effectiveness of microbial survival and death at different temperatures, food microbiologists can plot a thermal death time (TDT) line or curve from multiple D-values. By collating the D-values from several experiments at different temperatures, a semilogarithmic line is plotted, called the TDT line or curve (Figure 5-3). From the reciprocal of the slope of this line the z-value is derived. The z-value is useful because it predicts how much temperature change is needed to produce a 10-fold reduction in microbial thermal resistance. The time required at a given temperature to reduce a target microbial population to a specified level is called the F-value, also referred to as the TDT. For example, the widely accepted F-value in the canning of low-acid foods to destroy *C. botulinum* spores at 121°C (250°F) is 2.45 equivalent minutes with a z-value of 9.8°C (17.6°F) (Pflug and Gould 2000). Of course, the time necessary to destroy a microbial population, or reduce it to an acceptable level, depends on many factors. That is one reason the z-value must always be stipulated when citing the F-value. Using the previous example, the F-value is expressed as $F_{121}^{9.8}$, with the superscript representing the z-value and the subscript representing the given temperature of the F-value.

An important factor to consider when determining the F-value is the initial and final size of the target microbial population. The following formula is helpful in deriving the F-value to reduce a microbial population to the desired level:

$$F = D (\log n_1 - \log n_2)$$

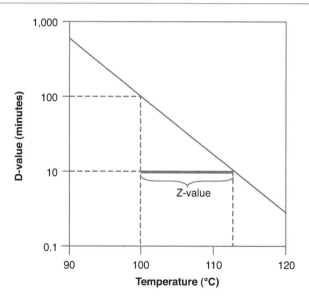

**Figure 5-3** Thermal Death Time Curve

where $D$ = the D-value, and $n_1$ = the initial number of cells, and $n_2$ = the final number of cells in the microbial population.

Although the traditional model of microbial death is exponential and plotted to yield a graphic straight line, recent evidence suggests that other models may provide a better prediction of microbial death rates. These alternative mathematical models yield sigmoidal-shaped curves or other deviations from the straight line (Fellows 2009). New computer technology and mathematical models provide more sophisticated predictions of microbial survival and death during heat treatment. This capability is particularly valuable because the various factors (Table 5-1) that affect microbial resistance to heat are considered in the predictions.

### Pasteurization by Heat

The introduction of pasteurized milk was a major milestone in public health. Prior to pasteurization, raw milk was a major contributor to the transmission of infectious diseases. Over the years, pasteurization has been utilized with a variety of products to destroy pathogens and spoilage microorganisms and to inactivate enzymes responsible for spoilage. Besides protecting public health, pasteurization has economic benefits because it permits products to be shipped greater distances and stored for longer periods without spoilage. Compared with other heat treatments, the energy requirements for pasteurization are much less, and the nutritional value and quality of the food are minimally affected. With the development of new processing technologies, the definition of pasteurization has been expanded to include several types of nonheat treatments. These new technologies are discussed later in the chapter.

The temperatures involved with conventional heat pasteurization are below 100°C (212°F). Treatments that heat foods above this temperature (e.g., UHT) are sometimes referred to as pasteurization, but these high-temperature treatments are better described as sterilization. Various combinations of temperature and time are used for pasteurization based on the thermal death times of the target microorganisms, as well as the food product's thermal properties.

Most foods that are heat pasteurized are liquid in nature, for example, milk, eggnog, juices, and sport drinks. Certain solid foods may also be subjected to heat pasteurization, but these foods often have additional "hurdles" such as lowered pH. For milk, one of the temperature–time combinations listed in Table 5-2 is necessary for pasteurization (Food and Drug Administration [FDA] 2009). The first temperature–time combination in Table 5-2 is called low-temperature long-time (LTLT) pasteurization, and the second time–temperature combination is called high-temperature short-time (HTST) pasteurization. These temperature–time combinations are sufficient enough to destroy *Mycobacterium tuberculosis* and *Coxiella burnetti*—the most heat-resistant non-spore-forming microorganisms. The vegetative cells of other pathogenic and toxigenic microorganisms are less heat-resistant, and thus, they are also expected to be destroyed at the same time–temperature combinations. On the other hand, microbial spores are not likely to be destroyed, and without additional control measures, the germination of microbial spores may occur after pasteurization.

In the spirit of performance-based regulatory standards, the FDA has established the 5-log pathogen reduction rule for juice producers (FDA 2009). Essentially, this standard requires the $10^5$ reduction of a "pertinent pathogen" in the juice product. The "pertinent pathogen" is defined

**Table 5-2** Pasteurization Temperatures vs. Times

| Temperature | Time |
|---|---|
| 63°C (145°F)[a] | 30 minutes[b] |
| 72°C (161°F)[a] | 15 seconds[c] |
| 89°C (191°F) | 1.0 second |
| 90°C (194°F) | 0.5 seconds |
| 94°C (201°F) | 0.1 seconds |
| 96°C (204°F) | 0.05 seconds |
| 100°C (212°F) | 0.01 seconds |

[a]If the fat content of the milk product is 10% or greater, or a total solids of 18% or greater, or if it contains added sweeteners, the specified temperature shall be increased by 3°C (5°F).
[b]Low temperature, long time (LTLT).
[c]High temperature, short time (HTST).

*Source:* FDA 2009.

as the most resistant pathogen most likely to occur in the juice. This typically is *Salmonella, E. coli* O157:H7, or *Cryptosporidium parvum.* Instead of mandating specific time–temperature combinations for heat pasteurization, juice producers are permitted to use innovative technologies or combinations of techniques to achieve the 5-log reduction. In many fruit processing plants, heat pasteurization is used because of its proven effectiveness and commercial availability of the necessary equipment.

### Heat Sterilization and "Commercial Sterility"

In 1804, the vacuum bottling factory of Nicholas Appert in Paris began the heat-treatment canning process. Over the next 50 years, technological advances in canning, thermodynamics, and production continued, eventually leading to the invention of a retort canning process in 1874 using a pressure cooker with live steam. Retorting is generally defined as the packaging of food in a container (can, glass, pouch, etc.) followed by sterilization, traditionally using pressurized steam and retention times based on F-values for specific temperatures. In recent years, methods of retorting using sterilization technologies besides steam have been developed.

Prior to sterilization, the air must be removed from containers of foods, a process known as exhausting (Fellows 2009). This is necessary to prevent the expansion of air and stress at the container's seams and seals, possibly resulting in loss of integrity, that is, leaking. An additional advantage of exhausting is the elimination of oxygen, responsible for corrosion within metal containers and oxidative damage to the food. After heat sterilization and cooling of exhausted containers, a partial vacuum is formed in the containers' headspace. Several methods are available for exhausting containers (Fellows 2009):

1. Filling the containers with hot food
2. Filling the containers with cold food followed by heating (80°–95°C) with the lid partially sealed to allow venting
3. Removing the air from containers using a vacuum pump
4. Using a blast of steam (steam flow closing) to carry away the air from the food surface immediately prior to sealing the containers

Heat sterilization technology used for retorting is based on saturated steam, hot water, or direct flame. With saturated steam, condensation on the outside of individual containers transfers latent heat to the food inside. Any air in the sterilizing retort can form an insulating barrier that will prevent adequate heating of the containers, possibly resulting in failure to achieve sterilization. Therefore, procedures and equipment must be in place to remove air from the retort equipment. With hot water sterilization, the heat is uniformly distributed and transferred to the containers, but the pressurization of air is necessary to permit the water to remain liquid at higher temperatures (e.g., 121°C). Flame sterilization involves exposing cans to direct flames with temperatures up to 1770°C. This results in extremely high rates of heat transfer, so the cans must be spinning at the time of sterilization, and flame sterilization is typically limited to smaller cans because of the generation of high internal pressures.

Many variations of equipment are used for retorting food products. A *retort* generally means a closed and pressurized vessel used to heat canned foods. Retorts are broadly classified on the basis of several characteristics: (1) the physical medium used for heating (water, steam, steam/air mixture), (2) methods for handling the containers (batch or continuous), and (3) whether the containers remain stationary or rotate during sterilization (still or agitated). When water is used as the heat transfer medium, the containers can be immersed, sprayed, or showered (cascaded). The batch method of container handling involves (1) loading the unpressurized retort through a door or lid; (2) sealing, pressurizing, and venting the retort; and (3) introducing the heating medium. The continuous method involves the containers moving continuously through the pressurized retort. Agitation or rotating of containers can be performed as a rolling motion or end over end, depending on the particular equipment type. Agitation ensures complete and uniform transfer of heat to the container and its contents. Whatever type of retorting equipment and process is used, the operation must be performed correctly to ensure commercial sterility of the containers' contents.

A major innovation for preserving foods involving sterilization is called aseptic packaging. Unlike retorting, aseptic packaging involves sterilizing batches of food before packaging it in individual containers. To maintain sterility, the package must also be sterilized, and the food product and package must be combined together in a sterile atmosphere. Although this approach may appear impractical, aseptic packaging is actually quite feasible, and it has many advantages over retorting. Automation of the sterilization and packaging processes results in greater productivity for food processors. The container materials most often used in aseptic packaging are laminates consisting of paper, polyethylene, and a thin film of aluminum. The resulting packages are low weight and can be formed as squares or other shapes that accommodate packing in crates, reducing the overall shipping costs of food products.

Aseptic packaging is used mostly for liquid foods, though it is also used for low-particle foods such as soups, cottage cheese, and baby foods. The most widely recognized application of aseptic packaging is for milk and juice products. These liquid foods are subjected to flash sterilization at ultrahigh temperatures (UHT) ranging from 130°–150°C for a few seconds. The application of UHT and aseptic technology involves greater complexity, and operators and maintenance staff are required to have higher skill levels. Figure 5-4 is a simplified diagram of one process used for aseptic packaging. Other variations of aseptic packaging are also used in the food and beverage industry.

The distinction between sterility and commercial sterility was briefly introduced earlier in this section. With commercial sterility, all vegetative cells and many spores of microorganisms in the food product are destroyed. Any spores that are not destroyed by thermal sterilization are inhibited by reduced pH and/or the presence of salt, nitrite, or other additives. Drying or reducing the $a_w$ of the food product is another hurdle used to inhibit spores. The most serious safety concern with commercially sterile foods is the growth of *C. botulinum* from surviving spores. In general, two approaches are used to ensure the destruction and/or inhibition of *C. botulinum*. The first approach involves sufficient heat to destroy the *C. botulinum* spores. This is necessary for low-acid (pH > 4.6) foods because *C. botulinum* is capable of growing at a pH above 4.6.

The traditional standard for thermal heating of low-acid foods is the 12D process, based on the D-values of *C. botulinum*. Assuming a heavy loading ($10^3$) of *C. botulinum* spores, a 12D reduction theoretically reduces the odds of a spore surviving to 1 in a billion. Of course, the time–temperature combination required for a 12D reduction depends on the specific characteris-

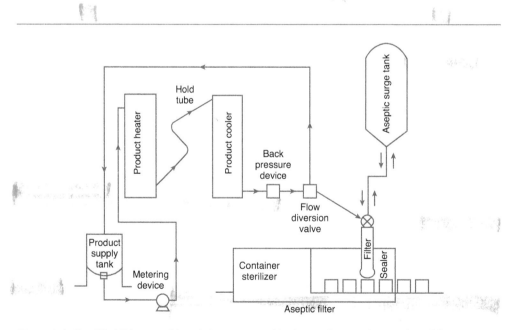

**Figure 5-4** Simplified Diagram of Aseptic Processing and Packaging System. *Source:* Adapted from FSIS, USDA

tics of the food. To compare different foods and the temperatures necessary to destroy *C. botulinum* spores, a standard F-value ($F_0$) is established for each food product. The reference temperature of 121°C (250°F) with a z-value of –7.7°C (18°F) is used as the benchmark. The $F_0$ value for a food product is the time in minutes required to destroy *C. botulinum* spores (i.e., commercial sterility) at the aforementioned reference temperature. The reference temperature can be converted to other temperatures of interest by using the appropriate D- and z-values.

A second approach to ensure inhibition of *C. botulinum* spores is the acidification of foods. For foods with an equilibrium pH ≤ 4.6, temperatures at or above the boiling point of water (100°C) should be sufficient to destroy vegetative cells and to inhibit surviving spores of *C. botulinum*. Whereas some foods may be naturally acidic, many foods are acidified using different methods. Acidification methods include blanching foods in an acidified aqueous solution; immersing blanched foods into acid solutions; direct batch acidification; adding measured amounts of acid to containers; and other methods. Whatever method is used, it is important that the equilibrium pH of ≤ 4.6 is attained throughout the food.

## Cooking and Other Heating Processes

Many food products undergo cooking processes prior to distribution and sale to consumers. Conventional cooking processes that involve baking, roasting, and frying are the most common. Other technologies based on dielectric (i.e., radiofrequency and microwave) and infrared (IR) radiation to heat/cook foods are also widely used. Another technology known as ohmic heating uses electricity and the electrical resistance of foods to generate heat. And some processes (e.g., extrusion) generate heat as a by-product that can be helpful in food preservation and pathogen destruction. The primary purpose of industrial cooking processes is to enhance the sensory experiences of eating the food product. Convenience ("heat and eat") is another attractive feature to consumers of precooked and RTE foods. But cooking processes are also used in the preservation and safety of foods by destroying microbial agents and inhibiting their growth.

Baking and roasting use heated air to remove moisture from foods and to form a desired texture (e.g., crust). This convective form of heat transfer is aided by the conductive transfer of heat from the pan or other container. Generally, the temperature on the outside of a food during baking reaches 100°C (212°F) for a considerable amount of time, which is sufficient to destroy most vegetative forms of microbial cells—including pathogens. The destruction of microbial agents within the food during baking and roasting depends on the amount of heat penetration. The removal of water during the baking process reduces $a_w$ and inhibits microbial growth, contributing to a longer shelf life of the product. The $a_w$ of a baked product along with other preservation hurdles (pH, additives, chilling, etc.) determine its expected shelf life. Most food safety issues associated with baked goods come from postbaking contamination by workers, equipment, and the air (Fellows 2009). Other potential sources of contamination with pathogenic or toxigenic microorganisms include the fillers used in baked products, particularly meat and cream fillings, which may also change the intrinsic parameters for microbial growth.

Frying is a common cooking process used by industry to impart flavor and texture to a variety of food products. Several methods of frying and a variety of oils are available for industrial cooking of foods. Consumer health concerns ranging from obesity to cancer over the fat content in fried foods have prompted many companies to carefully consider their frying methods and oils. Besides the fatty content of foods, the production of toxic compounds during frying has become a concern among consumers and regulatory agencies. Several complex chemical processes involving the temperatures and composition of foods influence the production of these toxicants. The discovery of acrylamide, a potential carcinogen, in several types of fried foods has led to considerable research in ways of reducing this toxic compound.

Frying involves high temperatures, approximately 170°–190°C, for a few minutes. The hot oil transfers heat to the food while simultaneously removing moisture, followed by the absorption of the oil to various degrees. The temperatures and times associated with frying are sufficient to destroy vegetative cells of microbial agents responsible for disease and spoilage, and the removal of moisture inhibits microbial growth. However, the core of the food must be sufficiently heated by either penetration with hot oil or heat conduction to ensure complete microbial destruction and the removal of moisture. The type of oil, frying time and temperature, and food composition influence the level of heat penetration and dehydration produced by the frying process.

An ancient process, the smoking of foods is sometimes considered a form of cooking as well as preservation. Actually, several types of smoking treatments are used in modern food processing, and not all of them use heat. Cold smoking and "liquid smoke" are used to flavor and color certain foods, and the microbicidal effects of these treatments are minimal. Smoking treatments that use heat are considered as either warm or hot smoking (Fellows 2009). Warm smoking is done at temperatures of 25°–40°C (77°–104°F), which are insufficient to destroy most microorganisms. For this reason, warm smoking is often combined with other curing treatments for food preservation. Because smoking is most often used to treat protein-rich foods of animal origin, the determination of PHF/TCS food status of a smoked product is critically important to food safety. And unless specifically treated to be a RTE food, cooking is necessary for smoked foods—especially those treated using cold, liquid, or warm smoking methods.

Hot smoking is done at temperatures of 60°–80°C (140°–176°F). Depending on the times and temperatures, hot smoking usually cooks the food and destroys most vegetative microbial cells. Along with heat treatment, the antimicrobial effects of hot smoking also occur from dehydration and chemical constituents in the smoke. A few chemical constituents such as formaldehyde are suspected carcinogens, and different techniques of hot smoking influence the relative abundance of these chemicals. Poor techniques may also result in insufficient times and heat penetration of foods to destroy pathogenic or toxigenic microorganisms adequately. To create hurdles to microbial growth, hot smoking is usually combined with other treatments. Whenever hot smoked foods are intended to be stored at room temperatures, the non-PHF/non-TCS food status must be confirmed.

Several forms of nonionizing radiation are used to generate heat (i.e., dielectric heating) for food processing. Microwave technology has become commonplace as a heat treatment. Depending on the power levels, dielectric properties of food, and duration of exposure, microwaves can be used for cooking, pasteurization, sterilization, and other purposes. Radio-frequency (RF) radiation is usually used for the drying and baking of food products. Infrared radiation is used mainly to improve the eating qualities of food products but can also be used to pasteurize the surfaces of foods. Some scant evidence exists that nonionizing radiation may produce biological effects unrelated to heating, but the main lethal effect of nonionizing radiation to microbial agents is attributed to the dielectric heating. As with other thermal treatments, the lethality of dielectric heating is related to the D-values of the microorganisms. Many studies have demonstrated the effectiveness of microwave heating on the destruction of pathogenic and toxigenic microorganisms. However, it is important that uniform heating of food is accomplished to ensure the thermal death of microbial populations.

Ohmic heating is used for foods with good fluidity and electrical resistance. To conduct electricity, the electrodes must be in good contact with the food as it passes through the ohmic heater. By rapidly generating a lot of heat, it is most useful as a pasteurization method for milk, juices, and viscous liquids. Along with the lethal effects of the heat, electrical currents also contribute to the destruction of microbial cells by causing membrane rupture and disruption of intracellular components.

## Cold and Freezing

Whereas canning methods of food protection have existed for more than 200 years, the freezing of foods did not become widespread until well into the twentieth century, after the availability of electricity. The demand for frozen foods increased even more during the 1970s through 1990s when consumers purchased freezers and microwave ovens. Freezing is very effective in preserving foods, and when done properly, freezing results in very small changes to the nutritional value and taste of foods. However, the costs of distributing and storing frozen or chilled foods are more compared with commercially sterile products. Furthermore, although heat treatment is an established method of pathogen destruction, cold treatment cannot be relied on for pathogen destruction.

Freezing preserves foods primarily by slowing microbial growth. Some microbicidal activity may occur and depends on the factors listed earlier in Table 5-1. Various types of microorganisms have different capacities for survival during freezing. Psychrotrophs and psychrophiles have a physiologic advantage for survival under freezing temperatures. Gram-negative bacteria such as *E. coli* and *Salmonella* species are more sensitive to extreme cold, whereas Gram-positive bacteria such as *Staphylococcus aureus* are more resistant. Bacterial and mold spores are virtually unaffected by freezing temperatures. Other factors such as the thaw rate of frozen foods are also very influential on microbial survival. Faster thaw rates tend to increase survival rates of bacterial populations, though the reason is not entirely clear. But slow thaw rates within the temperature "danger zone" permit the growth and multiplication of surviving bacteria.

Freezing may be used to destroy certain parasitic worms, though some species or serotypes of helminths are very resistant to freezing. Table 5-3 lists freezing temperatures and times required by federal regulations (9 CFR 318.10) to treat pork used in processed products. The purpose of these regulations is to ensure the destruction of *Trichinella* larvae (heat and curing methods of *Trichinella* larvae destruction are also permitted). Several species and serotypes of *Trichinella* larvae are known to be highly resistant to freezing and may survive for months or even years below −18°C (0.4°F). These freeze-resistant species and serotypes of *Trichinella* larvae are usually found in the striated muscles of carnivores (wolves, bears, foxes, etc.) from colder, northern latitudes (Dupouy-Camet and Murrell 2007). Cooking and/or other treatments are recommended to destroy the freeze-resistant species and serotypes.

Table 5-3  Alternate Periods of Freezing at Temperatures Indicated for the Destruction of Trichinae in Pork Used for Processed Food Products

| Maximum Internal Temperature[a] | | Minimum Time |
|---|---|---|
| Degrees Fahrenheit (°F) | Degrees centigrade (°C) | |
| 0 | −17.8 | 106 hours |
| −5 | −20.6 | 82 hours |
| −10 | −23.3 | 63 hours |
| −15 | −26.1 | 48 hours |
| −20 | −28.9 | 35 hours |
| −25 | −31.7 | 22 hours |
| −30 | −34.5 | 8 hours |
| −35 | −37.2 | ½ hour |

[a]Temperature measured in the center of the pork meat pieces. These temperatures and times are not applicable to other meats and wild game.

Source: 9 CFR 318.10

The cystircerci of *Taenia saginata* and *T. solium* in beef and pork, respectively, can be destroyed by freezing under commercial conditions similar to *Trichinella* larvae destruction (Gill 2006). The larvae (or metacercariae) of parasitic worms that infect fish can also be destroyed by commercial freezing temperatures, though the data are lacking for many helminths in fish to predict precise freezing temperatures and times. For food dishes where fish are eaten raw (e.g., sushi), the Food Code (Food and Drug Administration and Public Health Service [FDA and PHS] 2009) recommends the following freezing temperatures and times:

- The fish must be frozen and stored frozen at a temperature of −20°C (−4°F) or below for at least 168 hours.
- The fish must be frozen solid and stored frozen at −35°C (−31°F) or below for at least 15 hours.
- The fish must be frozen until solid at −35°C (−31°F) or below and then stored at −20°C (−4°F) or below for at least 24 hours.

The process of freezing foods begins with treatments to obtain the desired food quality and to affect the microbiology of frozen foods (Lund 2000). The carcasses of some animals are usually stored to achieve rigor mortis prior to freezing. This prevents the muscle tissue from contracting during freezing, called *cold shortening*. Fish are often bled, cleaned, and/or filleted prior to freezing. Most vegetables are blanched to inactivate enzymes, reduce the number of microorganisms, maintain color, displace air pockets, and facilitate packing. Foods that are consumed from a frozen state without cooking (e.g., ice cream, juice concentrates, fruits) are usually heat treated first to eliminate possible pathogens. For example, ice cream mix must be pasteurized or sterilized and rapidly cooled prior to the freezing process.

The heterogeneous composition of most foods means that freezing does not progress uniformly throughout the food product. The differences in solute concentration and other factors that determine thermal properties within foods also influence the temperature at which freezing occurs, as well as the rate of freezing. Whenever freezing takes place within a particular location of a food, it occurs in three temperature stages: (1) prefreezing, (2) freezing, and (3) reduction to the storage temperature (Lund 2000). Prefreezing begins when the food is subjected to cold temperatures, and it lasts until just before the formation of ice. The freezing stage is characterized by a constant temperature in the measured location of the food, as the heat transfers out of the food and the available water changes to ice. The final stage is the period of time when the temperature again starts declining, and it lasts until the storage temperature is reached.

Two key parameters are important to controlling the freezing process: (1) freezing time and (2) freezing rate. The freezing time starts with the prefreezing stage and lasts until the final storage temperature is reached. The freezing rate is the temperature difference (initial vs. final) divided by the freezing time. The freezing time and rate are both important to the food quality and productivity of the freezing process. The thermal properties of food discussed earlier are also important when freezing foods because heat transfer from the food to the surrounding cold medium must occur. Besides the thermal properties of the foods, which can vary greatly, the food containers and packaging also contribute to the freezing times and rates. The difference between the temperatures of the food and the surrounding freezing medium is particularly important to freezing time and rate.

Equipment and methods used for commercial freezing can be categorized on the basis of the freezing rates and/or the type of heat transfer medium. Commercial freezers fall into the performance categories of slow, quick, rapid, and ultrarapid based on the "ice front" movement rate in the food (Fellows 2009). On the basis of heat transfer medium, commercial freezers are categorized as either contact, air blast, or cryogenic freezers (Lund 2000). Contact freezers use plates, belts, or drums that are chilled with refrigerants and come in contact with the food product. Air blast freezers expose food to cold air using a number of techniques and enclosures, including rooms, tunnels, conveyor belts, and fluidized beds of air. Cryogenic freezers rely on liquid nitrogen or carbon dioxide as the freezing medium.

## CHEMICAL METHODS OF FOOD PROTECTION

### Conventional Food Preservatives/Additives

A great number of chemicals have potential as food preservatives and antimicrobial compounds, but a comparatively small number have been approved by the FDA as food additives. The problem with adding new compounds to the list of approved food additives is the potential toxicity to consumers, both acute and chronic. This is particularly important for antimicrobial compounds because these chemicals are chosen for their toxicity to microorganisms, and toxicity to other organisms (i.e., humans) is possible—unless proven otherwise. The FDA enforces strict rules for food additives, and adding compounds to the approved list requires an extensive review of the scientific data related to safety. Furthermore, a compound that demonstrates antimicrobial activity in the laboratory (*in vitro*) does not always have the same antimicrobial activity when added to certain foods.

Table 5-4 is a partial list of chemicals approved by the FDA as food additives, either as preservatives and/or antimicrobial compounds. The primary purpose for most of these chemicals is the inactivation or inhibition of microorganisms responsible for food spoilage—especially the fungi. Certain molds may produce mycotoxins, and although the inhibition of toxigenic molds is a benefit for food safety, the primary purpose of adding preservatives to processed foods is quality and preservation. Pathogenic or toxigenic bacteria may be inhibited to some degree by the chemicals listed in Table 5-4, but only sodium nitrite is specifically cited for food safety. Some of the compounds listed in Table 5-4 are called "natural" antimicrobials because they are derived from plant, animal, or microbial sources. Food processors do not rely solely on chemical food preservatives and antimicrobial compounds for the inactivation or inhibition of pathogenic/toxigenic microorganisms. Rather, they are typically used in combination with other technologies to provide hurdles.

Sodium nitrate ($NaNO_3$) and sodium nitrite ($NaNO_2$) have been used for many years as curing agents in meats. They help stabilize the red meat color, enhance flavor, and inhibit spoilage microorganisms. However, the greatest food safety benefit is the inhibition of *Clostridium botulinum* spores by nitrite ions, derived mainly from adding sodium nitrite and to a lesser degree from the reduction of nitrate ions. Under certain conditions, the nitrites can also inhibit the growth of other pathogenic and toxigenic bacteria (e.g., *L. monocytogenes*, *S. aureus*, *C. perfringens*), but nitrites are generally ineffective against bacteria belonging to the family Enterobacteriaceae, including *Salmonella* and *Escherichia*.

The relative inhibition of *C. botulinum* by nitrites depends on many factors, including its concentration, pH, temperature, and the presence of oxygen and other inhibitory compounds. For example, a synergistic effect of inhibition is observed under the conditions of low pH, anaerobic environment, and the presence of salt (Rahman 1999). After heating to temperatures of 105°–110°C, the effectiveness of nitrites increases 10-fold. This is called the Perigo effect or factor and is a result of the formation of other compounds, which have not yet been definitively identified. The Perigo effect is most important in canned meats containing nitrites during the heat treatment process.

Nitrates and nitrites can be converted to N-nitroso compounds, a class of potent carcinogens, after consumption (*in vivo*) or before consumption from high-heat cooking. Following several epidemiologic and laboratory studies, the presence of nitrates and nitrites in foods was suggested to increase the risk of certain cancers. Unfortunately, many of these studies have inherent weaknesses, and the strength of evidence is lacking to make definitive conclusions (Eichholzer and Gutzwiller 1998). Furthermore, vegetables also contain high levels of nitrates, and the detectable level of N-nitroso compounds in foods is generally very low. Nonetheless, the concerns raised by this controversy highlight the importance of performing risk assessments and risk-benefit analysis before regulatory approval of food additives.

Benzoic acid and the benzoate salts have been used for many years to inhibit molds and yeasts. At higher concentrations, these compounds can also be effective inhibitors of some bacteria. Benzoic acid is a weak acid, and its effectiveness is enhanced at lower pH values. In fact, benzoic acid

**Table 5-4**  Partial Listing of Chemicals Used/Proposed as Food Preservatives and Antimicrobial Additives

| Chemical Categories and Compounds | Primary Target Organisms | Example Food Applications |
|---|---|---|
| Ascorbic acid | Molds, bacteria | Fruit juices, meats, produce |
| Benzoic acid, benzoate salts | Yeasts, molds | Pickles, dressings, margarine, beverages |
| Propionic acid, propionates (e.g., calcium propionate) | Molds | Breads, grains, cakes, baked goods, some cheeses |
| Sodium nitrite, sodium nitrate | *C. botulinum* | Cured and canned meats |
| Sulfur dioxide and Sulfite-containing compounds (e.g., sodium metasulfite, potassium sulfite, sodium sulfite, potassium bisulfate, etc.) | Molds, yeasts, bacteria (including some gram-negative pathogens) | Alcoholic and nonalcoholic drinks, fruit and vegetable products, raw meat products, fish |
| Sorbic acid, sorbate salts (e.g., calcium sorbate, potassium sorbate) | Molds, yeasts, bacteria | Wide variety of foods, beverages, wines |
| Natural Antimicrobials | | |
| Animal-derived: chitosan, lactoferrin, lactoperoxidase, lysozyme | Bacteria | Cheese and other dairy products, cooked and processed meats |
| Plant-derived: allium, hydroxy-cinnamic acids, isothiocyanates, spices | Molds, bacteria | Fresh-cut fruits; proposed for meat, poultry, and fish products; vegetables |
| Microbial-derived: antibiotics (natamycin or pimaricin), bacteriocins (nisin) | Molds, bacteria | Cheese, canned foods, meat and fish |

*Sources:* FDA, Burt 2004, Davidson and Zivanovic 2003, Meyer 2003, Gould 2000, Rahman 1999.

and other weak acid preservatives (e.g., proprionate, sorbate) are typically added to acidic and acidified foods to enhance their effectiveness and to provide hurdles to microbial growth. Similar to benzoic acid, the sorbates are used primarily to inhibit the growth of molds and yeasts, but they are comparatively more effective against bacteria—including some pathogens. Important foodborne bacteria such as *S. aureus*, *Salmonella*, and *Vibrio parahaemolyticus* are effectively inhibited by sorbates at lower pH values (Jay et al. 2005). When combined with reduced nitrite, sorbates are also effective against *C. botulinum*, *S. aureus*, and spoilage bacteria in several types of cured meat.

Since ancient times, people realized that burning sulfur provided a purifying effect on foods and other objects. Actually, the burning of sulfur produces sulfur dioxide ($SO_2$), which enters microbial cells and inactivates them. In modern times, food processors use $SO_2$ directly as a gas or liquid, or it is generated in food products from the addition of sulfite-containing compounds. The most commonly used compound is sodium metasulfite ($Na_2S_2O_5$), followed by various sulfite salts (Gould 2000). Sulfites are added to foods and drinks as an antimicrobial preservative, mostly against molds and yeasts, but they are effective inhibitors of several *Salmonella* serovars and other Enterobacteriaceae (Jay et al. 2005). Besides their antimicrobial effects, sulfites are also used as antioxidants, enzyme inhibitors, antibrowning agents, and reducing agents in foods. Each specific function or purpose of sulfites depends on the concentration, and the concentration for a particular function can vary greatly for different foods. A drawback of adding sulfites to foods is that some individuals may experience an idiosyncratic reaction, possibly as a severe asthmatic response.

## Natural Antimicrobials

A great amount of interest in so-called natural antimicrobials has been generated over the years. One reason for this interest is to minimize the expensive toxicological testing for regulatory approval, as is required for synthetic chemicals. In addition, the public frequently perceives natural ingredients as safer compared with synthetic ingredients. Of course, this is not always true. Some of the most toxic substances known to humans come from natural sources. Additionally, many current food additives and antimicrobials originated from natural sources, but the synthetic production of these compounds has many benefits in terms of cost and product purity. Most important, if natural (or synthetic) antimicrobials are used in foods exclusively to control microbial agents of public health concern, the efficacy of these antimicrobials must be characterized and substantiated with rigorous scientific data. This includes any changes in antimicrobial efficacy from the storage and handling of food products. Notwithstanding these issues, the potential benefits of natural antimicrobials are significant—provided their applications and limitations are carefully considered.

Antimicrobials derived from animals consist mostly of enzymes and other proteins, along with a few small peptides. They include lysozyme, lactoferrin, chitosan, and lactoperoxidase. Lysozyme is an antimicrobial enzyme naturally found in tears, milk, eggs, insects, and fish. It is on the generally recognized as safe (GRAS) list and added to certain cheeses, frankfurter casings, and other foods. Lysozyme is most effective against Gram-positive bacteria, including spoilage bacteria and *S. aureus*, *C. botulinum*, and *L. monocytogenes*. Lactoferrin is also on the GRAS list and inhibits several spoilage and pathogenic bacteria. Among its approved uses, lactoferrin is applied as an antimicrobial spray on processed beef. Chitosan (not a protein) is produced commercially from chitin, a polysaccharide that is found in the exoskeletons of crustaceans and other arthropods, as well as other organisms in the nature. It is an effective inhibitor of several species of molds, yeasts, and bacteria, including several pathogenic and toxigenic bacteria. The efficacy of chitosan depends very much on its concentration, intrinsic and extrinsic parameters, and the presence of interfering constituents in the foods. The applications of chitosan include coatings on meat products and fruits, food additive/preservative, and incorporation into food packing materials (No et al. 2007). Chitosan has not been widely approved as a food additive in Western countries, but rather as a processing aid.

Lactoperoxidase is an enzyme found predominantly in milk but also detectable in other animal secreta. Actually, the antimicrobial effects of lactoperoxidase result from its catalysis of a reaction that produces hypothiocyanite (OSCN⁻) from the substrates thiocyanate (SCN⁻) and hydrogen peroxide ($H_2O_2$). The lactoperoxidase enzyme and the two substrates are collectively referred to as the lactoperoxidase system. The effectiveness of the lactoperoxidase system can be optimized or enhanced by the addition one or both of the substrates. The lactoperoxidase system is most promising as a means of preserving raw milk and other dairy products in developing countries. Because of a lack of quantitative data, the antimicrobial efficacies of the lactoperoxidase system for specific bacteria are difficult to model and predict (Meyer 2003).

Plant-derived antimicrobials originate from the flowers, fruits, leaves, stems, barks, or roots of plants. The chemical structures of plant-derived antimicrobials are diverse and can be grouped into several chemical classes or categories. Despite the great variety and abundance of antimicrobials from plants, few have been fully exploited for food protection. Some of the most promising plant-derived antimicrobials are *Allium*, hydroxycinnamic acids, isothiocyanates, and spices. *Allium* is the genus name for more than 800 species of plants related to the onion, such as garlic, shallots, scallions, leeks, and many others. An enzyme-catalyzed reaction associated with the ruptured cells of *Allium* yields several antimicrobial sulfur and phenolic compounds. These compounds contribute the ability of *Allium* to inhibit the growth and toxin production of several microbial species. Hydroxycinnamic acids (and related compounds) are derived from a variety of plants, some already used as foods (e.g., citrus fruits, carrots, celery). These compounds are frequently found as esters and sometimes as glucosides. Depending on the specific compound and its concentration, these compounds have been demonstrated to inhibit the growth of several microbial species, including several with public health significance. Isothiocyanates are naturally formed by the disruption of tissues from cruciferous vegetables and mustard family plants. They are potent inhibitors of molds, yeasts, and bacteria. The inhibitory and bactericidal properties of isothiocyanates appear effective against Enterobacteriaceae, particularly under wet conditions, and one potential application involves a sanitizing spray for fresh vegetables.

The plant-derived compounds with the greatest potential as food antimicrobials are associated with spices and their essential oils (Davidson and Zivanovic 2003). Spices and herbs have a long history of use dating back thousands of years, and early civilizations learned that these additives can help preserve foods and provide medicinal benefits. Conversely, depending on the dose, some chemical constituents of spices and herbs can be toxins or poisons (Barceloux 2008). A very long list of spices exists, originating from a wide variety of wild and domesticated plants. The process of extracting essential oils from spice plants is commonly done by steam distillation and to a lesser degree by liquid carbon dioxide. Some common essential oils with antimicrobial constituents are clove, cinnamon, oregano, thyme, caraway, sage, and black and red pepper. The chemical constituents of essential oils with antimicrobial properties are chiefly phenolic compounds, but the total number of individual constituents in essential oils can exceed 60 (Burt 2004). Some of the minor constituents in this mixture may play a significant role in the antimicrobial properties of essential oils, possibly through some synergistic effects with the other constituents.

Many scientific studies have documented the microbiostatic and/or microbicidal properties of spices and their essential oils. The affected microorganisms include spoilage molds, yeasts, and bacteria, and pathogenic/toxigenic bacteria. But for many reasons, caution is necessary whenever spices or their essential oils are proposed exclusively as a food protection measure. Most important, spicy foods normally do not contain sufficient concentrations of the chemical constituents to ensure complete antimicrobial effectiveness. Furthermore, pathogenic/toxigenic bacterial species differ in their resistance to various spices or herbs. In other words, generalizing the resistance of a particular microbial species to various spices (and vice versa) is not valid for actual applications. In fact, pathogen-contaminated spices and herbs have been responsible for numerous foodborne illness outbreaks. The applications of spices and their essential oils for food protection should be based on specific microbial challenge studies, and the applications should be in combination with other food protection technologies, in other words, the hurdle concept.

Antimicrobials derived from microorganisms can be divided into multiple categories, but the two most important are antibiotics and bacteriocins. Antibiotics are relatively wide spectrum against a range of microbial agents, and they generally have different microbicidal mechanisms compared with bacteriocins. Many different antibiotics are approved for veterinary use in livestock animals destined for human food, and the presence of antibiotic residues in foods is a major issue among some consumers and public health officials. The primary concern about antibiotics residues, whether from veterinary use or as a food additive, is the development of antibiotic resistance by foodborne pathogenic bacteria. For this reason, using antibiotics as food antimicrobials is very unpopular and faces regulatory approval difficulties. Despite this situation, several antibiotics have been used in foods since the 1950s. The most widely used antibiotic is natamycin (pimaricin). It is used primarily to prevent the growth of molds and yeasts in cheeses, dry sausages, and a few other foods. Natamycin is relatively ineffective against bacteria and, hence, is considered a food preservative rather than a food safety aid.

Bacteriocins are diverse groups of proteins or peptides produced by several species of bacteria, most notably the lactic acid bacteria (Galvez et al. 2008). These compounds differ greatly in their biological activity, biochemical properties, molecular weight, and modes of action. They are effective antibacterial compounds but relatively nontoxic to eukaryotic cells. Compared with therapeutic antibiotics, bacteriocins affect a limited range of target bacteria and often involve multiple mechanisms or modes of action. Such properties suggest the bacteriocins are less likely to promote bacterial resistance, but some scientists believe that the emergence of resistant pathogens is possible without using multiple hurdles to survival and growth (Davidson and Harrison 2002). Bacteriocins can be applied to foods as either a preparation (*ex situ*) isolated from industrial cultures or as starter cultures of bacteria that produce them upon growth (*in situ*). The large-scale preparation of bacteriocins has been difficult to achieve on an industrial level. The addition of starter cultures to foods (i.e., biocontrol) to introduce bacteriocins is often more feasible, but food compatibility and growth conditions for the starter bacteria must be carefully considered.

Nisin is the best-known bacteriocin with the longest history of approved use. It was first reported used in the 1950s to prevent the spoilage of Swiss cheese and received U.S. approval in 1988 for pasteurized cheese products (Jay et al. 2005). Nisin has since received approval for various food applications in more than 50 countries. Although it is effective against several types of spoilage bacteria, including some sporeformers, nisin is frequently ineffective against important strains of *C. botulinum*. In combination with other food protection technologies, nisin has been effective in inhibiting the growth of *L. monocytogenes*, and it has limited success in the inhibition of *E. coli* O157:H7, certain *Salmonella* serovars, and *S. aureus* in meat products (Galvez et al. 2008). Nisin does have an interactive effect with heat treatments, and the $F_o$ can be reduced for commercial sterilization when nisin is added to canned foods prior to retorting.

A great number of research reports have been published over the years on many bacteriocins, along with their proposed applications for food protection. Milk and dairy products are ideal foods for using bacteriocins or bacteriocinogenic starter cultures, and nisin and other bacteriocins are routinely used for this purpose. Studies have reported the use of bacterocin preparations in meat products with some degree of success in inhibiting spoilage and pathogenic/toxigenic bacteria. The perishable nature and pathogen contamination risk of seafood has made it the subject of research for using bacteriocins. A particularly interesting line of research is using bacteriocins to reduce the level of heat treatments for processed seafood. This would reduce the damage to seafood from high heat treatments. Many scenarios for using bacteriocins are proposed and plausible for fruits, vegetables, and juices. Foods such as bean sprouts and other raw vegetables that have been associated with disease outbreaks are good candidates for using bacteriocins in combination with other food protection technologies.

Despite all the research reports and proposed applications, the actual number of bacteriocins in commercial use for food protection is relatively limited. The reasons include bacteriocins' narrow range of effectiveness against target bacteria, incompatibilities among certain foods and their formulations, and difficulties with receiving regulatory approval. Nonetheless, bacteriocins offer many advantages over other food preservatives, and the interest in bacteriocins will likely continue to increase. The challenge ahead is determining the correct combination of bacteriocins with specific food systems and other food protection technologies to provide effective hurdles against bacterial survival and growth.

Before the natural antimicrobials discussed previously can be fully exploited for food protection, research in two areas must generate data and be interpreted to provide additional knowledge (Davidson and Zivanovic 2003). First, additional data must be generated on the spectrum of efficacy and specific food applications of natural antimicrobials. This entails determining which microorganisms are inhibited/inactivated by natural antimicrobials and which foods are compatible with using natural antimicrobials, particularly with regard to altered antimicrobial efficacies and consumer food quality issues. Antimicrobials may not have the same effectiveness in different foods, and antimicrobials may adversely alter the sensory characteristics of the foods. The second research area is determining the most effective combinations of natural antimicrobials with traditional food protection technologies. Most likely, for many reasons already discussed, natural antimicrobials will not be used alone as the sole means of food preservation and/or safety. The combination of natural antimicrobials with traditional food protection technologies is important to the hurdle concept of food protection.

## Food Contact Sanitizers/Antimicrobials and Fumigation Agents

Sanitizers for food contact surfaces and equipment are discussed in Chapter 4. In this section, the discussion focuses on the use of sanitizers or antimicrobial pesticides applied directly on foods or applied on surfaces for the purpose of sanitizing the food contact interface. Following passage of the Food Quality Protection Act (FQPA) in 1996, confusion and jurisdictional conflicts ensued between EPA and FDA over the definitions of "food additive" and "pesticide chemical." Under FQPA, certain antimicrobial compounds were defined as pesticides, which by extension changed the definition of a "pest" to include microorganisms. The jurisdictional conflicts were resolved by passage of the Antimicrobial Regulation Technical Corrections Act (ARTCA) of 1998. From a functional perspective, an antimicrobial pesticide regulated by EPA and a food additive regulated by FDA can both be food sanitizers. The primary distinction between an antimicrobial pesticide and a food additive used as a food sanitizer is the point where it is applied in the food handling chain.

Food sanitizers used on raw agricultural commodities (RACs) prior to entry into food processing facilities are considered antimicrobial pesticides. Under federal regulations, a food processing facility does *not* include structures or locations where RACs are simply washed, waxed, fumigated, and/or packed for shipping. Food sanitizers used in food processing facilities are regulated as food additives because the residues of the sanitizer will likely remain in the food product to some level. The aforementioned definitions and distinctions also apply to antimicrobial compounds other than sanitizers, such as antifungal agents. A specific exception to the regulations is the designation of ethylene dioxide and propylene dioxide (antifungal agents) as pesticides regardless of where they are used in the food handling chain.

Food sanitizers are used mostly to destroy pathogens and retard growth on the surfaces of fresh produce and meats. The desired efficacy of a food sanitizer is a 5-log reduction for particular pathogens of concern, though this level of efficacy is difficult to achieve in actual practice. Depending on the foods and potential sources of contamination, the pathogens of concern typically include important Gram-negative bacteria (e.g., pathogenic strains of *E. coli* and *Salmonella* serovars) and certain Gram-positive bacteria (e.g., *L. monocytogenes*). Food sanitizers are most effectively applied at strategic postharvest points in the food handling chain. Criteria for the selection of food sanitizers are based on the target pathogens, safety considerations for food workers and consumers, costs, subsequent pathogen-reduction measures, food quality deterioration issues, and other factors.

Acidified sodium chlorite is a sanitizer used for poultry, meats, seafood, and RACs. It is FDA approved as a secondary food additive and can be applied as either a spray or dip. This allows the advantage of a no-rinse application to foods. Table 5-5 lists approved uses of acidified sodium chlorite. The antimicrobial properties are the result of the oxidative effects of chlorous acid produced by the chlorite ion under acidic conditions. The chemical reaction between the sodium chlorite and acids to generate the chlorous acid mixture occurs instantly, and the effective shelf life of the mixture is generally less than 1 hour. Therefore, when used as a spray application for foods, the mixture must be prepared shortly before application. The antimicrobial effect is greatly influenced by the type of acids added, methods of spraying, and contact time on the meat surface. Acidified sodium chlorite has a good efficacy against *E. coli* O157:H7 and *Salmonella* serovars.

Calcium sulfate is combined with GRAS acids to produce a solution of acidic calcium sulfate. This mixture inactivates bacteria and is bacteriostatic. It currently has two approved applications in the United States: (1) a spray applied to RTE meats (e.g., hot dogs) prior to packaging, (2) a food additive to ground beef during the grinding process. Acidic calcium sulfate is beneficial for RTE meats because it aids in control of *L. monocytogenes* growth on meat surfaces within the package. The primary purpose of adding acidic calcium sulfate to ground beef is to lower the pH. This reduces bacterial counts in the product, an action that helps retard spoilage and possibly reduces the number of pathogens.

**Table 5-5** Allowed Uses of Acidified Sodium Chlorite Solutions

| Food Product | Application | ASC Solution ppm | ASC Solution pH |
|---|---|---|---|
| Poultry intact carcasses and parts, meat, organs, or related parts or trim | Spray or dip | 500–1,200 | 2.3–2.9 |
| Poultry intact carcasses and parts | Prechiller or chiller solution | 50–150 | 2.8–3.2 |
| Red meat, red meat parts, and organs | Spray or dip | 500–1,200 | 2.5–2.9 |
| Processed, comminuted, or formed meat food products | Spray or dip | 500–1,200 | 2.5–2.9 |
| Seafood[a] | Water or ice (use to rinse, wash, thaw, transport, or store) | 40–50 | 2.5–2.9 |
| Finfish and crustaceans[b] | Spray or dip solution (in processing facilities) | 1,200 | 2.3–2.9 |
| Raw agricultural commodities[c] | Spray or dip | 500–1,200 | 2.3–2.9 |
| Processed fruits and vegetables[d] | Spray or dip | 500–1,200 | 2.3–2.9 |

[a]Any seafood intended to be consumed raw shall be subjected to a potable water rinse prior to consumption.
[b]Treated seafood shall be cooked prior to consumption.
[c]Treated product shall be followed by a potable water rinse, or by blanching, cooking, or canning.
[d]Treated product shall be followed by a potable water rinse and a 24-hour holding period prior to consumption.

*Source:* Based on 21 CFR 173.325, compiled by USDA

Lactoferrin was identified earlier as an animal-derived antimicrobial added to foods. An activated form of lactoferrin (ALF, Activin) has GRAS status by FDA and is approved by USDA as an antimicrobial spray on beef carcasses and parts. The reported benefits of activated lactoferrin include interference with bacterial adhesion and colonization, inhibition of growth, detachment of microorganisms from biological surfaces, and the neutralization of endotoxin activity. Although information is limited regarding the efficacy of ALF compared with other chemical antimicrobials, it does appear to be effective against *E. coli* O157:H7, *Salmonella* Typhimurium, *L. monocytogenes*, and spoilage bacteria (Midgley and Small 2006).

Hydrogen peroxide ($H_2O_2$) is a weak acid but strong oxidizing agent. It is used on food contact surfaces for sterilization, but $H_2O_2$ is not allowed by itself as a sanitizer on foods in the United States unless combined with peroxyacids (Food Safety and Inspection Service [FSIS] 2010). Peroxyacetic acid is an equilibrium mix of several organic acids with $H_2O_2$ that is used mainly as a wash for meat/poultry carcasses and parts. Laboratory studies demonstrate significant log reductions of *E. coli* O157:H7 on beef carcass tissues. Unfortunately, these reductions have not been consistently achieved on beef carcasses in actual processing plants, and processors are recommended to conduct their own in-plant validations to determine intervention effectiveness (Midgley and Small 2006).

The most frequently used food sanitizers are solutions of organic acids. Most organic acid solutions consist of lactic and acetic acids. They are also made from formic, propionic, fumaric, citric, and other acids, and combinations of several acids. Organic acid solutions are most effective as carcass rinses at warm temperatures. However, they have a tendency to corrode equipment with increasing temperature. The efficacy of organic acid rinses against pathogens such as *E. coli* O157:H7 differs with the type and concentration of acids in the solution. In the United States, organic acid rinses are permitted on carcasses as a prechill intervention. In addition, lactic acid (up to 5% in solution) is permitted pre and post chill on livestock carcasses and beef/pork subprimals and trimmings, provided temperatures do not exceed 55°C (131°F). Scientists have raised concerns about the possibility of developing acid-resistant strains of bacteria in the future from using organic acid solutions. Increasing the acidity of solutions to ensure complete microbial kill is not feasible because of detrimental effects on the foods and corrosion of equipment.

Chlorine has a long history as a disinfectant for drinking water and, at higher concentrations, as a sanitizing solution for inanimate surfaces. It also is effective in reducing bacterial counts on livestock carcasses and certain other foods. But because chlorine is a powerful oxidant, the concentrations of chlorine in water rinses necessary for high log reductions of bacteria (200–500 ppm) are not suitable for meats and most foods. In addition, chlorine reacts with organic and inorganic compounds to form trihalomethanes (THMs), a class of carcinogenic compounds, and higher concentrations of chlorine can increase the formation of THMs. Chlorine sanitizing solutions are made primarily from calcium hypochlorite ($CaCl_2O_2$), sodium chlorite ($NaClO_2$), sodium hypochlorite ($NaClO$), or chlorine dioxide ($ClO_2$). The molecular forms of chlorine in solution do not exist as $Cl_2$ but rather as several combinations of compounds and ions.

Chlorine solutions for food applications are permitted by USDA in the meat industry with concentrations ranging from 5–50 ppm of free available chlorine ($HOCl$, $OCl^-$), depending on the specific application (FSIS 2010). Sodium and calcium hypochlorite are approved by FDA as indirect food additives, and they are permitted by EPA as antimicrobial compounds (i.e., pesticides) for postharvest applications on RACs such as fruit and vegetable crops. Chlorine dioxide is a gas introduced into water solutions and is regulated as a direct food additive. As such, FDA permits chlorine dioxide to be used in poultry processing and to wash non-RAC fruits and vegetables—provided the residual concentration of chlorine dioxide does not exceed 3 ppm in the water solutions (21 CFR 173.300). Chlorine dioxide is registered with the EPA as both a disinfectant and sanitizer, and in gaseous form as a sterilant.

Ozone ($O_3$) is a powerful oxidant gas and antimicrobial compound, capable of killing *Cryptosporidium parvum*, a protozoan pathogen with resistance to normal chlorine residuals in potable water. In fact, ozone is more effective than chlorine in the destruction of bacteria, viruses, and protozoans with a shorter contact time. It has the added advantage of leaving no residue after reacting with other constituents. Consequently, ozone is approved by FDA as a secondary direct food additive and can be used to treat, process, and store foods (21 CFR 173.368). This includes a variety of fruits, vegetables, poultry, and meat products. Selective use of ozone is recommended, however, because some foods (e.g., red meats) can suffer oxidative damage from it. Because ozone is unstable and rapidly decomposes, it must be generated on-site for applications, usually with an ozone generator. It is used on foods in either a gaseous state or aqueous solution, sometimes as a bubbling $O_3$ wash or dip rather than ozonated water.

Several other chemical compounds are approved and/or proposed as antimicrobial applications on foods. One such chemical is trisodium phosphate, normally found as an alkaline cleaning agent. This compound is GRAS approved by FDA for foods when used with good manufacturing practices (21 CFR 182.1778). Trisodium phosphate can be used as a spray or dip on unchilled chicken carcasses, and interim FSIS policy has permitted its use as a treatment for beef carcasses. A major disadvantage of trisodium phosphate is managing the resulting wastewater, which can lead to nutrient overload and eutrophication of natural waters. Other chemicals tested as food sanitizers or antimicrobial food contact agents include quarternary ammonium compounds and calcinated calcium. Additional chemical compounds are under development or undergoing testing for food industry applications.

The antimicrobial chemicals discussed previously are predominantly applied to foods as either sprays, washes, or dips. When chemicals are applied in a gaseous state to treat foodstuff (or other materials), it is usually referred to as fumigation. Several methods and chemicals can be used to fumigate foodstuff, and the choices are based on the target pests, type of bulk storage/packaging of the foodstuff, hazards to people and the public, potential for chemical changes or residues in the foodstuff, and other considerations. Most often, fumigations are used to eliminate vertebrate pests (rodents, birds, etc.), insects, and fungi. Sometimes, fumigation is used to control spoilage and pathogenic bacteria. There are several advantages to the fumigation of foodstuff, but the single greatest advantage is the permeation of the fumigant throughout the commodity—unlike liquid applications that treat only surfaces or minimally penetrate the surface. The disadvantages of fumigation include containment of the gases (i.e., fumigants), potential toxicity of the fumigant to nontarget organisms, and the requirements for special licenses or permits.

Several antifungal chemicals are used as fumigants on dried fruits, nuts, spices, cocoa powder, seeds, and other commodities. Two of the most widely used antimicrobial fumigants with similar modes of action are ethylene oxide and propylene oxide. Ethylene oxide is used mostly in the sterilization of medical instruments, devices, and disposable sterile products. To a lesser degree, it is also used to fumigate spices, other stored foods, and as a gaseous sterilant of food packaging materials. Ethylene oxide has been used for more than 40 years as a fumigant to control insects, fungi (molds and yeasts), and bacteria in foodstuffs. Other fumigant pesticides/antimicrobials used with foodstuffs are sulfur dioxide ($SO_2$), and ethyl and methyl formates. A considerable amount of research effort is being directed toward using natural antimicrobials as fumigants. Food irradiation has also been pursed as an alternative to fumigation, but the labeling requirements for irradiated foods is a negative marketing concern to food producers. Recently, in response to a series of salmonellosis outbreaks and recalls attributed to spices, the FDA has encouraged spice producers to better protect their products from contamination and/or treat them for salmonellae. The current best options for treating spices are either irradiation or fumigation. Both options have inherent advantages and disadvantages.

## MODIFICATION OF SELECT INTRINSIC AND EXTRINSIC PARAMETERS

Along with the application of heat or cold temperatures, modification of other extrinsic and intrinsic parameters of foods is used to control the growth of microorganisms. The longest established methods involve the reduction of water activity and pH. Since ancient times, people have dried foods to preserve them, using a variety methods ranging from sun and wind to smoke. The acidification of foods has also been used for centuries to preserve foods and to impart desired flavors. Over the nineteenth and twentieth centuries, as knowledge expanded from the physical and life sciences, engineers produced more sophisticated technologies that treated foods on an industrial scale. A relatively recent innovation involves modifying the atmospheres of foods in specially designed packages.

## Reduction of Water Activity in Foods

The concept of water activity ($a_w$) and its relevance to microbial survival and growth are discussed in Chapter 3. Since the late twentieth century, the relationship between $a_w$ and the death, survival, and growth of microorganisms has been extensively studied by microbiologists. Prior to defining this relationship in detail, the approaches to controlling microbial growth by reducing moisture content were not always reliable for food industry applications. Nowadays, the modification of $a_w$ is the basis of several technologies to protect foods, and $a_w$ is routinely used as an indicator of food protection in legal and guidance documents. The technologies for reducing $a_w$ are based on two principles: (1) reducing moisture content (i.e., dehydration) by heat or other extraction methods, including freeze drying and mechanical dewatering; and/or (2) reduction of free and available water by the addition of solutes that bind water molecules, referred to as osmotic dehydration.

### Dehydration Methods

The measured $a_w$ is critically important whenever drying is used as a method for food protection. Foods are generally categorized into low-, intermediate-, and high-moisture foods based on their $a_w$ values and overall moisture content by weight. Low-moisture foods usually have $a_w$ values between 0.00 and 0.60 with less than 25% moisture content; intermediate-moisture foods have $a_w$ values between 0.60 and 0.85 with moisture content between 15% and 50% (Jay et al. 2005). High-moisture foods have $a_w$ values well above 0.85, and at these values, the influence of $a_w$ in limiting the survival and growth of bacteria is diminished compared with other extrinsic/intrinsic parameters. In most cases, along with reducing the $a_w$ of foods, a combination of hurdles is employed to control microbial growth. The combined use of hurdles has become particularly important in recent years because consumer preferences have shifted toward foods with greater moisture content. A combination of hurdles with dried foods allows the retention of some moisture without compromising food protection.

Throughout the world, particularly in lesser developed countries where energy sources are limited, sun and wind exposure are the primary methods for drying foods. More recently, sophisticated solar dryers have become available, but only to those who can afford them. In industrialized countries, large-scale dehydration of foods is usually done by generating sources of heat or by a process called freeze drying. Dehydration of foods by hot air is accomplished using a variety of dryers: bin dryers, cabinet/tray dryers, fluidized bed dryers, conveyor dryers, impingement dryers, kiln dryers, rotary dryers, tunnel dryers, and other equipment (Fellows 2009). For liquid food products, spray dryers have become the preferred method of dehydration. These hot air dryers transfer heat mostly through convection and to a lesser degree through radiation and conduction by contact with hot trays or surfaces. Other dryers operate primarily through food contact with heated surfaces. The advantages of using contact/heated surface dryers are reduced energy costs and the capability to perform dehydration under anoxic conditions, thereby reducing oxidative damage to foods.

Some food drying technologies exploit nonionizing radiation to generate heat. Drying occurs from heating after the foods have been exposed to either microwave, infrared (IR), or radio frequency (RF) radiation. One advantage of using microwave and RF radiation dryers is the selective heating of moist areas in food while the relatively dry areas do not undergo much heating (Fellows 2009). This prevents overdrying foods to the point of adversely affecting taste and texture. Another advantage of using nonionizing radiation dryers is the reduced energy costs compared with hot air and heated surface dryers. The disadvantages of nonionizing radiation dryers include the initial investment costs for the equipment and the lower throughput or reduced productivity. An additional disadvantage is the nonuniform distribution and limited penetration of nonionizing radiation in bulk foods.

Freeze drying is a process where the foods are first frozen, followed by evaporation of ice from the foods through sublimation (Fellows 2009). But before sublimation can occur, the air pressure must be reduced (< 610 pascals) and then heat applied slowly to the frozen foods. The water vapor moves through the foods and is evaporated into the drying chamber. Compared with conventional drying, freeze drying is very expensive, and consequently, it is used only with foods that are easily damaged by conventional drying, for example, cooked and raw meats. Freeze dryers consist of a vacuum chamber and some type of heating device (e.g., heated shelves). Pumps are necessary to remove air from the vacuum chamber, and refrigeration coils convert the water vapor directly back to ice for removal from the dryer. The construction of freeze dryers is very sturdy, and the designs can be either bin, semicontinuous, or continuous (Fellows 2009). Both bin and semicontinuous freeze dryers have vacuum chambers that resemble cylindrical tunnels, but the semicontinuous freeze dryers have airlock doors at both ends of the cylinder to facilitate throughput. The continuous freeze dryers are designed to move trays of foods through different zones within a long vacuum chamber, and each zone has computer-programmable residence times and temperatures.

### Using Solutes to Control Water Activity

Like the drying and smoking of foods, ordinary salt (NaCl) has been used to preserve foods since antiquity. The relationship between salt content and $a_w$ is well established for most foods. Increasing the salt content of foods produces an osmotic pressure differential between the cytoplasm of microbial cells and the surrounding medium. Water diffuses from the microbial cells into the surrounding medium, where it becomes unavailable to the microorganisms, causing a loss of turgor in the cell membranes and shrinkage of the cells (plasmolysis). Microorganisms differ in their capacity to tolerate increasing salt concentrations before it interferes with growth and survival. One mechanism of this osmotolerance is the accumulation of low-molecular-weight solutes in the cytoplasm of microbial cells, counteracting the solute concentration in the surrounding medium. Generally speaking, fungi can tolerate relatively low $a_w$ values ($\sim$ 0.8–0.7), while most bacteria require higher $a_w$ values ($\sim > 0.9$) for growth and survival. Of course, there are exceptions to such generalizations. For example, *Staphylococcus aureus* is capable of growing at $a_w$ values of 0.86 or higher, though enterotoxin production occurs at higher $a_w$ values.

The minimum $a_w$ for the growth of microorganisms also varies with the type of solute used. Certain solutes bind the water molecules less tightly, and some solutes are capable of being transported into the microbial cytoplasm, where they have an equalizing effect on the osmotic pressure. Solutes that permit microbial growth at relatively high concentrations are called compatible solutes (Alzamora, Tapia, Welti-Chanes 2003). Many different foods can be the source of compatible solutes that permit microbial growth at lower $a_w$ values. Therefore, the type of food and solutes (naturally present or added) are important determinants of $a_w$ limiting microbial growth and survival. Other determinants are also important. Some solutes exert antimicrobial effects, and changes in other intrinsic and extrinsic parameters of microbial growth will alter the limiting $a_w$ values. The relationship between all these determinants and microbial growth/survival is complex to define and predict.

The most common solutes found in $a_w$ preserved foods are NaCl and sugars. A wide variety of products from meats to syrups has high concentrations of these solutes that act as preservatives and inhibit the growth of pathogenic and toxigenic bacteria. However, in an era of high blood pressure and obesity concerns, the reduction of salt and sugars in foods has become more common, along with consumer demand for minimally processed foods. For this reason, and as a margin of safety, the addition or retention of solutes is reinforced with a combination of hurdles. Lowered $a_w$ is rarely used alone in the modern food industry to control microbial growth. Additional hurdles include acidification, modified atmospheric packaging, adjusted redox potential, antimicrobial additives, competitive microorganisms, and temperature control.

## Acidification of Foods

As discussed earlier in Chapter 4, microbial growth is restricted between upper and lower levels on the pH scale. And microbial species have characteristic pH growth limits and optima that determine their ability to grow in foods. Of all the intrinsic parameters, pH is probably the most easily manipulated to control microbial growth. Foods can be treated to create either low or high pH (acidic vs. basic) conditions, but lower pH conditions are most frequently created with foods. The main reason is the inedibility of foods with a pH value above 9, the highest pH value of growth for most food-relevant microorganisms (Lucke 2003). Two basic methods are used to acidify foods. One method is by the addition of acidulants to foods. The other method involves the generation of acids through microbial activity. Fermentation is an example of using microbial activity to lower pH, but because this method involves the introduction of microorganisms, it is discussed separately under the section on biological controls.

Acidulants are not equal in their capacity to lower pH and to inhibit microbial growth. The relative acidic and basic properties of a substance are characterized by its $pK_a$, the negative logarithm of the acid dissociation constant. The substances often used as acidulants in foods have $pK_a$ values ranging between 3 and 5. Because foods typically have pH values ranging from 3 to 7, a significant amount of the acidulant is undissociated, meaning its ability to lower the pH in foods is less compared with stronger acids. But the $pK_a$ of an acidulant is not the only factor to consider. The lipophilicity (degree of affinity for lipids) of the undissociated form influences its ability to pass through the microbial cell membrane into the cytoplasm. Once inside the cytoplasm, the acidulant damages the cell by acidification, along with other possible mechanisms (Lucke 2003). Thus, some liphophilic acidulants are capable of inhibiting microbial growth without a major change in the food's pH value.

Benzoic, sorbic, and proprionic acids have relatively high lipophilicities and act primarily by entering the microbial cell cytoplasm. Along with acidification of the cytoplasm, the antimicrobial properties of these organic acids may involve other mechanisms. Accordingly, these organic acids are classified by FDA as food preservatives (i.e., antimicrobial food additives) instead of food acidulants. In comparison, acetic acid (e.g., vinegar) has only slight lipophilicity but also provides hydrogen ions in the food matrix, contributing to acidification. Because acetic acid is less liphophilic and has a history of safe use dating back thousands of years, it is not designated as a food preservative by FDA. Other organic acids used as food acidulants include citric, malic, tartaric, gluconic, and lactic acids. These organic acids have low lipophilicities.

Acidification of foods is typically performed in combination with other microbial growth hurdles. The principal reason is that many foods are inedible at pH values below 4.2, the lower limit where most pathogenic bacteria can survive and/or grow. Fortunately, even modest reductions in pH can impart stress on microbial cells, and additional hurdles (e.g., lowered $a_w$) are generally more effective in the presence of such stress. Another important reason is that pH changes can occur within parts of foods and under less-than-ideal storage, handling, and preparation practices. Additional hurdles provide an added margin of safety. A commonly used combination of hurdles is pH and $a_w$ modifications, as described earlier in Chapter 4, to determine the status of PHF/TCS foods. Heat treatments (e.g., pasteurization and commercial sterilization temperatures) are very often combined with the acidification of foods to destroy vegetative cells and control the germination of spores. Acidified foods also require less temperature and/or retention times to destroy vegetative cells and inactivate spores. This reduces energy costs and retains the desired sensory characteristics of foods.

## Vacuum and Modified Atmosphere Packaging

An important intrinsic parameter of microbial growth is composition of the local atmosphere, that is, the types and concentrations of gases present. Of primary concern is the concentration of oxygen ($O_2$) and carbon dioxide ($CO_2$). Obligate aerobes require a minimum level of $O_2$ to survive (e.g., *S. aureus*), whereas obligate anaerobes require an anoxic environment to survive (e.g., *C. botulinum* and *C. perfringens*). In between these two extremes exists a spectrum of microbial needs/tolerances of $O_2$ (e.g., microaerophilic, aerotolerant, facultative). In addition, high concentrations of $CO_2$ have an inhibitory effect on practically all microorganisms. This is common knowledge dating back to the early days of microbiology. Yet, the modification of local atmospheres to control microbial growth in foods did not become widespread until the advent of new packaging materials and automation technologies.

The terminology associated with the modification of local atmospheres is often confusing. Some commonly encountered terms are *hypobaric storage, controlled atmosphere storage (CAS), controlled atmosphere packaging (CAP), vacuum packaging (VP), modified atmosphere packaging (MAP), modified atmosphere storage (MAS)*, and *equilibrium-modified atmosphere (EMA)*. Each of the aforementioned terms has a unique definition based on the source of information. Practically speaking, the primary differences are whether the food atmosphere is contained within a room or a package and whether the atmosphere is continuously controlled over time or only initially modified. For the purposes of discussion, the term *MAP* shall be used to include all modifications to the atmosphere or headspace of packaged foods, including vacuumed spaces.

The primary purpose of MAP technology is to slow spoilage and extend the shelf life of foods while also maintaining safety (Ooraikul 2003). With vacuum packaging, air is removed by varying degrees from gas-impermeable packages and then sealed. The vacuum space usually changes in composition from the food tissue and microbial respiration that occurs. Other forms of MAP technology alter the concentration of gases and pressures in the packaging. Several types of gases have been experimentally used with MAP technology, but only three gases are widely used in commercial food processing. These gases are $O_2$, $CO_2$, and nitrogen ($N_2$). They are used singly or in various combinations to achieve the correct atmosphere/headspace in the MAP foods.

The presence of $O_2$ in the ambient atmosphere is approximately 21% by volume of air. For most MAP foods, $O_2$ is eliminated or reduced because it supports the growth of aerobic and certain facultative microorganisms, and it participates in chemical reactions with food components. On the other hand, excessive reduction of $O_2$ in fresh fruits, vegetables, and certain meats can result in undesirable aromas, tastes, or off colors. The gas $CO_2$ is naturally present at less than 0.05% by volume in the ambient atmosphere. Higher concentrations of $CO_2$ become bacteriostatic to aerobes, and hence, $CO_2$ is used as a food preservative by increasing its concentration in MAP foods. The bacteriostatic property of $CO_2$ is considerably enhanced under pressure and is greater with Gram-negative than Gram-positive bacteria. The third gas, $N_2$, is most abundant in the ambient atmosphere at 78% by volume. Because $N_2$ is relatively inert, it is used mostly to displace $O_2$ in MAP foods. It is also used as a filler gas to prevent the crushing or collapsing of packages.

Packaging materials are an integral component of MAP food technology. The nature of the food product determines what packaging materials are best suited for the application. Because foods require different mixtures of MAP gases for preservation or shelf-life extension, the permeability of package materials to $O_2$ and $CO_2$ are important selection criteria. The intended humidity and temperature storage conditions of the foods are also important to consider because the permeability of materials to different gases can change under these storage conditions. A wide variety of materials has been developed with different permeability to gases and water vapor. Sophisticated packaging systems have been developed in recent years that have selective permeability, removal, or generation of gases in MAP foods. One such innovation involves atmosphere modifiers consisting of sachets or surface coatings that actively modify the headspace atmosphere (Ooraikul 2003).

The selection of MAP technology for a particular food requires careful consideration of the microbial, physiologic, chemical, and physical factors involved (Ooraikul 2003). The microbial ecology of the foods is important to determine so that specific spoilage microorganisms can be targeted for inhibition, while pathogenic or toxigenic microorganisms are excluded opportunities for growth. For example, the elimination of $O_2$ in certain MAP foods inhibits the growth of aerobes, but the anaerobic condition also increases the risk of *C. botulinum* spore germination. The physiologic factors for consideration involve changes that take place in the plant and animal cells after harvest/slaughter. Fruits and vegetables undergo complex changes that alter their colors, odors, tastes, and consistency, as well as modify the local atmosphere (e.g., $CO_2$ and ethylene). Meats, poultry, and fish differ in their postmortem changes and rates (e.g., rigor mortis), and the microbiota present on the carcasses differ greatly. In turn, these differences affect the colors, tastes, odors, and overall spoilage rates of foods from animal tissues. The chemical factors for consideration involve mostly redox reactions of lipids, proteins, sugars, and other biomolecules. These reactions may cause rancidity or other undesirable changes. The physical factors for consideration include staleness, toughness, loss of juices, and so forth.

From a food safety perspective, the main concern about MAP foods is the creation of conditions that favor the growth of pathogenic or toxigenic microorganisms. The basis for this concern is two principles. First, the inhibition of common spoilage microorganisms may eliminate the microbial interference that holds pathogens in check, allowing them to multiply without competition. Second, modified atmospheres may provide pathogenic or toxigenic microorganisms with a favorable intrinsic parameter for growth. A great number of research studies have been conducted on these subjects with mixed results. In general, under atmospheres of high $CO_2$ concentrations, the growth of several foodborne pathogens is inhibited (Rao and Sachindra 2002). However, other parameters such as warm temperatures can override the inhibitory effect of high $CO_2$ concentrations. The greatest potential hazard with MAP foods is the growth of *C. botulinum* and the production of toxins. Many foods are naturally contaminated with *C. botulinum* spores from either soils or sediments, and the elimination or reduction of $O_2$ in MAP foods creates an anaerobic environment necessary for the germination of these spores. Fortunately, the safety of MAP foods appears to be comparable with other foods. But this may be the result of a combination of measures to reduce microbial contamination (e.g., pasteurization) and additional hurdles to reduce growth potential, in particular temperature controls. Whatever the variables involved, multiple hurdles are strongly encouraged and sometimes required in the United States with MAP foods.

## BIOCONTROL METHODS AND BIOTECHNOLOGY

The modification and exploitation of organisms to benefit societies has existed since the earliest days of humankind. The greatest technological leap forward in human history was the domestication of plants and animals, some 10,000 years ago. Through selective breeding, humans have modified plants and animals to make them yield more food and resist diseases and, in the case of work animals, provide a source of labor and power. Similarly, humans harnessed the microbial world to ferment raw materials and produce a variety of foods and beverages. Over the last century, monumental leaps have occurred in technology development from the biological sciences—particularly for medical, public health, and agricultural applications. Thus, the term biotechnology was coined in the twentieth century to describe the exploitation of biological systems and organisms to make products and for other technological applications. Unfortunately, the term *biotechnology* and related terms are often used imprecisely, and this has led to confusion, misconceptions, and overregulation (Miller 2007). Although the term *biotechnology* also includes chemicals and enzymatic systems derived from organisms, this subject was covered earlier in the section on natural antimicrobials. Therefore, this section briefly discusses the direct use of microorganisms as a method of controlling foodborne hazards (i.e., biocontrol). The subject of genetically modified organisms (GMOs) is very briefly introduced as well.

## Fermentation

The fermentation of foods dates back thousands of years, possibly as long as 8,000 years ago (Ross, Morgan, Hill 2002). Fermentation has been used over the centuries to preserve foods and make different types of food products and beverages. It was not until the golden age of microbiology that microorganisms were determined as responsible for fermentation. This led to the development of microbial starter cultures and the implementation of fermentation on an industrial scale. A wide variety of foods and beverages is now available to consumers thanks to the technological innovations associated with fermentation. They include breads, cheeses, sausages, yogurt, sauerkraut, sauces, fermented meats, wines, beers, liquors, and many other food products.

The process of fermentation basically involves the enzymatic conversion of carbohydrates in raw materials by microorganisms to compounds such as organic acids, alcohol, and carbon dioxide. In fact, food fermentations are often categorized by the main chemical products they produce (Fellows 2009). Specialized starter cultures of yeast and bacteria enhance the performance of fermentation, and they help ensure a consistent quality is maintained for industrial production. Yeasts are widely used to produce alcoholic beverages, while lactic acid bacteria are widely used to ferment various meats, vegetables, and dairy products. Commonly used yeasts include the genera of *Sacchoromyces, Aspergillus, Penicillium,* and many others. Commonly used lactic acid bacteria belong to the genera *Lactobacillus, Lactococcus, Pediococcus, Enterococcus,* and *Streptococcus.* In actual practice, complex mixtures of microorganisms are involved with many fermentations. Furthermore, during the fermentation process, the mix of microbial populations usually changes with the loss of substrate and changes in the intrinsic parameters (pH, $a_w$, Eh) of the matrix.

Fermentation preserves foods initially by a process known as microbial antagonism, followed by long-term changes in the intrinsic parameters of the food matrix. As the yeast or bacterial starter culture grows, it produces compounds that inhibit spoilage and pathogenic/toxigenic microorganisms. The most important compounds are organic acids (e.g., lactic acid) that lower the pH of the food matrix. Acidification of the food matrix is tolerated by the starter culture but is unsuitable for growth by other microorganisms, and with increasing fermentation time even becomes bacteriocidal. The fermentation microorganisms also produce several antimicrobial compounds that act by other mechanisms of action. These include lipophilic organic acids, $H_2O_2$, ethanol, and antibiotics. In addition, the lactic acid bacteria produce a class of compounds known as bacteriocins. As discussed earlier, the bacteriocins have become the subject of intensive research as antimicrobial food additives.

The survival of pathogenic/toxigenic bacteria has been extensively studied for food fermentations that involve lactic acid bacteria. In general, when food fermentation operations are *properly performed*, pathogenic and toxigenic bacteria are inhibited and will decline in numbers during storage, provided the intrinsic parameters of the food are unfavorable for survival (Adams and Nicolaides 1997; Nout 1994). High initial contamination levels with bacterial pathogens increase the risk of their survival during fermentation and storage. Concern also exists with the acid tolerance responses of *Salmonella* serovars, pathogenic *E. coli*, and *L. monocytogenes*. Additionally, enteric viruses can withstand many acids and remain viable during lactic acid fermentations. Hence, good sanitary practices must be a part of food fermentation operations.

The survival of pathogens following the fermentation of foods has been documented with reports of foodborne illness outbreaks. Sausages and salami often are fermented followed by dry-curing processes that may permit the survival of pathogens such as *E. coli* O157:H7 (Centers for Disease Control and Prevention [CDC] 1995a, 1995b; Tilden et al 1996). The parasitic nematode *Trichinella spirilis* may also survive sausage fermentation (Potter et al. 1976). Preventive measures include cooking or sufficiently heating the sausage to destroy any pathogens. Commercial food manufacturers heat treat sausages when distributed as RTE products. Infections from *Vibrio parahaemolyticus* are common in Japan and frequently linked to fermented raw fish (Nout 1994). Apparently, *V. parahaemolyticus* can readily survive these particular types of fermentation.

Cheeses made from raw milk have been responsible for outbreaks of *E. coli* O157:H7 infections, salmonellosis, campylobacteriosis, and other infections (CDC 2009, 2007b, 2000). The riskiest products are the soft cheeses. Since 1950, FDA has required manufacturers to use pasteurized milk for soft and fresh cheeses. Raw milk is permitted only when making certain aged cheeses. These cheeses must be aged for at least 60 days at temperatures greater than 1.7°C (35°F). The number of pathogens present in naturally aged cheeses decreases over time when stored at warm temperatures, partly because of lactobacilli that survive and continue to alter the intrinsic parameters. The growth of surviving pathogens is inhibited because of unfavorable intrinsic parameters (e.g., $a_w$, pH).

Fermented foods may become contaminated with chemicals and toxins unless appropriate precautions are taken. Contamination with mycotoxins and chemical pollutants is most likely associated with the raw ingredients. Although some toxins such as aflatoxin $B_1$ are reduced with lactic acid fermentations, little evidence exists that most toxins and chemical residues are reduced with fermentation (Nout 1994). Certain yeast starter cultures may also produce toxins, and toxic byproducts from fermentation can be produced, but the proper selection of starter cultures reduces this risk. The production of toxins by contaminating bacteria is a prime concern. Enterotoxins produced by *S. aureus* (and related staphylococci) must be prevented by eliminating contamination sources and ensuring that fermentation inhibits the growth of these toxigenic bacteria. The extrinsic and intrinsic parameters of food products following fermentation must also be controlled to inhibit the growth of staphylococci.

The greatest hazard of microbial toxins from fermented foods is associated with the growth of *C. botulinum*. The spores of this bacterium can contaminate raw ingredients or foods wherever soils and sediments are encountered. The production of botulinum toxins is quite possible if fermentation operations and the intrinsic parameters of food products are not properly controlled. Outbreaks of botulism have been associated with fermented tofu, fish, meats, and bean products (CDC 2007a; Sobel et al. 2004). The majority of these outbreaks originated from noncommercial sources (e.g., home prepared), where the fermentation operations are unregulated and less likely to be rigorously controlled.

In terms of relative risks, fermented foods are generally considered safer than many fresh foods, but they cannot be considered safer than canned or frozen foods. Nout (1994) has identified several risk factors associated with fermented foods. The countermeasures to these risks are summarized here:

1. Raw materials used for fermentation must be wholesome and minimally contaminated with chemicals, toxins, and pathogens.
2. Whenever possible or required, raw materials such as milk should be pasteurized.
3. Starter cultures should be optimized so that they are not toxigenic, while also being antagonistic to pathogens and having detoxifying capabilities.
4. Fermentation conditions must be controlled and equipment properly operated to ensure complete fermentation.
5. Storage and maturation conditions must not support pathogen survival and growth or toxin production.
6. Fermented foods should be cooked or heated prior to consumption to kill possible pathogens.

## Microbial Interference/Microbial Antagonism

The terms *microbial interference* and *microbial antagonism* are often used interchangeably. According to Jay et al. (2005), *microbial interference* is a more general term that refers to "nonspecific inhibition or destruction of one microorganism by other members of the same habitat or environment." *Microbial antagonism* refers to specific interference mechanisms between defined populations of microorganisms. For example, a starter culture (e.g., lactic acid bacteria) with known properties used in food fermentation to inhibit target microbial populations is one type of microbial antagonism.

Fermentation was discussed in the previous section; this section focuses on nonfermentation applications of microbial antagonism for food protection. The microbial cultures added to foods for the purpose of inhibiting or destroying undesirable microbiota are sometimes referred to as protective cultures or exclusion cultures.

The best-studied protective cultures consist of lactic acid bacteria. Many strains of lactic acid bacteria are well characterized and have been used safely for years with food fermentations. Thus, they represent excellent choices for microbial antagonism applications. Lactic acid bacteria inhibit spoilage and pathogenic bacteria by the production of compounds such as lactic acid, $H_2O_2$, bacteriocins (e.g., nisin), $CO_2$, and alcohols (Rodgers 2001). They also outcompete other microorganisms for nutrients and acidify the food matrix. Based on research studies, lactic acid bacteria appear very useful against *L. monocytogenes*, a particularly problematic pathogen to control in the food processing and storage environments. Experiments also demonstrate that particular strains of lactic acid bacteria can inhibit *Salmonella* serovars, *E. coli* O157:H7, *S. aureus*, *Aeromonas hydrophila*, and *C. botulinum* (Kostrzynska and Bachand 2006).

Protective cultures of lactic acid bacteria are already used commercially to reduce bacterial pathogens in produce and refrigerated, fermented, and cooked meats (Kostrzynska and Bachand 2006). Research studies suggest a number of other potential applications for protective cultures. One proposed application is the addition of protective cultures to cook–chill foods as a safeguard against temperature abuse (Rodgers 2003). The concept is that the protective culture lies dormant in the food unless the holding temperature exceeds safe limits. If unsafe temperatures occur, the protective culture responds by producing bacteriocins against high-risk pathogens such as *C. botulinum* and *L. monocytogenes*. This proposed application would be particularly useful in the food catering industry.

Before microbial antagonism technology can be applied to additional foods and scenarios, several research and regulatory issues must be tackled. From the research standpoint, a greater understanding of the antagonistic mechanisms involved with different species and strains (both protective cultures and pathogens) is necessary. This includes the identification and characterization of the many antimicrobial compounds produced by protective cultures. Antimicrobial compounds often interact with one another to inhibit pathogens, and such interactions can be difficult to study. Next, the practical aspects of using protective cultures in different foods must be researched. From the knowledge acquired by this applied research, the development of a "system" is necessary, that is, specifications for technical skills, equipment and culture materials, and procedures. Finally, the safety of the protective culture with regard to infective and toxic risks must be demonstrated.

In the United States, microorganisms added to foods are either classified as GRAS substances or food additives. A great number of bacteria are GRAS-recognized for specific food uses, many of them with a long history of use in food fermentation. For new bacterial strains, or with new intended uses of GRAS bacterial strains, the food company is obliged to submit a GRAS determination to FDA. The GRAS determination is made by qualified experts, usually a panel organized by the food company. Upon review of the submitted documentation, FDA issues a letter stating whether it agrees or disagrees with the GRAS determination. If the bacterial strain or its intended use is completely novel, FDA may classify it as a food additive, in which case a formal application and approval process are necessary. This would require the submission of efficacy and toxicological/safety data to FDA for evaluation.

## Biocontrol Using Bacteriophages

Bacteriophages, or simply phages, are viruses that parasitize bacteria. Phages are diverse in their morphological structures and have a high specificity for bacterial hosts. They attach themselves to bacterial cells and introduce their nucleic acids into the cytoplasm through a number of different mechanisms. Once the bacterial cell is infected, the phage's progeny are generated using the bacteria's metabolism. The progeny phages are then released from the bacterial cell through either continuous extrusion, without killing the bacterium, or lysis of the bacterial cell, resulting in death of the bacterium. Some phages incorporate their nucleic acid into the bacterial genome, or other genetic elements of the cytoplasm, and undergo a type of lysogeny or dormancy, called pseudolysogeny. Lytic phages induce bacterial cells to produce lysins, a group of enzymes responsible for hydrolyzing the cell wall and causing cell lysis. The lysins have different mechanisms of action that are specific to the phages and the phage–bacterial host combination. But before lysis can occur, a bacterial cell must be undergoing division (i.e., binary fission). In other words, phage-infected bacterial populations in the lag phase of growth do not undergo cell lysis.

The existence of phages has been known for more than a century, and they were investigated as a therapy to treat bacterial infections in humans before antibiotics became more feasible. The concept of using phages to control spoilage and pathogenic bacteria in foods dates back to research in the 1960s. However, it was not until 2006 that FDA first approved a mixture of phages for direct application on foods (21 CFR 172.785). Marketed under the trade name List-Shield (formerly known as LMP-102), this product consists of six different phages that lyse *L. monocytogenes*. It can be sprayed on RTE meats and poultry products, including luncheon meats, hot dogs, and other products with the risk of *L. monocytogenes* contamination. The company that sells this product cites a 99–100% reduction of *L. monocytogenes* contamination levels for various foods stored in a temperature range of 2°–42°C (35.6°–107.6°F). These temperatures are within the growth range of *L. monocytogenes*, which is also one of the few pathogens that can multiply under refrigeration temperatures.

The efficacy of phages has been demonstrated in research laboratories for many foodborne bacterial pathogens (Hudson et al. 2005). Unfortunately, the technical challenges to using phages as biocontrol agents in foods have been difficult to overcome for most of these pathogens. The factors involved with effective biocontrol include a myriad of conditions. First of all, sets of lytic phages that are specific to the target pathogens must be identified, mass produced, and purified for use. This poses the risk that toxic by-products may be produced along with the phage preparation. Even with a safe phage preparation, the number of phages and bacterial host cells must be above a critical threshold and contact one another in the foods to exert effective biocontrol. In addition, the conditions for phage infectivity and lysis of bacterial cells depend on factors such as pH, visible and UV light, osmotic pressure, density of nontarget bacteria, interfering chemicals, and temperature. Furthermore, pathogens must be actively multiplying in foods for lytic phages to destroy them, which is itself an undesirable condition. With respect to the latter condition, the control of pyschrotrophic bacteria under refrigeration temperatures may be the best applications of lytic phages.

Successful biocontrol in foods using phages involves complex factors that must be better understood. Research is needed on the efficacy of phages under different conditions and in various scenarios. Under an optimum set of conditions, phages can be effective biocontrol agents (possibly as a hurdle), but they are not applicable in all scenarios. Nonetheless, phages have other potential applications for food safety. For example, phages have been successfully used in laboratories to identify bacterial pathogens sampled from foods, and they have been successfully used as indicators of bacterial contamination on foods and in water. Another possible application of phages is to sanitize food contact surfaces. Perhaps the most feasible approach of exploiting phages is by adding their lysins directly to foods (Jofre and Muniesa 2000). Lysins could be derived en masse by industrial processes similar to other enzymes produced for the food industry. Hence, lysins would be another type of natural antimicrobial compound. As with all new technologies, however, the technical feasibility and economic factors must be favorable before the food industry adopts them. Ultimately, consumer acceptance or rejection will determine whether phages or lysins become commonplace as a food protection technology.

## Genetically Modified Organisms and Genetically Modified Foods

Since the earliest days of plant and animal domestication, some 10,000 years ago, humans have selectively bred organisms to enhance particular traits. This form of selection resulted in lineages of organisms that are genetically modified from the original wild species. With the advent of modern science and molecular biology techniques, the genetic modification of organisms has become possible within an extremely short period of time. Furthermore, genetic material can now be transferred across species, a process that is comparatively restricted in the natural world. The purpose of this section is not to review the many methods of genetic modification but rather to provide an overview of the potential food safety issues of this technology.

Over the past 30 years, the pace of creating genetically modified organisms (GMOs) has dramatically increased with advancements in molecular biology. GMOs include plants, animals, and microorganisms that are created by a variety of methods ranging from conventional breeding to genetic engineering. The methods of genetic modification are broadly categorized as either genetic engineering or nongenetic engineering. Genetic engineering (GE) uses methods either to introduce or eliminate specific genes from the genetic constitution of a cell. Recombinant DNA (rDNA) techniques are used to genetically engineer an organism. An organism created by rDNA techniques is also referred to as transgenic. In contrast, nongenetic engineering methods do not involve the rDNA techniques of cutting, copying, and reassembling strands of DNA. Instead, nongenetic engineering methods involve indirect or nonspecific modification of DNA, for example, simple selection, interspecies crossing, or induced mutagenesis.

The potential benefits of GMOs are enormous. With a growing world population and limited arable land, GMOs are considered by many scientists as the best hope of increasing agricultural productivity to feed undernourished populations. Genetically modified plants are already used throughout the world as food crops, and they offer the best prospect of increasing the food supply. Desirable characteristics of genetically modified plants include greater tolerance to stress (e.g., drought, disease, salt, insects), higher yields per acre, tolerance to herbicides, reduction of natural plant toxins, reduced need for soil tillage, and better nutritional and sensory quality. Genetically modified animals are very common in biomedical research, but they have not been used for agricultural purposes to the same extent as plants (International Union of Food Science and Technology [IUFoST] 2005). The primary reasons are technical challenges, expense, low rate of reproduction, and lack of public acceptance. Genetically modified microorganisms have been used for many years in industrial microbiology to produce a wide variety of chemical substances, including food additives and processing aids. Additional potential food applications include enhanced fermentation, production of antimicrobial food additives (e.g., bacteriocins) and targeted biocontrol of pathogens.

The safety issues of GMOs are not related to the methods of genetic modification but to the products produced by the genes (e.g., secondary metabolites, proteins). Modified genes may produce substances that are toxic, allergenic, and/or antinutrient. The food safety concern is the unintended—and possibly undetected—production of hazardous substances. Hopefully, these substances would be detected before the GMO is introduced into production and the marketplace. Of course, this assumes that such substances are detectable with current analytical methods and animal testing protocols. The prudent backup to this assumption is the ability to conduct postmarket epidemiologic surveillance of populations that consume GMOs. Properly designed and conducted epidemiologic studies may identify health effects from GMOs that laboratory studies have missed.

Regardless of the genetic modification methods used, the risks of GMOs as food sources will be challenging to assess. The principal reason is twofold. First, detecting potentially hazardous substances using conventional or targeted methods of analysis requires knowledge of which substances to analyze for. Second, using state-of-the-art analytical methods that inventory changes in genes, proteins, and metabolites (e.g., -omics) is limited by current knowledge to interpret these changes, particularly with respect to potentially hazardous substances produced. To complicate matters further, if any novel substances are detected, a complete risk assessment process with all the attendant uncertainties and costs must be performed (see Chapter 6). To help with these challenges, the National Research Council (NRC 2004) has ranked the likelihood of unintended effects by the genetic modification method, and it has proposed a framework to aid in determining such effects from genetically modified foods. In the future, to meet the demand of a growing and hungry world population, GMOs and genetically modified foods will continue to be introduced into our food supply. This progress must be accompanied by diligent assessment and management of the potential risks.

## FOOD PROTECTION BY IRRADIATION

Ionizing radiation has been studied for decades as a means of preserving and sterilizing foods, most notably for special purposes such as military rations and space mission meals. For several reasons, commercial use of food irradiation has been slow and has not yet reached its full potential as a food protection technology. One reason is consumer perception and concern that irradiated foods are unsafe. This perception is reinforced by the regulation of food irradiation since 1963 as a food additive by FDA. In contrast, WHO regulations define food irradiation as a simple process with specified conditions of use (Lagunas-Solar 1995). FDA also requires the labeling of irradiated foods, something which is not required for most food processing applications. Since the 1990s, efforts have been under way to educate consumers on the process and benefits of food irradiation.

Although consumer acceptance of food irradiation has been slow, perceptions are changing, and the allowable list of foods that may be irradiated has been slowly growing. The benefits of food irradiation have become acknowledged in the context of recent foodborne illness outbreaks. In 2008, following highly publicized outbreaks of *Salmonella* and *E. coli* O157:H7 from fresh produce, federal regulations permitted the irradiation of iceberg lettuce and spinach (21 CFR 179.26). Table 5-6 lists the permitted uses of food irradiation in the United States. All irradiated foods must be labeled with the Radura symbol (Figure 5-5) and the statement "Treated with radiation" or "Treated by irradiation." Many in the food industry believe that such labeling contributes to consumer uncertainty about irradiated foods. Over the years, proposals have been made to allow the modification or elimination of labeling requirements for certain food irradiation uses and to change the term *irradiation* to *pasteurization* for particular irradiation processes. To date, however, the labeling requirements have not been changed. Surveys have found that the majority of informed consumers were influenced more by the technology's effectiveness than by the terms used (Fox 2002).

The ionizing radiation portion of the electromagnetic spectrum has sufficient energy to detach electrons from atoms and molecules (i.e., ionization). The types of ionizing radiation are either subatomic particles (e.g., alpha particles, beta particles, neutrons) or electromagnetic waves (e.g., X-rays, gamma rays, high-frequency UV). Food irradiation is most often accomplished with

**Table 5-6** Permitted Uses and Limitations of Food Irradiation in the United States

| *Permitted Uses of Food Irradiation* | *Limitations of Use* |
|---|---|
| 1. For control of *Trichinella spiralis* in pork carcasses or fresh, non–heat-processed cuts of pork carcasses. | Minimum dose 0.3 kiloGray (kGy) (30 kilorad [krad]); maximum dose not to exceed 1 kGy (100 krad). |
| 2. For growth and maturation inhibition of fresh foods. | Not to exceed 1 kGy (100 krad). |
| 3. For disinfestation of arthropod pests in food. | Not to exceed 1 kGy (100 krad). |
| 4. For microbial disinfection of dry or dehydrated enzyme preparations (including immobilized enzymes). | Not to exceed 10 kGy (1 megarad [Mrad]). |
| 5. For microbial disinfection of the following dry or dehydrated aromatic vegetable substances when used as ingredients in small amounts solely for flavoring or aroma: culinary herbs, seeds, spices, vegetable seasonings that are used to impart flavor but that are neither represented as, nor appear to be, a vegetable that is eaten for its own sake, and blends of these aromatic vegetable substances. Turmeric and paprika may also be irradiated when they are to be used as color additives. The blends may contain sodium chloride and minor amounts of dry food ingredients ordinarily used in such blends. | Not to exceed 30 kGy (3 Mrad). |
| 6. For control of foodborne pathogens in fresh or frozen, uncooked poultry products that are: (1) whole carcasses or disjointed portions of such carcasses that are "ready-to-cook poultry" within the meaning of 9 CFR 381.1(b)(44), or (2) mechanically separated poultry product (a finely comminuted ingredient produced by the mechanical deboning of poultry carcasses or parts of carcasses)**.** | Not to exceed 3 kGy (300 krad); any packaging used shall not exclude oxygen. |
| 7. For the sterilization of frozen, packaged meats used solely in the National Aeronautics and Space Administration space flight programs. | Minimum dose 44 kGy (4.4 Mrad). Packaging materials used need not comply with Sec. 179.25(c) provided that their use is otherwise permitted by applicable regulations in parts 174 through 186 of 21 CFR. |
| 8. For control of foodborne pathogens in, and extension of the shelf life of, refrigerated or frozen, uncooked products that are meat within the meaning of 9 CFR 301.2(rr), meat byproducts within the meaning of 9 CFR 301.2(tt), or meat food products within the meaning of 9 CFR 301.2(uu), with or without non-fluid seasoning, that are otherwise composed solely of intact or ground meat, meat by-products, or both meat and meat by-products. | Not to exceed 4.5 kGy maximum for refrigerated products; not to exceed 7.0 kGy maximum for frozen products. |
| 9. For control of *Salmonella* in fresh shell eggs. | Not to exceed 3.0 kGy. |
| 10. For control of microbial pathogens on seeds for sprouting. | Not to exceed 8.0 kGy. |
| 11. For the control of *Vibrio* bacteria and other foodborne microorganisms in or on fresh or frozen molluscan shellfish. | Not to exceed 5.5 kGy. |
| 12. For control of foodborne pathogens and extension of shelf life in fresh iceberg lettuce and fresh spinach. | Not to exceed 4.0 kGy. |

*Source*: 21 CFR 179.26

**Figure 5-5** Radura Logo. *Source:* Courtesy of FDA

gamma rays from radioisotopes (Cobalt-60 or Cesium-137) and to a lesser extent by X-rays or electron beams. The deposition of energy from ionizing radiation into materials was traditionally measured in the unit of radiation absorbed dose, or rad. The rad has been replaced by the new International System (SI) unit of gray (symbol: Gy). In the context of food irradiation, one kGy is equivalent to the absorption of 1 kilojoule (kJ) of energy per kilogram of food. The kGy is the unit used to measure absorbed dose of radiation in foods; it should not be confused with the rem or sievert, which are derived using Quality Factors to account for biological effects from absorption of radiation.

The biological effects of ionizing radiation are based primarily on damage to DNA and to some extent RNA. This damage can occur from direct "hits" by the ionizing radiation that breaks the DNA/RNA strands. It also occurs indirectly by ionizing adjacent molecules that form free radicals and compounds that react with the DNA/RNA and other biologically important molecules. The magnitude of damage and biological effects from radiation are dose-related. Increasing doses of ionizing radiation to microbial cells result in greater damage to nucleic acids and other biological molecules. Microorganisms have different levels of resistance to radiation injury. One source of resistance is the microorganism's capacity to repair DNA damage, but increasing doses of radiation can overwhelm these repair mechanisms. Microbial cells with multiple copies of their DNA are also more resistant because redundant copies of DNA provide backup against the loss of critical genes. Other sources of resistance are related to the size and physiologic state of the microorganism. In general, smaller and simpler microorganisms require higher doses of radiation for destruction (Fellows 2009). Bacterial spores are more resistant than the vegetative cells of other microorganisms. Viruses are much more resistant compared with most foodborne bacteria and may not be destroyed with food irradiation (Fellows 2009; Monk, Beuchat, Doyle 1995).

The sensitivity/resistance of microorganisms to radiation is measured in a manner analogous to using D-values for thermal destruction. The $D_{10}$ value specifies the radiation dose necessary to reduce a microbial population to only 10% of its initial size, in other words, a 90% population reduction. The range of $D_{10}$ values for foodborne bacteria is from 0.04 kGy for sensitive bacteria to more than 10 kGy for hardy spores; viruses have $D_{10}$ values ranging from 2.4 kGy to more than 8 kGy (Monk et al. 1995). Individual $D_{10}$ values can vary significantly during irradiation under different environmental conditions involving temperature, presence of oxygen, pH, moisture content, and chemical composition of the food. Thus, the specific food or medium (often implicit of pH, moisture content, chemical composition, etc.) and the conditions of irradiation (temperature, vacuum or air) should be stipulated along with the $D_{10}$ value of a microorganism. Based on $D_{10}$ values and the specific purpose, commercial applications of food irradiation are often categorized as low dose ($\leq$ 1 kGy), medium dose (1–10 kGy), and high dose (> 10 kGy) (Fellows 2009). Most commercial applications use dose levels between 2 and 7 kGy to reduce microbial loads—including pathogens—and to extend shelf life (Lagunas-Solar 1995).

Terminology was developed in 1964 to describe food irradiation in terms of microbial quality and radiation dose (Jay et al. 2005). The dose range 0.75–2.5 kGy is referred to as radurization and is used primarily to reduce numbers of spoilage microorganisms on meats, poultry, seafood, produce, and certain grains. The next higher dose range, 2.5–10 kGy, is referred to as radicidation and is comparable to the pasteurization of milk, where non-spore-forming pathogens—except viruses—are destroyed or rendered undetectable by standard methods. Radicidation is used with a variety of meats, poultry, seafood, sprouts, and other foods. The highest dose range, typically 30–40 kGy, is used for radiation sterilization. This level of radiation treatment is called radappertization and is equivalent to commercial sterilization. Examples of foods that receive radappertization treatment include spices, herbs, and sterilized hospital meals.

An unfortunate misconception about food irradiation is the generation of radioactivity in foods. Food irradiation does *not* generate radioactivity in foods. A legitimate concern expressed by critics of food irradiation is the possible production of toxic compounds and the loss of nutrients. The use of ionizing radiation to treat foods has been extensively studied over the years, and so far, no credible evidence has been provided that irradiated foods are toxicologically unsafe. Based on radiation chemistry studies, the compounds produced by food irradiation are of less concern than from conventional thermal treatments. Similarly, the nutrient loss or degradation from food irradiation is comparable with other food treatments. Several prominent national and international organizations have supported food irradiation as safe and adequately nutritious at the dose levels currently used to achieve technical objectives (Fellows 2009).

Despite the general consensus that irradiated food is safe and nutritious, several credible concerns and limitations have been identified. Among them is the production of undesirable sensory properties such as tastes, odors, textures, viscosity, and so forth. For the most part, these undesirable sensory changes can be minimized by discriminating choices of which foods to irradiate and by carefully controlling the dose levels. Packaging materials represent a potential source of radiolytic products that can affect the sensory properties of foods and possibly the migration of toxicants into the food. A major advantage of irradiation is the treatment of prepackaged foods to prevent postprocessing contamination. Proper selection of packaging materials reduces the likelihood of producing radiolytic products. Studies have demonstrated that new materials and combined packaging methods (e.g., MAP) may enhance food protection.

Several potential problems with food safety management are possible with food irradiation. As discussed earlier, the conditions for food irradiation are important to the effectiveness of treatment.

Thus, the food irradiation process must be carefully monitored using the hazard analysis and critical control point (HACCP) system. Concern also exists that food irradiation could become a substitute for reducing bacterial loads on foods (e.g., sanitation) from existing programs such as Good Manufacturing Practices (GMPs). This would be a risky practice and negate the purpose of the hurdle concept. A related concern is the production of toxins (bacterial or mycotic) before food irradiation destroys the toxigenic microorganisms. In unusual situations, spoilage microorganisms could be destroyed while pathogens survive, and hence, foods appearing wholesome with long shelf lives may permit pathogen growth.

Food irradiation has the potential to significantly enhance food safety. Pathogenic and toxigenic microorganisms can be reduced or eliminated in high-risk foods with the proper application of ionizing radiation. If food irradiation use expands, its contribution to the reduction of foodborne illnesses could be a milestone in food safety. On the other hand, reliance on food irradiation for safety must not lead to complacency. Pre- and postirradiation steps such as cleaning, sanitation, time–temperature control, and so forth must not be summarily neglected or discounted. Perhaps the best management model for food irradiation is the milk pasteurization program that emphasizes both upstream and downstream food protection as well as testing to ensure the pasteurization process was effective. Education about the safety and benefits of food irradiation must also be forthcoming to instill consumer confidence in the technology.

## NEW AND EMERGING PHYSICAL PROCESSES OF FOOD PROTECTION

In the quest to satisfy consumer demands and remain economically competitive, food process engineers have responded with innovative technologies for food processing. In fact, over the past few decades, the rate of innovation in food processing has been accelerating (Bruin and Jongen 2003). Among the trends in consumer demands for foods are better taste, healthier choices, fewer additives, low prices, and convenience. Such demands have guided the food industry to produce minimally processed foods using a combination of hurdles and new technologies. The search for natural antimicrobials, covered earlier in this chapter, represents one major area of emerging technologies. Another major area is emerging physical processes of food preservation. Several of these physical processes are briefly described here.

High-pressure processing, or high hydrostatic pressure processing, involves subjecting foods to pressures on the order of $10^2$–$10^3$ megapascals (MPa) for seconds to minutes. At such pressures, the noncovalent bonds of proteins are altered. This inactivates enzymes in the food matrix—including critical enzymes of microorganisms, resulting in their injury and death. The antimicrobial efficacy of high-pressure processing is described as similar to pasteurization. In other words, when properly applied, the technology is effective in reducing the levels of vegetative microbial cells but relatively ineffective against spores, unless heat is also applied. Pathogenic bacteria have a wide range of sensitivity to hydrostatic pressures, and some strains of vegetative pathogens have resistance comparable to spores (Fellows 2009). The optimization of high-pressure processing depend on characteristics of the food (pH, $a_w$, etc.) and the operating parameters (time–pressure combinations, temperature, etc.). Therefore, the right combinations of foods, intrinsic/extrinsic parameters, operating parameters, and target microorganisms are important to standardize before using this technology for food protection. Currently, high-pressure processing has limited applications in the United States, but its applications may expand when used in combination with other technologies (i.e., hurdles).

Pulsed electric fields technology involves placing foods between two electrodes and subjecting them to short pulses of electric fields. The electric field pulses last for microseconds at field strengths of 25 to 70 kilovolts per centimeter (kV/cm), and a cumulative total of 20 to 100 electric pulses are given in a typical treatment (Bruin and Jongen 2003). Vegetative cells of spoilage and pathogenic microorganisms are most vulnerable to pulsed electric fields, while spores are considerably more resistant. The efficacy of this technology in the destruction of specific pathogens is difficult to generalize because the specific conditions and apparatuses used by different researchers do not permit direct comparisons (Fellows 2009). Additional research is needed to generate validated kinetic data and models of microbial inactivation. The application of pulsed electric fields technology is limited to liquid foods (juices, milk, soups, etc.).

Oscillating magnetic fields inactivate most microbial vegetative cells, though some microorganisms are not affected, and a few are actually stimulated to grow. Spores and enzymes do not appear to be affected by oscillating magnetic fields. Several hypotheses have been tested on the mechanisms of microbial inactivation, but the primary mechanisms are still not well understood. The principal advantages of oscillating magnetic fields are the reduction of microbial vegetative cells without significant loss of sensory and nutrient quality, reduced energy costs, and low equipment costs. There are also several disadvantages to this technology, and the specific applications remain uncertain.

Ultrasound technology causes cavitation within foods from the transmission of ultrasound waves, that is, rapidly alternating compression/decompression zones (Gould 2001). Cavitation (formation and collapse of microscopic bubbles) produces shock waves that generate heat and pressure, which in turn disrupt microbial cells and catalyze chemical reactions. The sensitivity of bacteria to ultrasound waves generally corresponds with their size, shape, and Gram stain. For example, large Gram-positive bacilli are more sensitive to ultrasound waves than are small Gram-negative cocci. Spores are quite resistant to ultrasound waves. Because many microorganisms are resistant to ultrasound waves, this technology has not been used commercially to preserve foods. But the efficacy of ultrasound waves can be significantly enhanced with the application of pressure and mild heat. The combination of ultrasound, pressure, and heat is called manothermosonication. This combination of technologies holds the promise of sterilizing or pasteurizing liquid products without causing significant thermal damage.

Pulsed white light and UV light are used to inactivate microorganisms on the surfaces of foods and packaging materials. Broader applications of this technology in the food industry are not feasible because these forms of nonionizing radiation have limited depth penetration. Irregular surfaces of foods may be problematic too. The pulsed white light used in food applications has "approximately 20,000 times the intensity of sunlight at sea level" (Fellows 2009). With appropriate applications and operating conditions, pulsed white light is capable of reducing pathogen levels by several logs on food surfaces, but its effectiveness with spores is questionable. In comparison, UV light at a wavelength of about 2,600 angstroms (Å) is a more powerful bactericidal agent. The principal disadvantage of UV light is the catalysis of oxidative reactions in foods that may cause rancidity and discoloration.

## REFERENCES

Adams MR, Nicolaides L. 1997. Review of the sensitivity of different foodborne pathogens to fermentation. *Food Control* 8(5/6):227–239.

Alzamora SM, Tapia MS, Welti-Chanes J. 2003. The control of water activity. In: *Food preservation techniques.* Zeuthen P, Bøgh-Sørensen L, eds. Cambridge, England: Woodhead Publishing.

Barceloux DG. 2008. *Medical toxicology of natural substances: Foods, fungi, medicinal herbs, plants, and venomous animals.* Hoboken, NJ: John Wiley.

Bruin S, Jongen TRG. 2003. Food process engineering: The last 25 years and challenges ahead. *Comprehensive Reviews in Food Science and Food Safety* 2(2):42–81.

Burt S. 2004. Essential oils: Their antibacterial properties and potential applications in foods—a review. *Int J Food Microbiol* 94(3):223–253.

Centers for Disease Control and Prevention. 2009. *Campylobacter jejuni* infection associated with unpasteurized milk and cheese—Kansas, 2007. *MMWR* 57(51):1377–1379.

Centers for Disease Control and Prevention. 2007a. Foodborne botulism from home-prepared fermented tofu—California, 2006. *MMWR* 56(5):96–97.

Centers for Disease Control and Prevention. 2007b. *Salmonella typhimurium* infection associated with raw milk and cheese consumption—Pennsylvania, 2007. *MMWR* 56(44):1161–1164.

Centers for Disease Control and Prevention. 2000. Outbreak of *Escherichia coli* O157:H7 infection associated with eating fresh cheese curds—Wisconsin, June 1998. *MMWR* 49(40):911–913.

Centers for Disease Control and Prevention. 1995a. Community outbreak of hemolytic uremic syndrome attributable to *Escherichia coli* O111:NM—South Australia 1995. *MMWR* 44(29):550, 1, 557–558.

Centers for Disease Control and Prevention. 1995b. *Escherichia coli* O157:H7 outbreak linked to commercially distributed dry-cured salami—Washington and California, 1994. *MMWR* 44(9):157–160.

Davidson PM, Harrison MA. 2002. Resistance and adaptation to food antimicrobials, sanitizers, and other process controls. *Food Technology* 56(11):69–78.

Davidson PM, Zivanovic S. 2003. The use of natural antimicrobials. In: *Food preservation techniques.* Zeuthen P, Bøgh-Sørensen L, eds. Cambridge, England: Woodhead Publishing.

Dupouy-Camet J, Murrell KD, eds. 2007. *FAO/WHO/OIE guidelines for the surveillance, management, prevention and control of trichinellosis.* Paris: Food and Agriculture Organization of the United Nations, World Health Organization, World Organisation for Animal Health.

Eichholzer M, Gutzwiller F. 1998. Dietary nitrates, nitrites, and N-nitroso compounds and cancer risk: A review of the epidemiologic evidence. *Nutr Rev* 56(4 Pt 1):95–105.

Fellows PJ. 2009. *Food processing technology: Principles and practices.* 3rd ed. Cambridge, England: Woodhead Publishing.

Food and Drug Administration. 2009. Grade "A" pasteurized milk ordinance (2009 revision). Rockville, MD: U.S. Public Health Service/U.S. Food and Drug Administration.

Food and Drug Administration. 2003. *Guidance for industry: Juice HACCP; small entity compliance guide.* Rockville, MD: U.S. Food and Drug Administration. Available from: http://www.fda.gov/Food/GuidanceComplianceRegulatory Information/GuidanceDocuments/Juice/ucm072637.htm.

Food and Drug Administration and Public Health Service. 2009. *Food code 2009.* College Park, MD: Department of Health and Human Services. Available from: http://www.fda.gov/Food/FoodSafety/RetailFoodProtection/FoodCode/ FoodCode2009/default.htm.

Food Safety and Inspection Service. 2010. *Safe and suitable ingredients used in the production of meat, poultry, and egg products.* Report nr FSIS Directive 7120.1, Revision 2. Washington, DC: U.S. Department of Agriculture.

Forsythe SJ, Hayes PR. 2000. *Food hygiene, microbiology and HACCP.* 3rd ed. Gaithersburg, MD: Aspen Publishers.

Fox JA. 2002. Influences on purchase of irradiated foods. *Food Technology* 56(11):34–37.

Galvez A, Lopez RL, Abriouel H, Valdivia E, Omar NB. 2008. Application of bacteriocins in the control of foodborne pathogenic and spoilage bacteria. *Crit Rev Biotechnol* 28(2):125–152.

Gill CO. 2006. Microbiology of frozen foods. In: *Handbook of frozen food processing and packaging.* Sun DW, ed. Boca Raton, FL: CRC Press.

Gorris LG. 2000. Hurdle technology. In: *Encyclopedia of food microbiology*. Vols. 1–3. Robinson RK, ed. London: Elsevier. Available from: http://knovel.com/web/portal/browse/display?_EXT_KNOVEL_DISPLAY_bookid=1870&VerticalID=0:

Gould GW. 2001. Symposium on "nutritional effects of new processing technologies." New processing technologies: An overview. *Proc Nutr Soc* 60(4):463–474.

Gould GW. 2000. The use of other chemical preservatives: Sulfite and nitrite. In: *Microbiological safety and quality of food*. Vols. 1–2. Lund BM, Baird-Parker TC, Gould GW, eds. Gaithersburg, MD: Aspen Publishers.

Hudson JA, Billington C, Carey-Smith G, Greening G. 2005. Bacteriophages as biocontrol agents in food. *J Food Prot* 68(2):426–437.

International Union of Food Science and Technology. 2010, March. *Biotechnology and food*. Report nr IUFoST Scientific Information Bulletin. Available from: http://www.iufost.org/sites/default/files/docs/IUF.SIB.Biotechnology.rev.pdf.

Jay JM, Loessner MJ, Golden DA. 2005. *Modern food microbiology*. 7th ed. New York, NY: Springer Science+Business Media.

Jofre J, Muniesa M. 2000. Potential use of phages and/or lysins. In: *Encyclopedia of food microbiology*. Vols. 1–3. Robinson RK, ed. Available at: http://knovel.com/web/portal/browse/display?_EXT_KNOVEL_DISPLAY_bookid=1870&VerticalID=0.

Kostrzynska M, Bachand A. 2006. Use of microbial antagonism to reduce pathogen levels on produce and meat products: A review. *Can J Microbiol* 52(11):1017–1026.

Lagunas-Solar MC. 1995. Radiation processing of foods: An overview of scientific principles and current status. *J Food Prot* 58(2):186–192.

Lucke FK. 2003. The control of pH. In: *Food preservation techniques*. Zeuthen P, Bøgh-Sørensen L, eds. Cambridge, England: Woodhead Publishing.

Lund BM. 2000. Freezing. In: *Microbiological safety and quality of food*. Vols. 1–2. Lund BM, Baird-Parker TC, Gould GW, eds. Gaithersburg, MD: Aspen Publishers.

Meyer AS. 2003. Antimicrobial enzymes. In: *Food preservation techniques*. Zeuthen P, Bøgh-Sørensen L, eds. Cambridge, England: Woodhead Publishing.

Midgley J, Small A. 2006. *Review of new and emerging technologies for red meat safety*. Report nr PRMS.083. North Sydney, Australia: Meat & Livestock Australia Limited. Available from: http://www.meatupdate.csiro.au/new/Review%20of%20new%20and%20emerging%20technlogies%20for%20red%20meat%20safety.pdf.

Miller HI. 2007. Biotech's defining moments. *Trends Biotechnol* 25(2):56–59.

Monk JD, Beuchat LR, Doyle MP. 1995. Irradiation inactivation of food-borne microorganisms. *J Food Prot* 58(2):197–208.

National Research Council and Committee on Identifying and Assessing Unintended Effects of Genetically Engineered Foods on Human Health. 2004. *Safety of genetically engineered foods: Approaches to assessing unintended health effects*. Washington DC: National Academies Press.

No HK, Meyers SP, Prinyawiwatkul W, Xu Z. 2007. Applications of chitosan for improvement of quality and shelf life of foods: A review. *J Food Sci* 72(5):R87–R100.

Nout MJR. 1994. Fermented foods and food safety. *Food Res Int* 27:291–298.

Ooraikul B. 2003. Modified atmosphere packaging (MAP). In: *Food preservation techniques*. Zeuthen P, Bøgh-Sørensen L, eds. Cambridge, England: Woodhead Publishing.

Pflug IJ, Gould GW. 2000. Heat treatment. In: *Microbiological safety and quality of food*. Vols. 1–2. Lund BM, Baird-Parker TC, Gould GW, eds. Gaithersburg, MD: Aspen Publishers.

Potter ME, Kruse MB, Mathews MA, Hill RO, Martin RJ. 1976. A sausage-associated outbreak of trichinosis of Illinois. *Am J Public Health* 66(12):1194–1196.

Rahman MS. 1999. Nitrites in food preservation. In: *Handbook of food preservation*. Rahman MS, ed. New York, NY: Marcel Dekker.

Rao DN, Sachindra NM. 2002. Modified atmosphere and vacuum packaging of meat and poultry products. *Food Rev Int* 18(4):263–293.

Rodgers S. 2003. Potential applications of protective cultures in cook-chill catering. *Food Control* 14(1):35–42.

Rodgers S. 2001. Preserving non-fermented refrigerated foods with microbial cultures—a review. *Trends Food Sci Technol* 12(8):276–284.

Ross RP, Morgan S, Hill C. 2002. Preservation and fermentation: Past, present and future. *Int J Food Microbiol* 79(1–2):3–16.

Sobel J, Tucker N, Sulka A, McLaughlin J, Maslanka S. 2004. Foodborne botulism in the United States, 1990–2000. *Emerg Infect Dis* 10(9):1606–1611.

Tilden J Jr, Young W, McNamara AM, Custer C, Boesel B, Lambert-Fair MA, Majkowski J, Vugia D, Werner SB, Hollingsworth J, et al. 1996. A new route of transmission for *Escherichia coli*: Infection from dry fermented salami. *Am J Public Health* 86(8 Pt 1):1142–1145.

Wesche AM, Gurtler JB, Marks BP, Ryser ET. 2009. Stress, sublethal injury, resuscitation, and virulence of bacterial foodborne pathogens. *J Food Prot* 72(5):1121–1138.

Zhao T, Doyle MP, Kemp MC, Howell RS, Zhao P. 2004. Influence of freezing and freezing plus acidic calcium sulfate and lactic acid addition on thermal inactivation of *Escherichia coli* O157:H7 in ground beef. *J Food Prot* 67(8): 1760–1764.

---

## USEFUL RESOURCES

Center for Food Safety, Food Irradiation. http://www.centerforfoodsafety.org/campaign/food-irradiation/
Environmental Protection Agency, Food Irradiation. http://www.epa.gov/rpdweb00/sources/food_irrad.html
Food Engineering Magazine. http://www.foodengineeringmag.com/
Food Processing Intelligence. http://www.fpi-international.com/
FoodProcessing.com. http://www.foodprocessing.com/index.html
Institute of Food Technologists. http://www.ift.org/
Intralytix, developer of ListShield, a bacteriophage additive to foods. http://www.intralytix.com/
History.com. *Modern Marvels* documentary DVD titles. Available from: http://www.history.com/
    "Bread"
    "Cheese"
    "Cold Cuts"
    "Fry It"
    "Ice Cream"
    "Milk"
    "Snackfood Tech"
Ozone Safe Food. http://www.ozonesafefood.com/
Purdue University, Center for Integrated Food Manufacturing. http://www.ag.purdue.edu/foodsci/cifm/Pages/default.aspx

# CHAPTER 6

# Risk and Hazard Analysis of Foods

## LEARNING OBJECTIVES

1. Define key terms related to the risk analysis of safe foods.
2. List and define the steps of risk assessment.
3. Identify and explain the different methods of identifying hazards in risk assessments.
4. Explain the relevance of hazard characterization and dose-response assessment to risk assessment.
5. Describe the contrasting differences of conducting risk assessments of microorganisms and toxicants.
6. Describe the risk management framework and the role of stakeholders.
7. Provide examples of risk management options used to protect the U.S. food supply.
8. Describe the history of the HACCP system and its adoption for food safety management.
9. Explain the differences between the HACCP system and risk analysis processes.
10. List and define the seven principles of the HACCP system.
11. Recognize the prerequisite programs of developing a HACCP plan.
12. Distinguish a critical control point from other events in a process flow.
13. Explain the relevance of critical limits in the control of food process hazards.
14. Recognize the purpose and types of verification procedures in the HACCP system.
15. Explain why recordkeeping is a necessary part of the HACCP system.
16. Identify the limitations of the HACCP system.
17. Describe how the HACCP system can be used in foodservice and retail establishments.
18. List the general categories of testing to protect the food supply.
19. Provide examples of food product testing to protect the food supply.

## RISK ANALYSIS AND FOOD SAFETY

The word *risk* has different meanings to different people. In business circles, *risk* is typically used to describe economic uncertainty or possible failure in an endeavor. To others, risk is the chance of harm to oneself, family, and friends. The connotations associated with risk arise from different perspectives, situations, and individual perceptions that are difficult to generalize. Even within the realm of public health and safety, different concepts of risk and its relevance to preventing harm and promoting health abound. Nevertheless, public health officials increasingly use the term *risk* when attempting to identify, evaluate, and control hazards in the environment, whether at work, home, or in public places. The steps involved in identifying, evaluating, and controlling hazards have been divided into three distinct but interrelated processes called risk assessment, risk management, and risk communication.

The widespread acceptance of risk assessment as a process for public health and safety is often credited to its endorsement in a landmark report by the Institute of Medicine (IOM) under the National Academies of Science (National Research Council [NRC] 1983). Known as the *Red Book*, this report recommends a clear distinction between the steps involved in identifying and evaluating hazards (risk assessment) and the options and decisions involved in controlling hazards (risk management). The purpose for such a distinction is to maintain objectivity—as much as possible—in the science-based decisions of risk assessment. In contrast, political, economic, and social factors influence the decisions involved in managing the risks from hazards. The definitions of risk assessment and risk management have changed somewhat over time, and various organizations and disciplines may define the processes differently.

As the importance of risk assessment and risk management became recognized, it also became clear that a third process—risk communication—was equally important. Barriers to effective risk communication are rooted in the different technical backgrounds, values, and perceptions of everyone involved, including scientists and the lay public. Without effective risk communication, the risk assessment and risk management processes are rendered ineffective. Consequently, the term *risk analysis* was defined to encompass all three processes. Not everyone agrees that risk analysis should include risk management and risk communication, but nearly everyone agrees on the importance of all three processes in controlling risks. For food safety purposes, the Codex Alimentarius Commission, a joint committee of the Food and Agricultural Organization (FAO) and the World Health Organization (WHO), established definitions of risk analysis terms (Codex Alimentarius Commission 2010). Table 6-1 lists a selected subset of these terms and definitions. These definitions are sufficiently broad to cover most aspects of risk assessment, risk management, and risk communication in food safety.

## Risk Analysis Processes

A committee under the IOM noted that the food safety community has a limited understanding of risk assessment concepts and science-based methodologies (Institute of Medicine [IOM] 2003). The committee also recommended that U.S. regulatory agencies use science-based strategies such as risk assessment to a greater extent to develop food safety criteria. This recommendation was strongly reinforced by additional recommendations by another IOM committee (IOM 2010). To implement these recommendations fully, food safety professionals require a greater understanding of risk-based and science-based methodologies. The following discussion is intended to introduce the student to the risk analysis processes. Additional training is necessary for those interested in pursuing a specialty in risk analysis.

**Table 6-1** Definitions of Risk Analysis Terms Related to Food Safety

| Term | Description |
|---|---|
| Hazard | A biological, chemical, or physical agent in, or condition of, food with the potential to cause an adverse health effect. |
| Risk | A function of the probability of an adverse health effect and the severity of that effect, consequential to a hazard(s) in food. |
| Risk Analysis | A process consisting of three components: risk assessment, risk management, and risk communication. |
| Risk Assessment | A scientifically based process consisting of the following steps: (i) hazard identification, (ii) hazard characterization, (iii) exposure assessment, and (iv) risk characterization. |
| Risk Management | The process, distinct from risk assessment, of weighing policy alternatives, in consultation with all interested parties, considering risk assessment and other factors relevant for the health protection of consumers and for the promotion of fair trade practices, and, if needed, selecting appropriate prevention and control options. |
| Risk Communication | The interactive exchange of information and opinions throughout the risk analysis process concerning risk, risk-related factors, and risk perceptions, among risk assessors, risk managers, consumers, industry, the academic community, and other interested parties, including the explanation of risk assessment findings and the basis of risk management decisions. |
| Risk Assessment Policy | Documented guidelines on the choice of options and associated judgments for their application at appropriate decision points in the risk assessment such that the scientific integrity of the process is maintained. |
| Risk Profile | The description of the food safety problem and its context. |
| Risk Characterization | The qualitative and/or quantitative estimation, including attendant uncertainties, of the probability of occurrence and severity of known or potential adverse health effects in a given population based on hazard identification, hazard characterization, and exposure assessment. |
| Risk Estimate | The quantitative estimation of risk resulting from risk characterization. |
| Hazard Identification | The identification of biological, chemical, and physical agents capable of causing adverse health effects and which may be present in a particular food or group of foods. |
| Hazard Characterization | The qualitative and/or quantitative evaluation of the nature of the adverse health effects associated with biological, chemical, and physical agents, which may be present in food. For chemical agents, a dose-response assessment should be performed. For biological or physical agents, a dose-response assessment should be performed if the data are obtainable. |
| Dose-Response Assessment | The determination of the relationship between the magnitude of exposure (dose) to a chemical, biological, or physical agent and the severity and/or frequency of associated adverse health effects (response). |
| *Exposure Assessment* | The qualitative and/or quantitative evaluation of the likely intake of biological, chemical, and physical agents via food as well as exposures from other sources if relevant. |

*Source*: Definitions from Codex Alimentarius Commission 2010

## *Risk Assessment*

The goal of risk assessment is to predict the probability of harm with the least amount of uncertainty. This goal is difficult to attain fully, but a rigorous approach based on scientific principles is necessary to assess risk problems. To this end, risk assessment consists of the following four steps:

1. Hazard identification
2. Hazard characterization and/or dose-response assessment
3. Exposure assessment
4. Risk characterization

Risk assessment is a widely accepted process for chemicals and other toxic agents in the environment—including foods. The overall paradigm of risk assessment is applicable to both microbial and toxic agents, despite the fact that significant differences exist between them. However, the use of risk assessment for microbial agents is relatively recent and still developing. The following discussions briefly examine the similarities and differences between risk assessment of microbial agents and toxic agents.

### Hazard Identification

The purpose of hazard identification is to determine whether a particular agent or situation constitutes a hazard, that is, an inherent property with potential for an adverse effect. For toxic agents, laboratory methods using animals (*in vivo*) and other biological systems (*in vitro*) have been the foundation of hazard identification. Laboratory methods can range from short-term bioassays to multiyear animal studies. The advantage of short-term (*in vitro*) bioassays is the low-cost, rapid screening of chemicals. Considering that thousands of new chemicals are introduced into commerce each year, the value of short-term bioassays is apparent. The primary limitation of short-term bioassays is their inability to consistently predict toxicity in whole animals and humans. This is because of the complex interactions of toxicants with organ systems and biochemical pathways (toxicokinetics, toxicodynamics, biotransformation, etc.). Studies using animals have a better ability to predict toxicity in humans, but they are limited by the physiologic/biochemical differences that exist between different species and humans. These differences can be significant in terms of toxicant metabolism and the induction of disease.

Laboratory methods are not the only source of scientific data for hazard identification. Epidemiologic studies provide direct evidence that an agent or situation is hazardous to humans. The vast majority of epidemiologic studies used to identify toxicants are observational rather than experimental. In observational studies, epidemiologists study human populations by dividing or stratifying them into different groups (i.e., cohorts).  One group has an exposure to potentially hazardous agents in their environment (including foods), while another group does not have similar exposures. The researchers compare the health outcomes of the exposed population to those of populations without the exposure. The association of an agent with an adverse health outcome provides the strong evidence for hazard identification. But the proof is not irrefutable; every epidemiologic study has some degree of unavoidable weakness that limits its ability to establish causation. Weaknesses in epidemiologic studies include small sample size, inability to verify/measure exposure to an agent accurately, and concurrent exposure to multiple agents (e.g., confounding exposures). Special study techniques and statistical analyses can minimize—but not completely eliminate—the weaknesses of epidemiologic studies.

A third source of hazard identification data is comparative and/or computational methods. These involve comparing the properties of a suspected agent with the properties of known hazardous agents. Comparative and computational methods help augment other hazard identification methods and add to the overall weight of evidence. These methods can be very sophisticated and data-intensive. For example, researchers use quantitative structure-activity relationship (QSAR) to compare the chemical reactivity and/or biological activities of different agents. Although useful for identifying trends or generating hypotheses for further research, QSAR's predictive ability is too limited to provide conclusive proof of a hazard. New comparative methods have emerged in recent years that involve assaying biological responses at the gene, protein, and metabolite levels (called genomics, proteomics, and metabolomics, respectively). The -omics technologies hold the promise of rapidly screening chemicals for potential toxicity, but their current applications are limited by the interpretation of massive data sets.

For microbial agents, hazard identification has its origins in infectious diseases control. Clinicians and epidemiologists have use scientific methods for more than a century to study infectious disease outbreaks and transmission. With the contributions of microbiologists and pathologists, the identification of pathogenic and toxin-producing microorganisms was established. The association of foodborne illnesses with a particular microbial agent provided documented evidence of a potential hazard. This was confirmed with clinical and laboratory research on the microorganism's infectivity or toxigenicity, growth requirements, and survival in foods. Nowadays, hazard identification is more challenging because of "changes in pathogens, foods, food distribution, food consumption, and population immunity" (Lammerding and Paoli 1997). In the future, surveillance programs for foodborne illnesses will play a greater role in the hazard identification of new microbial agents and hazardous foods.

## Hazard Characterization and Dose-Response Assessment

The second step of risk assessment is more quantitative in nature. Its purpose is to determine the relationship between the amount of agent in foods (i.e., dose) and the degree of harm in an individual, population, and/or subpopulation of individuals. Called hazard characterization, this step evaluates the range of possible health effects and the likelihood of disease among groups who consume the foodborne agent at different doses. For toxic agents, the dose-response relationship introduced in Chapter 3 is a critically important part of hazard characterization. The dose-response assessment of acute toxicity is comparatively straightforward to perform. With chronic toxicity, however, the dose-response relationship is usually not observable at lower doses, primarily because of limitations associated with biological variability and statistical power. In these cases, high-to-low dose extrapolation using mathematical models is necessary. Many different models exist for extrapolation, and the choice of which model to use is often controversial; regardless of the model used, various degrees of uncertainty exist for every extrapolation. This uncertainty is compounded when animals are used because humans may not respond in a similar manner. In addition, adjustments for the differences in dose and animal size must be taken into account for humans. An added extrapolation from animal-to-human is thus necessary to estimate the dose-response relationship. Together, the high-to-low dose and animal-to-human extrapolations contribute to the greatest uncertainty of dose-response assessments.

The concept of an infective dose for pathogens is introduced in Chapter 2. The relationship between the dose of pathogens and response in human hosts is complicated by factors such as host immunity/resistance and other susceptibilities, virulence factors among pathogenic strains, pathogen–immune system interactions, and other underlying biological processes. The food matrix also influences the dose-response by affecting pathogen survival and establishment in the host. Another important variable is the potential microbial growth in foods. Microbial growth in potentially hazardous foods (PHF)/temperature controlled for safety (TCS) foods can change exponentially under improper holding temperatures, causing an increase in the number microbial cells. In essence, this effectively changes the dose level. Conversely, antimicrobial treatments and pathogen destruction steps can reduce the number of viable microbial cells in foods. For example, heating a food prior to consumption may destroy a large number of microbial cells.

The most important difference in dose-response assessments between a toxic agent and pathogen is the absence of a no-observed-adverse-effect-level (NOAEL) for pathogens. Under the right circumstances, a single pathogen can cause an infection. Despite these challenges, according to a committee of the IOM, dose-response relationships for foodborne pathogens are important to pursue for more accurate risk assessments (IOM 2003). A recommended approach to derive dose-response relationships is to use multiple data sets that take into account the pathogen, host, and food matrix (Food and Agriculture Organization and World Health Organization [FAO and WHO] 2003). Researchers can then select and use math models for testing goodness-of-fit with the data, and then perform uncertainty analysis using several possible methods. In cases where insufficient data exist for a dose-response assessment—which include many pathogens and situations—researchers must perform hazard characterization with qualitative information or semi-quantitative ranking schemes.

### Exposure Assessment

Exposure assessment requires at least two dimensions of effort. The first dimension is determining which foods are potentially hazardous and their contamination level. The qualitative and quantitative methods used for this effort are quite different for each biological, chemical, and physical agent. The second dimension of effort is identifying the population and subpopulations at risk of eating the contaminated foods (i.e., exposed individuals); it also includes estimating the frequency and amounts of contaminated foods eaten (i.e., exposure level). This requires knowledge about the patterns of consumption and is related to the demographics of the population and subpopulations, as well as consumer preferences and behavior.

Determining which foods may be hazardous requires knowledge about the sources of foodborne agents. A wealth of historical information exists on the sources of classical foodborne agents. This is not true for new or emerging foodborne agents. They must be identified through epidemiologic surveillance and investigations and from laboratory-based sampling and monitoring of foods. Exposure assessment should include the entire farm-to-fork pathway to estimate the extent of possible contamination. Many processes and different scenarios along the pathway can exacerbate or, conversely, limit exposures to consumers. Cooking and other processes can destroy some toxicants and pathogens. On the other hand, food processing procedures may generate some toxicants, and pathogens may grow to greater numbers under conditions such as temperature abuse. The modification of intrinsic and extrinsic parameters influences microbial survival and growth, changing the ultimate exposure level at the consumer. Predictive microbiology is helpful in exposure assessment for determining the influence of different conditions on microbial survival and growth.

Exposure assessment of toxicants in foods is also complicated, particularly for chronic and low-level exposures. The complexity of chemical constituents in the food matrix is especially challenging. Natural and synthetic compounds in foods are extremely diverse and abundant. Some chemicals are desirable as nutrients, while others are undesirable, such as pesticides and mycotoxins. The first step to measuring exposure to toxic agents in foods is using the correct sampling procedures and analytical methods (Kroes et al. 2002). Careful planning and execution are necessary to obtain accurate measurements and reduce the variability. The sampling procedures must take into account the completeness and representativeness of the samples, not only within a particular food matrix but also between food lots and types and over time. Environmental factors (e.g., field and storage conditions), as well as processing methods of the foods, influence the concentration of chemicals in foods. After sampling is completed, laboratory scientists must carefully control the accuracy and precision of the analytical methods for quantitative estimates of exposure. They can encounter significant analytical variability between samples, over time, and from laboratory to laboratory.

Along with the prevalence and/or concentrations of agents in foods, the types and patterns of food consumption by different consumers are needed for a complete exposure assessment. Cultural differences, socioeconomic status, and numerous other demographic characteristics influence consumer preference and behavior. Characteristics of subpopulations in terms of age, sex, general health, disease status, and other factors are important to ascertain with respect to dietary patterns. Highly susceptible populations (e.g., hospitalized, elderly, young, unborn) are particularly important to identify with exposure to potentially hazardous foods. Data on dietary patterns come from four primary sources (Kroes et al. 2002): (1) food supply data, (2) household consumption surveys, (3) dietary surveys, and (4) duplicate diets (i.e., saving duplicate meals for analysis). In the United States, federal agencies use a variety of methods to collect data on the diets of Americans for risk assessments. Since 1961, the Food and Drug Administration (FDA) has periodically conducted surveys and analyses of the foods that Americans consume. Called the Total Diet Study, FDA collects food samples, or "market baskets," from four regions of the country (Egan 2002). These representative foods are then cooked (unless already ready to eat [RTE]) and analyzed for selected pesticides, industrial chemicals, elements, radionuclides, and nutrients.

### Risk Characterization

The purpose of risk characterization is to integrate the previous steps of risk assessment into a quantitative and/or qualitative estimation of overall risk. The goal is to accurately express the magnitude of risk with attendant uncertainties and provide input to the risk management process. Several approaches and formats are used to conduct and convey the risk characterization. Ideally, the risk should be conveyed as statistical probabilities for the occurrence and severity (i.e., consequences) of health outcomes for all segments of a given population. However, in practice, several data gaps often exist, and the variability is quite large, necessitating a more qualitative approach. In this regard, risk characterization can help identify important data gaps and focus scientific research to reduce variability and the overall uncertainty of risk. Still, it is important to remember that although uncertainty may be reduced, it is never completely eliminated, and a certain degree of risk will always be present in any food supply. Mitigating and reducing these risks are the primary objectives of food safety.

### Risk Management and Risk Communication

Under a congressional mandate, the Presidential/Congressional Commission on Risk Assessment and Risk Management was formed in 1994 to investigate the policy implications and appropriate uses of risk assessment and risk management. The commission recommended a framework, illustrated in Figure 6-1, for the risk management of environmental and public health risks (U.S. Presidential/Congressional Commission on Risk Assessment and Risk Management [Presidential/Congressional Commission] 1997). The commission's framework advocates an iterative process consisting of six stages that surround stakeholder engagement:

1. Define the problem and put it into context.
2. Analyze the risks associated with the problem in context.
3. Examine the options for addressing the risks.
4. Make decisions about which options to implement.
5. Take actions to implement the decisions.
6. Conduct an evaluation of the results of the action. (Presidential/Congressional Commission 1997)

The framework is intended to assist risk managers at various levels of the government as well as private business and members of the public. The central theme of the framework is risk communication through collaborative engagement of stakeholders throughout the risk management process. In the commission's report, stakeholders are defined as all those affected by the risk management problem—including the risk assessors, risk managers, and members of the public. The different risk perceptions and value systems of stakeholders are important to consider and reconcile for successful solutions to risk problems. This is accomplished by the engagement of stakeholders as early as possible in each stage of risk management. Effective risk communication methods are equally important. For example, in many cases, the information presented in risk characterization is often laden with scientific jargon and statistical data. Such information may need translation to more recognizable terms and concepts for communication with risk managers, and even more so for the general public.

The options and decisions for risk management are frequently controversial, and they rarely satisfy all the stakeholders' interests and preferences. Risk management options range

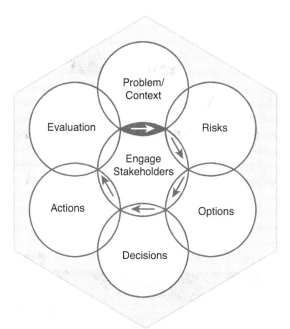

**Figure 6-1** U.S. Presidential/Congressional Commission's Risk Management Framework.
*Source:* Presidential/Congressional Commission on Risk Assessment and Risk Management 1997

from wait-and-see approaches to the strict regulation and enforcement of activities. In all cases, the risks must be balanced against the costs of controlling them. Furthermore, every risk cannot be totally eliminated or minimized with a finite amount of resources. Therefore, the relative risks of the problems are helpful for setting priorities, and a cost-effective analysis of each control option helps with the allocation of resources. The best risk management decisions also evaluate other factors such as legal, social, and cultural impacts. Once decisions have been made for managing the risk, they must be turned into actions that target the risk factors associated with the problem. Finally, evaluation (i.e., sixth stage) of the actions is necessary to ensure that they have indeed been effective. A "residual risk" is useful to evaluate the effectiveness of risk-reduction actions. This is the amount of risk remaining after controls have been put into place.

At the federal level of food safety, the best-known risk management actions involve the promulgation and enforcement of regulations. Several federal agencies, most notably FDA, U.S. Department of Agriculture (USDA), and the Environmental Protection Agency (EPA), promulgate food safety regulations. These regulations can be very prescriptive, that is, mandating specific procedures or technologies, or they can be performance-based, allowing for innovation and novel approaches. Whenever possible, performance-based standards are preferable because they may result in more cost-effective controls by using new technologies or redesigning processes. Most performance-based food safety standards in the United States are oriented toward process control and stability of food operations. Other performance-based standards put limits on the frequency and concentration of biological, chemical, and physical agents in foods. Such limits on agents in a medium (air, food, water, etc.) are called exposure standards.

The derivation of exposure standards starts with risk assessment data, particularly from the dose-response assessment step. A reference dose (RfD) is derived by EPA for many pesticides and chemicals from the dose-response data, after being modified with uncertainty factors. Using different methodologies, FDA develops acceptable daily intakes (ADI) for veterinary drug residues and other food additives. Although they are derived using different methodologies, the RfD and ADI are intended to represent the doses of a substance on a daily basis, usually over a lifetime of exposure, that are unlikely to cause adverse health effects. However, the RfD and ADI are not established exposure "standards" because they do not take into account feasibility, cost-effectiveness, and other considerations of risk management. The final exposure standard may deviate from the RfD and ADI after these considerations and other options of risk management are evaluated.

The exposure standards for foods in the United States are called tolerances and action levels (21 CFR 509.4). Tolerances are regulatory standards that place legal limits on certain agents in foods. Action levels are based on "informal judgments" that define safe limits for certain agents in foods. The primary legal difference between the two terms is the power of enforcement. Tolerances cannot be challenged in court, whereas action levels are not legally binding by the courts. Action levels, if violated, require more legal effort and procedures by the regulatory agency to uphold. Most of the current tolerances and action levels are designated for chemical residues. EPA establishes tolerances and action levels for pesticide residues, and FDA establishes tolerances and action levels for food additives, veterinary drugs, and unavoidable environmental contaminants. Because a large number of chemical substances are regulated in the food chain, not all existing tolerances and action levels are based on formal risk assessments.

The establishment of tolerances for microbial contaminants in foods is not a common practice in the United States. Instead, regulations emphasize sanitary standards and process controls to limit microbial contamination of foods. In a few cases, such as with *E. coli* O157:H7 in ground meat, a "zero" tolerance policy has been adopted by regulatory agencies; despite the good intention, this policy failed to reduce the rate of human illnesses attributed to *E. coli* O157:H7 (IOM 2003). One shortcoming with this policy is that it did not emphasize the testing of meats prior to grinding, which can mix potentially contaminated meats with uncontaminated meats. In addition, scientists often contend that zero tolerance cannot be definitively proven using sampling and analysis methods. The results of sampling and analysis are based on statistical data that represent the condition of a particular lot or other quantity of food. They do not guarantee the absence of a hazard, as some people may perceive. Another source of error is the ability of some microbial populations to grow and reproduce after sampling the food. In yet other cases, the pervasiveness of pathogenic or toxigenic microorganisms is so great that a zero tolerance is impractical or impossible to achieve without complete sterilization.

In lieu of legal tolerances, criteria for microbial contaminants are often established to monitor a food processing operation. The Food Safety and Inspection Service (FSIS) of USDA establishes criteria or performance standards for bacteria such as generic *E. coli* and *Salmonella* to measure the reduction and control of pathogens in food processing operations. These criteria are used in a manner similar to the guidelines published by the International Commission on the Microbiological Specifications for Foods (International Commission on Microbiological Specifications for Foods [ICMSF] 2002). The risk management strategy behind the use of criteria for microbial contamination is to ensure adequate control of a food operation or process. If statistically valid monitoring programs detect samples that exceed the criteria, the food operation or process is considered out-of-control, and action is necessary to identify and correct deficiencies that caused the excessive microbial contamination. Additional actions may involve the destruction or recall of foods deemed a public health threat.

Several countries and the international Codex Alimentarius Commission advocate the development of Food Safety Objectives (FSOs) to help with the risk management of hazardous agents in foods. The FSO is defined as the maximum allowable frequency and/or concentration of a hazardous agent in foods at the time of consumption (Codex Alimentarius Commission 2010). It is developed after the risk assessment process and during the examination of risk management options. The feasibility of attaining an FSO is confirmed before establishing it as a requirement for food products and/or processes. Although the U.S. government does not use the term *FSO* for risk management, federal regulatory agencies use other procedures to set and achieve public health goals in food safety.

A recent report by the IOM (2010) was critical of FDA's vision for food safety and recommended a modified approach to protect the food supply. Approximately 80% of the U.S. food supply is overseen by FDA, and the report strongly recommended the agency adopt a more risk-based approach to food safety. According to IOM, this will require organizational changes, a well-trained workforce in the risk-based principles of food safety management, and modernization of the legislative framework to provide FDA with the necessary legal authority. The report also states that risk communication is an integral part of a risk-based approach to food safety management, not only for communicating among stakeholders but also as a policy tool for achieving food safety (public health) objectives.

Risk communication is more than a dialogue among stakeholders. It is a multidimensional process that involves an exchange of risk information, consisting of risk messages (verbal and otherwise) that are crafted by the sender and interpreted by the receiver. In the broadest sense, risk communication includes food recalls, labels on food products, community outreach, briefings to lawmakers, regulatory enforcement communications, and food safety education of consumers. The interpretation of risk information is strongly influenced by people's beliefs, technical knowledge, hazard familiarity, control over risk and avoidance, and many other psychosocial factors. The source of risk information is particularly important with regard to credibility and trust. People responsible for risk communication must listen to and learn from their audience to craft risk messages effectively. Prudent approaches to risk communication require testing risk messages prior to their release. A misunderstood risk message undermines credibility and trust in future communication. Risk messages are used often with food safety in the form of food product recalls, consumer warnings, foodborne illness outbreak investigations, and education and training. These topics are covered again in Chapter 8.

## HAZARD ANALYSIS AND CRITICAL CONTROL POINT SYSTEM

The hazard analysis and critical control point (HACCP) system is actually a risk management tool that is tailored to individual food operations and/or processes. As part of the HACCP system, the potential hazards of food operations are identified and evaluated (i.e., the hazard analysis). Hazard analysis is the identification and evaluation of each hazard to determine the potential severity and probability of an incident or event (i.e., foodborne illness). The primary differences between the hazard analysis of HACCP and risk assessments are the scope and scale of risk problems. With respect to scope, risk assessments typically involve in-depth analysis of a particular agent, and the scale of the risk problem encompasses many food operations where the agent may be encountered. For example, a risk assessment at the federal level may involve the public health threat of *Listeria monocytogenes* in RTE foods from retail facilities. Risk assessment usually generates new knowledge about potentially hazardous agents, or it identifies gaps in knowledge where research is needed. In contrast, the hazard analysis of HACCP has a scope that utilizes existing knowledge about many agents. But the scale of a HACCP risk problem is restricted to specific food operations (e.g., canning operation in a particular plant), where the hazardous conditions and circumstances may be unique. The knowledge and information gained from risk assessments are often used as inputs to the hazard analysis of HACCP.

The HACCP system is a valuable aid to food safety management. After identifying and evaluating points in the food operation or process that are critical to controlling foodborne hazards (i.e., critical control points), process controls are developed and implemented. The critical control points are then monitored to ensure the controls are reliably maintained. The HACCP system is not a substitute for other preventive measures such as sanitary practices. Rather, it is a complementary system used in conjunction with other preventive measures and techniques, including current Good Manufacturing Practices (cGMPs) found in Title 21 of the Code of Federal Regulations, Part 110 (21 CFR 110).

### The Origins and Applications of HACCP

The HACCP system has its origins in the system safety program. A system is defined as components working together to accomplish tasks in a defined environment (Stephans 2004). The components that comprise a system include people, procedures, and plant and hardware. Systems engineering and safety are derived from military weapons development and complex endeavors such as space exploration, where failure of components could result in catastrophic events. System safety evolved to minimize these risks by identifying, analyzing, and controlling hazards associated with the system and its components. In the early days of manned space exploration, the risk of foodborne illness by astronauts was critically important to control for system safety. An astronaut suffering from foodborne illness is likely to be incapacitated, which could result in a catastrophic failure of the overall system during a mission. In 1959, the Pillsbury Company was contracted by the National Aeronautic and Space Administration (NASA) to develop foods that can be used for space missions (Sperber and Stier 2009/2010). Together with the U.S. Army Laboratories in Natick, Massachusetts, the three organizations worked to develop a new method of food safety.

The system safety program NASA used was based on the identification of critical control points (CCPs) for system failures. To integrate fully with the NASA system safety program, Pillsbury also identified CCPs in the manufacturing of safe food for space missions. Pillsbury later adopted the CCPs and the system safety approach in its own food manufacturing operations. The importance of using HACCP for food safety was publicly discussed in 1971 at a National Conference on Food Protection. About the same time, FDA was investigating the contamination of commercially canned goods with *Clostridium botulinum*. In an effort to identify where system failures occurred in the canning process, FDA requested Pillsbury to provide training to its inspectors on the HACCP system. In 1973, the FDA training program was published and represented the first time the term *HACCP* was used in a publication (Sperber and Stier 2009/2010). Over the next couple of decades, other commercial manufacturers began adopting and improving the HACCP system for food safety management, but federal regulators were slow to accept the new approach over traditional inspections. Eventually, FDA and USDA began mandating the use of HACCP for certain food operations. The Codex Alimentarius Commission also adopted voluntary guidelines on the application of HACCP for its member countries (Codex Alimentarius Commission 2003).

At the time of its introduction, the HACCP system represented a new approach to food safety. Previous food safety efforts involved identifying structural deficiencies and unsafe practices at the time of inspection. The HACCP system emphasized the systematic identification, analysis, and control of hazards during the processing of foods. Furthermore, the HACCP system prioritized food safety efforts by designating CCPs and establishing critical limits for each CCP; the monitoring of CCPs was necessary to ensure that deviations from the critical limits were not occurring, indicating the process was out-of-control. Audits could then be conducted of monitoring records to verify that the process was maintained in control, even when the inspectors were not physically present at the processing plant.

Although the HACCP system was primarily developed for food processing and manufacturing plants, it can also be applied to all parts of the food supply chain, including retail food preparation. The steps involved with the procurement, storage, cooking, and serving of foods are also amenable to the HACCP system of food safety management. Again, however, HACCP is not a substitute for good sanitary practices and other procedures that were discussed in Chapter 4. In fact, standard operating procedures (SOPs) for sanitary practices are a prerequisite for a HACCP system.

## The HACCP Principles, Plan Development, and Implementation

The guiding document for implementing the HACCP system is the HACCP plan. Several prerequisite activities and programs are absolutely essential for the development of a HACCP plan and its successful implementation. These include sanitary practices, equipment cleaning and sanitizing, pest control, procurement of food from safe sources, food worker hygiene and education, and the other principles of prevention discussed in Chapter 4. The development and use of SOPs for these activities are needed to ensure that all procedures are properly followed and effective. Furthermore, compliance with cGMPs is considered a prerequisite for the successful development and implementation of a HACCP plan (National Advisory Committee on Microbiological Criteria for Foods [NACMCF] 1997).

Along with the prerequisite programs, several preliminary steps are necessary before developing a HACCP plan. First, a HACCP team must be assembled with members who represent key operations and departments in the food plant and/or processes. The number and makeup of members will vary with the company's size but should include individuals knowledgeable about the processes (e.g., production engineers), quality assurance (QA) representatives, and appropriate food safety experts (e.g., food microbiologist). At least one individual on the HACCP team must be trained in HACCP principles from an approved source of instruction. The next step is for the HACCP team to describe in detail the food products and their production and distribution methods. This description includes the sources of raw materials, storage times and temperatures, processing steps, packaging materials, shipment methods, and other detailed information.

The final preliminary step is for the HACCP team to create a diagram of the process flow for the food product. The diagram helps to identify all "events" or "points" in the process, and it shows the relationship between events in the proper sequence. It is important for the team to annotate the duration of time for each event as well the time between events for later analysis. To ensure that the diagram is accurate, the HACCP team should subject it to a comprehensive review and verify it by a walk-through of the plant or process. In some situations, the team can group together multiple processes that are very similar to minimize paperwork later. Figure 6-2 is an example of a process flow diagram (Food Safety and Inspection Service [FSIS] 1999b).

After the HACCP team completes the preliminary steps, the team uses the principles of HACCP as guidance to develop a HACCP plan. Currently, seven principles or steps are involved with the HACCP approach:

1. Conduct a hazard analysis.
2. Identify the critical control points.
3. Establish critical limits for each critical control point.
4. Establish monitoring procedures.
5. Establish corrective actions.
6. Establish recordkeeping procedures.
7. Establish verification procedures.

### Principle I: Conduct a Hazard Analysis

Hazard analysis consists of two stages: (1) hazard identification and (2) hazard evaluation. The hazard identification stage involves determining which biological, chemical, and physical agents may be present and/or introduced into the process. The logical place to start is with the raw materials used to manufacture or prepare the food product. The reservoirs and/or sources of foodborne agents discussed in Chapters 2 and 3 are helpful in identifying potential hazards from raw materials. Additional information from literature searches, including documented risk assessments, is also necessary to ensure that the HACCP team uses updated knowledge for hazard identification. In some cases, an expert consultant may be necessary to help determine whether all the potential hazards have been identified. Next, using the process flow diagram developed in the preliminary steps, the team identifies additional points of food contamination with hazardous agents. It is important for the team to identify sources of secondary contamination from raw

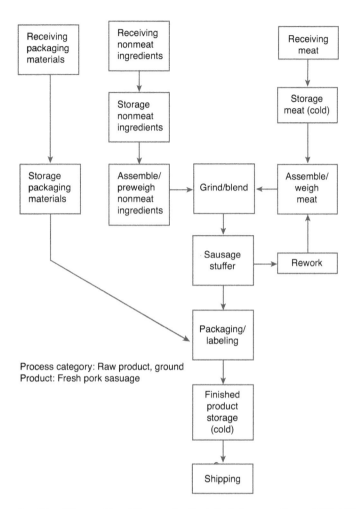

**Figure 6-2** Example of Food Process Flow Diagram for Fresh Pork Sausage. *Source:* FSIS 1999b

materials and cross contamination. Other primary sources of contamination may involve in-house food workers, machinery, dust, food contact surfaces, stored chemicals, and a number of other possible sources. Table 4-1 in Chapter 4 provides a summary of microbial sources, and Figure 3-1 in Chapter 3 provides an overview of toxicant sources.

The hazard evaluation stage consists of determining the risk magnitude in terms of severity and probability for each hazard. (Note: Some safety experts consider this to be a risk assessment of the hazard, typically used to derive a risk assessment code, or RAC.) In less quantitative terms, hazard evaluation involves determining the possible consequences and the likelihood of occurrence for each hazard. Differences can usually be discerned between hazardous agents and situations. For example, the consequences of staphylococcal enterotoxins (e.g., short-term gastroenteritis) are much less compared with those of botulinum toxins (e.g., neurotoxicity and death), and the likelihood of intoxication depends greatly on the different survival and growth conditions for the different bacteria (anaerobic vs. aerobic, pH differences, etc.). This simple example highlights the influence that the processes have on potentially hazardous agents. Thus, it is essential for hazard evaluation that the team perform a rigorous review of the conditions during processing. As much as practical, the HACCP team should collect and use qualitative and quantitative data. For infectious and toxigenic microorganisms, this means the intrinsic and extrinsic parameters of food materials should be evaluated at each point in the process flow. It is recommended that worksheets be used for the hazard analysis (Figure 6-3).

Guidelines are available (often in the form of questions) to assist in the hazard analysis for HACCP planning (FSIS 1999a; NACMCF 1997). Generic HACCP models are also available for certain food processes to aid in the development of a HACCP plan. However, these generic HACCP models are not turnkey programs in that they need modification to accommodate conditions for a particular process at a specific plant.

---

### HAZARD IDENTIFICATION/PREVENTITIVE MEASURE

PROCESS CATEGORY:

PRODUCT:

| PROCESS STEP | FOOD SAFETY HAZARD | PREVENTATIVE MEASURE(S) |
|---|---|---|
|  |  |  |

APPROVED BY: _____ Date: _____

**Figure 6-3** Example of Worksheet Used for Hazard Analysis. *Source:* FSIS 1999b

### Principle II: Identify the Critical Control Points

The hazard analysis may identify multiple events or points in the food process flow where a hazard is potentially introduced and/or exacerbated. For most of the points, the prerequisite activities and programs—if properly implemented—will minimize the risks for potential hazards. But a few of these events or points are absolutely critical to preventing a foodborne illness from consumption of the final product. These points in the process flow deserve special attention through dedicated monitoring, and hence, they are designated as critical control points (CCPs). The designation of a CCP can be tricky for some people to judge, and flow charts such as the one shown in Figure 6-4 are helpful in the decision making, though charts are not a substitute for expert judgment. It may be tempting to designate all points in the process flow as CCPs, but designating too many CCPs results in diluted priorities and necessitates dedicating excessive resources and paperwork to monitoring activities. Examples of CCPs include thermal processes (e.g., pasteurization, cooking, freezing, sterilization), time/temperature storage conditions, product formulation control, pH adjustment, and detection of contaminants such as metals.

When designating CCPs, a complete hazard analysis and careful review are needed. Specialized expertise may also be necessary to aid in determining whether points in the process flow are CCPs. Furthermore, CCPs for one particular plant or process may not be transferable elsewhere because the plant conditions and process flows may be different. As the decision chart in Figure 6-4 illustrates, CCPs have important characteristics. In general, CCPs require specific control measures that can be applied to eliminate or reduce the hazard(s). The effectiveness of the control measures should be measurable and accessible for monitoring, preferably by using instrumentation or automated sensors. If a subsequent point downstream in the process flow eliminates a particular hazard, then the upstream point where the same hazard may appear is less likely to be a CCP. This does not mean, however, that upstream safety precautions should be ignored; prevention principles require a combination of measures to ensure safety, and SOPs and periodic inspections are still necessary throughout the plant and process. The key difference is that the CCP should be steadfastly monitored for effective hazard control, and record-keeping of the monitoring efforts is necessary to ensure that no lapses occurred with the hazard control measures. Figure 6-5 is an example of a completed hazard analysis and designation of CCPs for the process flow diagram in Figure 6-2.

### Principle III: Establish Critical Limits for Each Critical Control Point

The effectiveness of hazard control measures at each CCP is measured against established critical limits. These are the minimum or maximum values for parameters at each CCP that must be controlled to prevent, eliminate, or reduce a food safety hazard to an "acceptable" level (NAC-MCF 1997). Many critical limits are related to the intrinsic and extrinsic parameters of microbial growth, but they may also include other biological, chemical, or physical parameters that can be qualitatively and/or quantitatively measured. Table 6-2 lists some examples of critical limits. Every CCP has at least one parameter or factor that is monitored to ensure hazard control measures are properly functioning.

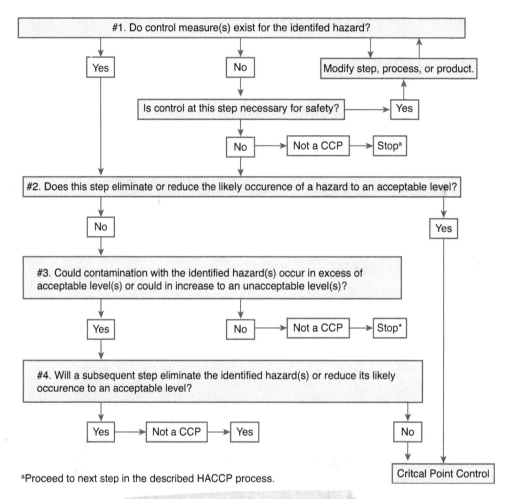

**Figure 6-4** Example of a Critical Control Point (CCP) Decision Algorithm or Tree. *Source:* Adapted from NACMCF 1997.

---

The HACCP team can derive critical limits from regulations, codes, published scientific studies, in-plant challenge studies, established historical information, and safety-related product specifications. Sometimes critical limits are derived from experts and/or professional or trade organizations. Whatever sources the HACCP team uses to derive the critical limits, they should be based on valid and credible sources, and they should be directly relevant to the hazard control measures at the designated CCPs. A critical limit should be exact and precise and should not be a range of possible values. Usually, a critical limit represents either an *upper limit* or a *lower limit* on a scale or continuum of values. Examples of these critical limits include values for temperature,

| Process Step | Food Safety Hazard | Resonably Likely to Occur? | Basis | If Yes in Column 3, What Measures Could Be Applied to Prevent, Eliminate, or Reduce the Hazard to an Acceptable Level? | Critical Control Point |
|---|---|---|---|---|---|
| Receiving—Meat | Bilogical: Pathogens—*Salmonella and* Other pathogens in pork trimmings | Yes | *Salmonella* may be present on incoming raw product. | Certification from suppliers that product has been sampled for *Salmonella* and meets performance standards. | 1B |
| | Chemical—None | | | | |
| | Physical—Foreign materials | No | Plant records show that there has been no incidence of foreign materials in products received into the plant. | | |
| Receiving—Nonmeat Ingredients/Packaging Materials | Biological—None | | | | |
| | Chemical—Not acceptable for intended use | No | Letters of guaranty are received from all suppliers of nonmeat ingredients and packaging materials. | | |
| | Physical—metal, glass, wood | No | Plant records demonstrate that foreign material contamination has not occurred during the past several years. | | |
| Storage (Cold)—Meat | Biological—Pathogens *Salmonella* | Yes | Pathogens are reasonably likely to grow in this product if temperature is not maintained at or below a level sufficient to preclude the growth. | Maintain product temperature at or below a level sufficient to preclude pathogen growth. | 2B |
| | Chemical—None | | | | |
| | Physical—None | | | | |

continues

**Figure 6-5** Example of Completed Hazard Analysis and Designation of Critical Control Points. *Source:* FSIS 1999b

| Process Step | Food Safety Hazard | Resonably Likely to Occur? | Basis | If Yes in Column 3, What Measures Could Be Applied to Prevent, Eliminate, or Reduce the Hazard to an Acceptable Level? | Critical Control Point |
|---|---|---|---|---|---|
| Storage—Nonmeat Ingredients/Packaging Materials | Biological—None | | | | |
| | Chemical—None | | | | |
| | Physical—None | | | | |
| Assemble/Preweigh Nonmeat Ingredients | Biological—None | | | | |
| | Chemical—None | | | | |
| | Physical—None | | | | |
| Assemble/Weigh Meat | Biological—None | | | | |
| | Chemical—None | | | | |
| | Physical—None | | | | |
| Grind/Blend | Biological—None | | | | |
| | Chemical—None | | | | |
| | Physical—Metal contamination | Yes | Plant records show that during the grinding process metal contamination may occur. | Maintenance of grinder blades and plates can preclude metal contamination. Routine examination during equipment breakdown. There will be a metal detector at packaging. | |
| Sausage Stuffer | Biological—None | | | | |
| | Chemical—None | | | | |
| | Physical—None | | | | |

**Figure 6-5** Continued

| Process Step | Food Safety Hazard | Reasonably Likely to Occur? | Basis | If Yes in Column 3, What Measures Could Be Applied to Prevent, Eliminate, or Reduce the Hazard to an Acceptable Level? | Critical Control Point |
|---|---|---|---|---|---|
| Rework | Biological—Pathogens Staphylococcus aureus | Yes | Use of rework can provide a medium for pathogen growth. | Rework left at the end of the day is condemned or used in a cooked product at the plant. | |
| | Chemical—None | | | | |
| | Physical—None | | | | |
| Packaging/Labeling | Biological: Pathogens—parasitic (Trichina) | Yes | Trichina has historically occurred in raw pork products. | Labels that clearly indicate this is a raw product, along with cooking instructions, and the safe food handling statement. | 3B |
| | Chemical—None | | | | |
| | Physical—Metal contamination | Yes | Metal contamination that may have come into the establishment with raw product or occurred during the grinding and stuffing process. | Functional metal detector is online in the packaging/labeling area to remove product with metal contamination. | 4P |
| Finished Product Storage (Cold) | Biological—Pathogens Salmonella Staphylococcus aureus | Yes | Pathogens are reasonably likely to grow in this product if temperature is not maintained at or below a level sufficient to preclude their growth. | Maintain product temperature at or below a level sufficient to preclude pathogen growth. | 5B |
| | Chemical—None | | | | |
| | Physical—None | | | | |
| Shipping | Biological—None | | | | |
| | Chemical—None | | | | |
| | Physical—None | | | | |

**Table 6-2**  Examples of Critical Limits and Monitoring Methods

| Critical Control Point | Potential Hazards | Hazard Control Measures | Critical Limits | Monitoring Methods |
|---|---|---|---|---|
| Evisceration of carcasses | Significant contamination of meat and equipment with pathogens can occur from leakage of gut material during evisceration. | Proper adjustment of evisceration equipment and presentation training of employees will reduce the level of contamination. Visual inspection of carcasses for fecal contamination. | Zero visible fecal contamination after processing; equipment kept properly adjusted; no gut breakage due to improper equipment adjustment; range of 20–50 ppm chlorine or other approved antimicrobial rinse on equipment and product. | Visible check (at least once per hour of production); check chlorine or other approved antimicrobial rinse at start-up and every 2 hours using documented random sampling procedures to demonstrate quality control. Designated quality assurance employee will record results in appropriate log. Equipment adjustment will be checked at start of each shift. |
| Receiving raw meat for making sausage | Salmonella may be on incoming raw product. | Certification from suppliers that product has been sampled for Salmonella and meets FSIS performance standards. | Supplier certification for Salmonella must accompany each shipment. | Receiving personnel will check each shipment for Salmonella certification. |
| Cold storage of meats | Bacterial pathogens may grow in this product if temperature is not maintained at or below the growth parameter. | Maintain product temperature at or below a level sufficient to preclude pathogen growth. | Raw product storage area shall not exceed 40°F. | Maintenance personnel will record raw product storage area temperature every 2 hours, initial/sign and date log. |
| Fermentation of semidry sausage | Possible growth of S. aureus, C. botulinum, C. perfringens, and Listeria monocytogenes. | Ensure pH of meat is reduced quickly below optimum growth range, and room temperature is not excessive. | The pH is reduced to ≤ 5.2 in ≤ 12 hours from start of fermentation. Room temperature is ≤ 90°F during shifts. | Production foreman logs start and stop times of fermentation process. Quality control collects 3 representative samples and measures pH, and records results. Production foreman measures room temperature each shift and logs the results. |
| Steam cooking of shrimp product | Insufficient time and temperature for pathogen kill. | Ensure product is cooked sufficiently to inactivate/destroy pathogens. | Minimum temperature of steam 210°F for ≥ 2.5 minutes. | Digital thermometer and timer with automated data logger. Cooker operator visually checks data logger each day. |
| Drying of salmon jerky using forced convection oven | Pathogen growth and/or toxin formation. | Ensure product is sufficiently dried to prevent bacterial growth. | Product thickness ≤ ¼ in. Drying time ≥ 5 hrs. Oven temperature ≥ 140°F. Product $a_w$ ≤ 0.85. | Foreman presets product slicer to ≤ ¼ in. Digital thermometer and timer with automated data logger. Foreman visually checks data logger each day. Quality control collects samples of each batch for $a_w$ testing and logging. |

NOTE: Critical limits are examples only and should not be used for specific processes.
Source: Adapted from FDA, 2001 and FSIS, 1999a.

time, pH, $a_w$, salt concentration, measurement of preservatives, available chlorine, and viscosity. Occasionally, critical limits are observations of an event or condition, in which cases the critical limit should be unambiguous and easily discerned, preferably as discrete events. Critical limits such as aroma and visual appearance may be used, but these critical limits are more subjective, and proper selection and training of employees are necessary to minimize variation in their observations.

### Principle IV: Establish Monitoring Procedures

Monitoring is a repetitive measurement or observation of CCPs that leads to corrective action whenever deviation occurs from the critical limits. Appropriate monitoring procedures are particularly important for modern food processing facilities, where thousands of food products may be produced in a matter of days, hours, or minutes. The loss of control at a CCP for even a short period of time can result in the distribution of unsafe food products on a disproportionately large scale. Thus, the HACCP team should carefully consider, plan, and implement the monitoring frequency. Whenever feasible, continuous monitoring using automated instrumentation is preferable. For example, the measurement of temperature using computer-controlled sensors and data management can detect deviations in real time, and such instrumentation is not subject to mistakes caused by fatigue and boredom of human observers. When continuous monitoring is not feasible, the frequency and method of monitoring must be adequate to detect when a CCP is out-of-control. Statistical sampling and data collection schemes are often necessary for sufficient confidence that deviations from critical limits will be detected. Furthermore, accurate measurements require the calibration and proper use of instruments. This entails the training of employees in monitoring procedures. To aid with the quality assurance of procedures, the development and use of SOPs for CCP monitoring are essential.

Traditional microbiological laboratory methods are rarely useful for monitoring CCPs because the turnaround time for results is too long before corrective actions can be initiated, if deemed necessary. In these cases, the measurement of chemical or physical parameters is often used as a surrogate indicator of microbial destruction and growth. Recently, new portable or on-site testing methods have been developed; these methods hold the promise of rapid turnaround times for results, provided they can be validated against traditional methods. For CCPs that require manual sampling procedures or observations, the results should be recorded in an accurate and reliable manner. The exact measurements or observations must be entered in a permanent record or log. Results recorded as dittos or "OK" are unacceptable entries.

### Principle V: Establish Corrective Actions

The purpose of establishing CCPs, critical limits, and monitoring procedures is to take corrective actions—when indicated—to prevent the distribution of unsafe food products. Corrective actions should be initiated whenever deviations occur from the established critical limits of a CCP, but the plans for corrective actions must be developed beforehand and documented in the HACCP plan. The HACCP plan should specify immediate procedures upon detection of deviations, and it must designate who is responsible for implementing the corrective actions, along with alternate designees. The HACCP plan must also stipulate the procedures for documenting any corrective actions taken.

To ensure compliance with federal regulations, FSIS regulators expect the following four questions to be addressed by the corrective actions (FSIS 1999a):

1. Has the cause of the deviation been identified and eliminated?
2. Will the CCP be under control after the corrective action has been taken?
3. Have measures to prevent recurrence of the deviation been established?
4. Do the corrective action procedures make sure that no product, which is injurious to health or otherwise adulterated because of the deviation, enters commerce?

The HACCP team needs to carefully develop a set of standardized corrective actions for all deviations from a critical limit. Various "what if" scenarios and tough questions are helpful in developing corrective actions, and historical information may also provide past "lessons learned" for corrective actions. The written procedures for corrective actions must be clearly understood and unambiguous for employees to follow. The plans for corrective actions should include where and how to obtain outside technical expertise for undetermined causes of deviations and what needs to be done in the interim while this expertise is being sought. Some of the most important decisions involve determining which products are affected by the deviations and the disposition of affected products. The HACCP plan should provide guidelines for these decisions and identify the person(s) responsible for making these decisions.

### Principle VI: Establish Recordkeeping Procedures

Although recordkeeping is disliked and considered a burden by many people, it is an essential part of the HACCP system. Studies show that without adequate recordkeeping, problems with products are likely to recur (FSIS 1999a). Procedures must be established for developing and maintaining records associated with the HACCP system. Recordkeeping should include documents related to development of the HACCP plan, especially the hazard analysis summaries, and ongoing operations, including CCP monitoring data logs. Often, to reduce the paperwork burden, food processing companies can integrate existing recordkeeping requirements for other programs with those for the HACCP system by making minor modifications or enhancements.

The records for a HACCP system do not have a mandatory format, though various sources provide examples of formats and the USDA offers the generic HACCP guidance documents. The central record is the HACCP plan, typically presented in summary tabular format, as illustrated in Figure 6-6 (Food and Drug Administration [FDA] 2001). However, FDA recommends the HACCP plan contain additional information on the HACCP team members and their assigned responsibilities; a description of the food product and its distribution, intended use, and consumers; and a verified process flow diagram (NACMCF 1997). This additional information is important, and if it is not included in the HACCP plan, it should be maintained with the other HACCP records.

Firm Name: _____     Product Description: _____

Firm Address: _____     Method of Distribution and Storage: _____

Intended Use and Consumer: _____

| (1) | (2) | (3) | Monitoring | | | | (8) | (9) | (10) |
| | | | (4) | (5) | (6) | (7) | | | |
| Critical Control Points (CCPs) | Significant Hazard(s) | Critical Limits for Each Preventive Measure | What | How | Frequency | Who | Corrective Action(s) | Records | Verification |
| | | | | | | | | | |
| | | | | | | | | | |

Page _____ of _____

**Figure 6-6** Example of Tabular Format for a HACCP Plan. *Source:* Adapted from FDA, 2001.

### Principle VII: Establish Verification Procedures

Verification procedures are needed to ensure that the HACCP system is effectively working as planned. For reasons related to technical complexity and management challenges, the effectiveness of a HACCP plan cannot be assumed without verification. USDA recommends three types of verification: validation, ongoing verification, and reassessment (FSIS 1999a).

Validation occurs during the initial phases of implementing the HACCP plan. It involves testing the assumptions and choices made during the preliminary steps and early stages of the HACCP principles. Two elements are necessary for validation. First, the decisions for choosing process controls and critical limits must be supported with valid scientific sources of information. In other words, the prescribed control of a particular hazard must be based on documented scientific facts—not assumptions. Examples of supporting scientific documentation include published processing guidelines, peer-reviewed articles in scientific journals, microbial challenge studies in pilot plants, in-house data from properly designed scientific studies, and regulatory performance standards.

The second element of validation involves in-plant observations, measurements, testing, or other procedures to ensure that the HACCP system is working as planned. This may require sampling the food product at strategic points (e.g., CCPs) and times throughout the process and sending the samples to a qualified laboratory for microbial testing or chemical/toxin residue analysis. The overall purpose of this validation is to ensure the HACCP plan works in actual practice, not just in theory. Because the prerequisite programs are also considered an essential part of the HACCP system, they may also require validation—especially if the prerequisite program is supposed to eliminate or reduce a hazard downstream in the process.

The purpose of ongoing verification, the second type of verification, is to ensure that the HACCP plan is being properly implemented on a day-to-day basis. This is different from monitoring CCPs for critical limit deviations; ongoing verification ensures that activities such as monitoring are actually being performed correctly. Activities ranging from instrument calibration to record-keeping are observed or audited to verify that personnel perform them as prescribed by the HACCP plan. It is particularly important for the HACCP team to verify the monitoring practices and corrective actions because these activities are critical to identifying and controlling out-of-control processes that may result in unsafe food products.

The third type of verification—reassessment—is a complete review of the HACCP plan, which should be performed at least annually, or whenever changes occur that require revising the hazard analysis or altering the HACCP plan. Changes in raw materials, processes, production levels, personnel, or plant conditions can lead to changes in the hazards addressed by the initial HACCP plan. Some of these changes may be obvious, whereas other changes may be subtle, possibly occurring over time. In either case, reassessment is necessary to ensure that the HACCP plan is up-to-date and not subject to oversights or omissions.

## Benefits and Limitations of HACCP

The major benefit of using HACCP is the systematic identification, analysis, and control of hazards associated with a food operation or process. If done properly, the hazard analysis portion of HACCP examines the entire process flow to identify points where hazards may exist. The identification and designation of CCPs prioritize food safety controls in the process flow. The establishment of critical limits, monitoring procedures, and corrective actions in the HACCP plan provides direction and guidance for food safety activities to minimize the risk of distributing unsafe food products. Finally, the recordkeeping and verification requirements of HACCP help to ensure continuity in the process control of food hazards; this also assists in the oversight of food safety activities by providing an auditable record that spans time, something that observations during periodic inspections cannot accomplish.

The primary limitation of HACCP is the standing requirement for other food safety programs. The HACCP system is not a standalone program. Other efforts such as sanitary practices, equipment cleaning and sanitizing, food worker training, pest control, waste management, facility construction, potable water supply, and cGMPs are necessary to ensure that the HACCP plan is relevant and adequate. Sole and blind reliance on the HACCP system can encourage complacency in other food safety programs, resulting in false assumptions and assurances underpinning the HACCP plan. Additionally, the HACCP system depends on current knowledge from scientific studies and risk assessments. The food processor must examine new knowledge about emerging hazards or circumstances that can exacerbate a hazard in the context of existing HACCP plans. Failure to keep abreast of developments in food safety could allow outdated control measures in the HACCP plan.

Other limitations of HACCP include different opinions of what constitutes a CCP. Not everyone agrees on which control points in a process flow are critical enough to be designated as CCPs. This is important because each additional CCP increases the burden of monitoring procedures and recordkeeping. In the past, CCPs were hierarchical and ranked by a number (CCP1 or CCP2), but recent approaches do not distinguish between different levels of CCPs: Either a control point is critical or it is not. Algorithms or decision charts such as the one shown in Figure 6-4 are helpful in determining a CCP. For control points that are not designated as critical (i.e., non-CCPs), food safety controls must still be in place and maintained, but constant monitoring and recordkeeping are not considered essential.

Many managers consider the time-consuming aspects and costs of recordkeeping some of the most unappealing aspects of the HACCP system. Yet, recordkeeping is crucial to monitoring the status of CCPs, as well as providing documented evidence that food products already distributed were safe. In the modern age of computers and data acquisition, the recordkeeping requirements can be streamlined, but the use of alternative recordkeeping procedures must be acceptable to food safety regulators, at least for the processes where a HACCP plan is mandatory. Different interpretations of "acceptable" records, particularly for verification or validation of the HACCP plan, can also be a source of dispute between regulators and industry.

Another limitation is the need for trained individuals to develop, implement, and maintain the HACCP system. If the appropriate expertise is not represented on the HACCP team, important hazards could be overlooked, underestimated in terms of risk, or inadequately controlled. For smaller food processors, the lack of specialized scientific expertise can be an obstacle to developing an effective HACCP plan. Before the HACCP plan can be implemented, personnel responsible for carrying out the plan must be trained in the proper monitoring methods and procedures. Training courses and guidance documents are available from a variety of sources, but differences in instruction and learning, along with turnover of personnel, can present challenges to training. If conditions associated with food processing change, the food processor may again need specialized expertise to reassess the HACCP plan. In cases where specialized expertise is not available from company resources, the food processor may need to make arrangements with consultants.

## HACCP and HACCP-Like Applications for Foodservice and Retail Establishments

Foodservice and retail establishments differ from food processing plants in a number of ways (Center for Food Safety and Applied Nutrition [CFSAN] 2005; Sun and Ockerman 2005). Most retail food establishments are not defined by a single product or commodity in a highly mechanized production facility. Instead, these establishments typically procure, store, display, prepare, and/or serve various foods. Examples of retail food establishments include restaurants, cafeterias, supermarkets, commissaries, convenience stores, church kitchens, mobile food carts, snack bars, catering firms, and day care centers. The operations of a retail food establishment typically involve a variety of production techniques, ingredients, recipes, and menu items. Other differences of retail food establishments include employees with diverse levels of education and experience, and often high levels of employee turnover. Retail food facilities may also have a small corporate structure, limiting the amount of resources available to provide food safety support.

The adoption of a formal HACCP system for foodservice and retail establishments can be daunting, or even considered as overkill by some people. Yet, the HACCP principles provide a systematic approach to food safety management that examines operations as a series of steps from start to finish, that is, process flows. By viewing retail food operations as a combination of process flows, retail food establishments can examine in detail the steps or points in each process flow for potential hazards and establish CCPs to help ensure food safety. Furthermore, many retail food process flows have steps in common with one another, and by focusing on these common steps or points, the establishment can more efficiently manage hazard analysis and control efforts. Thus, HACCP or HACCP-like approaches are valuable for food safety management in retail food facilities.

Although establishing a HACCP system by retail food facilities is voluntary, FDA encourages the development of a food safety management program based on HACCP principles (CFSAN 2005). For food preparation operations, three generalized process flows are described as being the most common:

1. Food preparation without a cooking step. An example process flow is as follows:
   **Receive → Store → Prepare → Hold→ Serve**
2. Food preparation with a cooking step. An example process flow is as follows:
   **Receive → Store → Prepare → Cook → Hold → Serve**
3. Food preparation involving complex steps and procedures, usually passing through the temperature "danger zone" more than once. An example process flow is as follows:
   **Receive → Store → Prepare → Cook → Cool → Reheat → Hot Hold →Serve**

Each of the preceding process flows has different potential food safety hazards, depending on the specific foods, procedures, and conditions encountered. From a fundamental perspective, a relationship exists between the points in the process flows and the foodborne illness risk factors introduced in Chapter 4. Table 6-3 shows this relationship for one process flow, along with notes

**Table 6-3** Relationship Between Process Steps and Risk Factors in a Food Preparation Process

| *Process Steps* →<br>*Risk Factors* ↓ | *Receive* | *Store* | *Prepare* | *Cook* | *Cool* | *Reheat* | *Hot Hold* | *Serve* |
|---|---|---|---|---|---|---|---|---|
| Food from unsafe sources | X | | | | | | | |
| Inadequate cooking | | | | X | | | | |
| Improper holding/ time and temperatures | | X | | | X | X | X | X |
| Poor personal hygiene | X | | X | | | | | X |
| Contaminated equipment/prevention of contamination | X | X | X | | | | | |

| Notes | |
|---|---|
| **Receive** | Foods may be contaminated from a variety of sources. |
| **Store** | Poor storage practices may lead to contamination of foods, and/or microbial growth may occur under favorable parameters. |
| **Prepare** | Cross-contamination and contamination from food workers and equipment are possible. |
| **Cook** | Microbial kill step. Inadequate cooking temperature does not destroy vegetative cells; adequate cooking temperature still does not destroy spores or heat-stabile toxins. |
| **Cool** | Improper cooling leaves food too long in temperature danger zone. |
| **Reheat** | Improper reheating leaves food too long in temperature danger zone and/or does not destroy vegetative cells. |
| **Hot Hold** | Improper temperatures for hot holding leaves food too long in danger zone. |
| **Serve** | Direct contact by food workers contaminate foods; too long at room temperature may allow microbial growth. |

describing the potential hazards. To minimize the overall risk of foodborne illnesses, food preparation operations should implement hazard control efforts at each point in the process flow. However, a few control points are considered critical (i.e., CCPs), and monitoring these CCPs to avoid deviations from critical limits or unsafe practices further reduces the risks. For example, correct cooking temperatures and times are important to pathogen destruction, and monitoring the cooking temperature/time of a dish helps ensure pathogen destruction. But because spores are not destroyed by conventional cooking, the time/temperature relationship spanning the cool–store–reheat–serve points or steps is also critical; the cumulative time in the temperature danger zone for all these points or steps must be monitored to ensure the total allowable time is not exceeded. For the points not considered as CCPs, the prerequisite programs and SOPs must be sufficient to prevent potential hazards.

One method of developing a HACCP plan is using recipe-based process flows (Bryan 1990; Snyder 2005). Recipes provide a list of ingredients and the steps involved with preparation of a menu item. By incorporating recipes into a process flow and connecting the steps as points in a diagram, food preparation operations can systematically perform the hazard analysis. More important, they can perform the hazard analysis before the actual process starts, resulting in an upfront prevention-oriented approach to food safety. The detail and depth of hazard analysis vary based on the size and complexity of the process flow. Often, the food preparation operation can group together several menus or menu items for similar hazards and the development of HACCP plans. The food establishment should list on a hazard analysis worksheet all points in the process flow with potential hazards. It should list specific preventive measures for each point, with reference to the appropriate SOP, if applicable; the food establishment should also designate CCPs.

## FOOD PRODUCT TESTING AND PERFORMANCE STANDARDS

Prior to widespread acceptance of HACCP principles, food product safety was based primarily on observations from inspections and some end-product testing for selected contaminants. At first glance, testing to detect contaminants in food products appears to be a viable strategy to ensure safety. After all, if a food product is tested and found to be contaminated with a hazardous agent, it can be prevented from being distributed or consumed. Testing food to detect contamination can be divided into three general categories (Kennedy 2008):

1. Testing prior to food leaving the farm or processing facility
2. Testing prior to food reaching the consumer
3. Testing to identify sources of contaminated food and/or to limit foodborne illness outbreaks

Unfortunately, testing foods to detect contamination has many limitations, both in practical terms and cost-effectiveness. The single greatest limitation is that testing cannot be accomplished for every food ingredient and/or item. In fact, the primary reason the HACCP system was developed for NASA was to attain maximum food safety without using most of the food for testing purposes (Sperber and Stier 2009/2010). Because not every food item can be tested for contamination, sampling schemes based on statistical approaches are essential. As an increasing amount of food is sampled and analyzed, greater confidence is achieved with the test results for food items in a particular lot. But the costs also increase with increased sampling and analysis, and additional food product is lost to testing. Furthermore, even statistically valid test results do not guarantee that every food item is uncontaminated. For many microbial contaminants, the magnification of contamination can occur in the food handling chain where favorable microbial growth conditions are encountered.

Another major limitation of testing is deciding which agents should be sampled and analyzed for. Many potential foodborne agents exist, and various agents can be introduced at numerous points throughout the food supply chain. In terms of analytical methods and laboratory protocols, each agent also has specific requirements. Testing for every possible agent is neither practical nor cost-effective. Targeted sampling strategies may be useful for certain agent–food combinations, but agent–food combinations can be complicated to determine and sometimes difficult to use for testing purposes. For example, the association of *E. coli* O157:H7 with hamburger meat is clearly established, but testing hamburger meat and having a zero tolerance policy have been mostly ineffective in reducing the rate of illness from this pathogen (IOM 2003). The primary reason is attributed to the timing of sampling. Food processors need to emphasize sampling the meat prior to grinding operations, before they grind together contaminated meat trimmings with uncontaminated meat trimmings. The downside of adopting this strategy is greater costs and more complicated sampling schemes, and the turnaround times for sampling results are typically too long for modern production levels.

Despite the limitations associated with food product testing, it will likely remain part of an overall risk management strategy, along with the HACCP system and enforcement of sanitary standards. The Food Safety and Inspection Service (FSIS) of USDA conducts surveillance of and/ or testing for certain pathogens and chemical residues in foods. The type of testing is different for various food product classes, and the reasons for testing may also be different. Under the pathogen reduction (PR)/HACCP rule, testing is required for generic *E. coli* at slaughter plants to verify the control of fecal contamination, and testing for *Salmonella* is required for selected raw meat and poultry products to ensure the performance of pathogen reduction measures (including HACCP). As part of a regulatory sampling program, FSIS also tests RTE meat and poultry products for the presence of certain pathogens such as *E. coli* O157:H7, *Salmonella*, and *Listeria monocytogenes*. This sampling program is not designed to detect statistically significant differences from year to- year, but as an aggregate, the data provide an indication of overall trends in pathogen control.

Under the National Residue Program, FSIS also tests for chemical residues in meat and poultry products intended for human consumption. The testing for chemicals includes agrochemicals such as certain antibiotics, sulfonamides, various other drugs, and pesticides. Along with agrochemicals, FSIS routinely tests for certain environmental chemicals and sometimes conducts special studies to test for chemicals such as dioxins. Whenever residue levels exceed established tolerances or action levels, the test results are shared with FDA and EPA, which are responsible for setting tolerances and action levels. From a risk management perspective, the testing for chemical residues by FSIS provides a structured process to evaluate selected compounds by food production class and to allow descriptive statistical analysis of trends. The National Residue Program can also be used to verify the effectiveness of chemical hazard control in HACCP systems implemented by the industry.

The implementation of testing programs by industry is driven by regulatory and voluntary standards. As mentioned previously, testing to monitor CCPs in a HACCP plan is useful when the turnaround times for results are relatively short. But even with long turnaround times for results, testing is useful to validate the effectiveness of a HACCP system. The ideal approach involves sampling and testing at various points throughout the food process flow. Unfortunately, the costs are often prohibitive to perform this type of extensive testing on a routine basis. Therefore, end-product testing is often performed, either as a voluntarily effort or as a mandatory requirement for some regulated food products. Because testing food product items is usually destructive, and 100% sampling rates are impractical, the sampling plan for end-product testing must be statistically based.

For microbiological testing of food products, sampling plans based on statistical schemes are available, and acceptance/rejection criteria have been established. The International Commission on Microbiological Specifications for Foods (ICMSF) published a document on the principles and specific applications for sampling and analysis (ICMSF 1986). To determine the acceptability of a food product or lot, ICMSF and other organizations establish microbiological criteria. ICMSF further categorizes the microbiological criteria into 15 cases that reflect the severity of hazard, sensitivity of the intended population, and the effects of handling/preparation on the hazard. A microbiological criterion for microorganisms is usually based on their enumeration (e.g., CFUs/g) within a subset of samples randomly chosen from a lot or batch of food product. For some microbial toxins or metabolites, the microbiological criterion is based on the quantity per unit(s) of mass, volume, area, or lot. Sampling plans are designed as either two-class or three-class plans. The two-class sampling plans have microbiological criteria that are more stringent compared with the three-class sampling plans, which have a tolerance range for microbiological criteria.

The sampling plans for microbiological testing of food products use letter specifications to represent the required number of samples and microbiological criterion for food product acceptance. The two-class sampling plans use the following letter specifications:

$n$ = The number of units (packages, cartons, carcasses, etc.) from a lot that must be sampled randomly and independently for analysis or examination.

$m$ = The microbiological limit or acceptance level, usually expressed as the number of bacteria per gram; a test sample is considered "positive" if it exceeds this limit.

$c$ = The maximum number of units (from the $n$ sample size) that may be positive, that is, the number of units that exceed the microbiological limit ($m$).

The three-class sampling plans are slightly different. The main difference is the allowance for marginal acceptance of a food lot. The letter specifications for three-class sampling plans are the following:

$n$ = The number of units (packages, cartons, carcasses, etc.) from a lot that must be sampled randomly and independently for analysis or examination.

$m$ = The microbiological limit for marginal acceptance.

$c$ = The maximum number of units (from the $n$ sample size) that may exceed the microbiological limit for marginal acceptance ($m$).

$M$ = The microbiological limit of maximum acceptance level for any single unit. The food lot is considered "marginally acceptable" if the microbiological limit ($m$) is exceeded for no more than $c$ number of units, but no single unit is allowed to exceed the $M$ level.

Table 6-4 lists examples of two-class and three-class sampling plans and microbiological criteria. Note for the frozen, cooked poultry meat that testing for *Staphylococcus aureus* is considered a three-class sampling plan, whereas testing for *Salmonella* is considered a two-class sampling plan. Under the three-class sampling plan, one sample out of the five taken from a lot may contain less than or equal to $10^3$ CFUs/g of *S. aureus* and still be considered acceptable. If the one sample is greater than $10^3$ CFUs/g but less than or equal to $10^4$ CFUs/g of *S. aureus*, the lot is considered marginally acceptable. Under the two-class sampling plan, no samples can contain *Salmonella* for acceptance purposes. With the three-class sampling plan for generic *E. coli* and frozen or cold-smoked fish, the lot is considered acceptable if three samples out of five are less than or equal to 11 CFUs/g; the lot is considered marginally acceptable if no more than three samples exceed 11 CFUs/g provided not even one sample exceeds 500 CFUs/g.

Food product testing is only part of an overall risk management strategy. It must be integrated with food safety programs such as the HACCP system, enforcement inspections, GMPs, training, and so forth. Effective food product testing requires an understanding of the capabilities and limitations of test methods and where in the food supply chain that testing will best mitigate the

**Table 6-4** Selected Examples of Food Sampling Plans and Recommended Microbiological Limits

| Food Products | Tests | Class Sampling Plan | n | c | m | M |
|---|---|---|---|---|---|---|
| Cooked poultry meat, frozen. | *S. aureus* | 3 | 5 | 1 | $10^3$ | $10^4$ |
| | *Salmonella* | 2 | 5 | 0 | 0 | - |
| Boneless meat, frozen (beef, veal, pork, mutton) | APC[a] | 3 | 5 | 3 | $5 \times 10^5$ | $10^7$ |
| Dried milk | APC[a] | 3 | 5 | 2 | $3 \times 10^4$ | $3 \times 10^5$ |
| | Coliforms | 3 | 5 | 1 | 10 | $10^2$ |
| | *Salmonella*, normal routine[b] | 2 | 5 | 0 | 0 | - |
| | | | 10 | 0 | 0 | - |
| | | | 20 | 0 | 0 | - |
| | *Salmonella*, for high-risk population[b] | 2 | 15 | 0 | 0 | - |
| | | | 30 | 0 | 0 | - |
| | | | 60 | 0 | 0 | - |
| Cereals | Molds | 3 | 5 | 2 | $10^2$-$10^4$ | $10^5$ |
| Fresh and frozen fish and cold smoked | APC[a] | 3 | 5 | 3 | $5 \times 10^5$ | $10^7$ |
| | *E. coli* | 3 | 5 | 3 | 11 | 500 |
| Frozen entrees containing rice or corn flour as a main ingredient | *B. cereus* | 3 | 5 | 1 | $10^3$ | $10^4$ |

[a]Aerobic plate count.
[b]Different values of *n* are based on the "case," that is, whether the intended use will decrease the hazard, cause no change, or increase the hazard.

*Source*: Data from ICMSF, 1986.

risks of foodborne illnesses. The capabilities and limitations of test methods are defined by their sensitivity, specificity, logistical burden of handling samples and equipment, turnaround time for results, maintenance and calibration requirements, and cost-effectiveness. In general, with currently available technology, an improvement in one capability worsens at least one other limitation. This tradeoff in capabilities and limitations may change in the future with advanced technologies, but for now, it is unavoidable.

Where to conduct food product testing is not straightforward. It requires detailed knowledge of the food supply chain. With an increasingly complex food supply chain, knowledge is distributed among a labyrinth of food producers, suppliers, distributors, and retailers. This is particularly problematic with the global food trade because an importing country cannot easily verify testing at the source in a foreign country. And testing imported foods in limited quantities for screening purposes is not a highly effective strategy. The most effective approaches to testing food products are based on risk- and science-based strategies.

### REFERENCES

Bryan FL. 1990. Hazard analysis critical control point (HACCP) systems for retail food and restaurant operations. *J Food Protection* 53(11):978–983.

Center for Food Safety and Applied Nutrition. 2005. *Managing food safety: A manual for the voluntary use of HACCP principles for operators of food service and retail establishments.* College Park, MD: U.S. Food and Drug Administration.

Codex Alimentarius Commission. 2010. *Codex Alimentarius Commission procedural manual.* 19th ed. Rome, Italy: Joint Food and Agricultural Organization/World Health Organization Food Standards Programme.

Codex Alimentarius Commission. 2003. *Recommended international code of practice—general principles of food hygiene.* Report nr CAC/RCP 1-1969, Rev.4- 2003. Rome, Italy: Joint Food and Agricultural Organization of the United Nations/World Health Organization Food Standards Programme.

Egan K. 2002, June/July. FDA's total diet study: Monitoring U.S. food supply safety. *Food Safety Magazine.*

Food and Agriculture Organization and World Health Organization. 2003. *Hazard characterization for pathogens in food and water; guidelines.* Report nr Microbiological Risk Assessment Series, No. 3. Rome, Italy: Food and Agriculture Organization of the United Nations.

Food and Drug Administration. 2001. *Fish and fisheries products hazards and controls guidance.* 3rd ed. Washington, DC: U.S. Department of Health and Human Services. Available from: http://www.fda.gov/Food/GuidanceCompliance RegulatoryInformation/GuidanceDocuments/Seafood/FishandFisheriesProductsHazardsandControlsGuide/default.htm.

Food Safety and Inspection Service. 1999a. *Guidebook for the preparation of HACCP plans.* Report nr HACCP-1. Washington, DC: U.S. Department of Agriculture. Available from: http://www.fsis.usda.gov/OPPDE/nis/outreach/models/HACCP-1.pdf.

Food Safety and Inspection Service. 1999b. *Generic HACCP model for raw, ground meat and poultry products.* Report nr HACCP-3. Washington, DC: U.S. Department of Agriculture. Available from: http://www.fsis.usda.gov/OPPDE/nis/outreach/models/HACCP-3.pdf.

Institute of Medicine. 2010. *Enhancing food safety: The role of the Food and Drug Administration.* Washington DC: National Academies Press.

Institute of Medicine. 2003. *Scientific criteria to ensure safe food.* Washington DC: National Academies Press.

International Commission on Microbiological Specifications for Foods. 2002. *Microorganisms in foods 7. Microbiological testing in food safety management.* New York, NY: Kluwer Academic/Plenum Publishers.

International Commission on Microbiological Specifications for Foods. 1986. *Microorganisms in foods 2: Sampling for microbiological analysis: Principles and specific applications is the only comprehensive publication on statistically based sampling plans for foods.* 2nd ed. Toronto: University of Toronto Press.

Kennedy S. 2008. Epidemiology. Why can't we test our way to absolute food safety? *Science* 322(5908):1641–1643.

Kroes R, Muller D, Lambe J, Lowik MR, van Klaveren J, Kleiner J, Massey R, Mayer S, Urieta I, Verger P, et al. 2002. Assessment of intake from the diet. *Food Chem Toxicol* 40(2–3):327–385.

Lammerding AM, Paoli GM. 1997. Quantitative risk assessment: An emerging tool for emerging foodborne pathogens. *Emerg Infect Dis* 3(4):483–487.

National Advisory Committee on Microbiological Criteria for Foods. 1997, August 14. *Hazard analysis and critical control point principles and application guidelines.* Washington, DC: U.S. Food and Drug Administration/U.S. Department of Agriculture. Available from: http://www.fda.gov/Food/FoodSafety/HazardAnalysisCriticalControlPointsHACCP/HACCPPrinciplesApplicationGuidelines/default.htm.

National Research Council. 1983. *Risk assessment in the federal government: Managing the process.* Washington DC: National Academy Press.

Snyder OP. 2005. Application of HACCP in retail food production operations. *Food Protection Trends* 25(3):182–188.

Sperber WH, Stier RF. December 2009/January 2010. Happy 50th birthday to HACCP: Retrospective and prospective. *Food Safety Magazine: Special Feature.*

Stephans RA. 2004. *System safety for the 21st century.* Hoboken, NJ: John Wiley.

Sun Y, Ockerman HW. 2005. A review of the needs and current applications of hazard analysis and critical control point (HACCP) system in foodservice areas. *Food Control* 16(4):325–332.

U.S. Presidential/Congressional Commission on Risk Assessment and Risk Management. 1997. *Framework for environmental health risk management. Final report, Vols. 1–2.* Washington, DC: Government Printing Office.

## USEFUL RESOURCES

Environmental Protection Agency. *Thesaurus of Terms Used in Microbial Risk Assessment.* http://www.epa.gov/waterscience/criteria/humanhealth/microbial/thesaurus/

Food and Drug Administration. Hazard Analysis and Critical Control Points (HACCP). http://www.fda.gov/Food/FoodSafety/HazardAnalysisCriticalControlPointsHACCP/default.htm

Food and Drug Administration. Total Diet Study. http://www.fda.gov/Food/FoodSafety/FoodContaminantsAdulteration/TotalDietStudy/default.htm

Foodrisk.org. http://www.foodrisk.org

International HACCP Alliance. http://www.haccpalliance.org/sub/index.html

Retail Food Alliance. HACCP Personal and Facility Certification. http://www.retailfoodalliance.com/html/cert.html

Risk World. http://www.riskworld.com/

USDA. *Guidebook for the Preparation of HACCP Plans and Generic HACCP Models.* http://www.fsis.usda.gov/Science/Generic_HACCP_Models/index.asp

USDA FSIS Data Collection and Reports. http://origin-www.fsis.usda.gov/Science/data_collection_&_reports/index.asp

USDA National Agricultural Laboratory. HACCP. http://fsrio.nal.usda.gov/nal_display/index.php?info_center=1&tax_level=1&tax_subject=614

USDA National Food Service Management Institute. Standard Operating Procedures. http://sop.nfsmi.org/

World Health Organization. About Microbiological Risk Assessment (MRA) in Food. http://www.who.int/foodsafety/micro/about_mra/en/

# CHAPTER 7

# Laboratory Methods for Food Safety

*1. Which steps in food processing and distribution are of most value in evaluating risks?*

*2. How can this information be incorporated into safety inspections to improve system integrity?*

*3. How can lab data as preventative measure help enhance investigation of disease outbreaks?*

**LEARNING OBJECTIVES**

1. Explain the safety reasons for conducting food testing.
2. List and describe the basic steps of food sampling and testing.
3. Describe why representative food sampling and sample handling are important.
4. Recognize different methods of food sample homogenization.
5. Identify the historical contributions of conventional microbial methods to food testing.
6. Describe the different outcomes and possible consequences of microbial injury.
7. Explain why microbial indicators are used with food testing, and recognize the attributes of an ideal indicator of microbial contamination.
8. Describe what constitutes coliform bacteria, and explain the advantages and limitations of using coliform bacteria for food testing.
9. Recognize noncoliform indicator organisms and biochemical indicators used with food testing.
10. Identify common methods of viable cell counts for food safety.
11. Distinguish the key differences between standard plate counts and other specific methods of viable cell counts.
12. Describe the basic principles of immunological laboratory methods for microbial identification and quantification.
13. Distinguish between the major types of immunological laboratory methods.
14. List and describe the enabling tools of modern molecular genetic and nucleic acid methods.
15. Explain why nucleic acid probes are important for identifying pathogenic microorganisms.
16. Describe important differences between Southern hybridization/blotting and other methods of nucleic acid analysis using probes.
17. Explain how subtyping microorganisms can help to control foodborne illnesses.
18. Describe what makes most genetic fingerprinting methods different from other nucleic acid methods.

19. Recognize the key differences in food testing between microorganisms, chemical residues, and toxins.

20. Explain why rapid food testing methods are preferred, and describe what factors influence the availability of rapid test methods.

## THE LABORATORY AND FOOD SAFETY

Table 7-1 lists the primary purposes for conducting food testing in three broad categories. The first category, introduced and discussed in Chapter 6, includes periodic testing of food products to monitor the effectiveness of good manufacturing processes (GMPs). Food testing is also required to validate hazard analysis and critical control point (HACCP) systems, and in some cases mandated by the U.S. government. The second category is predominantly a public health responsibility, performed by agency laboratories at the federal, state, and local levels of government. Food testing helps to identify the etiologic agents in foodborne illness outbreaks, determine the source(s) of contamination, and prevent further illnesses and recurrence of outbreaks. The third category includes federal monitoring programs to study trends in food contamination and, when necessary, take corrective actions to control contamination problems. Data from these monitoring programs and independent research can serve as input to risk assessment and risk management activities. More recently, concern about intentional contamination (i.e., terrorism) has expanded food testing to deter and detect threats to the food supply.

Although food testing is an important part of food safety programs, most types of food testing require laboratory equipment, supplies, facilities, and specialized expertise. For these reasons, a partnership between food safety programs and a support laboratory is critically important to establish. Laboratory services must be available for both routine and emergency situations. To ensure that these services are available when needed, food safety organizations must make arrangements beforehand in the form of contracts or other written agreements, depending on the organi-

---

**Table 7-1** Purposes for Performing Food Testing

- **Ensure Good Manufacturing Practices (GMP) and Safe Food Handling Processes**
  - Food/product quality
  - Protect public health (e.g., food safety and performance objectives)
  - HACCP applications (e.g., validation, monitoring)
- **Outbreak Investigation and Intervention**
  - Determine etiology and sources of agents
  - Take actions to prevent further illnesses and/or recurrences
  - Public Health knowledge—new threats
- **Regulatory Compliance and Other Applications**
  - Federal monitoring/pathogen reduction
  - Research on foodborne contaminants and risk assessments
  - Food defense: detect intentional contamination

---

zational relationship to the laboratory. Of paramount importance, the contract laboratory must be qualified to perform the specific procedures and tests that are anticipated by the food safety organization. The contract laboratory should also have arrangements with a network of other qualified laboratories to perform highly specialized or infrequently requested tests. Failure of the food safety organization to establish written arrangements with laboratories can result in crisis management that will worsen a situation, leading to an increased risk of foodborne illnesses and/ or higher costs of correcting unsafe conditions.

The requisites of any valid laboratory testing program are qualified technicians to perform the tests and a quality assurance program to help oversee the laboratory's performance. To become qualified, technicians must undergo specialized training and/or certification for each laboratory method. The technicians and laboratory staff should also be supervised by a professional with the appropriate scientific credentials. As for food safety professionals, their role in laboratory testing varies with assigned responsibilities. Often, their roles involve collecting and shipping food samples to the laboratory for testing. In other cases, food safety professionals may request specific laboratory tests and interpret the results. Under some circumstances, food safety professionals may be responsible for performing or supervising limited food testing in a laboratory setting.

The number of laboratory methods available to test for foodborne agents and physicochemical properties of foods may seem overwhelming. This is further complicated by methods that are constantly changing with new technology and techniques, many of which have not been validated or approved for use. Despite these challenges, food safety professionals should strive to have a basic understanding of laboratory methods. The purpose of this chapter is to provide an introduction to laboratory methods for food testing, with emphasis on the methods most relevant to food safety. Details on the procedures and techniques associated with laboratory methods are beyond the scope of this text. Students who are interested in food testing are encouraged to read the references listed at the end of this chapter and to seek training in specific laboratory methods of food testing.

## Overview of Food Testing

Figure 7-1 summarizes the process of food sampling and testing. The process starts by ensuring that sampling is done in a statistically representative manner and by ensuring food samples are properly collected, handled, and preserved for later analysis. The next step is preparing the food samples for analysis. This usually begins by homogenizing the food samples and, depending on the type of planned analysis, may also include more sophisticated approaches involving extraction and concentration. After sample preparation, laboratory scientists analyze the sample to detect and possibly quantify an agent. The detection of an agent can be visual, such as the presence of a microbial colony on an agar plate, or it can be instrumental, such as the measurement of fluorescence using a fluorometer. Test results can be reported as qualitative or quantitative, depending on the type of analysis. The final step is interpretation of the test results. Guidelines are necessary to assist food scientists to interpret the data as either positive or negative for qualitative analysis or to determine the level of significance for quantitative analysis. A broader scope of interpretation involves understanding the implications and limitations of test results. For example, does a particular test result indicate a potential health hazard to the public?

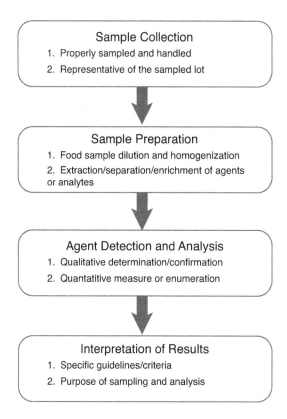

**Figure 7-1** Basic Steps Involved with Food Testing

## Food Sample Collection

Without representative sampling of foods, the results of testing are meaningless. As described in Chapter 6, statistical schemes or plans such as the ones offered by the International Commission on Microbiological Specifications for Foods (ICMSF) are available for end-product sampling of food lots (ICMSF 1986). Other documents provide sampling plans for regulatory investigations (Food and Drug Administration [FDA] 2010b). A more detailed discussion of sampling plans for foods is provided by Midura and Bryant (2001). When in doubt, the sampling of raw or finished food products should be based on expert advice from a statistician or from published sampling plans designed for a particular application. An important point to remember is that no statistically based sampling scheme can guarantee the detection of foodborne agents, but it can increase the opportunity of detecting them. In general, the probability of detecting agents is increased by more frequent sampling and by sampling additional sites from the food item and the lot. For foods in a production line, multiple sampling times increase the probability of detecting agents that occur in "slugs" or zones of contamination as they move along the production line.

Other practical considerations of sampling are where and how to collect the sample from the individual food items. Even with 100% testing of every food item, which is usually destructive and not feasible to perform, detection is not assured. Contaminants are rarely uniformly distributed in the food item. Often, they are found in particular compartments of the food matrix (i.e., biased distribution). With knowledge about the contaminating agent and its sources, strategies can be devised to sample compartments in food matrices. For example, the sampling of meat and poultry carcasses for certain bacterial pathogens (*E. coli* O157:H7, *Salmonella*, *Campylobacter*, etc.) is best accomplished by collecting surface samples from the carcasses because contamination occurs mostly from the intestinal contents during evisceration. On the other hand, ground meats are likely to have the bacterial contaminants mixed throughout the food product; surface sampling of ground meats is not as effective as is surface testing of intact meats. In the case of prions responsible for bovine spongiform encephalitis (BSE), the best place to sample is the brain and other central nervous system (CNS) tissues of cattle.

Chemical residues have a predilection to accumulate in certain tissues of the animals and plants prior to harvesting for human food. Lipophilic xenobiotics, for example, preferentially accumulate in adipose tissues and fats. Collecting samples from the fatty parts of food is thus a more effective strategy for these substances. On the other hand, veterinary drug residues are usually sampled from the liver and/or muscle tissues of carcasses. The reasons are related to the drugs' pharmacokinetics. The liver and muscles deplete drug residues at a slower rate compared with other tissues. Additionally, the risk of human exposure is greater with these tissues because they are edible portions of the carcasses. Therefore, when the source of the toxicant is associated with exposure to livestock, it is important for food safety professionals to understand the pharmacokinetics of drugs and other xenobiotics. For plant-based foods, pesticides and other chemical agents may have an affinity for particular parts of the plant, necessitating selective sampling from the food item.

If the distribution of harmful agents in the food matrix is unbiased or random, it is likely to approximate one of several probability distributions (Poisson, negative binomial, log-normal, etc.). In these cases, the variability or spread (measured by the variance) of values among subsamples from the food item strongly influence the confidence level of test results. Higher levels of variance in subsamples yield less confidence in the test results, and vice versa. Several techniques can be used to increase the confidence level (i.e., lower the variance) when sampling a food item (Jarvis 2000). One technique is to take larger analytical sample sizes from the food items. Another technique is to comminute or homogenize the sample prior to removing a subsample for analysis. This more evenly distributes the agents throughout the food matrix and sample, though for reasons discussed earlier, homogenization does not ensure unbiased distribution of some agents, particularly pesticides (Pellizari et al. 2003).

Once the sampling strategy and sample locations have been determined, proper technique is important to ensure that an adequate amount is collected and that extraneous contamination is prevented. The amount of sample necessary depends on the analytical method and the intersample variance of the agent. The sampling standard operating procedure (SOP) and laboratory protocol should specify the precise amount of sample, as well as collection techniques. Extraneous contamination with microbial agents can occur from poor aseptic technique, unsterile supplies, and careless sample handling. This can lead to false positives in test results, or the extraneous contamination can cause microbial interference during culturing. Problems in test results may also occur from extraneous contamination with chemicals. Contamination with some chemicals can inactivate the microbial agents targeted for identification/enumeration. For example, antimicrobial compounds in rinses or on food contact surfaces may contaminate the food sample and reduce the number of microorganisms prior to laboratory analysis. Thus, food safety professional must take care to ensure that the food is free of excessive sanitizers or other antimicrobial compounds prior to sample collection.

Not all samples are collected directly from the food products. Food scientists frequently perform environmental sampling where food products are produced. Recently, greater emphasis is has been placed on environmental sampling because recent foodborne illness outbreaks have been linked to environmental contamination with pathogens, including nonfood contact surfaces (FDA 2010b). Samples are routinely collected from food contact surfaces to determine the effectiveness of sanitary practices or sanitizing treatments. The data from this type of environmental sampling are also used to verify that sanitary GMPs are properly implemented in a food processing facility. Sometimes, foods are sampled indirectly from the materials that come in contact with them. This is particularly useful for conducting surveys of contamination. For example, the exudates or rinses from raw foods are convenient sources to survey contamination with certain microbial agents (Musgrove et al. 2003). With these types of surveys, the study design is critically important. And although the data from these surveys are useful for studying trends or making comparisons between different facilities, they are not designed to determine the level and frequency of contamination among food lots.

After food safety professionals collect representative types of samples properly, they must protect them from further contamination and deterioration during transport and storage. Sampling SOPs and laboratory protocols should explicitly state the precise method and procedure for handling samples. In most cases, samples are sealed in independent containers and kept refrigerated/chilled during transport to the laboratory. The colder temperatures inhibit the growth of microorganisms that could alter the microbial ecology, in turn affecting the analysis. Colder temperatures also slow chemical reactions that could produce products capable of interfering with the analysis. Unless the food samples are already frozen, in which case they should remain frozen during transport and storage, unfrozen foods should not be frozen. Freezing can destroy some pathogens (e.g., *Campylobacter*) and render them undetectable. Food safety professionals should transport samples as soon as possible to the laboratory, and unless stipulated differently in the protocols, the laboratory should analyze the samples within 36 hours of collection. Individual samples should be clearly identified with the sampling date, time, location, purpose, and other pertinent information. In certain cases—particularly for regulatory enforcement or compliance determination—a clear record of chain of custody for the samples is necessary (FDA 2010b).

## Preparation of Food Samples

Before the laboratory can analyze food samples, the samples must be properly prepared. Foods have different physical, chemical, and biological properties that characterize their makeup and determine the sample preparation requirements. Physically, food matrices are mixtures of solids, semisolids, and liquids in various proportions and with unique characteristics. Chemically, foods are composed of complex mixtures of carbohydrates, proteins, fats, and a multitude of other organic and inorganic compounds. **Biologically,** foods may have diverse **populations of microor-**ganisms that **make up a microbial ecosystem.** Additionally, foods composed of animal and plant tissues may continue to respire or undergo other biochemical changes. **Without appropriate sam-**ple preparation, **the physical, chemical, or biological properties of foods can interfere with labora-**tory methods of analysis. The procedure and steps of sample preparation are specific to each laboratory method and should be documented in the appropriate laboratory protocols and SOPs.

Preparation of solid food samples usually begins with dilution followed by homogenization. The traditional method of sample homogenization is with laboratory blenders. If the intended analysis is for microorganisms, laboratory technicians must take care that they use aseptic tech-niques when weighing and transferring sample portions to and from the blender. The implements and containers that contact the food sample (forceps, spatulas, spoons, pipettes, blender cup, etc.) should be sterile. The time and environmental conditions during sample preparation are also important because excessive times under favorable growth conditions can change the microbial population of the food sample. Conversely, harsh environmental conditions can inactivate or destroy microorganisms of interest. With laboratory blenders, high RPMs and excessive blending times can generate heat that destroys microorganisms. Laboratory scientists use several techniques to minimize heat generation during blending. These techniques include limiting blending times and adding chilled diluents to the blender cup (Midura and Bryant 2001).

Alternative methods to traditional blending have been developed over the past few decades to homogenize food samples. The Stomacher is an accepted method of sample homogenization. Food laboratories around the world have added the Stomacher as standard equipment to their inventory. Unlike the blender, the Stomacher homogenizes a food sample by a set of paddle-like cams that extrude, crush, and circulate the food. The food sample is within a sterile plastic bag during homogenization, so it never directly touches the paddles. Many solid food samples can be prepared without (or with minimal) dilution, and the Stomacher is programmable to accommo-date different times and speeds. Food samples with sharp or exceptionally hard pieces may not be suitable for the Stomacher because they can cause perforation of the plastic bag.

Along with the Stomacher, other paddle homogenizers have become available in the market-place. The Bagmixer works in a manner similar to the Stomacher. The primary differences include the following: the Bagmixer has a window that permits viewing the sample during homogeniza-tion; the paddles are adjustable; and the bags have a built-in filter that separates fibrous residues and other solids from a filtrate, which can be pipetted for subsequent analysis. The Smasher is another paddle homogenizer that first rapidly crushes the food sample with a strong pounding action, followed by a peristaltic blending action. The initial crushing/pounding action decreases the time required for food sample homogenization. The Smasher also has several levels of adjust-able speeds and times, and it has a collection chamber below the sample bag in case of leakage.

A third type of solid food sample preparation combines high-frequency vibration with shock waves and stirring. The Pulsifier uses an oval ring to transmit these forces to the sample and diluents contained within a plastic bag. Microorganisms are dislodged from the food and extracted into the diluents for subsequent analysis. The effectiveness of extracting microorgan-isms using the Pulsifier correlates highly with "stomaching" methods of extraction (Fung 2002). Unlike the blenders and paddle-type homogenizers, the food sample in the Pulsifier is minimally destroyed, and less food debris is transferred to the diluents and extract. This reduces the likelihood that food debris will interfere with microbial analytical methods—particularly with nucleic acid methods (e.g., polymerase chain reaction, or PCR).

Certain types of analysis require additional sample preparation following homogenization. Sample preparation is usually different between microbial and chemical agents, and the type of analysis determines the degree of sample preparation. Even at the level of individual microbial species and chemical classes, significant differences in sample preparation can exist. Generally, sample preparation involves the extraction and concentration of the agents or analytes prior to the analysis. Considering all the different agents and types of analyses, sample preparation requirements cannot be discussed for various combinations of agent and analytical method. Quite often, procedures for sample preparation are modified to accommodate specific purposes or food types. Whenever a question arises about sample preparation, the up-to-date requirements should be specified in the appropriate laboratory protocol.

## MICROBIOLOGICAL CULTURE AND STAINING METHODS

The development of microscopes laid the foundation of microbiology. Until microorganisms could be visualized, their existence was theorized but not actually confirmed. When Leeuwenhoek first observed microorganisms in 1675, the microscope became the indispensable tool of microbiology. Microscopes have become increasingly sophisticated over the centuries, even permitting the observation of viruses and molecules. Although many other technologies have also advanced the science of microbiology (e.g., PCR), the observation of microorganisms still provides compelling evidence of their presence in a particular medium or environment.

Another important accomplishment in the history of microbiology was the development of culture media to grow and study microorganisms in the laboratory. From the mid-nineteenth century through the early twentieth century, tremendous progress was made in developing different types of culture media, including the incorporation of agar to provide a solid matrix for microbial colonization. With a great variety of culture media containing different nutrients and substrates for biochemical reactions, the study of microbial metabolism—particularly among bacterial pathogens—became possible. Although sophisticated technology using nucleic acids has recently overshadowed culture methods in microbiology, culture methods have several advantages over nucleic acid analysis. Additionally, culture media are often needed to isolate and enrich the microorganisms of interest before other analytical methods are employed.

The components of culture media are often wide ranging, some well defined with high purity, whereas others are poorly defined but still essential for microbial growth (Holbrook 2000). The composition of culture media is critically important to meeting the nutritional requirements of different microorganisms. By manipulating the composition of culture media with various formulations, microbiologists can grow, isolate, and identify particular species or strains of microorganisms. In fact, culture media are generally described by their relative ability to support the growth of different microorganisms. The descriptive categories of culture media include the following (Yousef and Carlstrom 2003):

- Nonselective culture media
- Selective culture media

- Differential culture media
- Selective-differential culture media

The nutritional content of nonselective culture media is sufficiently rich to grow a wide range of microorganisms. Nonselective culture media are typically used to enumerate most microbiota from a food sample or to collect inocula from selected colonies for further testing or identification. Selective culture media are formulated with components that restrict the growth of microorganisms to those of interest, also known as the targeted microorganisms. Nontargeted microorganisms do not compete well against targeted microorganisms in selective culture media, usually because of components added to inhibit nontargeted microorganisms while simultaneously encouraging the growth of targeted microorganisms. Differential culture media are used to test for a distinguishing metabolic characteristic of particular microorganisms. This is usually based on a biochemical reaction with an associated change in some observable indicator (pH and color change, colony appearance, proteolysis, gas production, etc.). Some culture media are formulated with components that offer both selective and differential properties, that is, selective-differential culture media. These types of culture media provide an efficient means of selecting and differentiating targeted microorganisms among a complex microbiota. In the early days of microbiology, individual laboratories painstakingly made culture media from scratch. Nowadays, many types of prepackaged formulations and ready-to-use products are commercially available.

By the end of the nineteenth century, dyes became another essential tool for microbiologists (Guardino 2005). Microbiologists use dyes to stain microorganisms such as bacteria, making them directly observable under a light microscope. But equally important, microbiologists use different dyes to stain parts of microbial cells with certain biochemical constituents. This provides an added method of classifying microorganisms on the basis of stain retention, which also reflects the biochemical composition of cellular structures. The most widely recognized staining technique in microbiology is the Gram stain, developed in 1884 by Hans Christian Gram, a Danish bacteriologist. The Gram stain procedure is based on two dyes, crystal violet and a counterstain safranin. If the crystal violet dye is retained by a layer of peptidoglycan in the cell wall after alcohol treatment, the bacteria have a purple color and are designated as Gram-positive. Bacteria containing a secondary cell membrane made with a lipopolysaccharide layer do not retain the crystal violet dye. The counterstain safranin gives these bacteria a pink or reddish color, and they are designated as Gram-negative. In pathogenic and food microbiology, the Gram stain determination of bacteria is an important step in their classification and sometimes is used to infer the sources of contamination.

Over many years, testing schemes and procedures have been developed for the differentiation of bacteria based on traditional culture and staining methods (Holt 1994). Figure 7-2 illustrates a partial flowchart to identify a subset of selected bacteria—most of them with importance in food safety. This flowchart is not a definitive guide for identifying the bacteria but merely emphasizes the strategy involved in using differentiation methods. Of particular interest is the initial importance of the Gram stain and cellular morphology in differentiating bacteria. In actual practice, differentiation tests sometimes produce ambiguous results or false negatives and false positives. This may be because of biological variability within a species or procedural errors such as poor media preparation, faulty procedures, poor laboratory technique, and other causes. To minimize

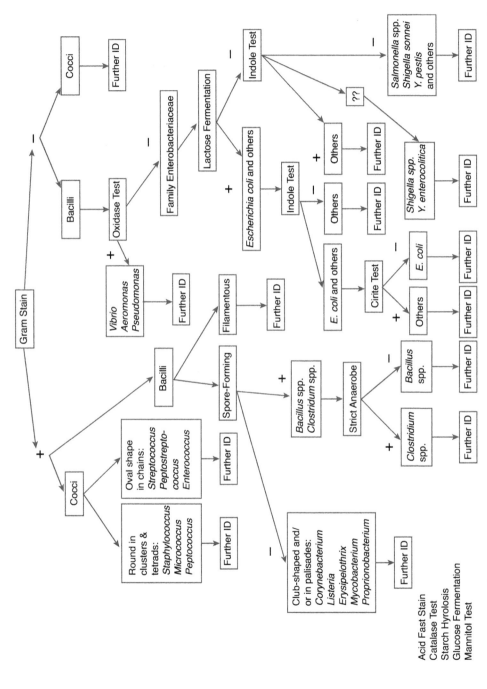

**Figure 7-2**  Flowchart Illustrating Differential Identification of Selected Bacteria. *Source:* Adapted from Holt, 1994. *Bergey's Manual of Determinate Bacteriology*

procedural errors, the laboratory technicians must be proficient in the methods used. Besides the obvious need for training and experience in the methods used, laboratory accreditation and quality assurance programs help ensure proficiency is maintained.

## Metabolic Injury, Resuscitation and Recovery, and Viable but Nonculturable Cells

Prior to the 1980s, bacterial cells were categorically considered to be either alive or dead based on the presence or absence, respectively, of growth in laboratory media. This simplistic view has been replaced with the recognition that many bacteria—including several foodborne pathogens—have a range of viability states, some of which cannot be detected by routine laboratory analysis. Stresses in the environment induce these viability states, which include adaptive responses, injury and recovery, and dormancy. Pathogenic bacteria in one of these viability states have many implications for laboratory testing and disease transmission. Therefore, it is important for food safety professionals to have a basic understanding of these viability states.

In the broadest sense, stresses to foodborne microorganisms include suboptimal changes in extrinsic/intrinsic parameters, antimicrobial treatments of foods or contact surfaces, and/or other unfavorable environmental conditions. Microorganisms that are subjected to stress may respond in several possible ways, depending on the type and degree of stress and the organism's physiology. The physiology of most microorganisms can tolerate mild stress. With extreme stress, microorganisms can experience a degree of shock or injury, possibly leading to death or other nonlethal responses. Stress-induced shock can trigger adaptive responses that enhance tolerance to the stress. Sometimes, the adaptation to one stress can enhance cross-protection for other stresses. With severe nonlethal injuries, time is required for repair and recovery, and the microorganism may enter a state of quiescence.

*Injury* to microorganisms implies damage to cellular or subcellular structures that causes some loss of function. Such injuries are not easily observed in the cells of microorganisms, but the loss of function associated with an injury is more easily ascertained. For example, injured microbial cells may not be able to grow and proliferate on culture media like their uninjured counterparts. Some scientists make the distinction between metabolic injury and structural injury on the basis of growth with different culture media and temperatures (Wesche et al. 2009). Jay, Loessner, and Golden (2005) describe microbial cells that are incapable of forming colonies on selective culture media as having undergone metabolic injury. Many scientists "consider metabolic and structural injury to be varying degrees of the same type of injury" (Wesche et al. 2009). In the final analysis, the distinction between metabolic and structural injury on the basis of colony growth may be a moot point because not all microbial cells in a given population will experience the same degree of injury. Microbial cells experiencing less injury can grow and produce colonies, whereas the microbial cells with severe injury may not.

Foodborne bacteria that have experienced nonlethal injury may eventually recover and resume growth and reproduction. The time to recovery depends on many factors—the most important being the degree of injury and the cellular repair mechanisms inherent to the bacterial strain. Several foodborne bacteria are also known to enter a state called *viable but not culturable* (VBNC). Bacterial cells in the VBNC state cannot be cultured using media in which they normally grow, but they remain viable and capable of resuming growth (Oliver 2005). Furthermore, pathogenic bacteria in the VBNC state retain their virulence. The resumption of growth for bacterial cells in the VBNC state depends on key changes in the environment that resuscitate them. The relative importance of VBNC pathogenic bacteria to the infection of humans is not clearly understood. From a food safety perspective, the presence of VBNC pathogenic bacteria is a concern with routine food testing programs because a negative culture test for pathogenic bacteria in the VBNC state is a false finding. Many laboratory testing protocols include a resuscitation step for VBNC and injured bacteria.

## Indicators of Microbial Contamination for Food Safety

A particularly difficult challenge with food testing is determining which pathogenic microorganisms to test for. Although a few important pathogens are targeted in certain food products, a great number of potential pathogenic and toxigenic microorganisms are potential contaminants. To test each food product for every possible microorganism of public health significance is impossibly time consuming and expensive. One solution to this problem is to identify an easy-to-use indicator of possible contamination with pathogens. Over the years, authors (Bonde 1966; Jay et al. 2005; National Research Council [NRC] 2004; Tortorello 2003) have articulated several biological and analytical attributes that an ideal indicator for pathogens have. The following list is a paraphrased summary of desirable attributes of an ideal indicator for pathogens:

- Its presence should correlate with the health risks.
- It should be quantifiable and present whenever the pathogens are present.
- Its survival or persistence in the environment should strongly parallel or exceed that of the pathogens.
- Its density in the environment (e.g., water and food) should be sufficient to detect with an easily sampled volume.
- It should be specific to and identifiable with the source of contamination (e.g., feces, host species).
- It should be easily distinguishable from other microbiota that may be present.
- The analytical method for its detection must be sensitive, precise, consistent, rapid, inexpensive, and logistically feasible.

Obviously, an ideal indicator does not exist. Tradeoffs are expected among the preceding attributes with different types of indicators and methods of analysis.

Indicators of microbial activity in foods are generally divided into two categories: (1) food safety and/or sanitary indicators, and (2) food quality indicators. The latter category of indicators is used to evaluate the shelf life and aesthetic acceptability of food products. This textbook does not specifically address quality indicators of microbial activity in foods. Instead, it introduces select indicators for food safety and sanitation. The following section emphasizes the detection of indicator organisms for food safety, though; some indicators are based on the detection of cellular components or metabolic activity of microorganisms (i.e., nonorganism indicators). A couple of these nonorganism indicators are discussed under biochemical indicator methods later in this chapter.

### Coliforms as Indicator Organisms

In the mid- to late nineteenth century, the usefulness of an indicator organism was recognized with water testing. During that time, Dr. Theodor Escherich discovered that a certain bacterium was nearly always present wherever human feces are found. The bacterium (now called *Escherichia coli*) belonged to a related group of bacteria that was dubbed "coliforms." Using conventional culture and staining techniques, coliforms could be identified faster and easier as a group rather than identifying each individual species. The presence of coliform bacteria became a practical indicator for the fecal contamination of water supplies, and over time, they were used for the same purposes with milk and other foods. Because enteric pathogens are generally associated with feces, coliforms were presumed to indicate the possible presence of enteric pathogens. But not all coliform bacteria originate from feces, so the distinction between total coliforms and fecal coliforms became necessary. The analytical difference between the two subgroups is based on culture requirements and the thermotolerance of fecal coliforms.

Coliform bacteria do not constitute a taxonomic group. Instead, they represent a functional categorization based on staining and culturing characteristics. Total coliforms are Gram-negative, non-spore-forming rods. They are aerobic or facultatively anaerobic and can tolerate the presence of bile salts. Total coliforms are also oxidase-negative and ferment lactose with the production of gas within 48 hours at a temperature of 37°C. Several genera of bacteria have these characteristics—particularly the genera *Escherichia*, *Enterobacter*, *Klebsiella*, and *Citrobacter*. With the exception of the genus *Escherichia*, several species from the other genera are also naturally found in plants and the environment. Among the species of *Escherichia*, only *Escherichia aerogenes* is established as a normal inhabitant of vegetation and occasionally the intestinal tract. Fecal coliforms are normally found in the intestinal tracts of most warm-blooded animals, and they have subtle characteristics that help distinguish them from other total coliforms. Nearly all fecal coliforms, for example, are capable of fermentation at the higher temperatures of 44.5°–45.5°C, while only a few nonfecal coliforms are similarly thermotolerant (Tortorello 2003). To distinguish definitively between total and fecal coliforms, additional testing is necessary. Over the years, the identification and enumeration of generic *E. coli* has become more feasible, and testing for generic *E. coli* has become an alternative to testing for fecal coliforms. Additionally, testing only for generic *E. coli* reduces the possibility of positive test results from thermotolerant coliforms of nonfecal origin.

The coliform bacteria have a long history of use as indicator organisms for public health protection. This long history and the accumulation of knowledge from coliform testing is the primary advantage of using coliforms as indicator organisms. Waterborne and foodborne disease outbreaks have been associated with positive test results for coliform bacteria. Likewise, the reduction of disease transmission has been associated with the absence of coliform bacteria in water and food. However, this relationship is not consistently observed. Coliform bacteria are still only indicators of contamination by pathogens, and their absence or presence in samples is not a definitive predictor of exposure to pathogens. The value of coliform testing for hazard evaluation of foodstuff depends on the specific application. Total coliforms are obviously less specific indicators of enteric pathogens compared with fecal coliforms, whereas generic *E. coli* is a much more specific indicator than are both subgroups of coliforms. Still, there is danger from overreliance on coliform and generic *E. coli* testing when evaluating food safety hazards. In most situations, the microbial indicator represents one of many factors to be considered when evaluating food safety hazards.

When interpreting coliform testing results, several generalizations about coliform bacteria as indicator organisms in foods are important to remember. First, the number of acceptable coliforms in foods is relative. Coliforms are encountered on several types of foods, but great numbers of coliforms and generic *E. coli* in any foods should cause concern. The presence of coliforms in foods is an indicator of sanitary practices, and great numbers of coliforms in food samples suggests poor or inadequate sanitation. As a minimum, the HACCP system should be used to identify points where sanitation or other measures can reduce the coliform count. For certain foods and beverages, such as bottled water and milk products, regulatory tolerances or limits on coliforms density have been established, which if exceeded deems the product unsafe for consumption (21 CFR 165.110 and FDA 2009). Similarly, federal/state regulations and guidelines specify allowable levels of fecal coliforms in certain seafood. And fecal coliform standards are established for shellfish harvesting waters to manage the hazards from runoff that may contain pathogens of fecal origin.

A second generalization is that coliforms are more likely to be encountered in raw or fresh foods because the habitat of several coliform species includes the outdoor environment. On the other hand, the presence of coliforms in processed food products may indicate poor process control. Moreover, the presence of coliforms or generic *E. coli* in food products that have undergone a pathogen kill step may be indicative of postprocessing contamination. Regulatory criteria based on generic *E. coli* (Biotype I) testing have also been established to verify process control with meat and poultry products (9 CFR 310.25 and 9 CFR 381.94). International guidelines and evaluation criteria are established for coliform and generic *E. coli* to assist with food end-product testing (ICMSF 1986).

A third generalization involves the unsuitability of coliforms and generic *E. coli* as indicators for specific pathogenic and toxigenic microorganisms. The association of enteric pathogens with fecal contamination depends on the health and carrier status of the contributing hosts. Some enteric pathogens of fecal origin are exceptionally robust and may survive longer in the environment than fecal coliforms and generic *E. coli*. Generally, coliforms are not suitable indicators for viruses, protozoa, and helminths. And although coliforms and generic *E. coli* are presumed to be associated with enteric pathogens, the natural habitat of many pathogenic and toxigenic microorganisms includes the environment. For example, pathogens such as *Listeria monocytogenes* and *Vibrio* species, along with several toxigenic bacteria (e.g., *S. aureus*, *Clostridium* spp.), are free-living in the environment. For these environmental microorganisms, fecal coliforms or generic *E. coli* are not helpful indicators.

### Other Indicator Organisms

Microbiologists have used and studied other microorganisms as food safety/sanitation indicators. The taxonomic family Enterobacteriaceae has about 20 genera that include *E. coli*, other coliform species, and several genera of foodborne pathogens. The identification and enumeration of Enterobacteriaceae as a group has been proposed as an alternative to coliform testing of foods (Tortorello

2003). As indicator organisms in food, the Enterobacteriaceae are similar to the total coliforms. In other words, they are not truly indicative of fecal contamination but are useful indicators of sanitation and process control. The Enterobacteriaceae differ collectively from the coliforms by their better survivability and ability to colonize in the environment, yet they remain sensitive to sanitizers. These attributes make Enterobacteriaceae particularly valuable to monitor the effectiveness of sanitary GMPs and HACCP prerequisite programs. Despite these potential advantages, the Enterobacteriaceae are not widely used in the United States as indicator organisms.

Since about 1900, several species of the genus *Enterococcus* have been studied and used as indicator organisms for water quality, and during the 1960s and 1970s, they were proposed as indicator organisms for foods (Jay et al. 2005). The enterococci comprise about 30 species of Gram-positive bacteria with habitats that include water, soils, vegetation, and the intestinal tracts of humans and animals. Some species of enterococci are used for fermentation of foods or as probiotics (Franz et al. 2003). Enterococci are widely distributed in nature, but a few species are most closely associated with intestinal tracts of animals or humans and fecal pollution. The most well-known species include *E. faecalis* and *E. faecium*. Compared with fecal coliforms, enterococci are less abundant in human feces, but they usually die off more slowly in water, making them more persistent indicators of fecal pollution. As such, enterococci are particularly valuable for monitoring recreational surface waters. Unfortunately, the use of enterococci as sanitary or safety indicators for foods is much less advantageous. The primary reason is that multiple possible sources of enterococci make them less specific indicators of fecal contamination, and their persistent survival in the environment does not fully convey the effectiveness of sanitary practices against pathogens. Additionally, valid methods for detecting generic *E. coli* are now much faster and more efficient, making the generic *E. coli* test much more feasible.

Several anaerobic bacteria belong to the gut microbiota of animals and humans, and some of these bacteria (e.g., *Bifidobacterium* and *Bacteroides* species) have significant potential as indicator organisms. The genus *Bifidobacterium* includes more than 25 species of bacteria, and they are found in very high densities in feces. In fact, their density is several orders of magnitude higher than *E. coli* (Jay et al. 2005). Moreover, the bifidobacteria can be differentiated to determine their origin from human feces, animal feces, or the environment. These attributes and others make the bifidobacteria good candidates as indicators for fecal contamination. Unfortunately, the analytical method for bifidobacteria is a major impediment to their adoption as indicator organisms. The bifidobacteria are strict anaerobes that grow quite slowly, with turnaround times for test results taking days, and the bifidobacteria are less likely to grow in foods with naturally high redox potential (Eh) values (e.g., vegetables). Nevertheless, laboratory methods have been developed and used to detect bifidobacteria in meat and meat products (Beerens 1998). Perhaps in the future, with nucleic acid test methods and automated technology, the bifidobacteria (or other bacteria) will become more feasible as sanitary indicators.

A recalcitrant problem in food processing plants is the colonization of *Listeria monocytogenes*. This important pathogen is relatively hardy and capable of growing in high salt concentrations and low temperatures. Once established in niche growth areas, *L. monocytogenes* can contaminate foods throughout the processing plant, even after foods have been subjected to lethal treatments for pathogens. Environmental sampling programs are helpful in controlling this pathogen, but conventional indicator organisms do not reflect the presence of *L. monocytogenes*. However, testing protocols for the genus *Listeria* are relatively fast and easy compared with species identification, and various *Listeria* species are more frequently encountered in the environment than *L. monocytogenes*. Thus, a test for environmental *Listeria* is an appropriate indicator for *L. monocytogenes*. By monitoring the processing plant for *Listeria* species, the effectiveness of sanitation practices can be verified, and problem hot spots can be identified and corrected in a timely fashion. Under the authority of federal regulations (9 CFR 430.4 and 21 CFR 110.80), environmental testing for *Listeria* is required in plants that produce ready-to-eat (RTE) food products. This requirement for *Listeria* testing has encouraged the development of commercially available test methods and kits.

Coliforms and pathogenic bacteria are themselves hosts to viruses, called *bacteriophages* or simply *phages*. Detection of phages is indicative of live or inactivated bacterial host cells. The abundance of phages is usually much greater than their bacterial hosts, and phages tend to survive better in the environment than their bacterial hosts. In fact, the survival of phages in the environment appears to parallel that of human enteric viruses (Muniain-Mujika et al. 2003). These attributes make phages promising indicators of contamination from feces and with pathogens—including enteric viruses. F+(male-specific) Coliphages, named after their host *E. coli*, have been studied as surrogate indicators of fecal contamination in foods such as meats and produce (Allwood et al. 2004; Hsu, Shieh, Sobsey 2002). Methods have also been developed for the detection of phages that infect *Enterococcus faecalis* (i.e., enterophages) as potential indicators of fecal pollution in water (Bonilla et al. 2010); this method may have applications in the future with food or shellfish harvesting waters. Other enterophages also have potential applications for shellfish sanitation; studies have shown the probability of detecting human enteric viruses in shellfish increases when phages specific to *Bacteroides fragilis* are detected (Muniain-Mujika et al. 2003).

Like other indicators, the biological and analytical attributes of phages represent a mix of tradeoffs. On the positive side, the turnaround time for results with phage testing is many hours shorter than with culturing the host indicator bacteria. On the negative side, sample preparation usually involves more elaborate steps (i.e., extraction and concentration of the phages), and the prepped sample must be analyzed using plaque assays incorporating log-phase bacterial hosts. Without a highly developed host cell system, nonindicator phages may cause plaques if their normal bacterial hosts are closely related to those of the host cell system. Newer technologies such as nucleic acid hybridization may offer easier analysis, but before phages are widely accepted as indicators, additional research, development, and validation are needed to improve testing methods and to fully characterize the relevance of specific phages in foods.

The final group of indicator organisms to be discussed is the heterotrophs. These microorganisms include a wide range of bacteria, yeasts, and molds. They are grown on nonselective culture media to obtain a viable cell count. For more than 100 years, viable cell counts of water, food, and other materials have been used to assess their quality and safety. The standardized testing methods for heterotrophs have changed over the years, and many procedural variations still exist in the literature. Test procedures have been called several different names over the years, with the most commonly cited names being *heterotrophic plate count*, *standard plate count*, *total plate count*, and *aerobic plate count*. Over the last two decades, the heterotrophic plate count has become the preferred name by drinking water authorities, whereas the other names are still used with certain applications (Reasoner 2004).

Compared with other indicator organisms, the heterotrophic microorganisms are loosely defined as a group. They typically include aerobic and facultative anaerobic mesophiles, both pathogens and nonpathogens, but typically exclude anaerobes, psychrophiles, thermophiles, and so forth. If desired, microbiologists can modify the test procedures and conditions to select for the groups typically excluded (Tortorello 2003). With food safety applications, plate counts of heterotrophic microorganisms are typically used as an indicator of bacterial loading and the effectiveness of sanitary practices and sanitizing rinses or treatments. Unless colonies are selected from the culture plate and subjected to additional testing, plate counts of heterotrophs do not distinguish between pathogens and nonpathogens, so they do not provide a direct indication of pathogen presence. Nevertheless, a large number of heterotrophic microorganisms on food contact surfaces or finished food products is indicative of an out-of-control process. Additional information on testing for heterotrophs is provided in the later section on standard plate counts.

### Biochemical Indicator Methods

The biochemical reactions of life produce compounds and energy changes that can be measured and used as an indicator of microorganisms. One of the most widely accepted biochemical indicator methods is adenosine triphosphate (ATP) bioluminescence. Because ATP is the source of energy in living cells, and because ATP disappears within 2 hours after cells die, the quantitative measurement of ATP provides an indicator of the mass and viability of cells. ATP bioluminescence can be accomplished using several techniques. Among the simplest techniques is the luciferin-luciferase system, the bioluminescent lighting system of fireflies. In the presence of ATP and oxygen, a two-step reaction by the enzyme luciferase transforms luciferin to oxyluciferin, AMP, and light. The amount of light produced is measured using a luminometer, and this measurement can be used to mathematically relate ATP levels to the biomass of cells, though it does not provide enumeration of microorganisms. The advantages of ATP bioluminescence for food safety include a rapid and quantitative method of estimating the microbial population or loading on food products or food contact surfaces.

Several different models of commercial ATP bioluminescent assays are designed to measure the ATP of microorganisms. Most of these assays incorporate reagents for cell lysis and filtration for removing somatic cell ATP. This is necessary to eliminate nonmicrobial ATP that may come from foods. ATP bioluminescent assays have been used to estimate bacterial contamination on the surfaces of meat and poultry carcasses, cantaloupes, and food equipment; and in drinking water and milk (Chen and Godwin 2006; Whitehead, Smith, Verran 2008). The rapidity of results from ATP bioluminescent assays make them valuable for HACCP system applications, especially if the system is automated for continuous monitoring. An important limitation of ATP bioluminescent assays is the nonspecific nature of their results. Unless ATP bioluminescence is coupled with other test methods (e.g., immunoassay), the measurement of ATP does not provide an indication of the microbial species present (Hunter and Lim 2010). Given this limitation, the best application of ATP bioluminescent assays is to monitor the efficacy of sanitary practices and antimicrobial treatments. For example, ATP bioluminescence assays could be used to monitor the food contact surfaces in a process to ensure effective sanitizing treatments.

Another biochemical indicator with a longer history of use does not measure the activity of microorganisms, yet it is considered important to the microbial safety of milk products. The milk from different animals contains variable amounts of an enzyme called *alkaline phosphatase* (ALP). This enzyme is deactivated at temperatures of 71.7°C with a duration of at least 15 seconds, a temperature slightly higher than the LTLT (low-temperature, long-time) method of pasteurization. Since the 1930s, the measurement of ALP activity has been used as an indicator of milk pasteurization and, by inference, the absence of pathogenic microorganisms. In reality, low ALP activity in milk does not guarantee the absence of pathogens. The reasons include the following: (1) the amount of ALP in raw milk is highly variable, including intra- and interspecies; (2) milk products can become contaminated with pathogens after pasteurization; and (3) ALP reactivation can occur over time, especially with milk pasteurized under HTST (high-temperature, short-time) conditions. Notwithstanding the previous reasons, whenever ALP activity exceeds the acceptable limit (currently 350 mU/L), improper pasteurization should be suspected, and the causes should be investigated immediately.

Over many decades, several methods and techniques were developed to measure ALP activity. These include the Scharer colorimetric method, introduced in 1938, and the Aschaffenburg and Mullen (A&M) method, introduced in 1949 (Payne and Wilbey 2009). Both of these methods are based on the enzyme-mediated (i.e., ALP) reaction of substrates that produce a colored compound, which is then measured using a color comparator or colorimeter. A more rapid and sensitive method has been developed based on a quantitative fluorometric technique (Klotz et al. 2008). With the fluorometric method, a nonfluorescent substrate is converted by ALP to a highly fluorescent product, and the results are measured using a fluorometer (AOAC International 1994). Because of the small amount of ALP in milk and high sensitivity of the fluorometric method, the results are expressed simply as milliunits per liter (mU/L). In 2005, the fluorometric method was mandated as the standard test system for dairy products in the United States, and the acceptable level of ALP in pasteurized milk was lowered from 500 mU/L to 350 mU/L (FDA 2009).

## Microscopic and Viable Cell Count Methods

For foodborne illness outbreak investigations, or surveillance activities, the precise identification and/or enumeration of pathogenic microorganisms are the primary goals. Similarly, the identification of species is necessary for monitoring programs aimed at pathogen reduction in foods. However, most routine microbiological examinations of foods involve monitoring indicator organisms, without necessarily identifying the particular species. Although not all inclusive, Table 7-2 lists some general microscopic and viable cell count methods for the aforementioned purposes. Newer methods and techniques are continuously being developed, but many of them are technological enhancements or combinations of those listed in Table 7-2.

### Standard Plate Count and Variations

The first method in Table 7-2 is the standard plate count, and variations thereof. Other terms that have been given for this method are the bacterial plate count, aerobic plate count, and het-

**Table 7-2** General Culture and Microscopic Methods of Viable Cell Counts

| Method | Description |
|---|---|
| Standard plate count and variations<br>　Conventional standard plate counts<br>　　Pour plating<br>　　Surface spread plating<br>　Spiral plate enumeration<br>　Redigel system | • Indicates the level of microorganisms in a product.<br>• Includes both nonpathogens and pathogens.<br>• Does not recover all microorganisms, for example, some anaerobes.<br>• Useful for quality control and possibly CCP monitoring. |
| Microscopic colony counts | Microcolonies are counted on a microscopic slide. |
| Agar droplets | Serial dilutions of agar droplets; colonies are counted with a 10× viewer. |
| Commercial matrix and culture medium systems (e.g., Petrifilm, SimPlate) | Homogenized sample is mixed with diluents and applied to the special material containing the culture medium. The results are read using a colony counter (Petrifilm) or measuring fluorescence in wells (SimPlate). |
| Membrane filter methods<br>　Coliform membrane filter method<br>　Direct epifluorescent filter technique (DEFT)<br>　Hydrophobic grid membrane filter (HGMF) | After being properly homogenized, the sample is drawn through a membrane filter that captures the microbes. Fluorescence or visible color changes are often used to identify coliform groups or specific species (e.g., DEFT). Special gridded filters allow MPN-type enumerations (e.g., HGMF). |
| Most probable number (MPN) | Statistical estimation of microbial numbers based on serial dilutions. |
| Nondestructive surfaces examination<br>　RODAC plates (and variations) | Touch agar on smooth surfaces and culture microbes. |
| Swab/swab-rinse methods | Swab rough surfaces for culturing. |
| Sticky film | Press surfaces with tape-like film and then culture microbes. |

*Source:* Compiled from Jay et al. 2005 and Fung 2002.

erotrophic plate count. Currently, the preferred term in water testing is the heterotrophic plate count, and many food microbiologists also prefer this term. This method is the most widely used in estimating the total number of viable cells in foods (Jay et al. 2005). Estimates of viable cells are based on counting the colony-forming unit (CFU), which represents at least one (or more) microorganism(s) capable of growing to form a visible colony. The conventional standard plate count starts with the blended or homogenized food sample, followed by serial dilutions with an appropriate diluent. The serial dilutions are then poured or spread on agar plates with a suitable culture medium, and after incubation at the correct temperature and time (e.g., 35°C for 48 hours), the plates are examined for colonies. Usually, only the agar plates with between 30 and 300 colonies are counted and reported as CFUs because this range of colonies is practical to count and because the colonies are less likely to spread or overlap one another, making it easier to discern individual colonies. To determine the density of viable microorganisms in the food, a simple mathematical calculation based on the amount of food and the appropriate dilution factor is used with the CFU count. Figure 7-3 provides an overview of a conventional standard plate count.

Several important points should be remembered about standard plate counts. First, the standard plate count estimates the total number of viable bacteria (or fungi with the appropriate culture medium). This includes both pathogens and nonpathogens, and unless colonies are selected for further testing, a distinction between them cannot be made. Second, only viable cells are detected. Some cells become metabolically injured before, during, or after sample collection. These microbial cells may not be detected with the standard plate count (see discussion on VBNC cells earlier). Third, although a nonselective culture medium is used, every culture medium has some degree of selectivity. Some species will not successfully compete with the other microbiota in the sample, or the culture medium may lack an essential nutrient or conversely contain an inhibitor. The conditions under which incubation occurs may also contribute to this

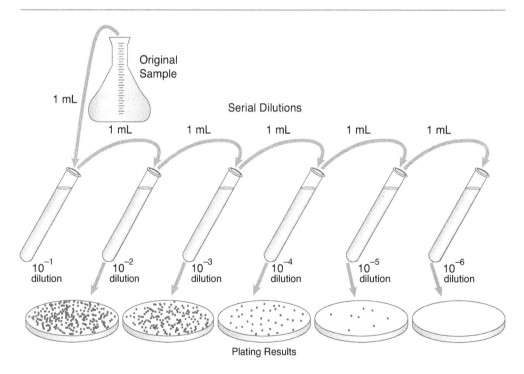

**Figure 7-3** Overview of a Conventional Standard Plate Count

selectivity. For example, strict aerobes usually encounter more favorable growth conditions on the surface of agar plates. And some microorganism (i.e., psychrotrophs) can be heat-sensitive to heated agar, or they may not grow as well at suboptimum temperatures during incubation. Finally, a problem occasionally occurs with "spreaders," that is, colonies that spread out and crowd other colonies, making the enumeration of CFUs difficult.

Technology provides automated alternatives to the conventional standard plate count. One such device is the spiral plater. This device works by dispensing liquefied sample on a rotating agar plate. As the agar plate rotates, the sample-dispensing stylus moves from the center toward the outer edge of the agar plate in an Archimedian spiral pattern. At the same time, the amount of dispensed sample progressively decreases toward the outer edge. In essence, this generates a systematic (or serial-type) dilution of the sample as it is deposited around the agar plate. After incubation, the colonies are counted in a zone where they are sufficiently spaced apart from one another. A calibrated grid determines the volume of sample dispensed in the colony counting zone, and the density of microorganisms in the sample is derived from dividing the CFUs by the dispensed sample volume. Of course, if the original sample was also diluted, the plating results must be adjusted by the amount of diluents added to the original sample.

The spiral plater has several advantages over the conventional standard plate count. The most obvious advantage is productivity. A trained technician can inoculate more than 50 agar plates per hour. Another advantage is the relative consistency in test results between different technicians. The automated plating performed by the device minimizes the potential for human error and individual differences in microbiological technique. A laser counter can be used to produce accurate results in seconds, and more recent versions of the spiral plater devices are fully automated, requiring the technician only to add the liquid sample (Fung 2002). The need for certain supplies (e.g., dilution bottles, pipettes) and auxiliary equipment is also minimized or eliminated. The overall agreement in results between the spiral plater and conventional standard plate count is considered favorable (Jay et al. 2005). Although the spiral plater has been used to test a variety of foods over the past 20 years, its major disadvantage is that solid foods must be fairly well liquefied to prevent particles from blocking the dispensing stylus.

The next two methods listed in Table 7-2 (microscope colony counts and agar droplets) are similar in principle to the standard plate count, but they are generally faster and require a microscope to count the very small colonies. Microscope colony counts involve spreading a very small mixture (0.1 mL) of liquid sample and agar over part of a glass slide. This is then incubated and afterward dried and stained. The microorganisms that reproduce appear as microcolonies and are counted using a microscope. The agar droplets method involves diluting food homogenate sample (1 mL) into a tube of melted agar. From this tube, a line of agar droplets is made onto the bottom of a sterile, empty Petri dish. A small portion of this tube (3 drops, each 0.1 mL) is also placed into a second tube of melted agar, from which another line of agar droplets in made onto the Petri dish. From the second tube of sample–agar mixture, a 3-drop portion is also transferred to a third melted agar tube. Again, a line of droplets from the third tube is placed onto the Petri dish. The overall transfer of inocula across tubes is equivalent to serial dilutions. After incubation for only 24 hours, the colonies are counted using a 10× viewer. The main advantages over the conventional standard plate count are a faster turnaround time for results and less time spent on the laborious procedures.

Several commercial systems have been developed that incorporate the culture medium within a matrix, onto which the sample can be introduced and then incubated. The Petrifilm system is composed of films that contain rehydratable nutrients, forming a plate about the size of a credit card. The sample is placed onto the film plates under a protective cover. After incubation, the colonies can be counted using an automated plate reader. Petrifilm plates are available with selective-differential culture media for several important groups of microorganisms, including total coliforms, *E. coli*, Enterobacteriaceae, *S. aureus*, and environmental *Listeria*.

Another type of commercial system is the SimPlate, consisting of a round plastic plate with 84 wells. The sample and culture medium are placed in the center of the plate and gently swirled around to fill the wells. Excess liquid is poured onto an absorbent pad, while the wells are designed to retain a precise amount of sample and culture medium. The plastic plate is incubated for 24 hours under 35°C temperature. The wells also contain specific biochemical substrates that produce a fluorescent signal when metabolized and exposed to a UV light. Based on the initial sample dilution and number of wells that produce a fluorescent signal, the most probable number (MPN) of microorganisms can be determined. SimPlate test kits are available for the total plate count, total coliforms, *E. coli*, yeast and mold counts, and *Campylobacter*.

### Membrane Filter Methods

Membrane filters were first developed in the 1930s, and almost immediately, they were used for research applications in microbiology. Over the years, a variety of practical applications in food and water protection have been developed using membrane filters. Typically, the membranes used for microfiltration have pore sizes ranging from 0.1 to 10 micrometers (μm). Pore sizes generally around 0.45 μm will retain bacteria. The primary advantage of using membrane filters is the ability to filter large volumes of sample to capture low densities of bacterial contaminants. Filters can be stained and examined directly using a microscope to count bacterial cells, but the addition of culture media allows the growth of colonies directly on the membrane filter. This demonstrates cell viability and facilitates the counting process. By using selective-differential culture media and special dyes or fluorescent markers, membrane filter methods can be efficient and effective tools in the identification and enumeration of different bacterial groups and/or species.

The most commonly performed membrane filter test is for coliform bacteria and generic *E. coli*—and the majority of these tests are performed to monitor water quality and safety. With food homogenates, the standard membrane filter is easily clogged, so these tests are best suited for liquid foods with low levels of particulate matter (FDA 2010a). To understand how the membrane filter method works, a summary of the procedures with the conventional membrane filter test for total coliform bacteria is provided here.

First, the appropriate amount of liquid sample is passed through the membrane filter with the assistance of a vacuum pump. The bacteria are captured on the membrane filter, which is then transferred to a dish containing a selective culture medium. For total coliforms, the culture medium typically consists of M-Endo medium or LES Endo Agar. Incubation is carried out at 35°C for 22–24 hours, and colonies with a pink to dark red color and green metallic surface sheen are counted. These results are considered presumptive and reported as CFUs/100 mL. To ensure the colonies are indeed coliforms, an additional two stages of confirmatory and completed testing are usually required. Confirmatory testing involves inoculating tubes of lauryl sulfate tryptose (LST) broth from selected colonies, and after incubation at 35°C for 48 hours, the LST tubes are checked for gas production. The LST tubes that are positive for gas production are used to inoculate tubes of brilliant green lactose bile (BGLB) broth for the completed testing stage. After another incubation period at 35°C for 48 hours, the presence of gas in BGLB tubes provides the confirmation of coliform bacteria. A separate "completed" test step can also be performed to test whether the coliforms are of fecal origin.

The conventional membrane filter test described here is designed to identify/enumerate only total coliform bacteria. Fortunately, several different formulations of culture media that now allow for the presumptive detection of total coliforms, fecal coliforms, and/or generic *E. coli* on the same membrane filter have become commercially available. Such culture media are usually sold as part of test kits or systems, and many of them are validated by AOAC International, a widely recognized and nonprofit association that publishes standardized methods for chemical and microbiological analyses.

One test system (i.e., ISO-GRID) includes a variation of the membrane filter known as the hydrophobic grid membrane filter (HGMF). The HGMF is used to test many different food products by first prefiltering diluted samples through a 5-μm filter to remove larger particles. The HGMF is constructed with 1,600 wax squares, and after the sample is filtered, the HGMF is placed on an agar plate containing the culture medium with special dyes. During incubation, microbial growth and colony sizes are restricted within the individual wax squares. The dyes are not absorbed by the HGMF, which provides better contrast for easier identification and enumeration of microorganisms. Rather than counting individual colonies, the 1,600 wax squares with growth are counted as colonies, and the microbes are enumerated using a statistically based MPN procedure; instruments are also available that count the squares in a matter of seconds.

The versatility of HGMF test systems provides additional advantages. Most test systems are made with interchangeable components that expand or enhance capabilities. For example, different commercially available culture media can be purchased to identify and enumerate other important foodborne microorganisms. Besides coliforms and generic *E. coli*, culture media are available for total bacterial counts, *Salmonella*, *Listeria*, *E. coli* O157:H7, yeasts and molds, and other microorganisms. Specialized culture media are also available to enrich the growth of selected microorganisms, resuscitate injured microorganisms, and perform confirmatory testing for *E. coli*. If properly validated and performed, HGMF tests produce results that are statistically equivalent to the golden standard methods of culturing.

A useful modification of the membrane filter method is the direct epifluorescent filter technique (DEFT). With this technique, the sample is filtered to entrap the microorganisms, and the microbial cells are then stained with a fluorescent dye. Using an epifluorescent microscope, a microbiologist can enumerate the total number of microorganisms. If the enumeration of a specific pathogen or indicator organism is desired, DEFT can be adapted using a fluorescent-antibody that binds to the target organism. The major advantage of using DEFT is the rapid turnaround for test results, approximately 30 minutes. This technique has been used for a variety of applications ranging from enumeration of *E. coli* O157:H7 in beef to assessing the efficacy of food irradiation (Arujo et al. 2009; Tortorello and Stewart 1994). A disadvantage of DEFT is the inability to determine the viability of microbial cells. However, a variation of the technique called *microcolony-DEFT* can determine cell viability. This is accomplished by placing the membrane filter on culture media and incubating it from 3 to 8 hours, followed by counting the microcolonies. Another variation combines DEFT and HGMF technologies to greatly enhance overall capabilities.

### Most Probable Number Culture Methods

Particles in homogenized food samples can clog membrane filters or interfere with accurate colony counts on agar plates. These problems are minimized by putting aliquots of sample in culture broth tubes for incubation. However, enumerating the microorganisms in broth tubes is problematic. The most probable number (MPN) culture method accomplishes enumeration in broth tubes by serially diluting the food sample and statistically estimating the microbial population by using a formula or lookup tables. The basic premise is that serial dilutions of the original sample decrease the sample population, and eventually some tubes will contain viable microbes (i.e., positive tubes) while others will not (i.e., negative tubes). Enumeration by MPN is based on several assumptions (FDA 2010a). The first assumption is that microorganisms in both the food sample and culture broth are randomly distributed and dispersed. Inocula transferred to other tubes are assumed to represent discrete sampling events that follow the Poisson distribution, where each "outcome" is either a positive or negative event. Another assumption is that every inoculum with even one microbial cell will produce growth, usually detectable by the production of gas or color change in the tube (i.e., positive result). Obviously, these assumptions are ideal and cannot be verified for every test. Nonetheless, because of their simplicity and agreement in results between laboratories, the MPN culture methods are very popular.

Figure 7-4 illustrates the basic procedure for the MPN culture method. In theory, the MPN culture method can be used for any pathogen with the appropriate selective culture broth. It is the preferred method for determining the densities of coliform bacteria. Any number of dilutions can be used to compute the MPN, but procedures often specify three or more serial dilutions based on a decimal series (e.g., $1.0 \rightarrow 0.10 \rightarrow 0.010 \rightarrow$ and so forth). Using more tubes per each dilution increases the precision of the test results; this also increases the amount of tubes and labor needed for each test. Confidence intervals or limits have become incorporated into lookup tables—usually for 95% confidence. In other words, there is 95% confidence that the actual density of microorganisms in the original sample lies within the confidence interval's upper and lower levels. The statistically based methodology of the MPN has been used since the early 1900s, and MPN-like procedures have been incorporated into the designs of newer and automated test systems (e.g., SimPlate and ISO-GRID HGMF). Thus, the MPN procedure is likely to remain a component of many quantitative test systems for microorganisms.

### Nondestructive Sample Collection and Culture Methods for Microbiological Examination of Surfaces

The surfaces of foods and equipment are often sampled to monitor the effectiveness of sanitary practices and pathogen prevention programs. One method for the surface sampling of foods is by excision (including scoring, scraping, and abrading) followed by sample preparation and

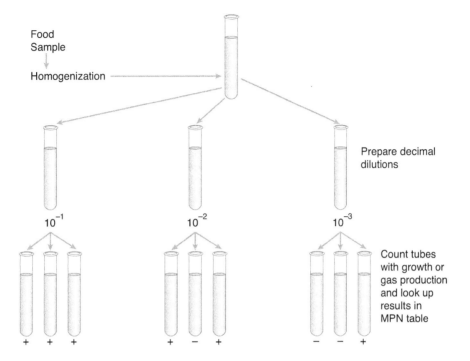

**Figure 7-4** General Procedure for a Most Probable Number (MPN) Analysis

analysis using standard methods. This method provides the most effective and reproducible testing results, mostly because it recovers nearly all the microorganisms attached to the surface (Capita, Prieto, Alonso-Calleja 2004). The disadvantages of this method include its invasive and destructive nature, the expertise required by the sampling technician, and time-consuming aspects. In comparison, nondestructive surface sampling is considered more practical and economically feasible, though it has several shortcomings.

Nondestructive sampling of surfaces poses special challenges because surfaces have physical characteristics that may interfere with effective sample collection. The surfaces of foods and equipment typically have different porosities, smoothness/roughness, shapes, moisture content, and firmness. In addition, different nondestructive techniques and materials are available and used to sample the surfaces. All these differences influence the overall recovery rate of microorganisms attached to the surface. Although some nondestructive methods may correlate with the excision method, the nondestructive methods do not recover all the microorganisms attached to the surface, and results tend to be more variable compared with the excision method. Additional concerns are the units to use in reporting the results (e.g., viable cells or CFUs per surface area). Several methods and techniques have been developed to facilitate the nondestructive sampling and analysis of surfaces. Some of the most common methods are briefly discussed in this section.

The oldest and most popular method of sample collection from a surface is by swabbing it. This method has changed somewhat over the years with refined techniques and materials, but the basic approach remains the same. First, a sterile and moistened swab is used to thoroughly rub a surface. A sterile template is usually placed over the surface to focus sampling in certain areas and to calculate the contamination/surface area ratio. Next, the swab sample is placed in a vial or other sealable container with a known volume of diluent. After being shaken, the diluent is used with a nonselective or selective culture medium to enumerate the microorganisms in a manner similar to the standard plate count. A major advantage of the swabbing method over other non-destructive methods is ability to sample rough or irregular-shaped surfaces. The shortcoming of this method is the high variability in results. When sampling meat and poultry carcasses, the recovery rate of bacteria using the swabbing method ranges from 0.01% to 89% compared with the excision method (Capita et al. 2004). Factors that contribute to this variability include the swab material, specific techniques used to sample a surface, and the degree of microorganism attachment to the surface.

Materials used for swabs include cotton, gauze, alginate, and polyester-bonded cloth. Some swabs are sponges made from cellulose or polyurethane. The more abrasive-type materials seem to improve recovery of microorganisms from a surface. Specific swabbing techniques also influence the recovery rates of microorganisms. For example, the wet-dry swabbing technique is considered more effective than the single swab technique is. With the wet-dry swabbing technique, a wet swab is first used followed by a dry swab, and both swabs are used for the sample preparation. Other variations in technique result from pressure applied during swabbing, timing of swabbing, and differences in technician skill and competency. These latter variations in technique can be minimized with detailed SOPs, technician training, and quality assurance programs. With regard to the degree of microorganism attachment to the surface, this phenomenon is complex and not fully characterized. Important determinants include the physicochemical properties of the surface, the microbial species present, and the stage of attachment (reversible or irreversible adhesion, penetration, biofilm development, etc.).

A convenient and established method of sampling environmental surfaces is the RODAC (Replicate Organism Direct Agar Contact) or contact plate. First described in the public health literature by Hall and Hartnett (1964), the RODAC plates are small plastic dishes into which a nonselective or selective culture medium with agar is poured. The main distinctions between RODAC plates and similar Petri dishes are the amount of agar and the plate design. RODAC plates are completely filled with culture media and agar to form a convex surface extending above the plate brim. After the agar is hardened, the RODAC plates can be pressed or rolled across a smooth surface to sample microbial contamination. The RODAC plates are designed to prevent the covers from contacting the agar, and they can be stacked together and placed directly into an incubator. Colonies that form on the agar surface are counted after the appropriate incubation period.

Best suited to monitor the effectiveness of sanitary practices, RODAC plates are designed to sample surfaces that are nonporous, firm, and smooth. When used to sample surfaces where detergents and sanitizers were applied, a neutralizer is necessary to avoid inhibiting growth on the agar. The disadvantages of RODAC plates include possible interference by spreader colonies on the agar and that they are not as effective with heavily contaminated surfaces. The recovery rate of microbiota from a surface with RODAC plates varies but represents a small percentage of the total, and the results are actually better when low numbers of microorganisms are encountered (Jay et al. 2005). In general, with smooth and nonporous surfaces, the RODAC plate method correlates well with swabbing surfaces for the recovery of microorganisms.

Several innovative methods have been developed over the years that are similar in principle to the RODAC plates. One such method involves using an "agar syringe." This device works by extruding a portion of agar beyond the end of a small barrel-shaped syringe, and the agar is pressed against the surface to be sampled. The agar end is then sliced off, put in a Petri dish, and incubated for the enumeration of colonies. A similar method called the "agar sausage" uses plastic tubing instead of a syringe device. More recently, an innovative adhesive tape and pop-up dispenser have been developed to sample the surfaces of meats (Fung 2002). After the sterile tape is pressed against the meat's surface, it is transferred to an agar surface for incubation. The viable cell counts using the adhesive tape method are highly correlated with the swabbing method.

## IMMUNOLOGICAL LABORATORY METHODS

Knowledge provided by immunology research has led to the development of several important laboratory methods for infectious disease control, as well as for food safety. The basic phenomenon underlying most of these methods is the binding of antibodies to antigens. This binding property has been quantified in terms of sensitivity and specificity. In general terms, *sensitivity* refers to the "minimum level of antigen or antibody that can be detected by a given test," whereas *specificity* refers to the "ability of a particular assay to distinguish one antigen from another" (Dick and Parrish 2007). Immunological laboratory methods are widely used and established technologies that have contributed immensely to the identification and characterization of pathogens. In turn, these methods provide an epidemiologic tool to study the incidence, prevalence, transmission, and sources of pathogenic agents—particularly foodborne pathogens. For this reason, food safety professionals should be familiar with the basic principles of immunological laboratory methods.

As described initially in Chapter 2, an antigen is any chemical substance that can evoke an immune response. The antigenic molecule can be alone or attached to another molecule. When a foreign antigen is introduced into an organism with a functioning immune system, specialized antibodies, also called *immunoglobulins* (Ig), are produced, and these antibodies can be extracted from the blood serum. These serum antibodies are further classified by isotype, with the most commonly measured isotypes designated as IgM and IgG antibodies. The IgM antibodies usually appear rapidly in the serum after an infection, peaking around 7–10 days, and they decline in abundance over several weeks. In contrast, the IgG antibodies are not detectable until about 4–6 weeks following an infection, and once the IgG antibodies appear, they persist longer than IgM antibodies. These differences in the timing and abundance of antibodies provide the clinician with important clues about the patient's stage of infection.

Antigens have special sites called *determinants* or *epitopes,* where specific and complementary antibodies bind. The illustration presented earlier, Figure 2-8, shows an antigen with several determinants and the typical locations of antigens associated with a bacterial cell. The strength of binding to a single antigenic determinant with the antibody's combining site is called the *antibody affinity.* Antibody molecules may also have a different number of binding sites for antigenic determinants. Similarly, antigens may have multiple determinants on the same molecule—either multiple copies of the same determinant and/or different determinants for other antibodies. When antigens or antibodies have multiple binding sites, they are referred to as *multivalent.* The overall stability of an antigen–antibody complex depends on the antibody affinity, multivalent nature of the reactions, and structural arrangements of the molecular parts. Together, these three factors determine the specificity of an antibody. In some cases, antibodies may bind to determinants on other antigens, forming a cross-reaction complex. The reason for cross-reactions may be that the other antigens have identical or structurally similar determinants to those on the target antigen.

Immunological laboratory methods exploit the high specificity of antibodies for their homologous antigens. Even in the presence of contaminating molecules, the multivalent interaction of antibodies and antigens is usually sufficient to form a precipitate. More sophisticated methods have been developed that involve immobilizing the antigens or antibodies on a surface and labeling them with enzymes, radioactive elements, or fluorescent molecules. These sophisticated methods offer greater sensitivity than earlier methods that rely on precipitation reactions. Furthermore, the sensitivity and/or specificity of tests can be manipulated by the use of monoclonal and polyclonal antibodies. Monoclonal antibodies are produced *in vitro* and consist of a homogeneous population of antibodies that will bind with only one specific type of determinant on the antigen. In comparison, polyclonal antibodies are derived *in vivo* (from animals), and they are a heterogeneous mix of antibodies that will bind with different determinants on the antigen. Both types of antibodies have advantages and disadvantages that differ with the particular application.

## Agglutination and Hemagglutination Inhibition Assays

Agglutination is when particles in a liquid suspension collect together and form clumps. If antigens or antibodies are immobilized on a particle, the presence of homologous antibodies or antigens in sufficient concentrations results in agglutination. This is the basis of the agglutination assay. Biological fluids are often assayed using polystyrene beads and latex particles coated with specific antigens or antibodies. If the homologous antibody or antigen is present, agglutination will occur, and the test result is considered positive. Agglutination assays are relatively fast and can be performed in a tube or on a microscope slide. Photometric detection and measurement of agglutination can also be performed. Because many antigens from bacterial pathogens are already attached to particles derived from cellular structures, agglutination methods are especially useful for serotyping applications (see serotyping as described in the next section).

Hemagglutination inhibition assays are used mostly for viral identification, and to a lesser degree for identifying or subtyping bacterial pathogens. Several types of viruses and bacteria have proteins that will agglutinate red blood cells (RBCs). If antibodies to the pathogen are available in the serum, they will bind with the antigenic proteins of the pathogen, which in turn inhibits agglutination of the RBCs. Thus, the presence of antibodies to the pathogen inhibits hemagglutination, indicating a possible infection, whereas the absence of antibodies permits hemagglutination, indicating an absence of infection.

## Serotyping

The importance of serotyping schemes for several pathogens is discussed in Chapter 2. The laboratory methods for serotyping involve using antiserum that contains the appropriate antibodies to detect homologous antigens. For particulate antigens, which include many of those associated with foodborne pathogens, agglutination methods can be used. The particulate antigens of bacterial pathogens are classified by location using the letters O, H, and K for the cell wall, flagellum, and capsule, respectively. For nonparticulate and soluble antigens, such as those associated with toxins, other methods must be used (e.g., gel diffusion). The combinations of different antigen–antibody complexes are used in serotyping schemes to differentiate pathogens into different strains and subtypes. Some serotyping schemes are also useful as markers of virulence (e.g., *E. coli* O157:H7).

Although serotyping is a useful tool for epidemiologic investigations and surveillance, it has several limitations. First, in the last couple of decades newer molecular methods that offer better discriminatory power to classify pathogens into different strains and subtypes have become available. Additionally, the antisera for specific pathogens must be maintained, and the availability of antisera for different bacterial pathogens is limited. Another limitation is the relatively higher expense of serotyping compared with other methods. Despite these limitations, the cumulative knowledge and historical momentum from serotyping have made it invaluable for foodborne pathogens such as pathogenic *E. coli*, *Salmonella* serovars, *Campylobacter* species, *Listeria* species, and others. In an effort to retain cumulative knowledge acquired from serotyping, many scientists are working toward linking the serotypes to genotypes (Ballmer et al. 2007; Wise et al. 2009). This is plausible in theory because the serotype is a phenotype based on expression of the organism's genes (though it does not account for environmental influences and posttranslational modifications). If successfully validated, PCR-based technologies could be used to rapidly ascertain the serotype, reducing the laboratory time from days or weeks to hours.

## Radioimmunoassays

When an antigen or antibody is labeled with a radioactive isotope, it can be easily detected with a radiation counter. By mixing a radiolabeled antigen or antibody with its unlabeled and homologous counterpart, a radiolabled antigen–antibody complex is formed. Antibodies are usually electrostatically attached to polymers to form a solid phase. After removing any unbound radiolabeled molecules, the remaining antigen–antibody complexes can be assayed using a radiation counter. This method is highly sensitive and can detect nanogram (ng) quantities of molecules. The downside of using radioimmunoassays is the difficulty of using radioisotopes under the tight restrictions of a radiation safety program.

The high degree of sensitivity with radioimmunoassays makes them particularly suited for detecting toxins (Jay et al. 2005). Radioimmunoassays have been used to detect staphylococcal enterotoxins, endotoxins, shellfish (algal) toxins, and other toxins. This method can also be used to detect bacterial cells in a matter of minutes. Although highly sensitive, the use of radioimmunoassays in food microbiology has declined substantially in favor of less-restrictive and more portable methods of analysis.

## Fluorescent Antibody Method

Instead of using radiolabels, the fluorescent antibody method employs a fluorescent molecule as a tag or label to an antibody. The fluorescence is then detected using a special fluorescent microscope. There are direct and indirect fluorescent antibody techniques. With the direct technique, the primary antibody is tagged with the fluorescent molecule. After the fluorescent-tagged antibody and homologous antigen bind together, any excess fluorescent antibody is removed or washed away, and the antigen–antibody complex is easily detected. Hence, the direct technique is used to detect an antigen of interest. With the indirect technique, the primary antibody is not tagged directly with the fluorescent molecule. Instead, an antibody to the primary antibody (i.e., anti-immunoglobulin) is tagged. When the antibody, antigen, and anti-immunoglobulin are incubated together, a complex consisting of all three compounds is formed. In contrast with the direct technique, the indirect technique is designed to detect an antibody of interest.

The indirect fluorescent antibody technique is used most often in clinical testing to diagnose infectious diseases. Major advantages of this technique are the ability to differentiate between IgM and IgG antibodies and its sensitivity and specificity for identifying viruses. Although fluorescent antibody techniques have been used extensively in the past in food microbiology, they have become less popular compared with newer molecular methods.

## Enzyme-Linked Immunosorbent Assay and Enzyme Immunoassay

Since it was first invented in 1971, enzyme-linked immunosorbent assay (ELISA) has undergone numerous modifications and has become one of the most widely used methods in biology and medicine. Known also as the enzyme immunoassay (EIA) and by other names, the ELISA procedure consists of multiple steps that bind antibodies to antigens and/or to other antibodies, followed by washing steps. One set of the antibodies or antigens is attached to a solid phase to prevent their removal, and any excess and unbound materials are removed during the washing steps. One set of the antibodies is also labeled with an enzyme that will produce a detectable signal when the appropriate chromogenic substrate is added. The resulting enzyme-mediated color change is measured using a spectrophotometer; the amount of target antibody or antigen present in the sample is a function of the color intensity.

Many variations of the ELISA exist, and different adjectives are used to describe these techniques based on the underlying principles of operation. Sometimes the adjectives can be confusing or misleading, and some authors use the terms interchangeably, adding to the confusion. Terms such as *direct, indirect, sandwich, double sandwich, competitive,* and *noncompetitive* are used. Figure 7-5 illustrates the general principle of a direct ELISA test for detecting an antigen of interest (i.e., target). Variations include the "sandwiching" of antibodies using other antibodies (i.e., anti-immunoglobulins). With classic ELISA techniques, one set of the antibodies must be linked with an enzyme capable of changing a colorless substrate to a colored product for detection. With some ELISA techniques, the target antibody must compete with the enzyme-linked antibody for binding sites; in these competitive ELISA tests, the amount of target antibody in the sample is inversely proportional to the color change. Regardless of the principles of operation, all ELISA techniques must undergo a lengthy optimization process before they can be used in practice. Fur-

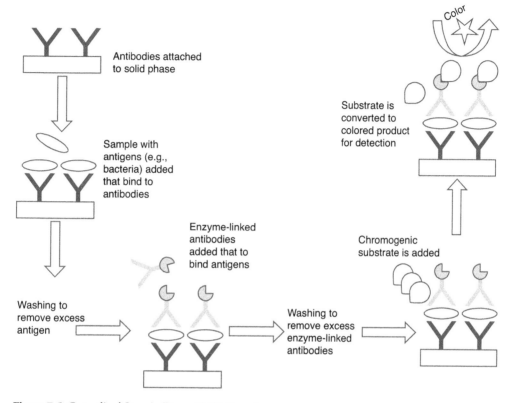

**Figure 7-5** Generalized Steps in Direct ELISA Procedure

thermore, the user of an ELISA test must be proficient in the procedures and should understand the underlying principles of its operation.

For infectious disease control purposes, the ELISA techniques are designed primarily to detect either antigen-specific antibodies or microbial antigens. The former technique is useful for diagnosing patients with an infectious disease because most people who are exposed to infectious agents produce antigen-specific antibodies. Microbial antigens, on the other hand, are associated directly with the pathogen. Thus, the ELISA technique that detects microbial antigens is used to identify pathogens in foods, and sometimes in certain clinical specimens of infected patients. Microbial antigens may also include toxins if they possess antigenic determinants. The detection limit of pathogens in foods using ELISA is $10^3$–$10^5$ CFUs/mL, while the detection limit of toxins in foods is a few nanograms (ng) or less per mL (Jay et al. 2005; Mandal et al. 2011; Radcliffe and Holbrook 2000). This means that the ELISA is particularly well suited for detecting toxins, whereas the detection of pathogenic bacteria in foods usually requires an enrichment step to increase cell numbers. Commercial ELISA test kits are available for common foodborne pathogens and toxins. However, these test kits are often designed for patient diagnosis and have been adapted for detecting pathogens in foods. A partial list of ELISA-based test kits is provided in Appendix 1 of FDA's *Bacteriological Analytical Manual* (FDA 2010a).

In recent years, ELISA-like techniques have been developed that amplify the detection signal or use different signal molecules. Instead of an "enzyme-linked" antibody, these newer assays may utilize fluorogenic, electrochemiluminescent, real-time PCR, and other molecular signaling "reporters" with the antibodies. Such assays are much more sensitive and quantifiable compared with traditional ELISA techniques, though many of them still need to be validated. Because these newer immunoassays lack an enzyme-linked reporter, they are not technically considered ELISA techniques. The term *enzyme immunoassay*, or EIA, is somewhat more inclusive of these types of assays.

## MOLECULAR GENETIC AND NUCLEIC ACID METHODS

The analysis of nucleic acids has played a role in the identification of microorganisms for many years, but this role has become increasingly important with advances in molecular biology and technology. Without question, the invention of polymerase chain reaction (PCR) and gene probes has revolutionized research biology and medicine, including the field of food microbiology, and these techniques will continue to make an impact in the future. Technologies that analyze nucleic acids are becoming faster, more high throughput, and cheaper to perform. More important, these technologies are proven to be highly reliable and useful in disease outbreak investigations and food safety.

The encoded instructions of life reside in the DNA and RNA. The flow of biological information is represented by a simple paradigm that has been around since the 1950s:

DNA is transcribed by mRNA → mRNA is translated into amino acid sequences by tRNA →
Amino acid sequences make up proteins that become phenotypic characteristics of an organism.

Research over the past several decades has added much to this simple paradigm. Scientists now understand more about the regulation of DNA transcription, posttranscriptional modifications of mRNA (e.g., alternative splicing), and posttranslational modifications of proteins. Any of these activities can influence the final gene products and overall phenotypic expression. The relevance of multiple genes on a phenotypic trait has also become recognized as more important. And the transfer of genes and mutations are better understood in terms of adaptation and survival. Finally, it is now recognized that the relationship between genes and the environment is not dichotomous; genes and the environment interact to alter phenotypic expression. This is facilitated by molecular tags on the DNA (e.g., methylation), and it permits short-term and reversible adaptations to environmental changes without altering the DNA's nucleotide sequence. Such modifications to the DNA are called *epigenetic mechanisms*.

The differences in species and strains of organisms can be traced to the nucleotide sequences of their respective genomes. The genome of an organism is the entire complement of hereditary information encoded in the DNA, or RNA for many viruses. For bacteria, the genome includes both the chromosomal DNA and plasmids—those small, circular segments of DNA present in the cytoplasm. Alterations in the genomes of bacteria can occur from mutations, mobile genetic elements (e.g., transposons), and genetic transfer between cells (e.g., transformation, transduction, conjugation). In the past, the sequencing of genes and plasmids were painstakingly slow and difficult to accomplish. Nowadays, automated sequencers are commonplace, and the entire genomes of many organisms have been sequenced. To date, more than 1,100 organisms' genomes have been sequenced and published, and more than 5,800 genome sequencing projects are in various stages of completion (Liolios et al. 2010). More than 4,172 of the sequencing projects involve bacterial genomes. Among these bacteria are several important foodborne pathogens.

Although several important advancements in molecular biology and technology have enabled the current capabilities, three tools stand out as critically important to the analysis of DNA and RNA. These tools are polymerase chain reaction (PCR) and other amplification chemistry, restriction endonucleases, and nucleotide sequence information and libraries. The invention of PCR enabled the amplification of extremely small quantities of DNA to larger quantities for subsequent analysis. The capability to amplify nucleic acids is a major advantage over using other macromolecules such as proteins, which require culturing organisms and separation techniques to produce sufficient quantities of material. Many variations of PCR currently exist, and other amplification chemistry methods have been developed over the years, but the conventional PCR methods are still widely used. Conventional PCR methods are performed using a thermocycler. This is a laboratory instrument that repeatedly cycles through programmed temperature stages to facilitate the PCR steps. A single cycle in conventional PCR consists of the following steps:

1. The sample piece of double-stranded DNA to be amplified is isolated and placed in the reaction vessel.
2. The vessel is heated to 95°C to disrupt the hydrogen bonds between the two strands of DNA, denaturing the DNA into two single strands. These two single strands of DNA represent the templates for amplification.
3. Primers consisting of single-stranded oligonucleotides (17–24 nucleotide bases) are annealed to complementary bases pairs on the single-stranded DNA. This requires a temperature range of 50°–60°C, depending on the nucleotide composition of the primers. Pairing between the primers and single-stranded DNA is highly specific and necessary for polymerase activity.
4. The temperature of the vessel is raised to 72°C to optimize polymerase activity. The enzyme *Taq* DNA polymerase is responsible for synthesizing new DNA by adding nucleotide bases that are complementary to those of the single-stranded DNA template. This results in two sets of double-stranded DNA identical to the original sample.
5. The preceding cycle (denaturation, annealing, and synthesis) is repeated many times to form a chain reaction. Each cycle doubles the amount of double-stranded DNA from the original sample. For example, 30 cycles produce more than 1 billion copies of the original sample DNA.

The discovery and use of restriction endonucleases (a.k.a. restriction enzymes) is another standout tool for the analysis of nucleic acids. These restriction enzymes are derived from bacteria that use them to "cut up" nucleic acids of invading bacteriophages. Restriction endonucleases cut double-stranded DNA at points where an exact sequence of four to six nucleotides exists. For example, a restriction endonuclease called EcoRI (derived from *E. coli*) cuts DNA wherever the nucleotide sequence GAATTC exists; the enzymatic cut by EcoRI actually occurs between the G and A of the sequence. Hundreds of different restriction endonucleases are commercially available and used to manipulate DNA. The availability of restriction endonucleases is analogous to having scissors capable of cutting DNA at precise locations. This allows scientists to cut the DNA strands at precise places for further analysis using DNA sequencing and by comparing different DNA fragment sizes.

The third standout tool for the analysis of nucleic acids is the availability of nucleotide sequence information and libraries. The nucleotide sequence of genes is important to identifying different species and strains of microorganisms. Furthermore, nucleotide sequence information is necessary to develop genetic probes and other tools for nucleic acid analysis. Massive amounts of data have been accumulated in computerized databases on the nucleotide sequences of genes and genomes. Multiple sources of sequence information exist, but the three most prominent sources are genome sequence databases, the National Center for Biological Information (NCBI), and independent collections of genotypic patterns and/or nucleotide sequences called *libraries*. Special computer programs have been developed to search for similarities among nucleotide sequences in databases, and a new discipline called bioinformatics has emerged to analyze and interpret the massive amounts of molecular biology data.

With knowledge about a particular nucleotide sequence from a species or strain of organism, scientists can naturally derive or synthesize a nucleic acid probe to detect that sequence. Essentially, a nucleic acid probe is a piece of DNA that anneals to the complementary nucleotide sequence in a target DNA or RNA. The resulting double-stranded nucleic acid is considered a hybrid, and the process of the probe and target strands combining together is called *hybridization*. Segments of DNA or RNA that are approximately 50 nucleotides long or less are called *oligonucleotides*. Nucleic acid probes can be the length of oligonucleotides or longer. Because the hybridization of two nucleic acid strands (probe and target) depends on their sequences being complementary, the specificity of the test probe is extremely high. As for the sensitivity of a test probe, it is greatly dependent on the amount of target nucleic acid present in the sample and the type of reporter group used to label the probe. Common types of reporters include radioisotopes and fluorescent or chemiluminescent compounds. Nucleic acid probes are used with several different methods to detect and subtype foodborne pathogens.

The three tools described here are essential to the molecular genetic and nucleic acid methods of analysis. In general, the nucleic acid methods used in microbiology are divided into two broad categories: (1) methods that require information about nucleotide sequences, and (2) methods for which detailed information about nucleotide sequences is unnecessary (e.g., fingerprinting methods). The following sections briefly describe several important methods and generalized steps associated with these two categories.

### Detection of Pathogenic Bacteria Using Nucleic Acid Gene Probes and PCR

To illustrate how nucleic acid probes can be used to detect foodborne pathogenic bacteria, the basic method of colony hybridization in FDA's *Bacteriological Analytical Manual* is described (see Figure 7-6). This test method starts with an aliquot of homogenized food sample spread across an appropriate agar culture medium. The culture plate is then incubated to produce visible colonies;

these colonies typically form a pattern over the plate's surface. Next, a solid support made of a membrane or filter paper is pressed against the culture plate to transfer portions of the colonies to the solid support. The colonial pattern on the culture plate is also captured as a mirror-type image on the solid support. The bacterial cells on the solid support are lysed to release DNA by subjecting them to a combination of high pH and temperature. This is accomplished with 0.5 molar NaOH and by using steam and/or microwave irradiation. The genomic DNA released by the lysed bacterial cells becomes denatured and affixed to the solid support.

At this point in the procedure, nucleic acid probes labeled with either a radioisotope (e.g., $^{32}$P) or a reporter enzyme are incubated with the denatured DNA on the solid support. The choice of probe depends on the species or subtype to be identified and availability of the desired probe. Table 7-3 is a partial list of nucleic acid probes available to detect pathogenic bacteria in foods. These probes are based on either the whole or partial sequence of select genes in the bacteria. During incubation, the gene probes hybridize with complementary nucleotide sequences of the bacteria's DNA. Any excess gene probes that do not hybridize are removed from the solid support with a washing step. The appropriate temperature and salt concentration is important during the washing step. The correct temperature is particularly important and usually determined from empirical observations. If washing temperatures are too high, they break the hydrogen bonds of the hybrid DNA. If the washing temperatures are too low, they cause some probes to misalign with the target DNA and form noncomplementary strands. The formation of noncomplementary strands can lead to false-positive test results.

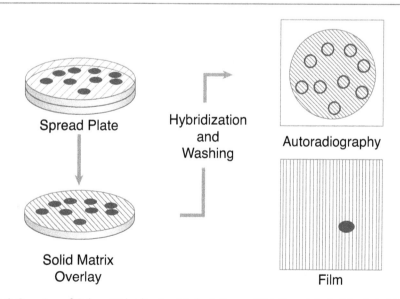

**Figure 7-6** Overview of Colony Hybridization Method. *Source:* FDA Bacteriological Analytical Manual

**Table 7-3** Some Gene Probes Used to Detect Pathogenic Bacteria in Foods

| Bacteria | Target |
| --- | --- |
| *Campylobacter jejuni* | r-RNA |
| *Escherichia coli* | Heat-stable toxin (ST) |
| | Heat-labile toxin (LT) |
| | Shiga-like toxins |
| | Invasive genes |
| | O157:H7 |
| *Listeria* species | r-RNA |
| *L. monocytogenes* | Listeriolysin O |
| | Major secreted polypeptide (*msp*) |
| *Salmonella* species | r-RNA |
| *Shigella* species | Invasive genes |
| *Staphylococcus aureus* | Enterotoxin B |
| *Vibrio cholerae* | Cholera enterotoxin |
| *V. parahaemolyticus* | Thermostable direct hemolysin (*tdh*) |
| *V. vulnificus* | Cytotoxin-hemolysin |
| *Yersinia enterocolitica* | Cytotoxicity/Sereny |
| | Invasive gene (*ail*) |
| *Y. pseudotuberculosis* | Invasive gene |

*Source:* FDA Bacteriological Analytical Manual.

The final steps of the procedure are detection of hybrid DNA and interpretation of the results. With radioisotope-labeled probes, a process called *autoradiography* is used. In this process, an X-ray film covers the solid support, and radioactive decay from the labeled gene probes causes the film to be exposed. The film is then developed, and the exposed portions appear as dark spots wherever a colony with hybrid DNA is located. The results are interpreted by assuming each exposed spot represents a CFU of the pathogenic bacterium. The final concentration of bacteria in the sample is determined by multiplying the CFUs by the appropriate dilution factor. In recent years, nonradioactive labels (e.g., fluorescent) have been used with gene probes; the images of the fluorescent signals can be captured using special digital cameras.

The direct detection of bacterial DNA in foods using nucleic acid probes is not practical, at least not at the present time. Large copy numbers of the target DNA are needed for detection whenever using nucleic acid probes. One solution to this problem is to amplify the copy numbers of target DNA using PCR techniques. But even with PCR-based amplification, an enrichment culture of the sample is often necessary first. After inocula are taken from the enrichment culture, the PCR is carried out in a thermocycler using the appropriate primers, DNA polymerase, and free nucleotides. Multiple cycles of PCR are performed (typically between 30 and 40 cycles) to obtain sufficient quantities of the target DNA. Before nucleic acid probes can be used to detect complementary sequences in the target DNA, some sort of solid support is needed to anchor either the probes or target DNA. This is necessary to prevent the loss of hybridized DNA during washing steps to remove excess probes and other materials. The types of solid support used include membranes (e.g., Southern blotting), dipsticks, bottoms of microtiter plates, and other objects or materials.

The Southern hybridization and blotting method has been used for many years to detect target DNA. First, sufficient quantities of target DNA are produced using PCR, and then the large segments of DNA are cut into smaller fragments using restriction endonucleases. The smaller DNA fragments are necessary for the next step—agarose gel electrophoresis, a laboratory technique used to separate molecules of different lengths and/or net charges. An electrical charge is passed through the gel matrix, and the DNA fragments are separated by their length across the gel. Shorter fragments move faster, while longer fragments move slowly. After separation in the gel, the DNA is transferred to a nylon membrane (i.e., the solid support) by a process called *blotting*. The DNA is normally denatured into single strands during the blotting process. The DNA becomes permanently attached to the nylon membrane by exposure to UV radiation.

Once the denatured and target DNA is permanently attached to the nylon membrane, the labeled probes are added. The nylon membrane is then incubated so that the probes will hybridize with the complementary fragments of DNA. Excess probe is removed by washing it from the membrane. Historically, radioisotope-labeled probes were most common, and autoradiography was used to visualize the presence of the probe-target DNA hybrids. More recently, probes labeled with fluorogenic or chromogenic compounds are preferred to radioactive materials. The results appear in "lanes" on the membrane, and the separated bands have the appearance of "ladders." The presence of the target DNA or genes is highlighted in the appropriate bands by the reporter molecules.

The obvious disadvantages of the colony and Southern hybridization methods are the time-consuming and laborious procedures involved. Fortunately, developments in technology have produced instruments that automate many of the procedures. In addition, kits are commercially available that have reduced the time for preparing reagents; these kits offer better quality control of laboratory procedures. Some of these instruments and kits have been validated for detecting foodborne pathogens, while many others are in the development stage and not yet commercially ready or available. Each year, scientific publications propose new genetic methods for the detection of pathogens—most of them for clinical purposes, with some adapted for food microbiology. Listing all of the proposed and available methods would be a great undertaking, and such a list would probably be outdated before it could be completed. For the purposes of introducing students to new molecular genetic technology, a few systems are briefly described here.

The BAX System by DuPont Qualicon is an example of PCR-based test systems. The latest version of the BAX System (Q7) utilizes highly specific primers, nucleic acid probes, and amplification chemistry called *real-time PCR*. Unlike traditional PCR, the technique of real-time PCR employs fluorescent dyes to quantify the amount of new DNA—called amplicons—produced during the cycles of PCR. By measuring the fluorescent signals emitted by the dyes, the PCR can be measured in real time (during the reactions) and quantitatively. In theory, the amount of DNA in the original sample is related to the exponential growth of the amplicons, and the fluorescent signal is directly proportional to the generation of amplicons. Along with quantification of the amplicons, a major advantage of real-time PCR is no need for post-PCR processing using agarose gels. Real-time PCR also has a much greater sensitivity of detection compared to using gels. When multiple types of nucleic acid probes are used together, the detection of separate species can be accomplished in the same sample (mulitplexing).

The BAX System standardizes and simplifies the molecular biology techniques for PCR-based analysis of foodborne pathogens. The apparatus in the system consists of a cycler/detector, computer workstation and software, heating blocks, and various supplies (PCR tubes and holders, pipettes, etc.). Reagents for the system come as assay kits for different pathogenic and toxigenic microorganisms. Assay kits are currently available for *Campylobacter* species, *E. coli* O157:H7, *S. aureus*, *Listeria* species and *L. monocytogenes*, *Salmonella*, and yeasts and molds. The basic procedure starts with taking a sample from an enrichment culture, lysing the cells, adding tablets that contain the PCR reagents and fluorescent dyes, and hydrating them for processing in the cycler/detector. After placement in the cycler/detector, the results are obtained on the computer in about 90 minutes.

Commercial kits are also available that utilize traditional PCR and nucleic acid probes. These test kits are considered end-point detection and generally have relatively lower precision and sensitivity compared with real-time PCR. The trend in the commercial sector seems to favor systems that incorporate real-time PCR with nucleic acid probes. Several companies in addition to DuPont Qualicon offer test systems for detecting foodborne pathogens based on real-time PCR. The TaqMan Pathogen Detection Kits by Applied Biosystems are popular because the protocols are very similar, and the company sells many different nucleic acid probes. Bio-rad has updated its previous line of test systems with the iQ-Check system and kits for foodborne pathogens. Whereas some variations exist in apparatus and procedures between companies, the test systems basically consist of a real-time PCR cycler and detector, computer hardware and software, disposable laboratory implements, and prepackaged reagents. Figure 7-7 is a generic overview of the procedures involved with real-time PCR detection of pathogens. A major advantage of the real-time PCR systems is a test turnaround time of 18–27 hours, compared with traditional culture methods that require 3–7 days. Kits are available for several important foodborne pathogens, particularly for those regulated under pathogen reduction programs and HACCP system verification.

One of the disadvantages of commercial PCR-based kits is the cost of purchasing the equipment and consumable supplies. Organizations with the technical capability and expertise can develop noncommercial methods for real-time PCR detection of foodborne pathogens. Research laboratories often develop their own methods and protocols for particular projects and studies. However, most noncommercial methods for real-time PCR detection have not been validated for applied and routine testing purposes. With initiative and determination, an organization can validate noncommercial methods, including real-time PCR detection of foodborne pathogens (Lofstrom et al. 2009). From a laboratory management perspective, however, the disadvantages of noncommercial methods must be weighed against the advantages of commercial methods. The disadvantages of noncommercial methods include a higher skill level of laboratory technicians, greater labor/time involved with mixing reagents and cleanup, and added laboratory quality assurance duties.

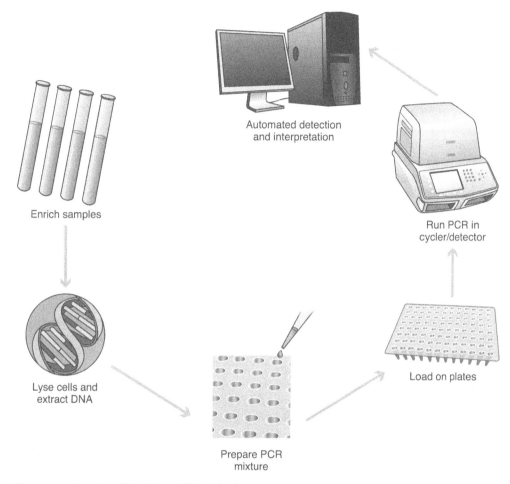

Automated detection
and interpretation

Enrich samples

Run PCR in
cycler/detector

Lyse cells and
extract DNA

Load on plates

Prepare PCR
mixture

**Figure 7-7** Overview of Real-time PCR Method

## Genetic "Fingerprinting" Methods

### Subtyping Microorganisms

Microorganisms originating from a single colony change from one another when separated into new and different habitats. These changes increase both with time and different environmental conditions. Some changes are phenotypic, meaning they can be observed using classical biological techniques, whereas many more changes are genotypic, occurring at the nucleotide sequence level of their genomes. In fact, most of the phenotypic changes are based on the underlying genotypic changes. New strains of microorganisms can evolve very quickly from genotypic changes. The term *strain* is relative, and it is often defined as any group of organisms at the subspecies level with some sort of common characteristics. Discerning and categorizing these different characteristics within a microbial species is the basis of subtyping. Over the past several decades, the molecular biology techniques have revolutionized subtyping.

The subtyping of pathogens has practical applications in epidemiology and microbiology. Small or subtle changes in an organism can be used to track the source of a pathogen in the environment and transmission among different hosts. Furthermore, small changes in one or a few genes of a pathogen can result in greater survival, virulence, and/or resistance to antibiotics. Most clinical laboratories do not routinely subtype pathogens below the species level. Epidemiologists usually request subtyping when an increase in the incidence of an infection or illness has been observed, indicating a possible epidemic. Several potentially large epidemics—including foodborne disease outbreaks—have been curtailed by timely subtyping of a microbial agent. Research microbiologists also perform subtyping to study the adaptation of pathogens to new habitats and potential disease reservoirs.

Before the advent of modern molecular biology, pathogens were subtyped solely on the basis of phenotypic characteristics. Serotyping is an example of phenotypic subtyping still used today for organisms such as *Salmonella* and pathogenic *E. coli*. Biotyping is another subtyping method based on metabolic functions and biochemical substrate tests. Although phenotypic subtyping is still useful for many purposes, the discriminatory power of molecular genetic methods is unsurpassed. With knowledge about the DNA and RNA sequences of pathogenic species, it is relatively straightforward to subtype on the basis of genotype. Unfortunately, knowledge about genotypes of foodborne pathogens is incomplete. Even with pathogens that have had their entire genomes sequenced, the gene changes (e.g., mutations) that occur between strains cannot be continuously updated in the genomic databases.

Despite incomplete knowledge of genotypes for foodborne pathogens, some molecular genetic methods can be performed without having the entire gene sequences. These are commonly called genetic *fingerprinting* methods. Several genetic fingerprinting methods and techniques have been developed, each with specific advantages and disadvantages. With the exception of phage typing, genetic fingerprinting methods are based on the specificity of restriction endonucleases. These enzymes cut up DNA at precise restriction sites where the nucleotide sequences match. The resulting DNA fragments are variable in strand lengths. Two closely related pathogens will have slightly different nucleotide sequences in their respective genomes—including the location of restriction endonuclease sites. The DNA fragments from the two pathogens will have a slightly different mix of strand lengths. After the DNA fragments are separated by strand length using gel electrophoresis and visualized using labeled probes or gel stains, the resulting patterns can be compared with one another and/or with libraries of other patterns.

The majority of genetic fingerprinting methods and associated techniques are known by a litany of acronyms derived from their technical names. The most widely known methods and techniques include the following:

Amplified-fragment length polymorphism (AFLP)
Bacteriophage (or phage) typing
Microarrays
Multilocus enzyme electrophoresis (MEE)

Pulsed field gel electrophoresis (PFGE)
Random amplification of polymorphic DNA (RAPD)
Restriction enzyme analysis (REA)
Restriction fragment length polymorphism (RFLP)
Ribotyping

Describing each of the methods and techniques listed here is beyond the scope of this book. Additionally, most of them are not routinely used in food microbiology, and some are likely to be superseded in coming years by new and more rapid molecular techniques. Therefore, the methods described in the following sections are selectively chosen based on their recent past and relative contributions to food safety.

### Bacteriophage Typing

Bacteriophages, or phages, are viruses capable of infecting bacteria and causing cell lysis. The host specificity of phages is highly refined, based on protein receptors and complementary nucleotide sequences of the phage and the host bacterium. Host specificity is so great among phages that they can be used to subtype bacteria below the species level. Therefore, a phage can be exploited as a natural nucleic acid probe. Phage typing has around for many years, and although all foodborne bacteria can be typed with phages, the practice of phage typing is more common with certain species (Jay et al. 2005). *Staphylococcus aureus* has the most extensive record of being phage typed, dating back to the 1950s. Other foodborne bacteria that are phage typed include *L. monocytogenes*, strains of toxigenic *E. coli*, and *Salmonella*.

To phage type bacteria, the isolate is treated with a panel of different phages, and the resulting pattern of cell lyses is characteristic of the bacterium's phage type. Maintaining a stock of bacteriophages is necessary for phage typing, and the procedure requires a fairly high degree of technical skill. For these reasons and others, phage typing has waned over recent years. Newer and innovative techniques have been published using phage typing. They include using phage mutants and phages with luminescent or fluorescent reporter genes (e.g., *lux* genes, green fluorescent protein gene). In one publication, a simple method of phage typing was described that can detect 1–10 living cells of *Salmonella* or *E. coli* O157:H7 in 3–5 hours (Ulitzur and Ulitzur 2006). The high degree of sensitivity, specificity, and short turnaround testing time demonstrated by this publication are very desirable characteristics for food testing. Before such methods can be adopted and used routinely for food testing, they need to be developed to demonstrate feasibility and validated against other accepted/approved methods.

### Ribotyping

Each ribosome in cells, where protein synthesis occurs, consists of a small and a large subunit. These subunits are complexes of proteins and ribosomal RNA (rRNA). Ribosomes and their subunits are physically characterized by sedimentation coefficients called Svedberg (S), which is determined by both the mass and shape. Prokaryotic organisms such as bacteria have a 70S ribosome with two subunits of 30S and 50S. The subunits also have several definable and phylogenetically important rRNA fractions designated as 16S, 23S, and 5S. Genes in the chromosome encode the rRNA transcripts used to make the ribosomes. The highly conserved nature of rRNA makes it an excellent chronometer of bacterial evolution and can be used to classify bacteria below the species level. The molecular method called *ribotyping* has been used to define and redefine many genera and species of bacteria. In the past, the methods for ribotyping bacteria were limited by the availability of technology. Manual ribotyping involves the following basic steps:

1. Nucleic acid probes are made by making complementary DNA (cDNA) probes from reverse transcription of rRNA or by making synthetic nucleic acid probes based on rRNA nucleotide sequences. The probes are labeled a reporter molecule or element, usually a radioisotope.
2. After the test bacterium is isolated and enriched using culture methods, its genomic DNA is extracted.
3. The extracted DNA is cut into various length strands using restriction endonucleases.
4. The DNA fragments are separated using an agarose gel and electrophoresis.
5. With Southern hybridization and blotting techniques, the separated DNA fragments are denatured and transferred to a membrane, and then fixed.
6. The labeled cDNA probes are complementary sequences to genes in the genomic DNA that encode the rRNA. These probes are used to form cDNA–DNA hybrids that can be visualized with the reporter on the membrane.
7. The pattern on the membrane filter is compared with a library of other patterns for similarity.

These days, ribotyping has been completely automated, and the entire analysis can be accomplished in less than 8 hours. Pavlic and Griffiths (2009) review automated ribotyping as a rapid method for food safety. The authors conclude that automated ribotyping is useful for subtyping pathogens such as *Listeria monocytogenes* and *Salmonella*, but they found automated ribotyping had less discriminatory power for *Campylobacter* species and *E. coli* subtypes. Although ribotyping is a useful tool for defining species and certain subtypes, it may not be a good indicator of traits such as virulence among pathogenic strains. In these cases, the detection of virulence genes in the bacterial genome is more useful.

### Pulsed Field Gel Electrophoresis

The utility of molecular subtyping was profoundly demonstrated in 1993 during a highly publicized outbreak of *E. coli* O157:H7 infections from hamburgers served at a fast-food restaurant chain (Bell et al. 1994; Swaminathan et al. 2001). Several different antigenic and genetic methods were used to subtype the *E. coli* O157:H7 isolates from infected patients. The method of pulsed field gel electrophoresis (PFGE) was particularly useful because it identified asymptomatic patients who were infected with the outbreak subtype (i.e., strain) of *E. coli* O157:H7. More important, the PFGE patterns of *E. coli* O157:H7 from the sampled lots of hamburger were identical to the outbreak strain—providing strong evidence of causation between the food and human cases of infection. Subsequently, several state health departments began requesting PFGE subtyping of *E. coli* O157:H7 from the Centers for Disease Control and Prevention (CDC) laboratory, and the number of requests soon overwhelmed the laboratory's capacity (Swaminathan et al. 2001). Starting in 1995, CDC selected several states to participate in a national molecular subtyping network for surveillance of foodborne bacterial diseases. The selected states were provided with standardized PFGE subtyping and pattern analysis technology. This network of states and CDC became known as PulseNet. Since then, PulseNet International, which extends to locations around the globe, has been established.

Today, PulseNet USA consists of more than 70 laboratories across the United States (Association of Public Health Laboratories [APHL] 2010). These laboratories are located under local, state, and federal public health and agricultural agencies, including CDC, FDA, and USDA. Since its inception, PulseNet has proved itself an efficient and effective tool to detect, investigate, and control foodborne illness outbreaks. The preferred molecular subtyping method of PulseNet is still PFGE. Standardized PFGE laboratory protocols have been developed for at least six foodborne bacterial pathogens: *C. jejuni*, shiga-toxin-producing *E. coli* (including *E. coli* O157:H7), *L. monocytogenes*, *Salmonella*, *Shigella* species, and *V. cholerae*. Bacterial isolates from patients, foods, and/or the environment are used to generate the PFGE patterns, which are then submitted to a national database and shared among participating laboratories. In 2008, a total of 48,195 foodborne pathogen isolates were subtyped using PFGE, and PulseNet detected more than 1,500 local clusters of foodborne illness (APHL 2010). This includes the detection of a nationwide outbreak of *Salmonella* serotype Typhimurium from peanut-containing products (Centers for Disease Control and Prevention [CDC] 2009). Although the patient cases came from 12 different states, the similar and unusual PFGE pattern among the isolates prompted further epidemiologic investigation. Peanut butter and peanut-containing products were confirmed by laboratories as the transmission vehicle when the food samples revealed a PFGE fingerprint pattern of *S*. Typhimurium that resembled the outbreak strain.

Figure 7-8 provides an overview of the PFGE method. The process starts by making a buffered suspension of bacteria from the culture. The bacterial suspension is mixed with molten agarose and poured into a mold to form a plug. Several gel plugs from the bacterial test culture are normally prepared. After the agarose solidifies, the gel plugs are put into a lysis solution to rupture the bacterial cells and release the DNA. Washing steps are performed to remove cellular debris and leave the DNA intact within the gel plugs. A piece of the gel plug is cut off and placed in a mixture of restriction endonuclease. The selection of restriction endonucleases in the mixture is critically important and depends on the specific protocol and species to be analyzed. In general, a restriction endonuclease is an infrequent cutter of DNA. This produces variable lengths of DNA strands that are quite large, and the number of DNA fragments is usually no more than 10–20. Most other fingerprinting techniques produce a greater number of DNA fragments with shorter strands.

The PFGE method usually does not require nucleic acid probes or Southern hybridization/blotting. The gel plugs containing the DNA fragments are placed into the wells of a larger agarose gel for electrophoresis. Unlike conventional electrophoresis techniques, PFGE applies electrical currents in varying pulses of time, and with alternating electrical fields occasionally changing the direction of migrating DNA fragments. The electrophoretic profiles are programmable and facilitate the movement of larger DNA fragments across the gel. Separation of the DNA fragments occurs according to size, with the smaller fragments moving faster and farther across the

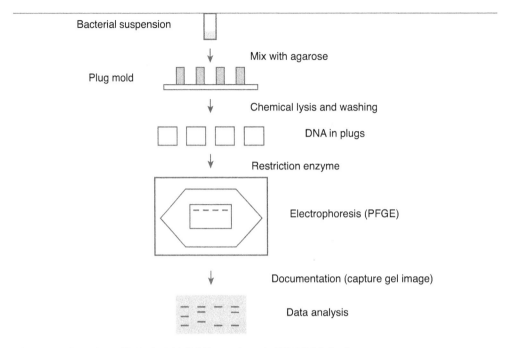

**Figure 7-8**  Overview of Pulsed-Field Gel Electrophoresis (PFGE) Method.
*Source:* CDC [http://www.cdc.gov/pulsenet/whatis.htm]

gel. The fragments also cluster together by similar size to form bands across the gel. The bands are visualized simply by staining the gel, and the pattern of bands are digitized with a computerized imaging system. Comparisons can be made between the fingerprint band patterns of different bacterial isolates to identify similarities. A database of band patterns and computerized search engines greatly enhance the utility of the PFGE method.

Although the PFGE method offers many benefits to food safety and public health, it has several practical disadvantages. One major disadvantage is comparing the results between different laboratories. Slight variations in materials and techniques between laboratories can make comparisons of the PFGE band patterns difficult. Standardized protocols and computer analysis software can minimize this difficulty, but the ultimate approach is to compare band patterns from isolates in adjacent lanes of the same gel (Francis et al. 2007). Additionally, unlike ribotyping, the PFGE band patterns do not provide a convenient measure of genetic relationships among isolates. Other disadvantages of PFGE are the costs, training, and time. The expense of purchasing PFGE apparatus is not trivial, and an upfront investment is necessary. Technicians who perform the laboratory procedures must have a certain level of technical skill and expertise because the process is not totally automated. And the time necessary to complete PFGE typically takes several days.

Considering the number of pathogen fingerprints in PFGE databases, and the widespread adoption of PFGE by many organizations, PFGE is likely to remain the gold standard for molecular subtyping of foodborne bacterial pathogens, at least for the foreseeable future (Gerner-Smidt et al. 2006). Yet, rapid advances are occurring in the field of genomics and molecular genetics, and technology is making new methods more feasible. Technologies to ascertain the nucleotide sequences of pathogens are becoming faster, cheaper, and more portable, and they offer greater comparability among results and between laboratories. Furthermore, these newer technologies can be used with important foodborne viruses and other organisms, as well as bacterial pathogens. Most likely, PFGE will be augmented and eventually substituted in PulseNet with other molecular subtyping methodologies that offer greater sensitivity, specificity, flexibility, speed, and portability. The preferred strategy of epidemiologists is to integrate these new methodologies into PulseNet and to harmonize them with PFGE data (Gerner-Smidt et al. 2006; Tauxe 2006).

## Microarrays

A great technological leap forward in biological research occurred in recent years with the development of microarrays, colloquially called "gene chips." Microarrays start with a solid support—the "chip"—often made of glass or silicon. Various types of ligands (oligonucleotides, cDNA, proteins, carbohydrates, etc.) that act as probes can be affixed to the chip. To capture target nucleic acids from a sample, oligonucleotides or cDNA are used as the probes. One or several fluorogenic (or sometimes colorimetric) dyes are used to label the target nucleic acids, and after hybridization with complementary probes on the chip, the fluorescent signals can be read using a special camera. The unprecedented capability offered by microarrays is the number of probes that can be affixed to and read on one chip. Different probes on the order of $10^4$ can be affixed to specific locations on one chip. This allows for the simultaneous detection and analysis of thousands of hybrids from a single sample. Special pattern recognition software and statistical tools are necessary to analyze the massive amount of data produced by such microarrays.

Currently, the majority of microarray applications is for basic biological and biomedical research. The two most common reasons for using microarrays are to measure gene expression and determine genotypes. Gene expression is measured by converting sample mRNA from the organism into cDNA and then analyzing cDNA hybridization with probes on the chip. Essentially, this procedure indirectly measures the up-regulation of genes by detecting which mRNA transcripts were produced and the relative quantity of transcripts. With genotyping applications, probes that represent different genotypes are affixed to the chip. When a sample of unknown DNA fragments is incubated with the microarray, the DNA fragments that are complementary to the appropriate genotype probes hybridize with them. The location of each genotype probe is exact, and computer software helps determine the genotypes from the sample. Pattern recognition or fingerprinting software can also be used to compare the results from other organisms.

The entire genome of a foodborne pathogen can be represented by probes on a single microarray, called a *high-density microarray*, but the costs of microarrays increase substantially with increasing numbers of affixed probes. The most common applications of microarrays with foodborne pathogens involve species and strain identification (Rasooly and Herold 2008). This can be accomplished with a limited number of probes to generate a signature pattern for the pathogen. Additional targets of interest with foodborne pathogens are virulence factors and antibiotic resistance. In total, the number of probes needed on a microarray for routine food microbiology testing is less than a few hundred, which is considered a low-density microarray. Commercial companies are not very interested in producing low-density microarrays, preferring instead to pursue the more lucrative markets of high-density microarrays. An alternative to commercial microarrays is to use a robotic spotter system to produce the chips, and scanners to read them. Obviously, purchasing this equipment and equipping a laboratory are not without difficulty and costs. Nevertheless, the costs of equipment necessary to produce microarrays are decreasing, which may encourage more laboratories and specialty vendors to produce low-density microarrays for routine testing purposes.

Some technical challenges must be addressed when using microarrays to test food samples (Kostrzynska and Bachand 2006). Food matrices vary greatly in complexity, and the microbiota of foods can be diverse. Ideally, samples from foods should require a minimal amount of preparation, and the analytical method should be able to detect and quantify low levels of several pathogens in a mixed microbial population. For the most part, before microarrays can be used to detect and characterize pathogens in foods, an enrichment step is necessary, and PCR amplification of genomic DNA from the isolates is needed. The probes on a microarray must also be optimized to recognize key gene sequences of important pathogens and to discriminate between different microorganisms. Finally, a considerable amount of technical skill is needed to perform the procedures necessary for running microarrays. These challenges must be addressed before microarrays become feasible alternatives to existing microbial testing methods. Research is ongoing to improve and validate microarrays for food testing applications.

The aforementioned problems are not insurmountable, and microarrays are expected to play an increasingly important role in food microbiology testing. After all, microarrays promise faster and more accurate identification and characterization of foodborne pathogens, including parasites and viruses. As microarrays become more commonplace in clinical settings and epidemiologic investigations, applications in food testing are likely to grow. An added incentive for using microarrays is food defense, that is, detecting and deterring agroterrorism and deliberate food contamination. Federal research funding in this area has bolstered efforts to produce faster and more accurate methods of detecting foodborne microorganisms.

## Detection of Viruses in Foods

The detection of viruses in foods is particularly problematic for several reasons. Like many bacterial pathogens, the number of enteric viruses in contaminated foods is relatively low, at least in comparison with the stool specimens of infected persons. Unlike bacteria, viruses cannot be easily cultured to enrich their numbers. Host cell culture systems are needed to culture and/or assay for viruses, and culture host cells for the most important foodborne viruses (e.g., norovirus, hepatitis A virus) are either not available or do not grow viruses well. Conventional methods to detect viruses in patients include electron microscopy, antigen-based assays, and antibody titer tests. These methods do not work well with foods, mostly because viruses are much less concentrated in foods. An exception to this generalization with foods is bivalve mollusks, which can concentrate viruses from polluted waters.

In the absence of convenient tests for enteric viruses in foods, indicator organisms are used to infer the likelihood of viral contamination, and epidemiologic analysis from outbreaks may incriminate certain foods. More recently, the availability of molecular genetic methods has made the detection of viruses in foods much more feasible. Since the 1990s, methods that utilize PCR-based assays for detecting viruses in foods have been published, particularly for shellfish. After extraction and concentration from foods, the viral nucleic acid can be amplified using reverse transcription coupled with PCR (RT-PCR) or a combination of reverse transcription and real-time PCR (rRT-PCR). Detection of the amplified nucleic acid can be accomplished with the appropriate probes and reporter molecules. The selection of PCR primers and probes is technically difficult for noroviruses because of their genetic variability. This technical problem must be tackled before virus sampling and detection methods can be standardized and validated for a variety of foods (Food and Agriculture Organization/World Health Organization [FAO/WHO] 2008). One possible approach to this problem is a combination rRT-PCR with primers and probes for multiple targets (multiplex PCR). Another approach is the customization of microarrays with multiple probes for different genetic variants of viruses.

## LABORATORY ANALYSIS OF CHEMICALS AND TOXINS

### Chemical Residues

As described earlier in Chapter 3, chemical residues in foods consist of pesticides, veterinary drugs, and other agrochemicals; industrial chemicals and pollutants; cleaning, sanitizing, and disinfecting compounds; food additives; by-products from heat treatments; chemicals from food contact surfaces and packaging; and naturally occurring metals from the environment. In the past, the detection of chemical residues was limited by the analytical methods, and the exposure limits were often based on detection limits. Over the past several decades, the sensitivity of analytical methods to detect chemical residues has far exceeded knowledge of their toxic effects at those levels. This created a dilemma for public health officials who can no longer establish a zero-tolerance policy for chemical residues in products and the environment. In other words, the detection limit of an analytical method is rarely the basis of establishing tolerances or exposure limits for chemical residues. Consequently, the analytical method of choice for chemical residues is a compromise between its detection limit and precision relative to the tolerance level, costs, and practicality. In many cases, regulatory requirements and guidance documents stipulate an analytical method for particular chemical residues. Otherwise, the choice of analytical methods is based on expert judgment. Whenever possible (or when required by law), a validated method is always preferred.

Sample preparation can be quite extensive for many chemical contaminants and food types. The target analyte (i.e., chemical to be analyzed) must be separated from the physical and chemical components of the food matrix without being destroyed in the process. Various extraction procedures and protocols have been developed based on natural properties of the analyte and the food (Curren and King 2002). Homogenization of the food sample is usually the first step and may involve grinding, mixing, crushing, mincing, pressing, chopping, and any number of reasonable techniques. Extraction of the organic analytes may involve partitioning, solvation, distillation, adsorption, or diffusion. A particular concern with analyte extraction is the coextraction of similar components in the food matrix that could interfere with analysis. Clean-up refers to the removal of coextracted components, and this may require additional extraction techniques to remove the undesired components. Another possible step with sample preparation includes concentration of the analyte.

The analysis of chemical residues in foods basically involves either classical wet-chemical methods or instrumental methods. The analysis can be qualitative (i.e., identification) or quantitative (i.e., "how much"). The modern laboratory is equipped with several types of analytical instruments that can detect chemicals down to the level of parts per million (ppm), parts per billion (ppb), or even lower. Table 7-4 provides examples of analytical methods for chemical residues in foods. This table represents a partial list of chemical residues and analytical methods prescribed by the USDA as part of the National Residue Program (Food Safety and Inspection Service [FSIS] 2009). Under the program, the Food Safety and Inspection Service (FSIS) collects samples from meat, poultry, and egg products at facilities inspected by federal officials. The samples are analyzed for certain veterinary drugs, food additives, and unavoidable environmental contaminants. The analytical results are compared against tolerances and action levels established by either FDA or EPA, and when samples exceed these levels, the analytical results are shared with FDA and EPA for regulatory compliance actions. The aggregate data are also analyzed to study trends in residue contamination and to enhance national control efforts.

Laboratory analytical methods for chemical residues usually involve several stages and combinations of techniques. Analytical chemists must ensure that the right approach is taken according to established laboratory protocols. The breadth of analytical methods and techniques for analyzing potential chemical hazards in foods is impossible to cover in this chapter and book. The International Union of Food Science and Technology (IUFoST) provides some generalized points for those seeking to analyze chemicals in foods (IUFoST 2011):

- Purpose of the analysis—it is important for those commissioning the analysis to be clear about the reasons for the analysis and how the result is to be used
- Sampling—samples should be representative of the product being analysed. Once taken, the samples should be handled, stored and prepared properly, so that they are not altered in any way that would affect the analysis
- Method suitability—the analytical method has to be fit for purpose - even if a method has been devised for the specific hazard in question, it may have to be adapted or modified for a particular foodstuff or to take into account other chemicals present that may interfere with the analysis
- Validation—following on from the above, the method, if it is new or modified, will have to be validated - i.e. tested to show that it works
- Quality control and standardisation—although the method itself has been shown to be fit for purpose, there needs to be evidence that it can produce consistent results over a period of time and in the hands of different analysts.

**Table 7-4** Analytical Methods and Proficiency Levels for Selected Chemicals Under the National Residue Program

| Compound Class | Compound | Analytical Method | | Minimum Proficiency Level[a] | |
|---|---|---|---|---|---|
| | | Determinative (quantitative) | Confirmatory (identification) | Determinative (quantitative) | Confirmatory (identification) |
| Antibiotics | Chloramphenicol | GC-ECD | GC-MS | 0.25 ppb (M)(B) | 0.25 ppb (M)(B), 0.30 ppb (M)(T) |
| | Desfuroylceftiofur cysteine disulfide | HPLC-UV | HPLC/MS-MS | 0.10 ppm | 50 ppb |
| | Tetracycline | Bioassay | HPLC | 0.40 ppm | 0.5 ppm |
| | Neomycin | Bioassay | HPLC/MS-MS | 2.5 ppm | 0.1ppm (K,M), 0.4 (L) |
| | Ciprofloxacin | — | HPLC/MS-MS | — | 25 ppb |
| Arsenicals | Arsenicals | AAS | AAS | 0.2 ppm | 0.2 ppm |
| Heavy metals | Cadmium | — | ICP/MS | — | 10 ppb |
| | Lead | | ICP/MS | | 25 ppb |
| Synthetic hormones | Diethylstilbesterol (DES) | GC-MS | GC-MS | 0.5 ppb | 1.0 ppb (L,M) |
| | | | GC-MS | 1.0 ppb | 1.0 ppb (L,M) |
| | Zeranol | GC-MS | | | |
| Sulfano-mides | Sulfapyridine | TLC | GC/ESI-MS | 0.08 ppm | 0.1 ppm |
| | Sulfadiazine | TLC | GC/ESI-MS | 0.08 ppm | 0.1 ppm |
| | Other sulfanomides | TLC | GC/ESI-MS | 0.08 ppm | 0.1 ppm |
| CHCs/COPs/PCBs | Aldrin | GC-ECD | GC-ECD | 0.10 ppm | — |
| | Chlorpyrifos | GC-ECD | GC-ECD | 0.10 ppm | — |
| | Methoxychlor | GC-ECD | GC-ECD | 0.50 ppm | — |
| | PCB 1260 | GC-ECD | GC-ECD | 0.50 ppm | — |
| | PCB 1254 | GC-ECD | GC-ECD | 0.50 ppm | — |
| | Toxaphene | GC-ECD | GC-ECD | 1.00 ppm | — |

[a]Minimum proficiency level: The minimum concentration of a residue at which an analytical result will be used to assess a laboratory's quantification capability. This concentration is an estimate of the smallest concentration for which the average coefficient of variation (CV) for reproducibility (i.e., combined within and between laboratory variability) does not exceed 20% (9 CFR 318.21).

AAS = atomic absorption spectroscopy, APCI = atmospheric pressure chemical ionization, B = bovine, CHCs = chlorinated hydrocarbons, COPs = chlorinated organophosphates, ECD = electron capture detection, ELISA = enzyme-linked immunosorbent assay, GC = gas chromatography, GPC = gel permeation chromatography, HPLC = high-performance liquid chromatography, K = kidney, L = liver, M = muscle, method detection limit = the lowest quantity of residue (or sample component) that can be reliably observed or found in the sample matrix by the analytical methodology used, MS = mass spectroscopy, NA = not applicable, PCBs = polychlorinated biphenyls, ppb = parts per billion, ppm = parts per million, RTE = ready to eat, SIM = selected ion mode, TBD = to be determined, TLC = thin layer chromatography, T = turkey.
*Source:* FSIS 2009.

- Measurement uncertainty—no method will ever give exactly the right result all the time—in fact, in any analysis the result obtained will only ever be an approximation (adequately close, if the method is suitable) to the 'true' answer. It is important to understand where the potential sources of error might arise, and which are the most significant, when interpreting the results.

## Analysis of Toxins

Toxins represent a special category for chemical analysis. Produced naturally by diverse groups of organisms, toxins vary greatly in molecular size and complexity. Furthermore, toxins do not occur in pure forms, and because most toxins are products of secondary metabolism, they can be difficult to separate and distinguish from the products of primary metabolism. If toxins occurred in pure form or are easily extracted, they could be identified rather easily with modern analytical instrumentation. With plant- and animal-derived foods, toxins can be an integral part of the tissues, perhaps partitioned in particular compartments. Toxins may also be contaminants in the food matrix as a consequence of microbial activity. Thus, the principal challenge of toxin identification and quantification is extracting and purifying these substances from the milieu of organic constituents in the food matrix.

Historically, microbial toxins have been detected in foods using bioassay and immunological methods. Table 7-5 lists the most common of these methods. Bioassay methods consisting of whole animals, parts of animals (e.g., ileal loops), and cell cultures can be used to detect toxins and/or to characterize their biological activity (Pimbley and Patel 1998). Even these days, many countries still require the mouse or rat bioassay methods to detect lipophilic marine toxins in shellfish (Gerssen et al. 2010). An advantage of bioassays is the detection of toxins that are not easily separated or identifiable in an extract, and the biological activity of combined toxins or toxins with mixed chemical structures can be ascertained. The obvious disadvantages of bioassay methods include animal care issues, costs, and turnaround time for results. Additionally, acute bioassay methods are not very helpful with rapid detection of toxins that represent chronic exposure hazards, such as aflatoxins and cancer.

Immunological methods, including variations of those discussed earlier for microbes, are simpler and less expensive, and they can be used to detect toxins with chronic exposure potential. These methods have been developed and refined over several decades for the detection and quantification of many different microbial toxins. Their effectiveness is a result of the highly specific nature of the antigen–antibody binding, where the toxin possesses an antigenic determinant(s) to the antibodies. Along with detection, the antibody's affinity for antigens helps separate the toxins from the sample while moving through a liquid, gel, or membrane. A key requirement, of course, for an immunological method is the availability of antibodies specific to the toxins. Several types of toxins require a carrier molecule to achieve immunogenicity, a necessary property to produce antibodies. While immunological methods have several advantages, they also have a limited detection range compared with newer instrumental methods.

Over the past two decades, the science of physical chemistry has advanced significantly, and new technologies have emerged that dramatically increase the sensitivity of toxin detection and quantification. Newer and more sophisticated extraction methods (e.g., supercritical fluid extrac-

**Table 7-5** Examples of Assay Methods Used for Microbial Toxins

| Microorganism | Toxin | Assay Method |
|---|---|---|
| *Staphylococcus aureus* | All enterotoxins | Rhesus monkey emesis |
| | A, B | Murine spleen cells |
| | A–E | ELISA and automated ELISA |
| | A–D | Reverse passive latex agglutination |
| *Bacillus cereus* | Diarrheagenic | Rabbit ileal loop, vascular permeability, guinea pig skin |
| | Diarrheagenic | Reverse passive latex agglutination, ELISA, microslide double diffusion |
| | Emetic | Rhesus monkey emesis |
| *Clostridium botulinum* | A, B, E, F, G | Mouse lethality |
| | A, E, G | ELISA |
| | A–E | Electroimmunodiffusion |
| *Clostridium perfringens* | Enterotoxin | Mouse lethality, mouse ileal loop, rabbit ileal loop, guinea pig skin, Vero cells |
| | Enterotoxin | Reverse passive latex agglutination, ELISA, microslide double diffusion, electroimmunodiffusion |
| Toxigenic algae | Okadaic acid and dinophysistoxins | Mouse or rat bioassay, ELISA |
| | Pectenotoxins | Mouse or rat bioassay |
| | Yessotoxins | Mouse or rat bioassay, ELISA |

*Source*: Gerssen, 2010; Pimbley and Patel, 1998.

tion, solid phase extraction, solid phase membrane extraction, immunoaffinity column) are showing significant promise in toxin recovery. Extraction methods are important because the greatest source of variability is from sampling and extraction procedures, at least for aflatoxins (Reiter, Zentek, Razzazi 2009). The separation phases of analysis have also improved with technologies such as thin-layer chromatography (TLC), high-performance liquid chromatography (HPLC), and very high pressure liquid chromatography (VHPLC) (Gerssen et al. 2010). When these separation methods are coupled with advanced detectors based on fluorescence and mass spectrometry, a powerful analytical instrument for toxin detection is possible.

Sophisticated laboratory instruments for toxin analysis are used predominantly for research purposes. Through research, these analytical instruments have identified several new toxins, especially among the marine toxins. However, these instruments are expensive, and they require highly skilled technicians and maintenance that are beyond the capabilities of most food laboratories. Therefore, to monitor or screen foods for toxins, the preferred methods of analysis are the faster, simpler, and less costly alternatives. The use of TLC with UV-visible light detection is popular because it is high throughput with low operating costs, and it easy to identify the targeted compounds (Turner, Subrahmanyam, Piletsky 2009). The trend also appears to be toward increasing use of immunological methods as a result of their rapid and simpler platform for toxin testing. A great many immunologic-based test kits for toxins have become commercially available in recent years. Many of these kits are already validated for routine screening purposes. Other laboratory methods are still used as a reference standard and for test result confirmation.

## RAPID METHODS AND EMERGING TECHNOLOGIES FOR FOOD TESTING

The emergence and availability of rapid methods to detect pathogens have been growing exponentially over the past several decades (Fung 2002). Each year, new techniques and methods are published in scientific journals, and new devices or kits become commercially available. The demand for more rapid test methods is driven mostly by the food industry's requirements. Consumers expect safe and wholesome foods from industry, and food recalls or foodborne illness outbreaks can be costly—even financially devastating—to a food company. To ensure that the raw materials and ingredients received by a supplier are good quality, food companies want to test the supplier's materials. Food companies are also mandated under HACCP rules to ensure that they provide safe food products, which necessitates monitoring and testing for foodborne agents. Waiting days or weeks for test results can halt production and/or reduce the quality (e.g., freshness) of food products. Rapid methods can help meet testing requirements without causing a loss of productivity or adding excessive costs. Public health officials can also benefit from rapid methods of food testing. With rapid methods, the etiologic agent and sources of foodborne illnesses can be determined more quickly, and corrective actions to prevent further illnesses can be initiated sooner.

The availability of rapid methods for food testing very much depends on the development of new technology. From a research and development (R&D) perspective, three interrelated factors are most influential on the emergence of new technologies: (1) federal R&D funding priorities, (2) the availability of enabling technologies, and (3) commercial incentives. The first factor was greatly influenced by recent historical events. In 1996, the Food Quality Protection Act of 1996 mandated the use of the HACCP system in certain segments of the food industry, and the pathogen reduction rules by USDA emphasized sampling to verify program effectiveness. This pushed R&D funding priorities toward rapid and cost-effective testing methods of detecting foodborne agents. A few years later, the biggest influence on R&D priorities was the terrorism events of September 11, 2001, and the anthrax letter mailings shortly thereafter. Following these events, the public and federal government turned their full attention to detecting, deterring, and thwarting terrorism acts. Along with changes in laws and administrative priorities, the R&D budgets and priorities of many federal agencies prioritized projects that could detect biological, chemical, or physical agents. Grants from federal agencies provided the funds necessary to advance the basic and applied sciences, and federal funding provided the capital for companies to develop new technologies that are considered too risky by investors.

The second factor, availability of enabling technologies, refers to technologies that permit engineers to develop entirely new systems, that is, devices or kits capable of performing particular tasks. Among the most important enabling technologies for food testing are molecular biology methods (e.g., PCR, gene sequencing), electronics and computer technology, and materials science/engineering. To develop more rapid methods for food testing, the basic steps of food sampling and testing (Figure 7-1) are examined, and enabling technologies are used to reduce the timeline of the entire process. For example, incremental improvements can be accomplished by streamlining sample preparation or by eliminating the need to culture microorganisms. The review of enabling technologies and their incorporation into systems for food testing is far beyond the scope of this book. Suffice to say, thousands of articles are published each year on this topic, and patents are filed every year on new enabling technologies or inventions. Some have already been incorporated into testing systems, while others have the potential for greatly improving food testing. Ultimately, the availability of rapid food testing methods depends on their engineering development, validation, and commercialization.

The third factor behind the development of technologies, commercial incentives, is the most powerful in terms of test availability. Market size and consumer demand are the basic driving forces of a free market economy. Businesses respond to these forces by providing products to meet the demand. The business market for clinical testing is lucrative, and rapid clinical tests are in increasing demand. In fact, a new market for medical point-of-care and treatment (POCT) devices has emerged with a multi-billion-dollar potential. Similarly, the biodefense industry has grown in response to the demand for better and faster detection technologies. It is no wonder that companies respond by producing commercially available technologies for these markets.

Although not as large as clinical testing markets, the food testing market is also rapidly growing. According to a market research report titled *Food Microbiology—2008 to 2013* (Strategic Consulting 2008), more than 738 million food microbiology tests were performed worldwide in 2008, with a total market value exceeding $2.06 billion. The report also projects continued growth in the food microbiology market. The reasons cited for market growth include increased food production, higher priorities for food safety, and increased regulation. These trends are also believed to increase the demand for more rapid test methods. Still, in 2008, 58% of the food microbiology tests performed worldwide was based on traditional methods, while the remaining 42% was based on immunologic and other molecular methods.

The emergence and commercial availability of rapid test methods for foods have been reviewed by several authors (Fung 2002; Ge and Meng 2009; Mandal et al. 2011). Table 7-6 lists the technological categories of most rapid test methods for foods. Whereas the number of rapid test methods for foods has increased, the number of commercially available methods is still proportionally small. One proposed explanation is the difficulty of preparing the food matrix for analysis (Brehm-Stecher et al. 2009). Several strategies have been suggested to reduce the time and activity required for sample preparation. Unfortunately, sample preparation of the food matrix remains challenging, particularly with certain types of foods. And even with new or automated sample preparation methods, the testing costs and complexity are likely to increase. Several years ago, one author with decades of experience in food testing technology made 10 predictions about

**Table 7-6** Technological Categories of Most Rapid Test Methods for Foods

| |
| --- |
| *Modified and automated conventional methods* |
| Biosensors |
|     Bioluminescence biosensor |
|     Impedimetry (electrical impedance) |
|     Piezoelectric biosensors |
|       Flow cytometry |
|       Solid phase cytometry |
|       Electronic nose |
| *Immunological methods* |
| Nucleic acid based assays |
|     DNA hybridization |
|     Polymerase chain reaction |
|     DNA micro assay (Gene chip technology) |

*Source*: Mandal et al. 2011.

the future of rapid test methods, though he acknowledged that predicting the future is very tricky (Fung 2002). His unique insights are offered here for the student to contemplate:

1. Viable cell counts will still be used.
2. Real-time monitoring of hygiene will be in place.
3. Polymerase chain reaction (PCR), ribotyping, and genetic tests will become reality in food laboratories.
4. Enzyme-linked immunosorbent assays (ELISA) and immunological tests will be completely automated and widely used.
5. Dipstick technology will provide rapid answers.
6. Biosensors will be in place for HACCP programs.
7. Instant detection of target pathogens will be possible by computer-generated matrices in response to particular characteristics of pathogens.
8. Effective separation, concentration of target cells will greatly assist in rapid identification.
9. A microbiological alert system will be in food packages.
10. Consumers will have rapid alert kits for pathogens at home.

## REFERENCES

Allwood PB, Malik YS, Maherchandani S, Vought K, Johnson LA, Braymen C, Hedberg CW, Goyal SM. 2004. Occurrence of *Escherichia coli*, noroviruses, and F-specific coliphages in fresh market-ready produce. *J Food Prot* 67(11): 2387–2390.

AOAC International. 1994. *Alkaline phosphatase activity in fluid dairy products: Fluorometric method.* Report nr AOAC Official Method 991.24. Gaithersburg, MD: AOAC International. Available from: http://www.aoac.org/omarev1/991_24.pdf.

Araujo MM, Duarte RC, Silva PC, Marchioni E, Villavicencio ACLH. 2009. Application of the microbiological method DEFT/APC to detect minimally processed vegetables treated with gamma radiation. *Radiat Phys Chem* 78:691–693.

Association of Public Health Laboratories. 2010. PulseNet: A critical food safety surveillance system. *Issues in Brief 1.*

Ballmer K, Korczak BM, Kuhnert P, Slickers P, Ehricht R, Hachler H. 2007. Fast DNA serotyping of *Escherichia coli* by use of an oligonucleotide microarray. *J Clin Microbiol* 45(2):370–379.

Beerens H. 1998. Bifidobacteria as indicators of faecal contamination in meat and meat products: Detection, determination of origin and comparison with *Escherichia coli. Int J Food Microbiol* 40(3):203–207.

Bell BP, Goldoft M, Griffin PM, Davis MA, Gordon DC, Tarr PI, Bartleson CA, Lewis JH, Barrett TJ, Wells JG. 1994. A multistate outbreak of *Escherichia coli* O157:H7–associated bloody diarrhea and hemolytic uremic syndrome from hamburgers. The Washington experience. *JAMA* 272(17):1349–1353.

Bonde GJ. 1966. Bacteriological methods for estimation of water pollution. *Health Lab Sci* 3(2):124–128.

Bonilla N, Santiago T, Marcos P, Urdaneta M, Domingo JS, Toranzos GA. 2010. Enterophages, a group of phages infecting *Enterococcus faecalis*, and their potential as alternate indicators of human faecal contamination. *Water Sci Technol* 61(2):293–300.

Brehm-Stecher B, Young C, Jaykus LA, Tortorello ML. 2009. Sample preparation: The forgotten beginning. *J Food Prot* 72(8):1774–1789.

Capita R, Prieto M, Alonso-Calleja C. 2004. Sampling methods for microbiological analysis of red meat and poultry carcasses. *J Food Prot* 67(6):1303–1308.

Centers for Disease Control and Prevention. 2009. Multistate outbreak of *Salmonella* infections associated with peanut butter and peanut butter–containing products—United States, 2008–2009. *MMWR* 58(4):85–90.

Chen FC, Godwin SL. 2006. Comparison of a rapid ATP bioluminescence assay and standard plate count methods for assessing microbial contamination of consumers' refrigerators. *J Food Prot* 69(10):2534–2538.

Curren MSS, King JW. 2002. Sampling and sample preparation for food analysis. In: *Sampling and sample preparation for field and laboratory: Fundamentals and new directions in sample preparation.* Pawliszyn J, ed. Amsterdam: Elsevier.

Dick J, Parrish NM. 2007. Microbiology tools for the epidemiologist. In: *Infectious disease epidemiology: Theory and practice.* 2nd ed. Nelson KE, Williams CFM, eds. Sudbury, MA: Jones & Bartlett.

Food and Agriculture Organization of the United Nations/World Health Organization. 2008. *Viruses in food: Scientific advice to support risk management activities.* Report nr Microbiological Risk Assessment Series No. 13. Rome: FAO/WHO.

Food and Drug Administration. 2010a. *The bacteriological analytical manual.* Online ed. Washington, DC: U.S. Department of Health and Human Services. Available from: http://www.fda.gov/Food/ScienceResearch/LaboratoryMethods/BacteriologicalAnalyticalManualBAM/default.htm.

Food and Drug Administration. 2010b. *Investigations operations manual.* Silver Spring, MD: U.S. Food and Drug Administration.

Food and Drug Administration. 2009. *Grade "A" pasteurized milk ordinance (2009 revision).* Rockville, MD: U.S. Public Health Service/U.S. Food and Drug Administration.

Food Safety and Inspection Service. 2009. *2009 FSIS National Residue Program scheduled sampling plans (blue book).* Washington, DC: U.S. Department of Agriculture.

Francis JS, Harrington SM, Carroll KC, Bishai WR. 2007. Molecular epidemiology and infectious diseases. In: *Infectious disease epidemiology: Theory and practice.* 2nd ed. Nelson KE, Williams CFM, eds. Sudbury, MA: Jones & Bartlett.

Franz CM, Stiles ME, Schleifer KH, Holzapfel WH. 2003. Enterococci in foods—a conundrum for food safety. *Int J Food Microbiol* 88(2–3):105–122.

Fung DY. 2002. Predictions for rapid methods and automation in food microbiology. *J AOAC Int* 85(4):1000–1002.

Ge B, Meng J. 2009. Advanced technologies for pathogen and toxin detection in foods: Current applications and future directions. *JALA* 14(4):235–241.

Gerner-Smidt P, Hise K, Kincaid J, Hunter S, Rolando S, Hyytia-Trees E, Ribot EM, Swaminathan B, PulseNet Taskforce. 2006. PulseNet USA: A five-year update. *Foodborne Pathog Dis* 3(1):9–19.

Gerssen A, Pol-Hofstad IE, Poelman M, Mulder PPJ, van den Top HJ, Jacob de Boer J. 2010. Marine toxins: Chemistry, toxicity, occurrence and detection, with special reference to the Dutch situation. *Toxins* 2:878–904.

Guardino RF. 2005. Early history of microbiology and microbiological methods. In: *Encyclopedia of rapid microbiological methods.* Vol. 1. Miller M, ed. River Grove, IL: DHI Publishing.

Hall LB, Hartnett MJ. 1964. Measurement of the bacterial contamination on surfaces in hospitals. *Public Health Rep* 79:1021–1024.

Holbrook R. 2000. Detection of microorganisms in foods—principles of culture methods. In: *Microbiological safety and quality of food.* Vols. 1–2. Lund BM, Baird-Parker TC, Gould GW, eds. Gaithersburg, MD: Aspen Publishers.

Holt JG, ed. 1994. *Bergey's manual of determinative bacteriology.* 9th ed. Baltimore, MD: Williams & Wilkins.

Hsu FC, Shieh YS, Sobsey MD. 2002. Enteric bacteriophages as potential fecal indicators in ground beef and poultry meat. *J Food Prot* 65(1):93–99.

Hunter DM, Lim DV. 2010. Rapid detection and identification of bacterial pathogens by using an ATP bioluminescence immunoassay. *J Food Prot* 73(4):739–746.

International Commission on Microbiological Specifications for Foods. 1986. *Microorganisms in foods 2: Sampling for microbiological analysis: Principles and specific applications.* 2nd ed. Toronto: University of Toronto Press.

International Union of Food Science and Technology. 2011. *Chemical hazards in food.* Report nr IUFoST Scientific Information Bulletin. Available from: http://www.iufost.org/sites/default/files/docs/IUF.SIB.ChemicalHazardsinFood.pdf.

Jarvis B. 2000. Sampling for microbiological analysis. In: *Microbiological safety and quality of food.* Vols. 1–2. Lund BM, Baird-Parker TC, Gould GW, eds. Gaithersburg, MD: Aspen Publishers.

Jay JM, Loessner MJ, Golden DA. 2005. *Modern food microbiology.* 7th ed. New York, NY: Springer Science+Business Media.

Klotz V, Hill A, Warriner K, Griffiths M, Odumeru J. 2008. Assessment of the colorimetric and fluorometric assays for alkaline phosphatase activity in cow's, goat's, and sheep's milk. *J Food Prot* 71(9):1884–1888.

Kostrzynska M, Bachand A. 2006. Application of DNA microarray technology for detection, identification, and characterization of food-borne pathogens. *Can J Microbiol* 52(1):1–8.

Liolios K, Chen IM, Mavromatis K, Tavernarakis N, Hugenholtz P, Markowitz VM, Kyrpides NC. 2010. The genomes on line database (GOLD) in 2009: Status of genomic and metagenomic projects and their associated metadata. *Nucleic Acids Res* 38(Database issue):D346–354.

Lofstrom C, Krause M, Josefsen MH, Hansen F, Hoorfar J. 2009. Validation of a same-day real-time PCR method for screening of meat and carcass swabs for *Salmonella. BMC Microbiol* 9:85.

Mandal PK, Biswas AK, Choi K, Pal UK. 2011. Methods for rapid detection of foodborne pathogens: An overview. *Am J Food Technol* 6:87–102.

Midura TF, Bryant RG. 2001. Sampling plans, sample collections, shipment, and preparation for analysis. In: *Compendium of methods for the microbiological examination of foods.* 4th ed. Downes FP, Ito K, eds. Washington, DC: American Public Health Association.

Muniain-Mujika I, Calvo M, Lucena F, Girones R. 2003. Comparative analysis of viral pathogens and potential indicators in shellfish. *Int J Food Microbiol* 83(1):75–85.

Musgrove MT, Cox NA, Berrang ME, Harrison MA. 2003. Comparison of weep and carcass rinses for recovery of *Campylobacter* from retail broiler carcasses. *J Food Prot* 66(9):1720–1723.

National Research Council. 2004. *Indicators for waterborne pathogens.* Washington, DC: National Academies Press.

Oliver JD. 2005. The viable but nonculturable state in bacteria. *J Microbiol* 43 Spec No:93–100.

Pavlic M, Griffiths MW. 2009. Principles, applications, and limitations of automated ribotyping as a rapid method in food safety. *Foodborne Pathog Dis* 6(9):1047–1055.

Payne C, Wibley RA. 2009. Alkaline phosphatase activity in pasteurized milk: A quantitative comparison of fluorophos and colourimetric procedure. *I J Dairy Tech* 62(3):308–314.

Pellizzari ED, Smith DJ, Clayton CA, Quackenboss JJ. 2003. Assessment of data quality for the NHEXAS—part II: Minnesota Children's Pesticide Exposure Study (MNCPES). *J Expo Anal Environ Epidemiol* 13(6):465–479.

Pimbley DW, Patel PD. 1998. A review of analytical methods for the detection of bacterial toxins. *Symp Ser Soc Appl Microbiol* 27:98S–109S.

Radcliffe DM, Holbrook R. 2000. Detection of microorganisms in food—principles and application of immunological techniques. In: *Microbiological safety and quality of food.* Vols. 1–2. Lund BM, Baird-Parker TC, Gould GW, eds. Gaithersburg, MD: Aspen Publishers.

Rasooly A, Herold KE. 2008. Food microbial pathogen detection and analysis using DNA microarray technologies. *Foodborne Pathog Dis* 5(4):531–550.

Reasoner DJ. 2004. Heterotrophic plate count methodology in the United States. *Int J Food Microbiol* 92(3):307–315.

Reiter E, Zentek J, Razzazi E. 2009. Review on sample preparation strategies and methods used for the analysis of aflatoxins in food and feed. *Mol Nutr Food Res* 53(4):508–524.

Strategic Consulting. 2008, January. *Food Microbiology—2008 to 2013.* Available from: http://www.researchandmarkets.com/reports/1071788/food_microbiology_2008_to_2013.

Swaminathan B, Barrett TJ, Hunter SB, Tauxe RV, CDC PulseNet Task Force. 2001. PulseNet: The molecular subtyping network for foodborne bacterial disease surveillance, United States. *Emerg Infect Dis* 7(3):382–389.

Tauxe RV. 2006. Molecular subtyping and the transformation of public health. *Foodborne Pathog Dis* 3(1):4–8.

Tortorello ML. 2003. Indicator organisms for safety and quality—uses and methods for detection: Minireview. *J AOAC Int* 86(6):1208–1217.

Tortorello ML, Stewart DS. 1994. Antibody-direct epifluorescent filter technique for rapid, direct enumeration of *Escherichia coli* O157:H7 in beef. *Appl Environ Microbiol* 60(10):3553–3559.

Turner NW, Subrahmanyam S, Piletsky SA. 2009. Analytical methods for determination of mycotoxins: A review. *Anal Chim Acta* 632(2):168–180.

Ulitzur N, Ulitzur S. 2006. New rapid and simple methods for detection of bacteria and determination of their antibiotic susceptibility by using phage mutants. *Appl Environ Microbiol* 72(12):7455–7459.

Wesche AM, Gurtler JB, Marks BP, Ryser ET. 2009. Stress, sublethal injury, resuscitation, and virulence of bacterial foodborne pathogens. *J Food Prot* 72(5):1121–1138.

Whitehead KA, Smith LA, Verran J. 2008. The detection of food soils and cells on stainless steel using industrial methods: UV illumination and ATP bioluminescence. *Int J Food Microbiol* 127(1–2):121–128.

Wise MG, Siragusa GR, Plumblee J, Healy M, Cray PJ, Seal BS. 2009. Predicting *Salmonella enterica* serotypes by repetitive sequence-based PCR. *J Microbiol Meth* 76:18–24.

Yousef AE, Carlstrom C. 2003. *Food microbiology: A laboratory manual.* Hoboken, NJ: John Wiley.

---

## USEFUL RESOURCES

AOAC Method Validation. http://www.aoac.org/vmeth/oma_program.htm

Bacterial Microarray Group (BμG@S). http://www.bugs.sgul.ac.uk/

FDA *Bacteriological Analytical Manual (BAM).* http://www.fda.gov/Food/ScienceResearch/LaboratoryMethods/BacteriologicalAnalyticalManualBAM/default.htm

GOLD: Genomes Online Database. http://www.genomesonline.org/

MedlinePlus. Laboratory Tests. http://www.nlm.nih.gov/medlineplus/laboratorytests.html

National Center for Biotechnology Information. http://www.ncbi.nlm.nih.gov/

National Center for Biotechnology Information. Microbial Genomes. http://www.ncbi.nlm.nih.gov/genomes/MICROBES/microbial_taxtree.html

National Center for Biotechnology Information. A Science Primer. http://www.ncbi.nlm.nih.gov/About/primer/

Rapid Micro Users Group. http://www.rapidmicro.org/

Rapidmicrobiology.com. http://www.rapidmicrobiology.com/

U.S. Department of Agriculture. Food Safety and Inspection Service. Accredited Laboratories. http://www.fsis.usda.gov/Science/Accredited_Laboratories/index.asp

U.S. Department of Agriculture. Food Safety and Inspection Service. Data Collection and Reports. http://origin-www.fsis.usda.gov/Science/Data_Collection_&_Reports/index.asp

U.S. Department of Agriculture. Food Safety and Inspection Service. Guidebooks & Methods, Microbiology Laboratory Guidebook. http://www.fsis.usda.gov/Science/Microbiological_Lab_Guidebook/index.asp

U.S. Environmental Protection Agency. Pesticides: Analytical Methods & Procedures. Index of Residue Analytical Methods (RAM). http://www.epa.gov/oppbead1/methods/ram12b.htm

# CHAPTER 8

361-424

# Safety Management
# of the Food Supply

## LEARNING OBJECTIVES

1. Explain why a farm-to-fork perspective is necessary with safety management of the food supply.
2. Describe animal feeding operations (AFOs and CAFOs) and the potential problem areas related to environmental protection, public health in general, and food safety in particular.
3. List and explain the key strategies aimed at reducing the carriage and shedding of pathogens in farm animals.
4. Explain why animal feed is important to animal health and food safety, and recognize the types and sources of possible contaminants in animal feed.
5. Describe the major issues with manure management, and explain how manure management practices can affect food safety.
6. Recognize critical steps to control pathogen contamination levels of raw meats and poultry in the slaughter process.
7. List the ways that eggs can become contaminated with *Salmonella enterica*, and describe how to reduce or control contamination of eggs with *S. enterica* and other pathogens.
8. Describe the sources and types of potential hazards with milk and dairy products, and explain why milk is one of the safest food products available today.
9. Compare and contrast the differences between wild-caught and farm-raised fish in terms of preharvest food safety measures.
10. Compared with other types of seafood, explain why the biological and nonbiological factors of consuming molluscan shellfish make them inherently riskier in terms of foodborne hazards.
11. Describe specific programs and types of harvest controls used with molluscan shellfish to minimize the risks of infections and intoxications.
12. List and describe the different ways preharvest crops can become contaminated with harmful biological and chemical agents.

13. Discern the differences between the potential hazards and control options of sewage sludge versus manure when applied to food crops.

14. Identify the major food safety risks of pesticide practices for applications on crops, and describe the types of control strategies used to minimize these risks.

15. Explain why prevention of mycotoxin production and the elimination of mycotoxins are difficult in the food supply chain, particularly in lesser developed countries.

16. Describe the primary and secondary strategies of mycotoxin control in foods.

17. Explain the purpose of food processing, and recognize the major descriptors of processed and fresh foods.

18. List and describe the major food safety management tools for processing foods.

19. Recognize and explain the major food safety issues with the transport and distribution of foods.

20. Explain the traditional public health rationale for vigilant oversight of retail food establishments.

21. Describe the principal risk management strategies to protect the public health from foodborne hazards at the retail level, and explain how risk management is shared between federal, state, and local levels of government.

22. Describe how inspection scores are used to measure and convey the risks of foodborne illnesses at retail establishments, and explain the strengths and limitations of scoring systems.

23. Recognize the differences in food safety knowledge and actual practices of consumers at home.

24. From the material provided in the text, provide a strategy for developing food safety messages and educational programs for consumers.

25. Provide an overview of federal agencies, statutes, and regulations designed to protect the U.S. food supply.

26. Explain industry incentives or motivation to implement new or novel food safety practices without government mandate or intervention.

27. Define food terrorism and agroterrorism, and briefly explain why the food supply is vulnerable to acts of terrorism.

28. Explain the purpose of the CARVER + Shock program, and recognize key food defense issues identified by the SPPA Initiative.

29. List and describe the roles and relationships of key components in a food safety management system at the national level.

## THE FARM-TO-FORK PERSPECTIVE

Americans are fortunate to enjoy an abundant, diverse, affordable, and safe food supply. This is made possible by modern agricultural technology and methods, along with a fully developed network of food processors and distributors. Foods are available to consumers as a variety of choices, from fresh foods to highly processed foods that are ready-to-eat (RTE). Most Americans are unaware of the steps involved with bringing these food products to market. Yet, whether purchasing groceries or eating at a restaurant, consumers implicitly trust that their food is safe. Such trust is easily lost when foodborne illness outbreaks or contaminated foods are reported in the mass media. And although the government is usually held accountable for ensuring a safe food supply, the provision of safe food is a responsibility that involves everyone along the entire food supply chain. The purpose of this chapter is to provide an overview of the food supply chain with respect to food safety management. The role of government, industry, and consumers in food safety management is also briefly covered.

The current concept of food safety management encompasses a continuum of activities starting with producers and ending with consumers. This concept is cleverly characterized as the farm-to-fork or farm-to-plate continuum (Institute of Medicine [IOM] 2009). Figure 8-1 is a simplified diagram and illustration of the farm-to-fork continuum. There are good reasons for viewing food safety management with a farm-to-fork perspective. First, harmful agents can contaminate foods anywhere along the farm-to-fork continuum, though certain agents are more likely to be introduced at particular points. Contamination with harmful agents can originate from raw agricultural products, equipment, facilities, ingredients or additives, processes, packaging, transport vehicles, pests, food workers, and other sources. Second, many harmful agents can persist throughout the food supply chain despite being subjected to various processing and preparation steps. Examples of agents that can withstand harsh processing conditions are various microbial toxins, chemicals, and spores from bacteria such as *Clostridium perfringens* and *Bacillus cereus*. In the case of fresh or minimally processed foods, pathogens may be transported more or less directly from the farm to the consumer. Third, bacterial pathogens can multiply to infectious dose levels under favorable growth conditions during the storage and transport of foods. Although most bacterial pathogens are easily destroyed by cooking temperatures (e.g., *Campylobacter* spp.), heavy pathogen loading of foods increases the risk of cross-contamination hazards during food storage, handling, and preparation.

The most effective hazard control actions for foods are implemented across the farm-to-fork continuum. Certainly, careful food preparation and cooking practices reduce the risks for several types of food hazards, but these risks are compounded by unsafe practices earlier in the food supply chain. Reducing the frequency and/or level of contamination with harmful agents in foods before they reach the consumer is also likely to reduce the incidence of foodborne illnesses. This rationale is supported by epidemiologic surveillance and food monitoring data, and by risk modeling studies of food contamination (Centers for Disease Control and Prevention [CDC] 2010b; International Commission on Microbiological Specifications for Foods [ICMSF] 2006; Schroeder et al. 2005). Some potentially harmful agents are unavoidable or infeasible to eliminate in foods, and tolerances or action levels are necessary to establish. Although not explicitly stated, tolerances and action levels for harmful agents imply an acceptable level of risk to the potential hazards. Targeting strategic points along the farm-to-fork continuum with specific controls can maintain or reduce contamination levels with harmful agents at or below established tolerances and action levels.

Safety management of the U.S. food supply has been the subject of several Institute of Medicine (IOM) reviews and reports (IOM 2010, 2009, 2006, 2003, 1991; Institute of Medicine and National Research Council [IOM and NRC] 1998). Although the specific purpose of each report is different, several overarching themes are apparent in the recommendations of the reports. The most encountered theme is the need for a risk-based approach to food hazards—supported by scientific research and facts. In other words, risk assessment methodologies should be used to generate information for decision making, priority setting, and ultimately risk management of

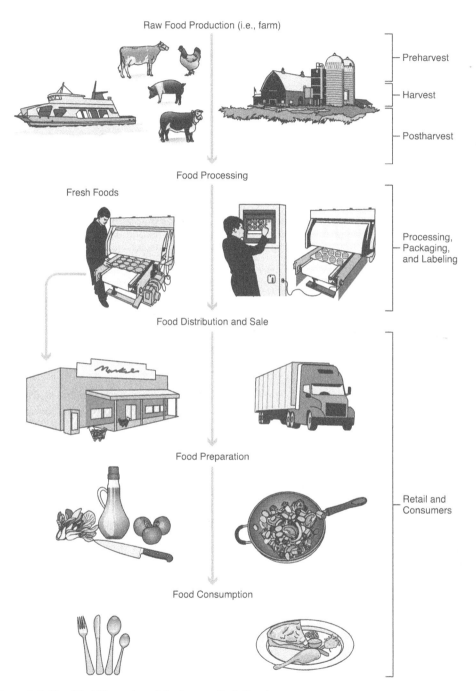

**Figure 8-1** Simplified Illustration of the Farm-to-Fork Continuum

food hazards. Although some older risk management policies for protecting the food supply are still applicable (e.g., pasteurization, sanitation), others have become outdated, less effective, or even counterproductive. The nature of food hazards is changing—particularly with regard to emerging infections and possible terrorism. New food technologies, products, and distribution systems have also changed the risks of many potential hazards. A risk-based approach is thus necessary to manage food safety in light of an increasingly complex food supply and emerging threats. Other themes in the IOM report recommendations include greater authority for food regulatory agencies, better coordination among federal and state agencies, more transparency and stakeholder involvement with food safety programs, due consideration of technical feasibility in controls, and the avoidance of barriers to free trade.

## FOOD PRODUCTION: PREHARVEST, HARVEST, AND POSTHARVEST OPERATIONS

### Industrial Farms for Animal Production

The raising of livestock for food has changed dramatically over the last 40 years. During this time, the number of family farms declined greatly, while the number industrial farms increased (Pew Commission on Industrial Farm Animal Production [PCIFAP] 2008). Industrial farms for animal production are characterized by larger operations with a higher density of animals that are usually fed onsite rather than by free ranging or grazing. This trend is most evident in the hog industry by the decline of individual farm operations and the increased inventory of hogs (Figure 8-2, A and B). Similar trends have occurred in the production of eggs, poultry, and cattle. From a business standpoint, higher densities of animals yield greater productivity at less cost per head of livestock. From a public health and environmental standpoint, higher animal densities produce problems related to animal health, waste disposal, water and air pollution, animal–human disease transmission, emerging pathogens, antibiotic resistance of pathogens, and other occupational and environmental hazards (Gurian-Sherman 2008; PCIFAP 2008). For the purposes of regulating pollution discharges, certain industrial farms are designated by the Environmental Protection Agency (EPA) as animal feeding operations (AFOs) and/or concentrated animal feeding operations (CAFOs) (National Pollutant Discharge Elimination System 2010). An AFO is generally considered any operation where animals are confined, fed, and/or maintained on a lot or in a facility for 45 days or more during the year, and the premises are not used during the growing season for vegetation, crops, forage, or postharvest residues. The CAFOs are designated and regulated based on size thresholds and other criteria. Table 8-1 lists the size thresholds for large, medium, and small CAFOs.

### *Preharvest/Preslaughter Food Safety Considerations with Animal Production*

From a food safety perspective, the primary problems with AFOs/CAFOs are related to maintaining good animal health and manure disposal. Animal health is important because even small changes in animal health can significantly influence the rate of foodborne infections in humans (Singer et al. 2007). Many animals have subclinical infections, and changes in animal health can increase both carriage rates and pathogen shedding. If properly managed, concentrated animals can be kept healthy with good veterinary care, adequate nutrition, and sanitation. However, the

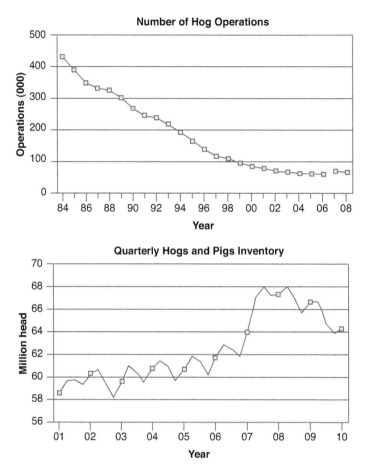

**Figure 8-2** Number of Hog Operations and Quarterly Hogs and Pigs Inventory in the United States.
*Source:* USDA-NASS

control of infectious diseases in CAFOs is difficult because pathogen transmission is potentially enhanced throughout a CAFO compared with lower density animal operations (Gurian-Sherman 2008). This includes pathogenic *Escherichia coli*, *Salmonella*, *Campylobacter* species, and other foodborne pathogens. CAFOs also facilitate the back-and-forth transmission of zoonoses between animal populations and human workers. Such exchanges promote mutations of pathogens, creating the opportunity for the emergence of more virulent strains. Some of these new strains may emerge as new foodborne pathogens, while others may emerge as a range of new respiratory viruses (e.g., H5N1 a.k.a. avian influenza or bird flu).

Several intervention strategies have been proposed and applied to reduce the carriage and shedding of zoonotic pathogens in animals (Callaway et al. 2004; LeJeune and Wetzel 2007).

**Table 8-1** Size Thresholds for Designating Concentrated Animal Feeding Operations (CAFOs)

| Animal Sector | Size Thresholds (number of animals) | | |
| --- | --- | --- | --- |
| | Large CAFOs | Medium CAFOs[a] | Small CAFOs[b] |
| Cattle or cow/calf pairs | 1,000 or more | 300–999 | Less than 300 |
| Mature dairy cattle | 700 or more | 200–699 | Less than 200 |
| Veal calves | 1,000 or more | 300–999 | Less than 300 |
| Swine (weighing over 55 pounds) | 2,500 or more | 750–2,499 | Less than 750 |
| Swine (weighing less than 55 pounds) | 10,000 or more | 3,000–9,999 | Less than 3,000 |
| Horses | 500 or more | 150–499 | Less than 150 |
| Sheep or lambs | 10,000 or more | 3,000–9,999 | Less than 3,000 |
| Turkeys | 55,000 or more | 16,500–54,999 | Less than 16,500 |
| Laying hens or broilers (liquid manure handling systems) | 30,000 or more | 9,000–29,999 | Less than 9,000 |
| Chickens other than laying hens (other than a liquid manure handling systems) | 125,000 or more | 37,500–124,999 | Less than 37,500 |
| Laying hens (other than a liquid manure handling systems) | 82,000 or more | 25,000–81,999 | Less than 25,000 |
| Ducks (other than a liquid manure handling systems) | 30,000 or more | 10,000–29,999 | Less than 10,000 |
| Ducks (liquid manure handling systems) | 5,000 or more | 1,500–4,999 | Less than 1,500 |

[a]Must also meet one of two "method of discharge" criteria to be defined as a CAFO or may be designated.
[b]Never a CAFO by regulatory definition, but may be designated as a CAFO on a case-by-case basis.
*Source*: EPA

These strategies fall into three basic categories: (1) exposure reduction, (2) exclusion, and (3) anti-pathogen (LeJeune and Wetzel 2007). Exposure reduction strategies emphasize limiting the introduction of pathogens into a herd or flock. Exposure reduction strategies include isolation of new or sick animals; restriction of access by visitors, wild animals, and pests; good sanitation and the elimination of disease reservoirs in the local environment; reduction of animal density; good water and feedstuff quality; and hygienic feeding operations (Codex Alimentarius Commission 2004a). The quality of animal feedstuff is particularly important in exposure reduction (Davies et al. 2004), and this topic is covered in greater detail in a later section.

Exclusion strategies are based on microbial interference and colonization resistance (see Chapter 2). The inoculation of animal intestinal tracts with antagonistic bacteria is an example of an exclusion technology called *competitive exclusion* (Callaway et al. 2004). The bacteria used in competitive exclusion are nonpathogenic, and once established in the gut, they prevent or minimize the colonization of pathogenic bacteria. Competitive exclusion agents are used routinely to minimize *Salmonella* colonization in chicks, but the net benefits, particularly with other animal species, are not consistently observed; this inconsistency may be related to differences in quality control of cultures, concurrent and incompatible treatments, or simply biological variability in animals and bacteria (Callaway et al. 2004). Other exclusion strategies include probiotics and prebiotics (LeJeune and Wetzel 2007). Probiotics are preparations of individual species or mixtures of antagonistic microorganisms (bacteria and/or yeast) that are fed to animals. Probiotic preparations differ from competitive exclusion agents by the origin and types of microorganisms and by the antagonistic mechanisms in the animal intestinal tract. Microorganisms in probiotic preparations may not originate from animals, and the probiotic microorganisms may or may not colonize the intestinal tract but nonetheless alter the microbiota of the intestine. Unlike competitive exclusion agents and probiotics, prebiotics are actually organic compounds added to feeds, not viable microorganisms. Prebiotics are basically nutrients that only certain beneficial or antagonistic bacteria can digest. Even the host animal cannot digest or utilize the prebiotics. By providing nutrients that only certain bacteria can digest, a shift in the microbial ecology of the intestine occurs, allowing the population of beneficial bacteria to flourish and limiting the proliferation of pathogenic bacteria.

Anti-pathogen strategies include vaccinations, bacteriophage therapy, and antimicrobial compounds. Vaccination is the ultimate strategy of controlling—possibly eradicating—certain animal diseases. Vaccines have been developed for certain strains of *Salmonella* in poultry, swine, and dairy cattle (Callaway et al. 2004), but an efficacious vaccine against *E. coli* O157:H7 in cattle is currently unavailable (LeJeune and Wetzel 2007). Besides the great costs involved with developing vaccines, which can be prohibitive, several technical challenges make the development of vaccines difficult for enteric pathogens (LeJeune and Wetzel 2007). To develop a vaccine, the antigens that distinguish a pathogenic strain must be identified; this is complicated by the many molecular mechanisms of disease caused by different strains of enteric pathogens. Additionally, to be most effective, immune responses to enteric pathogens should occur in the gut, but the intestinal mucosa is specialized, and achieving sufficient immunity is difficult using conventional vaccine technology. Hopefully, in the future, emerging vaccine technology will provide more opportunities for the vaccination of animals against enteric bacterial pathogens. As for bacteriophage therapy, the administration of bacteriophages to animals has been the subject of research for many years, but real-world applications of bacteriophages have been limited because of variability in efficacy (Callaway et al. 2004). Additional research is needed before bacteriophages can meet the challenges of routine use.

The anti-pathogen strategy most frequently employed is administration of antimicrobial compounds. Therapeutic administration of antibiotics is done to treat animals with infections, and antibiotics are administered or fed to animals as a prophylaxis against infections and/or to promote growth (Mathew, Cissell, Liamthong 2007). Although therapeutic and prophylactic use of antibiotics in animals can reduce the carriage rates and shedding levels of pathogenic bacteria, the use of antibiotics may promote the development of antibiotic-resistant strains of pathogens, particularly if the antibiotics are improperly used. With therapeutic use of antibiotics, the most important practices to limit the emergence of resistant strains are antibiotic selection and optimal dosing (Prescott 2008). Of all the antibiotics issues, however, the most controversial is the use of antibiotics to promote animal growth. This practice raises serious concerns about transmitting antibiotic-resistant strains of pathogens to humans through foods (see related discussion in Chapter 3). Other compounds besides antibiotics are also used as an anti-pathogen strategy. For example, the addition of sodium chlorate in food or water has been shown to reduce certain Enterobacteriaceae in cattle and pigs; like many experimental antimicrobials and therapies, however, this compound has not been approved for routine applications in the United States (LeJeune and Wetzel 2007).

Other potential problems with maintaining good animal health are related to treatments with various veterinary drugs, pesticide use, and animal feeding. As discussed in Chapter 3, a variety of veterinary drugs are used to maintain animal health and to promote growth—including hormone-like compounds. If correctly administered, most animal drugs are unlikely to become residues in the tissues of food animals, but drugs are not always administered correctly. Some may be administered as "extra-label" or by untrained individuals (Government Accountability Office [GAO] 1992). Animals are also treated internally or externally with insecticides to control ectoparasites such as lice, ticks, and biting flies. Insecticides administered internally are regulated by the Food and Drug Administration (FDA) as veterinary medications, while externally applied insecticides are regulated by EPA. Failure to follow regulations and guidelines for the proper use of insecticides in/on livestock can result in residue contamination of the animal's tissues. The safest and most effective control of ectoparasites involves a combination of pesticides and environmental modifications called integrated pest management (IPT).

## Animal Feed

The farm-to-fork continuum of food animal products starts with the feedstuff (Crump, Griffin, Angulo 2002). Animal feeds are potential sources of biological, chemical, and physical agents, some of which can find their way into the human food chain. Formulations of modern animal feeds include renderings (from slaughter by-products), antimicrobials, and other drugs or chemicals. Renderings pose the risk of being contaminated with enteric bacterial pathogens or prions. When renderings are blended with animal feed, pathogens can be transmitted to animals, increasing the risk of human infections via the food chain (Crump et al. 2002). Feedstuffs blended with renderings are usually heat treated, but periodic surveys of finished feed often detect viable pathogens (Crump et al. 2002). The contamination of feed with *Salmonella enterica* is partly responsible for the global spread and increased incidence of salmonellosis in agricultural animals, particularly among chickens (Crump et al. 2002; Molbak, Olsen, Wegener 2005). Renderings from animal tissues are also believed responsible for the spread of bovine spongiform encephalopathy (BSE) prions among cattle. Unlike bacterial pathogens, prions are not usually destroyed by heat treatments. Preventive measures for prions include the strict exclusion of brain and spinal cord trimmings or parts from the renderings.

Animal feed may become contaminated with and spread zoonotic pathogens by means other than renderings. Incidental contamination of feed with pathogens occurs during transport and on-farm storage and mixing prior to animal feeding (Codex Alimentarius Commission 2004a; Davies et al. 2004; LeJeune and Wetzel 2007). Important contamination sources of pathogens in feedstuff on the farm are manure and pests such as rodents. Over the years, several studies have also suggested that ruminant animals have higher carriage rates and shedding levels of enteric pathogens when fed grains rather than forage or roughage. For example, feedlot (i.e., CAFO) cattle are fed grain-based diets so that they efficiently reach market weight, and some studies have found these cattle shed higher levels of *E. coli*, including pathogenic strains. In a recent review of this subject, the authors conclude that grain-based diets indeed contribute to pathogen shedding, though the magnitude of effects is varied (Callaway et al. 2009). More important, they conclude that switching from grain-based to forage diets reduces the shedding of generic *E. coli* and *E. coli* O157:H7 in cattle. However, the authors acknowledge that switching feedlot cattle to hay prior to slaughter is impractical. They recommend additional research to determine why and how the microbial ecology of bovine intestinal tracts changes with different diets. Such research could lead to better formulations of animal feed that can reduce the shedding and/or carriage rate of zoonotic pathogens.

Animal feed is vulnerable to unintentional contamination with industrial chemicals, agrochemicals, and toxins (Codex Alimentarius Commission 2004a). Sources of industrial chemicals are usually pollution sources. Feedstuff can also become contaminated with industrial chemicals by poor processing and storage practices. This occurred in 1973 when livestock feed was accidently mixed with flame retardant by a Michigan production plant. The flame retardant contained polybrominated biphenyls (PBBs) and was mistakenly used as an additive to the feed. Livestock at approximately 1,000 farms were subsequently fed the contaminated feed. Farmers first noticed health effects with their livestock, but the problem could not be attributed to any particular source. A farmer by the name of Rick Halbert conducted his own experiment using the contaminated feed and observed a variety of health effects and deaths among his dairy herd (Reich 1983). Unfortunately, a year would pass after the contamination incident before officials confirmed and acknowledged the source of the problem. By that time, the contaminated feed had been used for millions of chickens and thousands of cattle, pigs, and sheep. All of the affected animals and food products, including eggs and milk products, were destroyed, with the total costs reaching hundreds of millions of dollars (Reich 1983). Tragically, thousands of people, most belonging to families of the quarantined farms, were exposed to the tainted food products. This cohort of exposed people has been followed for years by epidemiologists who also measured their blood PBB levels; an elevated risk and dose-response relationship of certain cancers has been observed in the cohort (Hoque et al. 1998). The original events surrounding the Michigan PBB incident were dramatized in a film (*Bitter Harvest*) and a book (*The Poisoning of Michigan*).

Carryover of chemical residues into food products is possible from animal feed contaminated with chlorinated pesticides and certain environmental chemicals. The persistence of these chemicals in animals and animal-derived foods depends on the physicochemical properties and metabolic fates of the individual compound (Kan and Meijer 2007). Pesticides and compounds such as dieldrin, aldrin, DDT, hexachlorobenzene, polychlorinated biphenyls (PCBs), and dioxins have high accumulation potential in animals and carryover into food products. Polycyclic aromatic hydrocarbons (PAHs), which are pollutants from combustion sources, are highly persistent in the environment and animal tissues, and carryover into food products is possible in areas with high levels of pollution. Heavy metals (Pb, Hg, Cd, etc.) and arsenic in feedstuff most likely target the liver and kidneys of animals, and the carryover risks are greatest if humans consume these organs (Kan and Meijer 2007). Because the concentrations of pesticides and environmental chemicals vary by location and land use, the source of materials used for animal feed is important to protect and control as much as possible. Strategies for preventing the contamination of animal feed involve proper pesticide usage, surveys around forage crops, and periodic testing of feedstuff.

Mycotoxins represent a significant problem with animal feeds. Several types of mycotoxins are encountered in animal feeds and pastures. When consumed by livestock in sufficient quantities, the mycotoxin-contaminated feed can cause a multitude of animal health problems (Bhat, Rai, Karim 2010). The toxic effects can range from irritation of the animal's gastrointestinal tract to death in severe cases. Other toxic effects from mycotoxins include poor nutrient absorption, immunosuppression, and organ dysfunction. Any of these toxic effects can make animals more susceptible to zoonotic and opportunistic infections, thus increasing the chances of transmitting pathogens through the food chain. Several mycotoxins in feeds (or their metabolites) also have the potential for carryover in animal-derived foods, including meat, milk, and eggs. The most serious concern with carryover from animal feed is with an aflatoxin $B_1$ metabolite $(M_1)$ in milk (Bhat et al. 2010; Kan and Meijer 2007). Consequently, federal action levels are established by FDA for aflatoxins in animal feed and for the $M_1$ metabolite in milk.

## Manure Waste Management

*Manure* is a term used to describe the excrement produced by animals. The amount, physical consistency, and composition of manure produced by agricultural animals are influenced by animal breed, age, health condition, diet, and many other factors. Overall, agricultural animals produce a much greater amount of excrement per mass or weight than humans do. To fully appreciate the differences, a rough comparison of excrement generated by animals and humans is helpful. The amount of excrement produced by humans is highly variable. A reasonable estimate is 3.72 pounds of excrement per person per day (GAO 2008a). Assuming the average human weighs 150 pounds, the estimated amount of excrement produced per thousand pounds of human weight is nearly 25 pounds (25/1,000). By comparison, Figure 8-3 illustrates the average amount of waste produced per animal for several types of livestock. These numbers are derived from the typical mass (i.e., weight) of livestock and estimates of manure produced per 1,000 pounds of live animal mass (American Society of Agricultural Engineers [ASAE] 2003). When these estimates of manure are multiplied by the CAFO thresholds listed in Table 8-1, it becomes quite apparent that manure management is a big issue with animal production. For example, the minimum threshold for a large dairy cattle CAFO is 700 head; this equates to the CAFO producing over 42 tons of manure per day (120.4 lbs/day × 700 head ÷ 2,000 lbs/ton).

The major concern with CAFOs and manure management is pollution of the environment, principally surface and ground water, and to a lesser extent the air and land. Depending on the treatment types and degree, manure can damage the environment by nutrient overload, excessive biochemical oxygen demand, and contamination with a variety of chemical and biological agents. The latter category includes veterinary drug metabolites and zoonotic pathogens. Humans can be exposed to hazardous agents in manure through different environmental media and exposure pathways. Exposure pathways of greatest concern are waterborne, foodborne, and airborne. The principal foodborne hazards from manure are zoonotic pathogens. The species of pathogens present in manure are influenced by animal species and health, climate, indigenous or endemic diseases, and feed source. They include multiple species of bacteria (*Salmonella* serotypes, pathogenic

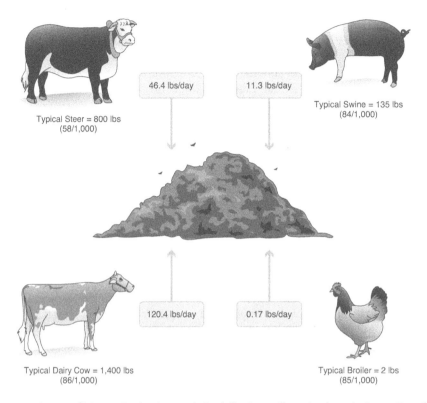

**Figure 8-3** Estimates of Manure Production per Animal (lbs./1,000 lbs. animal mass). *Source:* Data from ASAE 2003

---

strains of *E. coli*, *Campylobacter* spp., *Yersinia* spp., *Listeria* spp., etc.), protozoans (*Cryptospordium parvum*, *Giardia lamblia*, etc.), parasitic worms, and a few viruses (Rogers and Haines 2005).

Survival of zoonotic pathogens in manure depends on many factors. The single most important factor is the hardiness of a particular pathogen in the environment outside its host. Other critical factors are the composition of the manure and environmental conditions. These are somewhat analogous to the intrinsic and extrinsic parameters of food discussed in Chapter 4. In other words, factors such as temperature, nutrient content, microbial competition and predation, water content, pH, UV light, and so forth are key to the survival of pathogens in manure (Rogers and Haines 2005). Generally speaking, manure is a nutrient-rich medium that protects pathogens from exposure to UV light, desiccation, and similarly harmful environmental effects. Thus, in addition to enhancing survival, the storage of manure under favorable growth conditions may actually promote the multiplication of pathogens. With common foodborne bacterial pathogens, survival can range from 2 days for *Campylobacter* species in swine manure to 630 days for *E. coli* O157:H7 in sheep manure (Rogers and Haines 2005). Survival of pathogens on the farm is further complicated by recent revelations that some bacterial pathogens may live within free-living protozoa (Bleasdale et al. 2009; Young, Davis, Dirita 2007).

Manure containing viable pathogens increases the risk of foodborne disease transmission in several ways. First, infected animals in a herd or flock, especially in CAFOs, can spread pathogens to uninfected animals through manure, increasing the percentage of infected animals entering the human food chain. Second, contamination of animal hides or feathers with manure increases the opportunity for carcass and meat contamination during slaughter. Third, farm or food/slaughter workers can become infected from contact with manure, and the infected workers can contaminate human food, especially if they practice poor personal hygiene. Fourth, infected animals can gain access to and deposit manure in field crops destined for human consumption. Fifth, untreated or inadequately treated manure may be applied as fertilizer to crops for human consumption. Finally, water can become contaminated with manure and subsequently contaminate foodstuff. This occurs when runoff from manure contaminates crops, and when manure-contaminated water is used for irrigation or for washing produce and other agricultural commodities. Another possibility is manure contamination of animal watering sources, transmitting infections to uninfected livestock.

For animal producers, especially AFOs/CAFOs, an essential part of protecting the human food supply is a manure management plan. This entails the design and operations to collect, store, treat, and utilize the manure generated by animal production (ASAE 2003). The frequency of collecting and removing manure from animal feeding operations and farms depends on the number and density of animals present. Although it is impossible to maintain CAFOs in immaculate conditions, frequent removal of manure and periodic disinfection of pens or other animal containment facilities reduces overall pathogen loading, as well as minimizes the proliferation of pests and disease vectors. Collection of manure is also important to good feed hygiene because it reduces the potential for contamination of animal feedstuff. Storage of manure prior to treatment and/or utilization is important to manage in terms of runoff control, pest control, and preventing contamination of animals, feedstuff, and agricultural commodities.

Manure management systems in the United States are generally categorized as either passive or active (Rogers and Haines 2005). Passive systems involve minimal handling or manipulation of the manure and are most applicable to non-CAFOs. Handling or manipulation with passive systems is typically limited to moving and storing manure and applying it to land. Passive systems may also include lagoons or other storage methods, vegetated buffer zones, and the separation of animals by age or size to manage manure production and removal. Over time and with normal decomposition processes, the hazardous agents in manure are inactivated or attenuated with passive management systems. In contrast, active systems of manure management involve treatment processes to accelerate decomposition and/or change the hazardous characteristics of manure. This includes the inactivation of pathogenic microorganisms. Active systems are necessary for most CAFOs because the volume of manure that these operations produce is tremendous compared with historical farming methods. Examples of active systems include composting, aerobic and anaerobic digesters, and mixing lagoons. Active systems require much more human operator attention along with more upfront capital and greater operating costs.

Manure management poses a dilemma for public health officials and resource conservation proponents. With a growing global population, the recycling of nutrients in manure to fertilize crops is critically important, especially in lesser develop countries (Cliver 2009). On the other hand, excessive amounts of certain nutrients (e.g., N, P, and K) can migrate to waterways, where they can cause environmental problems such as algal blooms and eutrophication. Other chemical constituents in manure can migrate to waterways and groundwater and cause public health concerns. These include antibiotics, hormones, and veterinary drugs or their metabolites. Similarly, pathogenic microorganisms can be transferred to waterways, poorly protected wells, and food crops where they pose a risk of transmission to human populations. One possible solution to the pathogen problem is disinfection of manure, but certain disinfection processes can degrade the nutrient quality of manure for fertilizer applications (Martens and Bohm 2009). Hence, the environmental and public health risks of different manure treatments must be balanced in the context of social benefits, costs, and food production requirements. To more prudently control the hazards from CAFOs and with manure management, additional research is needed to generate data for risk assessment and the development of risk management strategies (Cliver 2009; Environmental Protection Agency [EPA] 2004).

### Livestock Slaughter Process

For the purposes of continuity, the slaughter process or animal "harvesting" (a term preferred by some producers) is discussed here rather than in the section on food processing. In addition, the slaughter process represents an important transition point from the farm to additional food processing and/or retail sales. Figure 8-4 shows a generic process flow diagram for beef slaughter. Variations of this diagram are encountered among beef producers, and significant differences exist between beef slaughter and other meat and poultry slaughter process flows. For example, instead of hide removal, pork carcasses are usually dehaired, and poultry carcasses are defeathered. To present an overview of food safety issues with the slaughter process, this section provides a generic introduction. Students who are interested in details about specific slaughter processes and practices are encouraged to look up the references and additional resources at the end of this chapter.

The animal holding and transport conditions prior to slaughter influence the spread of pathogens (Collins and Wall 2004). Animals become stressed when tightly confined together during holding and transport. As a consequence, animals may lose a significant percentage of their body weight through defecation, which then contaminates the floors and walls of pens and vehicles with manure. Several zoonotic pathogens are also shed in feces at a greater rate in stressed animals (Bach et al. 2004; Collins and Wall 2004; Dewell et al. 2008). In tight confinement, the hides or feathers of animals become contaminated either directly or indirectly with the manure and any potential pathogens. Some animals also suffer motion sickness during transport, and animals such as pigs are more likely to vomit. Hence, animals may arrive at the slaughter plant with more external contamination than when they were on the farm. Because most pathogens can survive in dried manure for several days, including on hides and feathers, the potential of contaminating finished carcasses during slaughter is increased.

Animal handlers can practice several preventive measures to minimize the contamination of hides and feathers with manure and pathogens. Handling practices that precondition animals or minimize stress may help reduce excretion and pathogen shedding. The correct timing of feed withdrawal prior to transport has been shown to reduce animal excretion, but other studies also find that this increases stress and pathogen shedding, and gastrointestinal breakage is sometimes more common among poultry during evisceration (National Advisory Committee on Meat and Poultry Inspection [NACMPI] 2008). Switching to more compatible diets prior to transport is

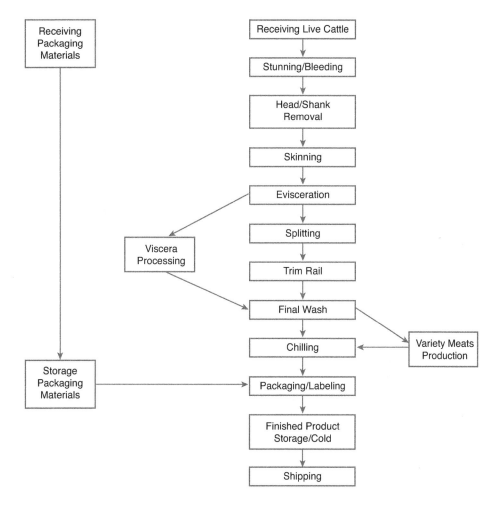

**Figure 8-4** Generic Process Flow Diagram for Beef Slaughter. *Source:* USDA, 1999a

being studied as an alternative to feed withdrawal. Another simple but effective measure is to clean and air-dry holding pens/crates and transport vehicles between lots of livestock. This minimizes the direct contamination of additional animals in successive trips. Limiting the holding times of animals prior to transport and slaughter also reduces pathogen shedding and manure production, and animals are less likely to become grossly contaminated when held for shorter periods in pens or crates. Another reason for limiting holding times is that animals frequently lay down after tiring, increasing contact with the contaminated floors and walls.

Upon arrival at the slaughter plant or abattoir, any sick or significantly contaminated animals should be culled from the shipment lot and holding pens. A small percentage (~18%) of meat producers test hides prior to slaughter (RTI International 2005), probably to survey the microbial loading of animals from different farms or sources. If washing is used to clean and calm down animals, it is best done in advance of slaughter to permit drying because washing animals immediately before slaughter has been shown to be less effective (NACMPI 2008). The reasons for this may stem from wet animals spreading contamination, or perhaps the added moisture contributes to pathogen survival.

The next step is stunning and bleeding the animal. Proper techniques for stunning/bleeding animals are very important to the humane treatment of animals, but they are not the most vulnerable points for bringing contamination into the slaughter plant (NACMPI 2008). Nevertheless, cuts or punctures of animals can introduce pathogens into the bloodstream and underlying tissues, so the bleeding instruments should be used and maintained in a sanitary manner. The next major steps to reduce external contamination of postmortem animals involve scalding treatments or rinses followed by skinning, dehairing, or defeathering.

The skinning/dehairing/defeathering and evisceration steps are critically important to controlling pathogen contamination of the finished carcasses and meats (NACMPI 2008). In healthy animals, the underlying muscle and fat tissues are considered sterile for practical purposes. However, as the outer layer of skin, hair, or feathers is removed, the edible portions of an animal become vulnerable to contamination with pathogens. This can occur from any number of transport modes. Airborne contamination occurs from particles, dust, and dried manure. Contact contamination can occur between animals (direct contact) and from contaminated surfaces, equipment, gloves, or hand tools (cross-contamination). Contamination can also be spread from an animal's skin, hair, or feathers to itself during the removal process (self-contamination). Proper methods and techniques, along with good sanitary practices, are necessary to minimize contamination of the carcasses. Automated or mechanically assisted methods on production lines often increase the likelihood of carcass contamination compared with skilled manual removal of skin, hair, or feathers.

Evisceration is a critically important step because the gastrointestinal contents of infected animals are likely to contain high densities of different pathogens (NACMPI 2008). Expulsion of the contents or tears in the gut can spread large numbers of pathogens around the plant, contaminating other carcasses, worker gloves and clothes, equipment, and tools. For larger animals, important procedures known as bunging are usually performed first. This involves cutting around the anal region and tying and/or bagging the rectum (i.e., bung) in a manner to prevent release of the intestinal contents. Similar procedures are used for the esophagus to prevent expulsion of the stomach contents. Evisceration methods and techniques vary greatly from plant to plant, and the degree of automation differs based on animal size and production volume. Larger carcasses such as beef and swine require more manual skill, whereas chicken broilers are frequently eviscerated in a fully automated manner. Even with larger carcasses such as swine, commercial systems are available for semiautomated and robotic evisceration. Good techniques by workers and properly operating equipment can minimize puncturing or ripping of the viscera. But occasional breaching of the viscera is expected. In these cases, workers must know how to remove the contamination and/or affected carcasses, and they must follow proper procedures for sanitizing or disinfecting tools and equipment. Most operations, especially poultry plants, utilize sanitizing rinses after or as part of the evisceration process. These rinses usually consist of hot water and/or approved chemical solutions. (See the section titled "Food Contact Sanitizers/Antimicrobials and Fumigation Agents" in Chapter 5.)

Following the final rinses, the carcasses are rapidly chilled and moved to refrigerated storage rooms to prevent the growth of pathogens and preserve product quality. The time interval from bleeding to chilling should be monitored and controlled to minimize the potential growth of pathogenic and toxigenic bacteria. Critical limits for time intervals are established on the basis of pathogen modeling, and they are influenced by the degree of contamination/decontamination of the carcasses. An example of a critical time limit for pork and beef carcasses is provided in the model hazard analysis and critical control points (HACCP) plans by the Food Safety and Inspection Service (FSIS), which states that the time interval from bleedout to start of chilling must be within 1 hour (Food Safety and Inspection Service [FSIS] 1999a, 1999b). The time necessary for the product to reach chill temperature is also important. Examples of critical limits for chill time are within 24 hours for pork and beef to reach 40°F or lower temperatures (FSIS 1999a, 1999b). For poultry products, the HACCP model uses a critical limit that all poultry products must reach a temperature of 40°F or less within 4 hours from bleeding (FSIS 1999c).

Processing plants use various chilling methods and parameters. Some rapidly cool the carcasses with a blast chiller and transfer the carcasses to a refrigerated storage room. Poultry producers frequently use immersion methods to cool carcasses rapidly, though the levels of pathogens and sanitizer/disinfectant in the immersion solution can influence the contamination level among carcasses (NACMPI 2008). Although carcass temperatures should be maintained below the suboptimal growth range of most pathogens (≤ 41°F), certain pathogens (e.g., *Listeria monocytogenes* and *Yersinia enterocolitica*) are more capable of growing and multiplying under refrigeration temperatures. For these pathogens, the total hours under refrigerated storage are important to monitor, and the modification of other extrinsic parameters (e.g., gases in room or packaging) will limit their growth.

Fabrication involves cutting the carcasses into parts. This can be performed at the slaughter plant or at different departments or facilities. In the past, carcasses were delivered to the neighborhood butcher, where they were made into choice cuts for customers. Butchers were even responsible for the slaughtering process. Whereas butchering is still performed to varying degrees, modern production plants fabricate most of the carcasses into primal or wholesale cuts of meat. These primal cuts may be shipped to other establishments for retail cutting into cooking or serving portions, or the retail cutting may occur at a production facility and be sold as prepackaged meats. Tenderization and grinding of meats may occur at production facilities too. The meat departments of many supermarkets and local grocers often cut meats, but more and more supermarkets are purchasing meats portioned and prepackaged from the wholesaler. Regardless of who performs the fabrication, attention to time/temperature controls, protection from contamination, and sanitary practices are paramount to minimizing the risks of foodborne illnesses.

Sanitary practices and dressing procedures are important early and throughout the slaughter process to minimize contamination and cross-contamination. Insanitary practices and careless dressing procedures upstream of the process can contribute to failures of pathogen control steps further downstream through pathogen loading. Practices to reduce pathogen loading include cleaning and sanitizing carcasses after hide removal, before evisceration, after dressing procedures, and with the commencement of fabrication (Sofos 2009). Methods of cleaning and/or sanitizing carcasses may involve a combination of hot water or steam, detergents and food sanitizing chemicals (see the section titled "Food Contact Sanitizers/Antimicrobials and Fumigation Agents" in Chapter 5), and spot removal of contamination (e.g., trimming or vacuuming procedures). The tools and surfaces that come in contact with carcasses need to be routinely cleaned and sanitized. Sterilizer pots are used most often to sterilize hand tools employed during slaughter and processing operations (RTI International 2005). Sanitary practices are also necessary to prevent cross-contamination from contact between carcasses, overspray from wash/rinse processes, ruptured guts, and the accumulation of dirt or other debris in the slaughter or processing plant. Approximately 75% of meat slaughter/processing plants and 71% of poultry slaughter/processing plants use a cleanup shift of workers to clean and sanitize the plant each day (RTI International 2005). Using a dedicated cleanup shift of workers is recommended over other options of cleaning and sanitizing the plant each day.

### Egg Production

Over the past few years in the United States, approximately 90 billion eggs with a dollar value exceeding $6 billion were produced annually; this volume of eggs was produced by an inventory of approximately 340 million egg-laying hens (National Agricultural Statistics Service [NASS] 2010). Obviously, eggs represent an important source of protein in the American diet as well as a major industry product. Eggs also represent a potential source of foodborne bacterial pathogens—particularly *Salmonella enterica* serovar Enteritidis. Annual estimates of human *Salmonella* Enteritidis infections from shell eggs have ranged as high as 276,500 (Schroeder et al. 2005). Moreover, recent outbreaks have highlighted how contaminated shell eggs can transmit salmonellosis around the country (CDC 2010a). To assist in managing the risks of salmonellosis, specific standards within the *Code of Federal Regulations* (CFR) have been promulgated to prevent *Salmonella* Enteritidis in shell eggs (21 CFR 118). Although egg producers with less than 3,000 layers (or egg producers who sell their eggs directly to consumers) are exempt from several provisions of these regulations, all egg producers should prudently follow the principles of prevention behind these regulations.

Shell eggs can become contaminated with *S.* Enteritidis by several possible modes. One mode involves external contamination of eggs through direct or indirect contact with the feces of infected chickens or with the feces from other infected hosts. A second mode of contamination occurs when eggs pass through the cloaca of infected hens. In both the aforementioned modes, internal contamination of the eggs is also possible through cracks or pores in the shells. A third mode of contamination is transovarian transmission from the infected hen. This latter mode of contamination occurs before the egg shell is formed. Thus, the egg becomes internally contaminated without any outward appearances of contamination. Preventive measures such as removing damaged eggs and washing/sanitizing the shells of eggs help eliminate external contamination, but such measures are ineffective against internally contaminated or infected eggs. If the infected eggs are fertile and hatch, the chicks will also be infected with *S.* Enteritidis. Infected chicks can then spread *S.* Enteritidis to other chickens and flocks.

In 1996, several federal agencies began collaborating on a health risk assessment of *S.* Enteritidis in shell eggs; they also identified and evaluated strategies to reduce the health risks (Schroeder et al. 2005). Over the following years, additional research and rule-making activities culminated in the current regulations on preventing *S.* Enteritidis in shell eggs. Along with good sanitation and protection of animal health, the current regulations emphasize a written prevention plan, biosecurity, testing of eggs and the local environment for *Salmonella*, and recordkeeping. Biosecurity is essentially a program designed to prevent chickens from coming in contact with *S.* Enteritidis by controlling or limiting access to them and by not allowing them to be relocated to potentially contaminated sites, including employees' homes (21 CFR 118.3). Biosecurity measures entail controlling visitors, domestic and wild animals, and pests and includes practices such as disinfection of equipment and poultry houses to prevent cross-contamination. To ensure preventive measures are working and to take corrective actions if necessary, environmental sampling and testing for *S.* Enteritidis is required at prescribed intervals (21 CFR 118.5). Whenever an environmental test is positive for *S.* Enteritidis, the eggs from an affected flock must either be diverted from production for treatment, or the eggs must be subjected to an *S.* Enteritidis testing plan. If egg testing is chosen as the alternative, an algorithmic list of actions is followed based on egg testing results for the life of the affected flock. Diverted eggs can be distributed and sold provided they have been subjected to a treatment that results in a 5-log reduction of *S.* Enteritidis, for example, pasteurization.

Eggs may be sold to processors as ingredients for other foods, including egg products, or they may be sold as shell eggs to retail establishments and consumers for preparation and consumption. Under USDA regulations and the Egg Products Inspection Act (EPIA), an *egg product* is considered eggs with the shell removed, or parts of eggs (e.g., yolks, whites), possibly blended with non-egg ingredients (7 CFR 57). This does not include historical food products where eggs are added in small proportions as ingredients. Because egg products can become easily contaminated with pathogenic or toxigenic microorganisms and support rapid microbial growth, they are required by EPIA to be pasteurized before leaving the official plant. Additional regulatory standards are established for sanitary practices and refrigeration at plants or other "egg handlers." For trace back purposes, the egg product containers must be properly labeled with the official plant number and other required information. In an era of global food trade, the importation of eggs and egg products is also regulated (7 CFR 57, 9 CFR 590).

Most raw shell eggs undergo a degree of processing before being shipped and sold to consumers. Regulations governing the inspection and voluntary grading of eggs provide detailed information on the minimum processing requirements for shell eggs (7 CFR 56, 9 CFR 590). Under these regulations, eggs are examined using a method called candling to grade the quality and to remove cracked or otherwise defective eggs. Although the term *candling* implies the use of a candle or other light source to view through the eggs, nowadays industrial egg packers use automated scanners to candle eggs. The reduction of microbial contamination on the shell eggs is accomplished by proper washing, sanitizing rinses, and drying before packaging. Minimum requirements for water quality and temperature, sanitizing chemicals, equipment, and other relevant conditions for these steps are covered in the regulations. Although not mandatory, whole eggs may also be pasteurized to destroy pathogens within the egg. However, most egg producers do not pasteurize their shell eggs, probably because some consumers claim to dislike the taste of pasteurized eggs. Finally, to prevent the growth of *S.* Enteritidis, temperature control is important for storing and transporting shell eggs. Eggs must be stored at an ambient temperature of 45°F or less within 36 hours after lay (21 CFR 118.4). However, if shell egg processing does not occur within 36 hours after lay, in which case the eggs should have been chilled, the eggs may be held "at room temperature for no more than 36 hours just prior to processing to allow an equilibration step to temper the eggs" (21 CFR 118.4).

### Dairies

Milk and dairy products constitute a major part of the American diet. Remarkably, approximately 185 billion pounds of milk are produced in the United States each year (NASS 2010). Many of the same issues discussed earlier with livestock apply to dairy farms, but milk is a unique commodity that poses greater risks if not properly protected. First, milk is a secretion "harvested" directly from another species and mixed together in great volumes, and as such, milk is greatly affected by the health and veterinary care of each animal. Second, milk is consumed by many individuals, in particular children, who are more susceptible to certain infections and the effects of toxicants. On the dairy farm, milk can become easily contaminated with pathogenic and/or toxigenic microorganisms. In addition, various toxicants or veterinary drugs in cows may contaminate the milk. More than 80 drugs used for veterinary applications may leave residues in the milk (GAO 1992), and as discussed earlier, mycotoxins or other toxicants in feeds may carry over in the milk. Hence, compared with other types of animal agriculture, operations at dairy farms are especially important to manage.

With regard to pathogenic bacteria, dairy farms can harbor several important genera such as *Salmonella*, *Campylobacter*, pathogenic strains of *Escherichia coli*, *Streptococcus*, *Listeria*, *Staphylococcus*, *Mycobacterium*, *Yersinia*, and others (Oliver, Jayarao, Almeida 2005). Most of these pathogens are associated with intestinal infections or environmental reservoirs (see Chapter 2), but many are also associated with extraintestinal infections of cows, including the mammary glands and udders (e.g., mastitis). This means that milk may become inoculated with pathogens from direct or indirect contact with manure or other environmental sources, as well as from excretions in the milk of infected cows. The overall abundance of these pathogens on the farm and their prevalence in milk depend on numerous factors (Oliver et al. 2005). Most notably, factors such as animal density (e.g., CAFOs), manure management, sanitation, animal health, feed sources, and sanitary milking techniques greatly influence the prevalence of pathogens and their levels of contamination in the milk.

Milk was considered a major vehicle for transmitting infectious diseases in the early twentieth century. Since then, it has become one of the safest foods to consume. This accomplishment mostly results from the pasteurization of milk, along with sanitary handling, packaging, and distribution of dairy products. Milk pasteurization and dairy processing plants are often located near the farm, but separating the dairy farm environment from the dairy processing plant is extremely important to prevent postpasteurization contamination. Another important point with regard to pasteurization is bacterial loading. Pasteurization is most effective when the raw milk is not heavily contaminated. Furthermore, staphylococcal enterotoxins in milk are not destroyed by pasteurization. For this reason and others, the sanitary standards of dairy farms are important to maintain. To enforce such standards, dairy farms should be inspected by a regulatory agency at least every 6 months (FDA 2009). Testing of raw milk is also performed to ensure bacterial limits are not exceeded and to identify problems with dairy production.

All dairy farms must have a milking parlor, stable, or barn that is constructed and maintained in a manner to facilitate manure removal and good sanitation. Milkhouses are used to cool and store milk prior to shipment. Along with effective cooling devices and holding tanks, these facilities must be plumbed with potable water and drains to permit cleaning of the facility and milk containers. Isolation and containment of milkhouses are important to prevent the entry of flies and other pests and to prevent other sources of contamination. Transfer of milk to milkhouses and to milk tank trucks must be done in a sanitary manner and without exposure to the surrounding environment. Specific details and additional requirements for dairy farms, processing plants, and associated facilities are contained in the Grade "A" Pasteurized Milk Ordinance (FDA 2009).

In recent years, raw or unpasteurized milk has become popular among some consumers, despite the fact that raw milk has been responsible for numerous foodborne illness outbreaks (CDC 2007). Federal law prohibits interstate sales of packaged raw milk, but the sale of raw milk is allowed to some extent within 29 states (Oliver et al. 2009). Testing requirements for raw milk in these states vary, but a testing program is not an effective safeguard compared with pasteurization. To be safe, raw milk must be effectively protected from pathogens on the farm and during storage and distribution. This is very difficult to accomplish and verify, particularly on dairy farms where the presence of pathogens may be widespread, and strict adherence to good sanitary practices is challenging. Furthermore, infected animals may be asymptomatic but still shed pathogens in their feces or excreted milk. Through a combination of strict preventive measures, the risks to consumers of raw milk can be reduced, but such measures are more difficult to enforce, and the risks are still greater without pasteurization.

## Seafood and Aquaculture

*Seafood* is a traditional term given to food animals and plants harvested from the sea or marine environment. It has also become a catchall term that includes freshwater fish. Much of the world depends on seafood as a source of animal protein, and the demand for seafood has increased in the United States over the past several decades, in part because of the touted health benefits of eating fish. A distinction is usually made between finfish and shellfish. The former is characterized as free-swimming with fins, while the latter is characterized by a shell or exoskeleton. For marketing purposes, shellfish usually include the squids and octopi, even though they do not have exoskeletons. Shellfish are further distinguished as crustaceans and mollusks. Crustaceans include lobsters, crabs, shrimp, and crawfish. Mollusks include clams, oysters, mussels, scallops, and similar species.

Seafood is either wild caught or farm raised (i.e., aquaculture). Wild-caught fish come from commercial fisheries and recreational fishermen. In 2004, the U.S. fisheries caught approximately 5 million tons of fish from inland and marine waters, which ranks third behind China (16.9 million tons) and Peru (9.6 million tons) (Food and Agriculture Organization [FAO] 2007). Yet, despite this amount, the United States imports 84% of its seafood, and half of the imported seafood is from aquaculture (National Oceanic and Atmospheric Administration Aquaculture Program [NOAA Aquaculture Program] 2010). The production levels of wild-caught fish have steadily increased over the decades, and some scientists predict that this cannot be sustained and that eventually a global collapse of many species will occur (Worm et al. 2006). Aquaculture or farm-raised fish production has also increased, and this growth has permitted the per capita consumption of fish in the world to remain fairly constant, despite a growing global population. In the future, a combination of marine ecosystem management and greater aquaculture production will be needed to meet the demands of the increasing global population.

### Wild-Caught Fish

Catching or harvesting fish from the wild is quite different from animal agriculture. The most important difference is that the wild environment of fish cannot be managed or controlled as well as the farm environment. Human population activities (e.g., pollution) and ecosystem perturbations in the wild greatly affect seafood safety. The best examples of this are marine biotoxins, which are considered a major health threat among wild-caught seafood. Toxins are naturally produced by dinoflagellates and other toxigenic algae in local waters, and these toxins often bioaccumulate in the tissues of certain finfish and shellfish. Sometimes, particularly when algal blooms occur, the toxins bioaccumulate to unsafe levels. When consumed by humans, the contaminated fish can cause severe intoxications (e.g., ciguatera, DSP, NSP, PSP, ASP). Although algal blooms occur naturally in ecosystems, the frequency of harmful algal blooms has been increasing as a result of pollution such as nutrient loading, thus also increasing the frequency of fish contaminated with marine biotoxins (Glibert et al. 2005).

Another phenomenon exacerbated by human activity is the bioaccumulation of mercury in the tissues of top predator fish. Mercury cycles through the environment from natural sources, primarily the earth's crust, volcanoes, and oceans. During cycling, mercury is transformed into many different chemical and physical forms, with the most toxic form being methyl mercury ($CH_3Hg$). The amount of mercury cycling in the environment has increased greatly as a result of human activities, chief among them are coal-fired power plants, mining operations, chlor-alkali plants, and more recently electronics waste. As a consequence, the levels of methyl mercury in some species of fish are unnaturally high, and the FDA and EPA recommend precautions for pregnant women and those of child-bearing age, nursing mothers, and young children (FDA and EPA 2004).

Anthropogenic (i.e., human-activity) sources are responsible for a variety of different toxic chemicals in the environment. Several toxic metals and persistent organic pollutants such as PAHs, dioxins, PCBs, and certain pesticides can remain in the environment for years. The fate or sink for most environmentally persistent chemicals is the sediment and water column of aquatic ecosystems. Once there, these chemicals can enter the food chain through the processes of bioaccumulation and biomagnification. The aquatic species most likely to be affected are benthic organisms, including shellfish, and top predatory fish. Both types of fish are heavily consumed by humans. Depending on the types of chemicals and local environment, seafood can be a primary source of exogenous chemicals in the human diet. In most cases, the health risks from consuming seafood contaminated with exogenous chemicals are from chronic exposures, and health risk assessments are conducted to establish tolerances.

Not all pollutants that pose hazards to seafood are chemicals or toxicants. Pollution from inadequately treated sewage and runoff from manure release high levels of bacterial, viral, and protozoan pathogens into local waters where fish are caught or harvested for human consumption.

Although finfish and crustaceans are likely to become contaminated with human/zoonotic pathogens in feces-polluted waters, the greatest risk is with bivalve mollusks. These shellfish are filter feeders, and by filtering polluted waters, they concentrate the pathogens within their bodies. Additionally, molluscan shellfish such as oysters are frequently eaten raw, without a cooking or kill step to inactivate possible pathogens. Outbreaks of norovirus infections, hepatitis, campylobacteriosis, salmonellosis, shigellosis, and other infections have been associated with consuming raw shellfish. Finfish are sometimes eaten raw (e.g., sushi), and they can be a source of bacterial infections (e.g., salmonellosis), as well as parasitic worms.

Even without human interference or influence, wild-caught fish may be infected or contaminated with pathogenic microorganisms and parasites that originate in the aquatic ecosystem. Bacteria of the genus *Vibrio* are natural inhabitants of brackish estuarine waters, and they often become part of the microbiota in the intestinal tracts of shellfish. Several species of vibrios are associated with gastroenteritis and life-threatening complications after consuming shellfish and to a lesser degree finfish. Bacteria such as *Aeromonas hydrophila* and *Plesiomonas shigelloides* have been associated with gastroenteritis and fish consumption, but the ecological aspects of these bacteria are less understood. Some marine bacteria are responsible for the production of scombrotoxin shortly after the death of certain fish species. Finally, several parasitic worms are known to infect freshwater and marine fish, and humans can become secondary hosts to these zoonotic parasites. Examples include the tapeworm *Diphyllobothrium latum* and the nematode *Anisakis simplex*. Both of these parasitic worms have complex life cycles that involve multiple intermediate hosts in the aquatic ecosystem.

Preharvest control of hazards associated with wild-caught fish is not straightforward. With seafood hazards that are caused or exacerbated by human activity, the long-term solution is to control pollution sources and emissions. But this solution is broad in scope and requires the concerted action of many organizations and groups, and such actions do not eliminate persistent chemicals in the environment from past practices. For naturally occurring seafood hazards, the harmful agent is a part of the aquatic ecosystem. Under these circumstances, actions to eliminate the harmful agent may somehow alter the ecosystem, and actions that alter the ecosystem are often unpredictable and possibly detrimental. Thus, compared with animal agriculture, the options for preharvest interventions for hazards are limited. Most preharvest interventions involve a mixed strategy of testing the local fish or waters for contamination, fishing advisories, commercial fishing restrictions, and consumer education.

The regulation of wild-caught fish is inherently complicated by characteristics of the seafood industry. Regulations by several federal agencies govern fishing vessels and methods and areas, and these regulations are enforced by maritime authorities. Pollutants and contaminants in the environment that may affect aquatic life and human health fall under the purview of EPA. Consequently, EPA assists other federal agencies with identifying chemicals in the environment that could accumulate in seafood. However, the majority of seafood entering the U.S. marketplace is imported, and the harvest sites of imported fish are very difficult to ascertain or confirm, much less to determine the chemical hazards in the harvesting waters. As an imported commodity, imported fish are inspected by Customs and Border Protection and the National Marine Fisheries Service, but primarily for detecting fraud (GAO 2009). Nevertheless, under the Seafood Inspection Program, the U.S. Department of Commerce offers a variety of inspections to the seafood industry on a fee-for-service basis. These inspections emphasize sanitation and seafood product evaluation, grading, and documentation. Certificates are issued on the basis of these inspections for a variety of purposes, including certification that a seafood product meets an importing country's requirements.

Regardless of its origin, seafood entering the U.S. food supply and interstate commerce is directly regulated by FDA under the Federal Food, Drug, and Cosmetic Act and the Public Health Service Act (IOM 1991). The principal regulatory power of FDA is rooted in tolerances, action levels, and a less precise but broader authority to deem food products as adulterated and injurious to health. But establishing tolerances or action levels for every potentially harmful agent in seafood is not feasible, and based on sampling and analysis, the enforcement of such tolerances and action levels is too resource intensive. This burden is partially alleviated by the introduction of the seafood HACCP regulation in 1995. Under the HACCP regulation, seafood processors must conduct a hazard analysis and implement a written HACCP plan whenever one or more hazards may be present (21 CFR 123.6). As part of the hazard analysis, the source of fish must be considered for the presence of biological, chemical, and physical agents. In the HACCP plan, steps must be taken to reduce or eliminate any potential hazards from harmful agents. The seafood regulations also have special requirements for imported seafood (21 CFR 123.12) and source controls of raw molluscan shellfish (21 CFR 123.28).

The control of hazards in molluscan shellfish has a long history compared with other types of seafood. The National Shellfish Sanitation Program (NSSP), administered by FDA, has its beginnings dating back to a U.S. Public Health Service conference in 1925. Early in the twentieth century, public health officials recognized the high risk of infectious disease after raw molluscan shellfish were consumed. To reconcile differences between FDA, state officials, and the shellfish industry, the Interstate Shellfish Sanitation Conference (ISSC) was established in 1982. FDA has a Memorandum of Understanding (MOU) with the ISSC, and FDA advises the ISSC on shellfish protection and sanitation. Among other activities, the ISSC and FDA jointly publish guidelines and a Model Ordinance for the control of molluscan shellfish (Interstate Shellfish Sanitation Conference and Food and Drug Administration [ISSC/FDA] 2007). This publication provides guidance ranging from preharvest protection to shipping and postharvest processing. As participants in the NSSP and members of the ISSC, individual states are obliged to enforce provisions of the Model Ordinance as a minimum in their own state and local ordinances.

The Model Ordinance and guidelines for the control of molluscan shellfish are exceptionally comprehensive in scope. They require surveys for potential sources of pollution that may affect shellfish beds and the monitoring of shellfish harvesting waters for microbial contamination. Sampling strategies for monitoring shellfish harvesting waters are based on adverse pollution conditions and/or systematic random sampling. Under the former strategy, water sampling locations and frequency are based on point sources of pollution and variations resulting from seasonal changes, rainfall, stormwater runoff, and other adverse events. The systematic random sampling strategy is preferred for shellfish harvesting waters subject to nonpoint sources of pollution or for areas remotely located from pollution sources. Depending on the characteristics of different shellfish harvesting waters, the Model Ordinance allows individual states to use either the fecal coliform or total coliform standard to evaluate water sample test results. Whenever the coliform standard is exceeded, the shellfish harvesting area is placed in a closed status until the water quality has improved to an acceptable level. During a closed status, shellfish cannot be harvested from the affected area. In most jurisdictions, this restriction does not necessarily apply to finfish because of the presumption that finfish will be sufficiently cooked by the consumer to kill any pathogens prior to consumption.

Early in its inception, the primary purpose of the NSSP was to protect molluscan shellfish from contamination with pathogens. With increasing concerns about chemical pollutants and marine biotoxins in shellfish, the NSSP and ISSC have included protective measures against these hazards in their Model Ordinance and guidelines. However, the protective measures against toxic substances are not as comprehensive as those against pathogens, probably because the toxicity of these substances is more dose-dependent, that is, dependent on the tissue contamination levels as well as the frequency and quantity of shellfish consumption. For chemical pollutants, the protective measures are based primarily on sanitary surveys of shellfish growing beds and waters and on the level of suspected toxicants in the shellfish tissues. This strategy obviously requires a sampling program of shellfish from the harvest areas. Tolerances and action levels are established for several metals, pesticides, and chlorinated hydrocarbons (e.g., PCBs), as well as a few marine biotoxins. The guidelines for marine biotoxins recommend collecting water and/or shellfish samples during harvesting times for laboratory analysis. These guidelines apply only to areas with a history of toxin-producing microorganisms and during times when marine biotoxins are likely to appear. Standards for evaluating sample results are specified for only three types of marine biotoxins, specifically those responsible for neurotoxic shellfish poisoning (NSP), amnesic shellfish poisoning (ASP), and paralytic shellfish poisoning (PSP). States are also required to develop contingency plans for emergency response in the event of shellfish toxicity.

### Aquaculture and Farm-Raised Fish

Aquaculture for human food involves raising finfish or shellfish in a contained environment until they reach market size, or it may involve rearing fish in a hatchery and releasing them into the wild for later harvest. Different types of aquaculture systems are designed to accommodate the species raised and the availability of local resources. Typical systems consist of ponds, raceways, tanks, pens, and/or cages. They can be either freshwater or saltwater systems, and they may have a recirculating or nonrecirculating water flow. Among countries of the world, the United States ranks only 10th in total aquaculture production (NOAA Aquaculture Program 2010). As of 2005, the total number of farms in the United States that produce food fish was estimated at 1,847 (NASS 2002/2005). These aquaculture farms produce only 5% of the U.S. seafood supply. As the world population and demand for seafood increases, the supply of wild-caught fish will become limited and may even decline. In the future, the world will increasingly depend more on aquaculture and farm-raised fish to meet the demand.

The primary issues with aquaculture farms are related to the environmental conditions, quality of feedstuff, and fish density and health. Compared with wild-caught fish, the environment of farm-raised fish must be directly managed to ensure that conditions are favorable to good growth and health of the fish. Several types of agrichemicals are used to aid in controlling environmental conditions in certain aquaculture systems. Frequently used agrichemicals include fertilizers to grow phytoplankton for fish food, water treatment compounds, pesticides (e.g., algicides and herbicides), disinfectants, and veterinary drugs (Food and Agriculture Organization, Network of

Aquaculture Centres in Asia–Pacific, World Health Organization [FAO/NACA/WHO] 1999). As with other farming operations, the proper selection and use of agrichemicals in aquaculture is essential to avoid contamination of fish tissues with chemical residues. Indeed, several agrichemicals are banned from use in aquaculture by numerous developed countries because they pose a potential risk to human health (Sapkota et al. 2008). To assist U.S. farmers and states with the selection and use of drugs, vaccines, and pesticides for aquaculture purposes, a federal subcommittee has put together a useful guide (Federal Joint Subcommittee on Aquaculture 2007).

Other sources of chemicals include pollutants in the environment near the aquaculture farm or facility. Discharges or emissions from nearby factories and transportation sources pollute surface waters, air, and soil. Conventional farms are a potential source of pesticides from runoff and overspray. Industrial or transportation accidents can release hazardous chemicals into the environment, though this type of contamination is usually obvious. In some geographic regions, metals and metalloids are abundant naturally in the earth's crust, and these elements may enter other environmental media through geochemical processes (Sapkota et al. 2008). Chemicals such as metals and persistent organic pollutants enter the aquaculture system from contaminated water sources or from atmospheric deposition of airborne pollutants. Such pollutants are insidious because of their chronic toxicity and ability to bioaccumulate in fish. A recent study analyzed fish fillets from several markets for polychlorinated biphenyls (PCBs) and polybrominated diphenyl ethers (PBDEs) (Hayward, Wong, Krynitsky 2007). In general, the fillets of farm-raised Atlantic salmon had higher levels of these contaminants than the fillets of wild-caught Pacific salmon. However, much higher levels of PCBs and PBDEs were found in the fillets of wild-caught bluefish and rockfish (i.e., striped bass) than in the salmon fillets, regardless of origin. The likely explanation for this finding is that bluefish and rockfish migrate and feed along industrialized coasts, where the persistent organic pollutants are more concentrated in the food web. In comparison, farm-raised salmon are contained in net cages not far off the coast and given feed for their nutrition. Closer proximity to the coast and/or possible contaminants in the feed may explain why higher concentrations of PCBs and PBDEs were found in the farm-raised salmon compared with wild-caught salmon.

As with terrestrial species of livestock, the feed used for farm-raised fish is an important component of animal health, and ultimately human health via the food chain. The types of feed used in aquaculture range from waste materials to specially formulated feeds. In some regions of the world, feces-contaminated wastewater or human excreta/manure is added to ponds as fish feed. Although inexpensive, this practice is risky because foodborne transmission of pathogens to humans can occur through contamination of fish tissues or by pathogen concentration in molluscan shellfish (Sapkota et al. 2008). With more intensive methods of aquaculture, greater productivity is achieved using formulated feeds, but this is not without potential problems. The ingredients and additives of formulated feed are potential sources of mycotoxins, chemicals, and veterinary drugs in farm-raised fish. Mycotoxin and chemical contamination of feed ingredients is usually inadvertent, while veterinary drugs are added to protect the health of fish. Over the years, multiple studies have detected chemical and veterinary drug residues in farm-raised fish that have been traced back to the feed (FAO/NACA/WHO 1999; Sapkota et al. 2008). Standards for acceptable contaminant levels and safe ingredients in animal feeds are developed by FDA's Center for Veterinary Medicine. Because the rearing conditions of imported farm-raised fish are unknown, FDA conducts some limited testing for a few contaminants on imported fish. In 2007, FDA detained several types of farm-raised fish and implemented a broad import control on farm-raised fish imported from China because of detection of drugs in the fish not approved for use in the United States.

Aquaculture fish populations raised under high densities are more vulnerable to infection and parasitism compared with fish in the wild. The greatest concern is with parasitic worms. Many different types of trematodes, nematodes, and cestodes are common in fish species, and research studies have found parasitic worms are sometimes more numerous in aquaculture systems than in natural ecosystems (Sapkota et al. 2008). Millions of people in the world are infected as secondary hosts with parasitic worms from consuming fish and aquatic plants (FAO/NACA/WHO 1999; Reilly and Kaferstein 1999; Sapkota et al. 2008). This problem is most prominent in eastern and southeastern Asia, where the most medically important parasites are indigenous, and where people prefer to eat raw or rare fish. Parasitic worm infection from fish consumption is not recognized as a major public health problem in most regions of the world because fish is usually cooked before consumption, which destroys the parasites. Thorough cooking of fish is the best safeguard against parasitic worms for the consumer because controlling parasites in the aquatic environment is inherently difficult, particularly with "open" aquaculture systems.

Open aquaculture systems are either located in the natural environment, or they receive and return water from and to the natural environment with little or no treatment. Consequently, farmed fish in open aquaculture systems are potentially exposed to parasites and other contaminants in the natural environment, and conversely, farmed fish may introduce novel parasites into the surrounding natural environment, along with organic and chemical wastes from the fish farm. In contrast, "closed" aquaculture systems usually treat and recycle the water. Many closed aquaculture systems consist of tanks located within buildings or other climate-controlled structures. This means the aquaculture operator exerts greater control over the environment of the farmed fish.

The bacterial species and populations present in aquaculture systems are determined by several factors. They include the design of an aquaculture system (e.g., recirculating vs. flow-through, fresh or salt water), water source and quality, uneaten feed, fish wastes, disinfectant use, and so forth. Of course, not all bacterial species in aquaculture systems/aquatic environments are human pathogens. Bacteria with potential as human pathogens are classified as either indigenous or introduced (Reilly and Kaferstein 1999). Indigenous bacterial pathogens include *Aeromonas hydrophila*, *Plesiomonas shigelloides*, and several species of *Vibrio* (in brackish or marine water). Other indigenous bacteria include environmental microbes belonging to the genera *Clostridium*, *Bacillus*, and *Listeria*. Nonindigenous pathogenic bacteria are introduced from sources involving humans, animals, wastes and wastewater, and runoff. The greatest concern is with feces-related contamination that introduces pathogenic Enterobacteriaceae and other enteric bacteria such as *Campylobacter*. Aquaculture systems should be protected as much as possible from the introduction of human pathogens, but postharvest food safety practices are critically important to preventing illnesses from both introduced and indigenous pathogens.

## Food Crops

Whether grown for animal feed or human consumption, crops must be protected against contamination with harmful biological, chemical, and physical agents (Codex Alimentarius Commission 2003c). The first consideration for preharvest crop safety is a site survey of the planned field or orchard. Past and current uses of the site and surrounding areas should be investigated to determine if the land or adjacent areas are potentially contaminated. Environmental sources such as wastewater treatment plants, factories, solid or hazardous waste sites, mining operations, animal production, power plants, transportation corridors, pesticide usage, and other potential sources are important to note. These sources also provide clues about the types of harmful agents that may be present. Contamination of the soil and/or crops can occur from airborne deposition, runoff, flooding, leaking tanks or lagoons, access by domestic and wild animals, and the leaching of buried materials. Whenever necessary or when doubt exists, testing should be performed to determine the presence of contaminants.

Water supplies are vital to agriculture for multiple purposes (Codex Alimentarius Commission 2003a; FDA Center for Food Safety and Applied Nutrition 1998). Crop irrigation probably represents the largest volume of water used from a source. This is significant because contaminated irrigation water has been implicated in numerous outbreaks of foodborne illnesses involving fresh vegetables and fruits. Water is also used for mixing agrichemicals and washing fruits and vegetables. It is important to match the planned uses of water with the appropriate sources and required quality. Sources of water may be ponds, waterways, canals, groundwater, reclamation from irrigation or treatment facilities, and municipal supplies. The baseline quality of water is very different with each of these sources, and a water quality assessment is necessary to help determine if potential hazards exist. However, water quality is not static and can change intermittently as a result of rainfall, storms, floods, drought, treatment failures, and so forth. Once the appropriate source and quality of water are determined to be acceptable, the water source must be protected from point and nonpoint sources of pollution, and a reassessment of water quality should be performed periodically and after events that may affect water quality.

### Applying Biosolids (Sewage Sludge) and Manure to Crops

The application of manure to fields was discussed earlier as an important resource conservation measure for the production of food. A similar situation exists with the disposal of biosolids produced by municipal wastewater treatment plants (i.e., sewage sludge). Of course, the greatest concern with applying sewage sludge to agricultural land is the potential for transmitting human pathogens to farm workers and to consumers via the food chain. But pathogens are not the only concerns with sewage sludge. Several toxic metals (As, Cd, Cu, Pb, Hg, Mo, Ni, Se, Zn) and organic compounds are associated with sewage sludge, and these elements and compounds could enter the human food chain. In many lesser developed regions of the world, human waste is either minimally treated or untreated before being applied as fertilizer to croplands. This practice is responsible for the transmission of several bacterial, viral, protozoan, and helminthic diseases to the local populace. Sometimes, the human pathogen–contaminated produce from these countries is imported into developed countries, but more likely, visitors from developed countries consume the pathogen-contaminated produce while traveling abroad.

The application of sewage sludge to land, including for feed and food crops, is regulated in the United States by the EPA (40 CFR 503). Under EPA regulations, standards are established for pathogen reduction and concentrations of toxic metals in sewage sludge. Pathogen reduction of sewage sludge is categorized as either Class A or Class B, where the class determines the application scenarios for sewage sludge. Class A pathogen reduction essentially means the sewage sludge is unrestricted for land applications because the sludge has been treated sufficiently to destroy virtually all pathogens. In contrast, treatments for Class B pathogen reduction are less efficacious, and restrictions are imposed on land application of this sewage sludge to allow for natural decomposition processes to inactivate pathogens. Several treatment processes can be used to reduce pathogens in sewage sludge (see Appendix B of 40 CFR 503), and regulatory criteria have been established for several reduction alternatives to attain either Class A or B pathogen reduction status. For Class A reduction alternatives, criteria are based on allowable limits for indicator bacteria (i.e., < 1,000 fecal coliforms MPN per gram of dry weight solids) and certain pathogens and/or on treatment processes involving combinations of time, temperature, pH, and other parameters that will most likely destroy human pathogens. For Class B reduction alternatives, the sewage sludge must have undergone treatment processes to significantly reduce pathogens, or the fecal coliforms analyzed in the sludge must not exceed $2 \times 10^6$ MPN or CFUs per gram of total solids (based on dry weight). Additionally, Class B sewage sludge has the following restrictions (40 CFR 503.31):

(i) Food crops with harvested parts that touch the sewage sludge/soil mixture and are totally above the land surface shall not be harvested for 14 months after application of sewage sludge.

(ii) Food crops with harvested parts below the surface of the land shall not be harvested for 20 months after application of sewage sludge when the sewage sludge remains on the land surface for four months or longer prior to incorporation into the soil.

(iii) Food crops with harvested parts below the surface of the land shall not be harvested for 38 months after application of sewage sludge when the sewage sludge remains on the land surface for less than four months prior to incorporation into the soil.

(iv) Food crops, feed crops, and fiber crops shall not be harvested for 30 days after application of sewage sludge.

(v) Animals shall not be grazed on the land for 30 days after application of sewage sludge.

In contrast with sewage sludge, manure is less rigidly regulated with respect to cropland applications. Most existing regulations are aimed at preventing pollution of waterways under the Clean Water Act. Nonetheless, the volume of manure produced by CAFOs can exceed the biosolids produced by local municipalities, and manure contains many zoonotic pathogens that may be transmitted through the human food chain. The application of manure to farmland is predominantly governed by good agricultural practices (GAPs), which are voluntary guidelines for protecting fruits and vegetables from foodborne microbial hazards (FDA Center for Food Safety and Applied Nutrition 1998). Table 8-2 lists the recommended practices for applying manure to vegetable and fruit croplands.

**Table 8-2** FDA Guidelines for Manure and Animal Feces to Minimize Microbial Food Safety Hazards for Fruits and Vegetables

Manure Handling and Application

- Manure storage and treatment sites should be situated as far as practicable from fresh produce production and handling areas.
- Consider barriers or physical containment to secure manure storage or treatment areas where contamination from runoff, leaching, or wind spread is a concern.
- Consider good agricultural practices to minimize leachate from manure storage or treatment areas contaminating produce.
- Consider practices to minimize the potential of recontaminating treated manure.

Untreated Manure

- Consider incorporating manure into the soil prior to planting.
- Applying raw manure, or leachate from raw manure, to produce fields during the growing season prior to harvest is not recommended.
- Maximize the time between application of manure to produce production areas and harvest.
- Where it is not possible to maximize the time between application and harvest, such as for fresh produce crops that are harvested throughout most of the year, raw manure should not be used.

Treated Manure

- Avoid contamination of fresh produce from manure that is in the process of being composted or otherwise treated.
- Apply good agricultural practices that ensure that all [manure] materials receive an adequate treatment.
- Growers purchasing manure should obtain a specification sheet from the manure supplier for each shipment of manure containing information about the method of treatment.
- Growers should contact state or local manure handling experts for advice specific to their individual operations and regions.

Animal Feces

- Domestic animals should be excluded from fresh produce fields, vineyards, and orchards during the growing season.
- Where necessary, growers should consider measures to ensure that animal waste from adjacent fields or waste storage facilities does not contaminate the produce production areas.

*Source*: FDA, 1998.

Mounting evidence suggests that pathogen internalization occurs with fruits and vegetables from sources such as manure, municipal biosolids, and contaminated water. Apparently, pathogens can become incorporated into the tissues of fruits and vegetables, where they may survive for extended periods of time and are protected from sanitizers (Doyle and Erickson 2008). This phenomenon has been observed with several foodborne bacterial pathogens in lettuce, spinach, cabbage, cantaloupes, parsley, carrots, tomatoes, apples, and other produce (Beuchat 2006; Doyle and Erickson 2008). Pathogen internalization studies and foodborne illness outbreaks over the past decade or more have raised serious concerns about applying manure and other potentially contaminated materials to food crops. Unfortunately, many unanswered questions remain about the relative importance of different pathogen sources and the mechanisms involved with pathogen internalization by plants. Several ecological and mechanistic issues associated with pathogen internalization have been identified for additional research (Lynch, Tauxe, Hedberg 2009; Teplitski, Barak, Schneider 2009). Perhaps with data and knowledge obtained from additional research, the application guidelines for manure and biosolids to food crops will be modified in the future.

### Pesticide Use

Agrichemicals are used in great volumes with modern farming operations. Whereas any improperly used chemical on the farm can pose a potential hazard, pesticide usage and residues on crops raise the greatest concerns for protecting the food supply against chemical contamination. Scientists actively debate the risks of low-level, mixed, and cumulative exposures to pesticides in the food chain (Boobis et al. 2008). This makes setting tolerances and action levels for these chronic hazards difficult, and the underlying scientific issues must be addressed through periodic risk assessments. From the standpoint of acute and catastrophic risks, however, the greatest concern is with foodborne poisonings/intoxications from unapproved uses or misapplications of pesticides, such as occurred in California during the 1980s with watermelons and the pesticide aldicarb (Goldman et al. 1990). As mentioned in Chapter 3, approximately 78% of all conventional pesticides produced are used for agricultural purposes (Kiely, Donaldson, Grube 2004). Considering the volume and types of pesticides used in agriculture, the regulation of pesticides and pesticide use is crucial to safety management of the food supply.

The regulation of pesticides in foods is complicated by the overlapping jurisdictions and involvement of EPA, FDA, and USDA (see Chapters 1 and 3). Pesticide registration, use, and the establishment of tolerances in/on raw agricultural commodities (RACs) are regulated by EPA. Yet, FDA can also establish action levels and tolerances for pesticides in foods as additives whenever RACs are used in processed foods. Regulatory monitoring of pesticide residues in foods is accomplished primarily by USDA and FDA. The primary difference between the agencies' monitoring programs is the point of sampling in the food supply chain. The sampling of RACs and several processed foods is carried out by USDA (and by states through agreements), whereas FDA performs sampling of commodity foods closer to the point of consumer purchase. The FDA is also responsible for pesticide sampling and monitoring of imported foods.

Pesticide application on agricultural lands is regulated by a two-pronged approach: (1) pesticide approval, registration, and labeling requirements, and (2) certification of pesticide applicators. Under the Federal Insecticide, Fungicide, and Rodenticide Act (FIFRA) and EPA regulations, pesticides must be registered for specific crops and application methods (40 CFR 152). Furthermore, pesticides must be scrupulously labeled with use directions; application rates and concentrations; safety, health, and environmental precautions; and other relevant information (40 CFR 156.10). Certain pesticides and formulations are registered and labeled as "restricted use," meaning they can be applied only by certified pesticide applicators. For agricultural purposes, commercial and private applicators may apply restricted use pesticides. A private applicator is "a certified applicator who uses or supervises the use of any pesticide which is classified for restricted use for purposes of producing any agricultural commodity on property owned or rented by him or his employer or (if applied without compensation other than trading of personal services between producers of agricultural commodities) on the property of another person" (40 CFR 171.2).

Good pest management strategies can minimize the amount of pesticides applied to crops. These strategies not only reduce the potential exposure of human populations to pesticides, but they also reduce the costs of purchasing and applying pesticides to crops. In addition, judicious application of pesticides can reduce selection pressures that create pesticide-resistant pests, as well as prevent the destruction of beneficial organisms, including crop pollinators (e.g., bees). A long-established set of strategies for pest control is called integrated pest management (IPT). These strategies basically involve monitoring pest populations and setting thresholds to determine when to apply pesticides and also using nonchemical controls based on knowledge of the pest's biology. The Natural Resources Conservation Service (NRCS 2010) recommends the "PAMS" approach to IPT, which stands for Prevention, Avoidance, Monitoring, and Suppression. Some nonchemical methods of control include crop rotations to disrupt pest life cycles, using biological controls such as natural predators, and spot treatments and weeding to prevent pest proliferation.

Several technological advances have greatly helped implement IPT strategies. Precision farming is one technological advance increasingly used to apply both fertilizers and pesticides. Based on the Global Information System (GIS), precision farming allows a farmer to precisely locate trouble spots in fields where customized quantities of agrichemicals are applied. Another technological advance is improved pesticide applicator equipment, allowing greater precision, less waste, and less pesticide drift during applications. For example, applicator sprays can be controlled to generate uniform droplet sizes for a particular application. Additionally, new pesticides based on naturally produced compounds and biochemical regulators (also called biopesticides) can target specific pests and/or certain life cycle stages of pests. Biopesticides tend to be used in smaller quantities and degrade more quickly compared with conventional pesticides. Finally, the development of genetically modified organisms or crops (GMOs) has produced strains that are more resistant to pests, thus reducing dependency on chemical pesticides. Unfortunately, as discussed previously, some consumers summarily reject GMOs as a human food source, even if research and risk assessments determine that GMO foods are reasonably safe.

### Mycotoxins Control

The ubiquitous nature of fungi means that mycotoxin formation is possible anywhere in the food supply chain. To make matters worse, approximately 400 potential mycotoxins are formed by more than 100 types of filamentous fungi (i.e., mold) species (Kabak, Dobson, Var 2006). Thus, the prevention of mycotoxin formation in food commodities is a formidable challenge, and the complete elimination of mycotoxins in foods is not feasible. Preventive efforts have focused mostly on a few classes of mycotoxins with significant toxicity and occurrence in human foodstuff and animal feeds. Important mycotoxin classes include aflatoxins, ochratoxins, ergot alkaloids, fumonisins, trichothecenes, patulin, and yellow rice toxins (refer back to Chapter 3 and Table 3-3 for more details). Mycotoxins have been responsible for acute toxicity (mycotoxicosis) and large food-borne disease outbreaks around the world, sometimes with very high mortality and morbidity, but the most widespread concern is with chronic toxicity from consuming low levels of mycotoxins in foods. Furthermore, the economic losses from mycotoxin contamination of agricultural commodities are a major concern for companies and countries. Approximately 99 countries around the world have some type of legal limits, tolerances, or action levels for selected mycotoxins in human foods and/or animal feed (FAO 2004). For these countries, products that exceed the legal limits for mycotoxin contamination are not allowed to be imported, sold, or distributed.

Strategies have been developed to prevent or reduce mycotoxin formation during the preharvest, harvest, and postharvest phases of crop production and storage. However, a boilerplate plan for all agricultural products is not possible because of differences in climate, agronomic practices, crop types and varieties, and postharvest infrastructures throughout the world. Customized plans for preventing mycotoxin formation should be developed for individual farming operations, product storage, processing, and distribution systems. Of the known mycotoxins, the formation of a particular mycotoxin is not restricted to a particular agricultural commodity or food. It all depends on the presence of the toxigenic mold species and favorable intrinsic and extrinsic parameters for mold growth and toxin formation. That said, some toxigenic mold species and mycotoxins are more problematic in certain food products (see Table 3-3 in Chapter 3). Animal-based foods (e.g., dairy, egg, and certain processed meat products) are sometimes contaminated with mycotoxins, but most often, mycotoxins are encountered in plant-based foods such as grains, nuts, and fruits (Institute of Food Science and Technology [IFST] 2009). For example, mold species of the genus *Aspergillus* are frequently associated with aflatoxin production in products containing corn, peanuts, and tree nuts. Similarly, the mycotoxin patulin, produced by mold species of *Penicillium* and other genera, is commonly encountered in moldy fruits and juices. The production of trichothocenes (e.g., T-2, DON) by *Fusarium* and other genera is particularly problematic in products derived from corn, wheat, barley, oats, and other grains.

Preharvest intervention strategies for mycotoxin formation are aimed at preventing or minimizing the infection of crops with toxigenic molds. A good starting point is to ensure that the seeds for planting are not infected or contaminated (IFST 2009). Improper storage conditions of seeds may allow mold contamination and growth, resulting in the infection of developing plants with toxigenic molds. Other preharvest interventions include genetically resistant varieties of crops (e.g., GMOs), good agronomic practices, and biological and chemical controls. Selecting strains of crops known to thrive well in a particular climatic region can help ensure good plant health and resistance to mold infections. Good agronomic practices involve knowing when to plant, irrigate, and harvest crops. They also include carefully chosen methods for crop rotation, tillage of the soil, spacing of plants, and soil treatments such as pH adjustment and fertilizer application (Codex Alimentarius Commission 2003b). The overarching goal of these agronomic practices is to prevent toxigenic molds from surviving in the fields, while also minimizing stress on the crop plants, making them more resistant to infection by toxigenic molds (Kabak et al. 2006). Crop rotation helps by avoiding contact of susceptible crop types with plant debris from a previous year's crop that may have been infected with a particular mold species. The timing and type of soil tillage influences the survival and death of toxigenic molds in the soil. When permitted by weather and prevailing environmental conditions, the proper moisture content of soils should be maintained by the right amount of irrigation and drainage to enhance crop resistance and discourage mold growth. Effective pest control (including insects and weeds) also reduces stress on crop plants and lessens the likelihood of introducing toxigenic molds.

Biological control of mycotoxin production is accomplished by the application of antagonistic or competitive bacteria, yeasts, or molds (Kabak et al. 2006). These microorganisms produce antimicrobial substances against toxigenic molds and/or outcompete them for resources (Cleveland et al. 2003). Some strains of molds introduced to crops are the same species as the toxigenic molds, but the introduced strain is atoxigenic (e.g., atoxigenic *Aspergillus flavus*). By belonging to the same species, the atoxigenic molds can gain a foothold advantage in occupying the niches before the toxigenic molds can. For effective preharvest control, the timing and manner of application are important considerations when using atoxigenic molds (Kabak and Dobson 2009).

Chemical control of mycotoxin production is basically the application of fungicides. With new fungicides constantly being developed, there are many different types of fungicides that can be applied to crops, each designed for specific target fungi and methods of application. Most fungicides are intended to control plant diseases of economic importance, but some fungicides are very effective against toxigenic molds. On the negative side, the application of fungicides to crops is an added expense, and if improperly used, chemical residue from the fungicide remains in the food product. Therefore, only registered fungicides should be used, and these fungicides should be used for registered purposes only and according to label instructions.

The harvesting stage of crop production is critical to preventing mycotoxin formation throughout the rest of the food handling chain. Controlling moisture and minimizing mold spore loading are the primary objectives during harvest that will limit mycotoxin production (Codex Alimentarius Commission 2004b, 2003b; Kabak et al. 2006). Timing of the harvest is the first step to accomplishing these objectives. Crops should be harvested at optimum maturity—unless it would cause crops to be exposed to extreme conditions of heat, moisture, or drought (Codex Alimentarius Commission 2004b). Historically, allowing grain crops such as rye to remain in the fields too long led to the growth of *Claviceps purpurea* and the formation of ergot alkaloids, causing deadly epidemics of ergotism. As much as practical, the harvested portion of the crop (grains, fruits, vegetables, nuts, etc.) should be prevented from contacting the soil and becoming damaged. Excessive contamination with soil increases spore loading, and damaged crops (bruised, broken, crushed, etc.) are more likely to support the growth of molds. Proper farm equipment maintenance and farm worker techniques are important to minimizing damage to the crops. Efforts to separate loads of harvest in the field by quality help reduce the spread of toxigenic molds to the entire crop. For example, diseased plants should be separated from healthy ones, and moisture level zones or spots in fields should be separated into different loads (Kabak et al. 2006). To further minimize spore loading and moisture content, the transport containers or vehicles should be clean, free of pests and debris, and dry (Codex Alimentarius Commission 2003b).

For most crops, the moisture content should be reduced immediately after harvest to the recommended level for storage. Under constant relative humidity and temperature, the moisture content of grains and nuts will differ by the amount of oil in the seed, with the oilier seeds having less moisture content (Kabak et al. 2006). The recommended moisture content depends on the type of crop and the predominant toxigenic molds of concern. Generally, the desired moisture content for most grains is less than 14–15% ($<\sim 0.70$ $a_w$) to prevent the growth of certain toxigenic molds such as *Fusarium* species (Bhat et al. 2010; Codex Alimentarius Commission 2003b; Kabak et al 2006; Magan and Aldred 2007). To reduce moisture content, some crops require mechanically assisted drying prior to storage. This represents a problem for many regions of the world where high humidity exists and drying equipment or facilities are unavailable. In many countries, sun drying is commonly performed, but mycotoxin production (e.g., aflatoxins) is still likely if dried grains are stored under moist or humid conditions. Monitoring the moisture content of stored commodities and the relative humidity helps ensure that storage conditions are not conducive to mold growth.

Postharvest storage temperature is another important parameter that influences the growth of toxigenic molds. Aflatoxins and ochratoxin A are produced in the temperature ranges of 12°–40°C (53.6°–104°F) and 10°–25°C (50°–77°F), respectively (Bhat et al. 2010; Kabak et al. 2006). Local weather conditions and seasonal temperatures are important considerations when storing raw agricultural commodities. Higher temperatures are obviously encountered year-round in tropical and subtropical regions of the world, where the majority of the lesser developed countries are also located. As much as possible, proper and uniform temperatures should be maintained in storage areas, perhaps with the assistance of ventilation or aeration. This requires monitoring the temperature at fixed and representative locations in the stored commodities. Temperature monitoring also helps to identify infestation problems. Metabolic activity from microbial growth and active pests results in increased temperature of stored grains, and a "temperature rise of 2°–3°C may indicate microbial growth and/or insect infestation" (Codex Alimentarius Commission 2003b).

The major mycotoxins of concern with fresh fruits and vegetables are patulin, ochratoxin, and tenuazonic acid (Moss 2008). With fresh fruits and vegetables, spoilage molds usually damage the commodity sufficiently to be rejected before a health hazard from mycotoxins becomes a serious problem (Moss 2008). Mycotoxin problems are more frequently associated with the processed products such as juices, wine, ketchup, and dried fruits (Bhat et al. 2010; Moss 2008). The principal reasons are related to the quality of raw commodity used for processed food and the storage and processing conditions. Surface-injured and bruised fruits are more vulnerable to toxigenic mold penetration and growth, and these aesthetically unpleasing fruits are used for processed products rather than sold on produce stands. With a combination of sufficient time, moisture, and warm temperatures, toxigenic molds can grow and produce mycotoxins that remain in the processed product. Ideally, fruits should be cooled to below 5°C (41°F) within 3–4 days, and the optimum storage temperatures should be achieved within another 2 days (Kabak et al. 2006). Additional control measures to retard mold growth can also be employed when storing fruits and vegetables. Some of these measures are briefly described here.

Other parameters besides moisture content and temperature are modifiable/controllable to inhibit the growth of toxigenic molds. Atmospheric modification of storage spaces has been demonstrated to retard the growth of toxigenic molds and limit the production of mycotoxins (Magan and Aldred 2007). By modifying the oxygen levels and/or by adding carbon dioxide and/or nitrogen, aerobic and microaerophilic fungi can be inhibited. This method has been successfully used for reducing alfatoxin production in peanuts and mold growth in apples (Kabak et al. 2006). Adding antimicrobial constituents, including preservatives and fungicides, is another strategy for inhibiting the growth of toxigenic molds. However, this strategy must be carefully employed with stored products to avoid toxic chemical hazards in the final products (Magan and Aldred 2007). Fumigation is a practice where the pesticide or antimicrobial is used as a gas in an enclosed space. Because of high toxicity, a great number of fumigants have become prohibited or restricted-use pesticides in the United States. Less toxic substances are being explored as fumigants to control mold growth in stored agricultural commodities, including food-grade preservatives (Barberis et al. 2010). Naturally derived extracts from plants and spice oils are promising as postharvest treatments (including as fumigants) for spoilage and toxigenic molds, with minimal toxic effects on humans (Kabak et al. 2006).

Because mycotoxin production is difficult to prevent fully in foods, a secondary strategy is to eliminate them prior to purchase or consumption. Removal or inactivation of mycotoxins has been studied as an intervention strategy, mostly during the processing steps of foods and animal feeds. Approaches to mycotoxin removal or inactivation rely on the use of chemical agents, microbial agents, and physical processes such as heat treatments (Bhat et al. 2010). The chemical agents include oxidants, acids, bases, reducing agents, adsorbents or sequestration agents, and various compounds with different chemical properties. These chemical agents are intended to destroy, inactivate, or extract the mycotoxins. This is different from preservatives, which are aimed at inhibiting microbial growth and/or toxin production. The disadvantages of chemical agents are the possible introduction of additional toxic hazards, reduction of the food's nutritional value, and undesirable changes in the food's sensory properties (Kabak et al. 2006). An alternative approach is to exploit the biochemical reactions of microorganisms and biologically derived molecules. Mycotoxins can be degraded or detoxified biochemically (i.e., biotransformation) by the action of bacteria, fungi, or purified enzymes (AFSSA et al. 2009). In the laboratory setting and with certain foods, adding certain microbial species and strains to foods has resulted in the biotransformation or binding of mycotoxins, making them less toxic or unavailable for absorption in the intestinal tract. For several practical reasons, this has not become a widespread practice in human foods or animal feeds, and additional research is needed before this biotechnology can be fully exploited (AFSSA et al. 2009; Kabak and Dobson 2009).

Several physical processes can reduce but not completely eliminate mycotoxins in foods. Physical cleaning and sorting processes are effective in separating moldy and damaged materials from agricultural commodities; this also removes the most heavily mycotoxin-contaminated portions before blending or other operations mix everything together (Bullerman and Bianchini 2007; Drusch and Ragab 2003). Washing is effective in reducing levels of various mycotoxins in grains and fruits (Kabak et al. 2006). Of course, washing also adds moisture content that could contribute to toxigenic mold growth, so it is best performed right after storage and just before additional processing steps. Heat treatments are common steps in the processing of foods. The heat stability of individual mycotoxins is related to their chemical structures, heating temperatures and duration, and characteristics of the food matrix (water content, pH, heat penetration, etc.). In general, mycotoxins are heat-stabile when subjected to pasteurization or conventional cooking temperatures of 80°–121°C (Bullerman and Bianchini 2007; Kabak et al. 2006). Degradation of mycotoxins is possible with higher temperatures and heating durations, but excessive heat degrades food quality and nutritional value. One type of heat treatment called *extrusion processing* is relatively more effective in degrading several types of mycotoxins (Bullerman and Bianchini 2007).

Ionizing and nonionizing (e.g., UV) radiation has also been used for nonthermal degradation of mycotoxins, as well as antimicrobial/antifungal treatments (Bhat et al. 2010; Kabak et al. 2006). The efficacy of mycotoxin degradation using ionizing or nonionizing radiation depends on many factors related to the energy levels of radiation and characteristics of the food matrix.

## FOOD PROCESSING AND DISTRIBUTION

### Food Safety and Processing

For millennia, foods have been processed for preservation purposes and/or to add flavor, texture, and other desirable characteristics. In the last 100 years, the proportion of total food consumed by Americans that is factory processed has grown to more than one-half. Nowadays, with a wide range of available technologies, modern food processing is much more sophisticated and can be designed to meet changing consumer preferences. The traditional aims of food processing still include preservation, nutrient fortification, and consumer appeal in terms of color, texture, taste, and smell. More recently, however, consumer preference has driven the food industry to produce a greater variety of products with emphasis on convenience, wholesomeness, fresh taste, and healthy choices (Morrison, Buzby, Wells 2010). Regardless of consumer preferences, Americans expect and assume these processed and packaged foods are safe.

Food processing starts with raw materials and finishes with a food product. "All food processing involves a combination of procedures to achieve the intended changes to the raw materials. Each of these unit operations has a specific, identifiable and predictable effect on a food and the combination and sequence of operations determine the nature of the final product" (Fellows 2009). Food process engineers and technologists design the process to produce the final product. Food products are usually classified by type, but differences in opinion exist on the definitions of the various food types. For the purposes of clarity, the following definitions are derived from Rahman (1999):

*Raw foods:* These are considered foods in their most primary state, shortly after harvesting or slaughter. Raw foods may have undergone postharvest washing or sizing, but otherwise they have not been processed.

*Fresh foods:* These are essentially raw foods that may have undergone postharvest washing, curing, or other minor treatments prior to storage in cold rooms or modified atmospheric spaces. Fresh foods maintain their harvested integrity without any noticeable changes in physical, chemical, or microbiological quality.

*Minimally processed foods:* These foods retain the texture, taste, and smell of fresh foods, and they may have undergone slicing, dicing, cutting, or other preparatory steps prior to packaging. Minimally processed foods are not treated using conventional or severe processing methods (e.g., canning, freezing, drying), but they may have been pasteurized or subjected to other "hurdles" to maintain freshness or quality and to extend refrigerated shelf life.

*Preserved foods:* These foods have been processed with preservation methods such as canning, freezing, drying, or other technologies to greatly extend storage times. Some preserved foods are processed in a manner that does not outwardly change their individual characteristics, making the food product easily recognizable from its raw predecessor. Examples include frozen vegetables and meats, or similarly, basic foods preserved using commercial sterilization technologies (e.g., retorting).

*Manufactured foods:* In essence, these foods have been processed to the degree that they no longer resemble the raw materials. Examples include sausages, cured meats, jams, and processed dishes or meals.

*Formulated foods:* These foods are characterized by the complete mixing and processing of ingredients to create fairly homogeneous textures and shelf-stable products. Examples of formulated foods include breads, cakes, biscuits, tortillas, and ice cream.

*Derivatives:* These are made from raw materials through refinement, purification, and additional processing. Many derivatives are used as ingredients in manufactured and formulated foods. Examples of derivatives include sugars, starches, oils, and fats. Further processing of derivatives is often done with chemical, physical, and microbiological treatments to create secondary derivatives.

Other important classifications of foods are ready-to-eat (RTE), not-ready-to eat (NRTE), and shelf stable. Simply stated, a RTE food does not require additional preparation or cooking prior to consumption. Fully prepared meals at home or in restaurants from raw materials are considered RTE. In this era of modern food processing, a variety of foods is manufactured and distributed to retailers as RTE. These RTE foods may be reheated or otherwise prepared for palatability, but they do not require a "kill" step or complete cooking prior to consumption. Examples of processed RTE foods include hot dogs, certain cured sausages, frozen entrees, canned meals, and deli-type (fresh) dishes prepared with fully cooked ingredients, or foods that have been cleaned, prepared, and intended to be eaten raw (e.g., cut fruits, salads). Conversely, NRTE foods require additional preparation or cooking for safety reasons prior to consumption. Common examples of NTRE foods are raw meats, poultry, and fish. Certain convenience and minimally processed foods may also be NRTE, meaning the consumer must further cook the food product sufficiently to ensure safety and/or edibility. For certain NRTE foods, federal regulations require labels on the food package that describe safe handling and cooking instructions (9 CFR 317.2 and 9 CFR 381.125).

Shelf-stable products are foods that have been treated in some manner to allow safe storage at room temperatures. Most NRTE foods and several types of RTE foods are *not* shelf stable. For example, hot dogs and deli meats are considered RTE, but they still require storage under refrigeration to prevent the growth of pathogenic or toxigenic microorganisms. As described in Chapter 4, foods that require time/temperature controls are considered to be potentially hazardous foods or temperature controlled for safety (PHF/TCS) foods (FDA and Public Health Service [PHS] 2009). Several food processing technologies described earlier in Chapter 5 are used to make shelf-stable products, and when several barriers to microbial growth are combined together, it is referred to as the hurdle concept or technology.

To make a safe food product, processors must start with knowledge about the potential foodborne agents (i.e., those covered in Chapters 2 and 3). This includes harmful agents that may be present in raw materials and those that may be introduced by the process itself, including from the facility, equipment, operations, packaging materials, procedures, and workers (Wallace 2006). The operations and objects illustrated in Figure 8-5 represent potential sources of harmful agents

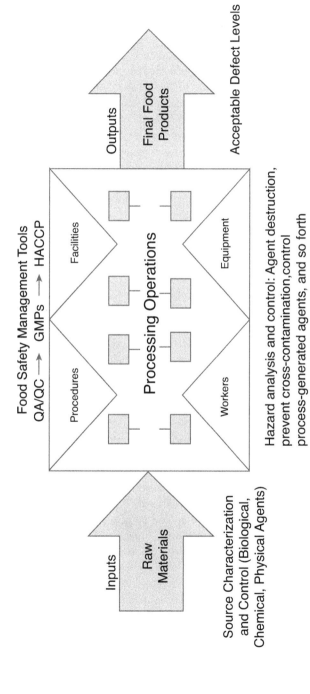

Food Safety Management Tools

QA/QC ⟶ GMPs ⟶ HACCP

Outputs

Final Food Products

Acceptable Defect Levels

Facilities

Processing Operations

Equipment

Procedures

Workers

Hazard analysis and control: Agent destruction, prevent cross-contamination, control process-generated agents, and so forth

Inputs

Raw Materials

Source Characterization and Control (Biological, Chemical, Physical Agents)

**Figure 8-5**  Diagram of Food Processing Inputs, Outputs, Operations, and Food Safety Management Tools

that may be introduced during food processing. Along with knowledge of potential foodborne agents, food processors must understand whether different treatments or operations will exacerbate, reduce, or eliminate hazards associated with these agents. For established operations, information is available from a variety of published and in-house documents, regulations, and subject matter experts. For novel operations, the effects on foodborne agents may be unknown or uncertain, and research is necessary to determine the effects of treatment. Even with knowledge about operations and their effects on foodborne agents, individual situations should be considered unique until verification testing confirms the expected/predicted outcomes. Several factors may not be immediately obvious, particularly with complex operations, and verification testing is necessary to ensure that factors have not been overlooked or have unexpectedly altered the process outcome.

Process control is necessary to minimize variations in food product quality, produce a safe product, and optimize efficiency and productivity (Niranjan, Ahromrit, Khare 2006). It involves measuring key processing parameters (e.g., temperature, mass, pressure, flow rates, pH, moisture, viscosity) and manipulating these parameters to maintain or correct process behavior. Measurement of processing parameters requires various sensors, along with procedures for their maintenance and calibration. Manipulation of parameters involves adjusting valves, machinery speed, energy input, and other actions. Methods of process control can be manual or automated, or a combination of both. Maintaining process control is critically important because an out-of-control food process can result in more than a poor quality product. It can result in a public health crisis. With modern food production volumes and distribution networks, a hazardous food product can cause widespread outbreaks of disease. Such events have unfortunately occurred multiple times over the past several decades.

Several food safety management tools are available—and in many cases mandated by law—to assist food processors and manufacturers (Jouve, Stringer, Baird-Parker 1998). The underlying management tool that most food businesses use is the quality assurance (QA) and quality control (QC) programs. Standards for QA/QC management programs are published by the International Organization for Standardization (ISO), a powerful nongovernment organization whose standards form the basis for many international treaties and laws in countries. Generic standards for quality management applicable to all business processes are found under the ISO 9000 family of documents. These standards emphasize the procedures, monitoring, recordkeeping, output defect detection, corrective actions, and continual improvement of industrial processes, regardless of the product produced. More recently, in 2005, the ISO published a new international standard specific to the food industry titled ISO 22000:2005, *Food Safety Management Systems—Requirements for Any Organization in the Food Chain*. This standard emphasizes interactive communications, system management, and HACCP and its prerequisite programs. It was developed cooperatively with the Codex Alimentarius Commission and is supposed to make Codex's HACCP Code (Codex Alimentarius Commission 2003c) easier for organizations to implement (Frost 2005). Additional standards in the ISO 22000 family are expected sometime in the future.

The QA program is an overarching program that includes the safety and nonsafety quality aspects of the product. QC operations are specific techniques and activities of process control necessary to "ensure that food is suitable for human consumption and that food packaging materials are safe and suitable" (21 CFR 110.80). The QA program utilizes generic food safety management tools and the HACCP system (a specific food safety management tool). Generic food safety management tools are also known as HACCP prerequisite programs. When used for food processing, they are sometimes referred to by different names, including *good manufacturing practices* (GMPs), *good production practices* (GPPs), and *good hygienic practices* (GHPs). Sometimes, distinctions are made between these different prerequisite programs. In other parts of the food supply chain, prerequisite programs include good agricultural practices (GAPs), good distribution practices, and good trading practices. In the United States, the concept of GMPs has been incorporated into regulations (29 CFR 110) as current GMPs (cGMPs). All food companies involved with the manufacturing, packing, or holding of human food must comply with the cGMPs regulations. Among the topics covered by cGMPs are personnel (food workers), building and facility design, sanitary operations, equipment and utensils, and production and process control. This provision also mandates appropriate precautions to prevent production procedures from contaminating food, regardless of the source. Furthermore, cGMP regulations require testing as necessary to identify possible contamination of food, whether from sanitation failures or from other sources.

Of all the food safety management tools, the HACCP system is best suited for controlling a specific process as it relates to food safety. By diagramming a specific process flow and conducting a hazard analysis of each operation or point, the HACCP system identifies critical control points required to produce a safe food product. With the development of a HACCP plan, process control is enhanced by establishing critical limits, monitoring procedures, and corrective actions. It should be remembered, however, that a HACCP plan is insufficient without the prerequisite programs, which constitute the foundation of any HACCP plan. Steps to developing a HACCP plan were discussed previously, and the student is referred to Chapter 6 for additional details. Use of the HACCP system has been endorsed and adopted by many organizations, but to date, regulations in the United States mandate the HACCP system only for the seafood industry (21 CFR 123.6), meat and poultry plants (9 CFR 417), and juice processors (21 CFR 120). Nevertheless, the HACCP system is widely used by many food processors, and its application has been extended to other parts of the food handling chain.

## Transport and Distribution of Foods

An important but sometimes overlooked aspect of food safety is food distribution and transport. Foods are transported across the country and around the world, both as processed food products and raw agricultural commodities. During transport activities and interim storage periods, foods are susceptible to contamination and unsafe practices that may lead to foodborne illness outbreaks. This problem was highlighted by a series of news reports in 1989 about trucking companies hauling foods in trucks that had previously hauled garbage or chemicals, a practice known as "backhauling" or "cross-hauling" (GAO 1990; Office of Inspector General 1998). In response to public concerns and a GAO report (GAO 1990), Congress passed the Sanitary Food Transportation Act (SFTA) of 1990. Despite passage of this act, additional problems with food transportation continued to be identified. Most notable among them was a salmonellosis outbreak of 224,000 people linked to a truck cross-hauling pasteurized ice cream premix and unpasteurized liquid eggs (Hennessey et al. 1996). Tragically, other incidents involved the deceased bodies of stowaways found in cargo ships carrying cocoa beans and raw sugar (Office of Inspector General 1998). In 2005, Congress passed the Sanitary Food Transportation Act of 2005 (2005 SFTA), which gave

FDA broad regulatory authority over the transportation of human and animal foods. A notice of rulemaking, a precursor to federal regulations, was published in April 2010 on implementing the 2005 SFTA, along with a guidance document for industry (FDA 2010a).

Existing FDA regulations already cover unsafe transport practices for human and animal foods, but they are distributed among many different sections and specific topics (FDA 2010a). Generally speaking, the major concerns are the contamination of foods with biological, chemical, and physical agents during storage, packing, unpacking, and transport; and poor refrigeration or temperature control. Foods are vulnerable to contamination from improper packing, poor sanitation, inadequate vehicle cleaning, backhauling of potentially hazardous/infectious loads, pest infestations, improper pesticide applications, leaking containers and vessels, infected workers, and other sources. Temperature abuse is another serious problem with transporting foods, particularly with PHF/TCS foods. This may occur from improperly operating refrigeration units, open cargo doors, poorly insulated/sealed cargo areas, inadequate temperature monitoring/adjustment, packing cargo in a manner that limits cold airflow, and excessive storage times on loading docks or other unrefrigerated areas. Considering the large number of interstate food shipments, such problems are difficult to discover by inspectors. Some states have taken innovative approaches to tackle this problem by partnering law enforcement agencies with public health officials. During 2006, Michigan State Police reported 22 cases of illegal and unsafe food transportation, of which several were considered serious health hazards (Powers 2007). The type of unsafe food transportation practices encountered on the highways is poignantly described below by Captain Powers:

> Raw poultry hanging from the roof inside the cargo area of a straight truck, juices dripping onto open boxes of produce below. The outside temperature on this sunny afternoon is 80 degrees, while the temperature inside the fly infested cargo box is 70 degrees plus. Juices from the rotting raw food is dripping out onto the pavement from under the rear cargo box doors. This truckload of rotting food is destined for a restaurant in your community. (Powers 2007)

The food distribution network in the United States is complex, consisting of multiple levels of distributors, processors, and retailers (see Figure 8-6) (GAO 2004). To protect public health, procedures are necessary to recall hazardous food products throughout this distribution network. Food recalls are classified by FDA and USDA according to their level of severity (GAO 2000). Class I recalls are considered the most serious: Eating food with a Class I recall classification exposes individuals to a reasonable probability of serious adverse health consequences or death. Foods typically associated with Class I recalls are contaminated with a pathogen or other potent agent, and/or they have been implicated in a foodborne illness outbreak. For example, food products contaminated with *Listeria monocytogenes*, *E. coli* O157:H7, or an undeclared severe allergen are likely to receive a Class I recall classification. Class II recalls involve food products that have a remote possibility of causing adverse health consequences, or the health consequences are considered temporary or medically reversible. Class III recalls involve food products that violate federal rules or regulations, but they are unlikely to cause adverse health consequences. Amazingly, except for infant formula, FDA and USDA do not have the authority to order food recalls, at least not currently (GAO 2008b). For the most part, recalls are voluntary actions by companies. By going

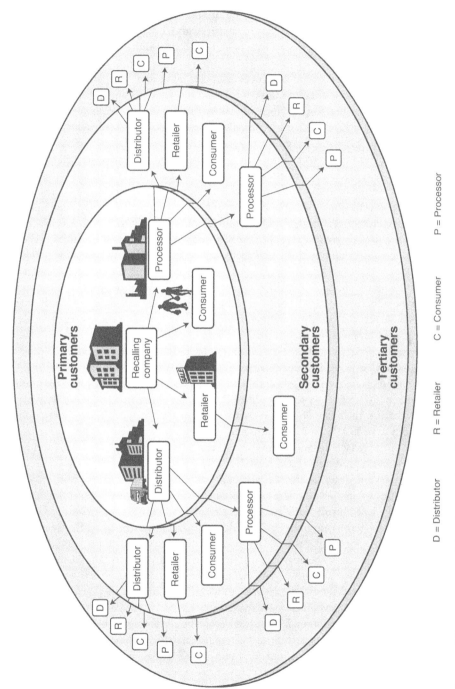

**Figure 8-6**  Downstream Food Distribution Chain Illustrating Multiple Levels of Distributors, Processors, and Retailers. *Source:* GAO, 2004

through the courts, FDA can seize, condemn, or destroy foods that are adulterated or misbranded, but this authority is limited in scope compared with recall authority. At the time of this writing, Congress is considering legislation (the FDA Food Safety Enhancement Act) that would give FDA recall authority.

The complexity of the food distribution network poses a twofold problem for public health officials. First, food recalls are difficult to implement fully in a timely manner. Second, determining the source of contaminated foods and/or ingredients implicated in a foodborne illness outbreak is time-consuming and costly, both in terms of excessive morbidity/mortality and industry financial losses. The congressional Government Accountability Office (GAO) reported that food recalls are often issued after the recommended shelf life of fresh foods such as bagged lettuce and ground meat, suggesting that they were already consumed or discarded (GAO 2004). Among all food recalls, the recovery rate of food products was surprisingly low, about 36–38%. One reason cited for this situation is the long turnaround times for food testing results. By the time food testing results identify/confirm contamination, the food product is likely to have been distributed. Other reasons cited for low recovery rates of recalled foods include the difficulties of tracking food products in the distribution network and the lack of recall verification by regulatory authorities and industry.

Whenever a foodborne illness outbreak occurs, public health authorities must attempt to discover the sources of foods associated with the outbreak, an activity called *trace back*. Failure to discover the food source can result in increased morbidity and mortality because the food product cannot be stopped and recalled from further distribution. *Trace forward* is an activity aimed at discovering where foods were distributed; this is important to recalling all contaminated products from the distribution network. For example, an outbreak of salmonellosis caused by only one peanut supplier resulted in the recall of more than 3,900 peanut-containing products by more than 200 companies (Wittenberger and Dohlman 2010). Trace back to a specific food source is also necessary to narrow the scope of recall and reduce economic damage to the industry. Following an outbreak of *E. coli* O157:H7 infections and blanket recommendations not to eat bagged spinach, the sale of all spinach dropped nearly in half compared to the previous year, causing significant losses to spinach producers (Calvin 2007).

Over the past several years, multistate and nationwide foodborne illness outbreaks have focused attention on the importance of trace back and trace forward capability throughout the food handling chain. A patchwork set of statutes and regulations requires some sort of traceability for most food products, but a comprehensive and uniform tracing system currently does not exist (McEntire et al. 2009). One statute, the Bioterrorism Act of 2002, amended the Food, Drug, and Cosmetic Act to include recordkeeping that will help trace food products. Under the law, "persons (excluding farms and restaurants) who manufacture, process, pack, transport, distribute, receive, hold, or import food" must keep records "to identify the immediate previous sources and the immediate subsequent recipients of food, including its packaging." The law also requires the registration of facilities "engaged in manufacturing, processing, packing, or holding food for consumption in the United States." Shortcomings of the law are the exclusion of farms and restaurants, and recordkeeping that is limited only to "immediate" sources and "immediate" recipients of foods, not the entire food supply chain. For any trace back investigation to be effective, every facility in the food supply chain must comply with the recordkeeping requirements. Therein lies the problem. In a sampling of food products, the Inspector General of the Department of Health and Human Services (DHHS) discovered that only 5 of 40 food products could be traced back "through each stage of the food supply chain" (Office of Inspector General 2009).

As part of the Food and Drug Administration Amendments Act of 2007, FDA was mandated to create a Reportable Food Registry. Essentially, this law requires registered food facilities to submit an electronic report if a food product is believed to be a serious hazard to humans or animals. The registry requires information about the hazardous food to assist in its traceability, such as lot numbers, universal product codes (UPC), brand names, label information, and so forth (McEntire et al. 2009). Additional information required to be submitted is the immediate sources and immediate recipients of the food product. Compared with past practices, the principal advantage of the Reportable Food Registry is the rapid (i.e., electronic) submission of essential data for trace back and trace forward investigations and recalls. Again, however, to effectively trace back and forward in the distribution of food products, each facility in the food supply chain must be compliant with federal recordkeeping requirements. There is hope in the future for a more comprehensive food product tracing system. Under contract with FDA, the Institute of Food Technologists conducted an in-depth review of issues, practices, technologies, and costs of traceability in the U.S. food supply chain (McEntire et al. 2009; Mejia et al. 2009). Hopefully, the findings and recommendations of this project will aid in the development of a cost-effective system for tracing food products.

## RETAIL FOOD ESTABLISHMENTS, INSTITUTIONAL FOODSERVICES, AND HOME PREPARATION

### Retail Food Establishments and Institutional Foodservices

Consumers have the option of buying groceries and prepared foods from a variety of sources. Based on the analysis of food purchasing patterns, consumer preferences have changed dramatically over the past century and even over the last several decades. Currently, approximately 42% of every dollar spent on food by American households is for food away from home (Economic Research Service [ERS] 2008). More than 1 million food establishments serve food in the United States and its territories (FDA 2010b). This includes meals at fast-food and full-service restaurants, schools, hotels, delicatessens, hospitals, and other facilities. Among the foods purchased by consumers for home preparation, approximately one-half is processed or packaged foods rather than fresh foods. It appears the most important factors influencing the food buying trends are increasing income levels and convenience (Morrison et al. 2010; Stewart et al. 2004).

Retail food establishments include privately owned foodservice facilities as well as grocery stores. The vast majority of Americans obtain their food from retail food establishments. According to the Bureau of Labor Statistics (BLS), in 2008, there were 546,300 privately owned foodservice and drinking establishments in the United States that provided 9.6 million jobs (Bureau of Labor Statistics [BLS] 2009a). Approximately 39.4% and 46.7% of these establishments are full-service restaurants and limited-service (fast-food) facilities, respectively. The remaining 13.9% of establishments consist of special foodservices (e.g., caterers, mobile canteens) and alcoholic beverage places (e.g., bars, pubs, taverns). The BLS also estimated a total of 85,200 grocery stores were located in the

United States during 2008, providing a total of 2.5 million jobs (BLS 2009b). Approximately 30% of these groceries are considered convenience stores that employ only 6% of the grocery store workforce. Supermarkets are large grocery stores that are known by various chain names. Several supermarket chains have begun offering prepared foods, sometimes with tables and seating for eating, and to-go meals, as well as fresh and packaged/processed foods. Many warehouse clubs and supercenters have also begun selling food and groceries along with general merchandise.

Institutional foodservice establishments include cafeterias or other foodservices in schools, colleges and universities, hospitals, nursing homes, day care centers, prisons and jails, and similar facilities. Institutions may contract with retail organizations to provide foodservices in their facilities rather than using in-house staff. Some institutions provide meals to residents in their homes (e.g., meals-on-wheels). An important distinction between most retail food establishments and some institutional foodservices is the type of patrons served. Institutional facilities such as hospitals, nursing homes, and schools serve food to a larger proportion of people who are more susceptible to foodborne diseases compared with the general population. An outbreak of foodborne illness among older adults, children, and sick persons can have much more serious consequences in terms of morbidity and mortality. For this reason, institutional foodservice establishments must carefully follow food safety and sanitation practices.

A key question related to consumer choice is "What are the relative risks of foodborne illness with different sources of foods and meals?" In a multiyear review of reported foodborne illness outbreaks in the United States, approximately 52% were associated with retail food service establishments (i.e., restaurants, delicatessens, cafeterias, hotels); 18% were associated with home meals; 4% were associated with schools; 4% of food sources were unknown; and the remaining 22% of outbreaks were associated with various other sources (Jones and Angulo 2006). The most recently available data on where food was consumed in reported outbreaks are illustrated in Figure 8-7. Although useful, data from reported outbreaks do not tell the whole story because most foodborne illnesses are believed to be from unreported outbreaks or sporadic cases (Mead et al. 1999). Surveys of consumers imply that restaurants or eating out are also responsible for the largest proportion of sporadic foodborne illness cases, but authors of such studies acknowledge many limitations exist with self-reported surveys (Jones and Angulo 2006). Regardless of the reported statistics, foodservice establishments historically and rationally represent a high public health priority. Anytime people gather in large numbers to consume food and drink, the transmission of infectious disease is a possibility, which can then lead to secondary disease transmission and extended outbreaks in the community. One infected food worker can thus transmit disease to a large number of people. If the establishment handles a great volume of meals, even a brief lapse in food safety practices can cause an outbreak of disease.

Regulation and inspection are the principal tools used to protect the public from foodborne hazards at the retail level of the farm-to-fork continuum. Inspections are conducted of foodservice and retail food establishments to identify violations of regulations and for enforcement actions. Federal authorities such as FDA have jurisdictional authority to inspect foodservice facilities, but with more than a million of these facilities located throughout the United States, FDA would not be able to inspect even a significant portion of them. Therefore, FDA relies on the cooperation of more than 3,000 state, local, and tribal agencies to regulate and inspect foodservice and retail food establishments (FDA 2010b). States differ somewhat in the content of their

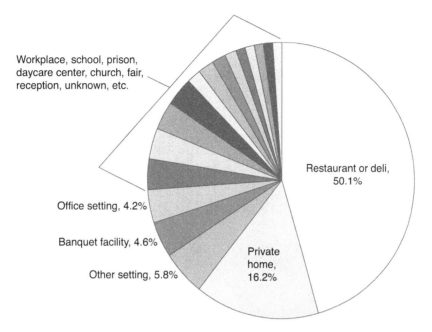

**Figure 8-7** Percentage of Reported Foodborne Illness Outbreaks in United States by Place Where Food Was Eaten, 2007. *Source:* Data from CDC

regulations and the organization of enforcement activities. In an effort to promote a high standard of uniformity across the nation, the U.S. Public Health Service started in 1934 to recommend a series of model regulations and ordinances for operations that provided food directly to consumers. In 1993 and subsequent years, the *Food Code* became the "model code and reference document for state, city, county and tribal agencies that regulate restaurants, retail food stores, vending operations and foodservice operations in institutions such as schools, hospitals, nursing homes and child care centers" (FDA and PHS 2009). The principles of prevention covered in Chapter 4 were derived in large part from the *Food Code.*

As part of its mission, FDA began a series of studies to measure the effectiveness of food safety programs at the foodservice and retail food level. Known as the Retail Food Factor Studies, they were based on periodic (5-year interval) surveys of selected institutional foodservice, restaurant, and retail food facilities (FDA 2004). The data were based on observations by inspectors using specific provisions from the *Food Code* related to foodborne illness risk factors (see Chapter 4). In the 2003 survey, an additional risk factor was added for potential contamination of food with toxic or unapproved chemicals. For each applicable *Food Code* provision, inspectors assigned ratings of either In Compliance, Out of Compliance, Not Observable, or Not Applicable. Results of these studies are used to measure trends in the occurrence of foodborne illness risk factors and to assist regulators and industry in setting priorities for improving food safety behavior and practices. Figure 8-8 summarizes the Out-of-Compliance results by risk factors and facility types.

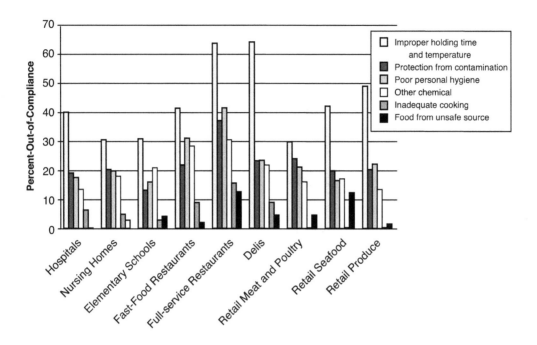

**Figure 8-8** Summary of Out-of-Compliance Foodborne Illness Risk Factors by Food Establishment Type, 2004. *Source:* Data from FDA, 2004

The model *Food Code* includes a form with an optional block for assigning a score to the inspection results. Most states use inspection scores as a snapshot of the facility's compliance with food safety regulations and ordinances. Many states also require posting inspection scores in the food facility and/or releasing them to public media outlets (e.g., Internet, newspapers, TV, radio). The popular belief is that inspection scores inform the public of risks and provide an incentive for businesses to comply with food safety regulations. Despite widespread use of food safety/sanitation scores, the value of inspection scores as a predictor of foodborne illness risks is questionable. Studies of inspection scores or violations and correlation with foodborne illnesses have yielded mixed results, and many methodological problems make objective assessments difficult (Jones et al. 2004). Several reasons may be responsible for the inconsistent observations of inspection scores and foodborne illness risks. One possible reason is that inspection scores do not adequately convey high-risk violations (i.e., foodborne illness risk factors). Another possible reason is related to differences in judgment, experience, and/or qualifications of inspectors. The frequency of inspection is also believed to influence the risk of foodborne illness, but evidence is lacking to make meaningful conclusions (Jones and Grimm 2008). Not surprisingly, consumers have unrealistically high expectations of the food safety inspection and scoring systems (Jones and Grimm 2008).

Training food workers in food safety and sanitation is considered a primary principle of prevention (see Chapter 4). Requirements for the training of food workers vary by state. Some states mandate formal training of all food workers, while other states provide incentives such as adding points to the inspection score for food worker training. Most experts agree that training food workers is important to providing the knowledge necessary to follow sanitary, hygienic, and safe practices with regard to food handling. But the supervision of food workers and the management of food operations are even more important to adherence with food safety practices. Managers are responsible for the entire operation of the food facility, and the safety culture fostered and oversight provided by management are critical elements in reducing the risk of foodborne illnesses. It seems logical, therefore, that managers should be well trained in the principles of food safety, and a manager's knowledge of food safety should be reflected in the facility inspection scores. Most states require food safety certification of a supervisor, manager, owner, or other responsible individual of the food facility or kitchen (Alamanza and Nesmith 2004). Certification training is offered by different trade organizations and private companies, and the examinations required for certification vary greatly by state. Past studies of the relationship between the presence of certified managers and inspection scores have had mixed results, but a recent study found a positive relationship between certified kitchen managers and the reduction of violations related to the foodborne illness risk factors; this study also identified several areas of needed improvement (Cates et al. 2009).

## Home Preparation of Food

Although it may be difficult to prove scientifically, home-prepared meals probably contribute much more to foodborne illnesses than is suggested by disease and outbreak statistics. Consumers frequently blame bouts of gastrointestinal illness on restaurant meals, but studies have shown that consumers generally have limited knowledge of food safety, and they often practice poor food safety at home. The vast majority of past research studies on consumer food safety (~75%) were survey-based, using either self-administered questionnaires or interviews (Redmond and Griffith 2003). Results of individual surveys about consumer knowledge of food safety vary. Overall, the majority of studies indicate that consumer knowledge is inadequate to minimize the risk of foodborne illness (Redmond and Griffith 2003). Table 8-3 summarizes key aspects of food safety knowledge from past surveys of U.S. consumers. Other research methods used to obtain information on consumer food safety are observational studies and focus groups. Observational studies are considered to be better indicators of actual consumer behavior than surveys are (but they are more difficult and expensive to perform). When the results of observational studies and surveys were compared, the actual observations of consumers' food safety practices generally did not correspond with surveys of the consumers' food safety knowledge, self-reported practices, and attitudes (Redmond and Griffith 2003). Most (but not all) of the actual food safety practices were worse than indicated by the surveys. If this generalization could be extrapolated to the entire population, which cannot be done for reasons of good science, then home-prepared food may indeed be the major source of all foodborne illnesses.

A useful method of evaluating the results from many different studies is called meta-analysis. Unlike a single quantitative study, meta-analysis is a statistical method that combines multiple

**Table 8-3** Selected Results of Surveys and Observational Studies of Consumer Food Safety Practices in U.S. Homes

| Food Safety Issues | Selected Results of Surveys and/or Observational Studies in the United States |
|---|---|
| Adequate cooking | An estimated 80–93% of consumers lack knowledge of correct heating temperatures. |
| | Most consumers (76%) reported that they do not regularly use a thermometer to measure the doneness of meat or poultry. |
| | Observations of consumers revealed most (95%) did not use a thermometer when cooking meat or poultry. |
| | 18–24% of consumers were observed using internal cooking temperatures that were too low. |
| Separation of raw and cooked foods/cross-contamination | An estimated 20–22% of consumers lack knowledge of separating cooked and raw meats during food preparation. |
| | 51% of consumers said they used the same surface to cut uncooked and cooked meat or poultry. |
| | Approximately 25% of consumers said they used the same cutting board for cutting raw meat or chicken without cleaning it before cutting cooked meat. |
| | 67% of consumers stated they washed or changed cutting boards after cutting up raw meat or poultry. |
| | Between 19% and 20% of consumers reported not washing a cutting board with soap or bleach after using it to cut raw meat or chicken. |
| | Between 25% and 71% of consumers were observed using improper cross-contamination procedures. |
| Refrigeration and cooling of foods | An estimated 40–56% of consumers lack knowledge of correct refrigeration temperatures. |
| | Between 24% and 47% of consumers were observed using improper cooling procedures for leftover foods. |
| Handwashing and drying | An estimated 14–21% of consumers lack knowledge of proper handwashing and drying. |
| | Between 66% and 76% of consumers reported they washed their hands after handling raw meat and poultry, and between 72% and 93% of consumers said they almost always washed their hands after handling raw meat and poultry. |
| | Approximately 19–20% of consumers reported they did not use (or routinely use) soap when washing their hands after handling raw meat or chicken. |
| | 44% of consumers reported they consistently forgot to wash their hands prior to meal preparation. 45% of consumers were actually observed attempting to wash their hands before food preparation. |
| | Between 29% and 57% of consumers were observed to neglect handwashing. |
| Consumer perception of home as an Important location for food "poisoning" | Only a small percentage of consumers thought the home was the most likely place for the mishandling of food (16%) or attributed the home as a source of foodborne illness (17%). |

*Source*: Redmond and Griffith 2003

studies together to improve statistical power (Egger and Smith 1997). Although sometimes controversial, meta-analysis has gained acceptance by many in the scientific community as a means of assisting in policymaking, so long as the meta-analysis is properly performed and utilized (Hoffert 1997). Meta-analysis is particularly useful in evaluating differences between individual studies and identifying data gaps for future research. Although rarely used to evaluate consumer food safety practices, one study by Patil Cates, and Morales (2005) used meta-analysis methods with 20 individual studies to estimate the risky food safety practices of consumers by demographic categories. Results of the meta-analysis found that consumer knowledge of good hygiene practices exceeded reported practices by 10% across the entire study sample. In other words, knowledge of good hygiene practices did not necessarily translate into actual behaviors and practices. The largest differences in knowledge and reported poor practices of consumer food safety were among individuals with "more than a high school education (25.6%), men (24.9%), and mid-age adults (21.8%)" (Patil et al. 2005). Correlations with other unsafe food practices and demographic characteristics were also identified, but the differences in knowledge and actual implementation of safe food practices was most remarkable. The authors recommend additional research to determine why food safety knowledge does not always translate into safe consumer behavior. This begs the question: Do consumers consciously or subconsciously choose not to adhere to good food safety practices? Answers to this question could greatly help with future risk communication and educational efforts.

Whereas the government regulates most segments of the food industry, the government's role in consumer food safety practices is limited mostly to educational initiatives (Redmond and Griffith 2003). Several sources of educational materials are available to consumers who wish to find it. In the United States, a great amount of consumer educational material on food safety is available on the Internet from federal and state agencies, nonprofit organizations, and some private companies (see Useful Resources at the end of this chapter). Public, private, and commercial organizations offer food safety seminars and outreach programs. Labels that provide safe cooking and handling precautions for consumers are placed on NRTE meats, poultry, and egg products. Clinicians may offer counseling about disease-specific food safety practices to individuals considered at high risk for serious consequences from foodborne diseases, such as pregnant women, the very young and very old, and the immunocompromised (Acheson and Fiore 2004; Kendall et al. 2003).

From the information discussed here, it should be apparent that food safety education of consumers is not a straightforward issue. Food safety messages and education do not necessarily translate into food safety practices. As with other educational programs, psychosocial factors influence the effectiveness of education, particularly with respect to personal risks and risky behavior. Simply sending a message or making information available about food safety is not sufficient. For example, in a large survey of selected states, only 51% of consumers reported seeing a safe food handling label on retail packages of raw or partially cooked meats and poultry products, and only 79% of these consumers remembered reading the label, of which only 37% changed their meat preparation practices after reading the label (Yang, Angulo, Altekruse 2000). The effectiveness of food safety education must be evaluated to ensure that it results in changes in knowledge and behavior. Experienced health educators recommend organizing and evaluating the effectiveness of food safety educational programs for consumers around five key behavioral constructs, which are epidemiologically important to preventing foodborne illnesses:

1. Practice personal hygiene.
2. Cook foods adequately.
3. Avoid cross-contamination.
4. Keep foods at safe temperatures.
5. Avoid food from unsafe sources. (Medeiros et al. 2001)

Part of food safety education is generating effective messages, as measured by changes in knowledge, attitudes, behaviors, and practices of the message recipients. This is applicable to all people involved in the farm-to-fork continuum, from food workers to the public. In recent years, food safety messages have been designed and evaluated in the context of risk communication, a discipline that is intertwined with risk assessment and risk management. Unlike traditional health communication models, risk communication takes into account the perceptions and relevance of risks to individuals and involves an exchange of information. Several authors (Jacob, Mathiasen, Powell 2010) outline and describe the development of effective food safety messages based on risk communication theory. The first step is to understand the target audience. This requires determining consumer knowledge and attitudes, sociocultural factors, and recognizing individual perceptions. As part of this first step, communication media should be identified that will best convey the food safety message to the target consumers, for example, printed materials, radio, TV, Internet, or other sources of information. The next step is to craft reliable messages in a timely manner, taking advantage of teachable moments such as news stories about food hazards or outbreaks. Messages should take into consideration the audience's lifestyle and use interesting narratives in place of statistically laden statements. Combining messages with social marketing strategies is also helpful in gaining the attention of consumers, and whenever possible, messages should be reinforced with multiple strategies and communication media. A third step or consideration in crafting food safety messages is ensuring clarity of content. Messages should be the right length, use clear language, and include graphics where appropriate. It is critically important to ensure that messages are consistent with one another and with other authoritative sources. Finally, messages should be tested before distribution to consumers. After distribution, the effectiveness of these messages should be evaluated using the most relevant and best-available evidence.

## FOOD SAFETY LAWS AND INDUSTRY INCENTIVES

More than 15 federal agencies have responsibilities for safety of the U.S. food supply. Table 8-4 lists the federal agencies with major roles in food safety. The authority and responsibilities of these agencies are rooted in multiple federal statutes that were passed in response to historical food safety concerns (see Appendix A). This division of authority and responsibility among multiple agencies has been the subject of criticism over the years (GAO 2005; IOM 2006). The primary concerns are unnecessary duplication of efforts, causing inefficiency and a burden to industry, while simultaneously permitting inconsistencies in oversight of the food supply chain (GAO 2005). For example, FDA and USDA both inspect at least 1,451 of the same domestic

**Table 8-4**  Federal Agencies' Food Safety Responsibilities

| Department and/or Agency | | Responsible for |
|---|---|---|
| U.S. Department of Agriculture | Food Safety and Inspection Service | All domestic and imported meat, poultry, and processed egg products |
| | Animal and Plant Health Inspection Service | Protecting the health and value of U.S. agricultural resources (e.g., animals and plants) |
| | Grain Inspection, Packers and Stockyards Administration | Establishing quality standards, inspection procedures, and marketing of grain and other related products |
| | Agricultural Marketing Service (AMS)[a] | Establishing quality and condition standards for dairy, fruit, vegetable, livestock, meat, poultry, and egg products |
| | Agricultural Research Service | Conducting food safety research |
| | Economic Research Service | Providing analyses of the economic issues affecting the safety of the U.S. food supply |
| | National Agricultural Statistics Service | Providing statistical data, including agricultural chemical usage data, related to the safety of the food supply |
| | Cooperative State Research, Education and Extension Service | Supporting food safety research, education, and extension programs in the land-grant university system and other partner organizations |
| Department of Health and Human Services | Food and Drug Administration (FDA) | All domestic and imported food products except meat, poultry, or processed egg products |
| | Centers for Disease Control and Prevention (CDC) | Protecting the nation's public health, including food-borne illness surveillance |
| Department of Commerce | National Marine Fisheries Service | Voluntary, fee-for-service examinations of seafood for safety and quality |
| Environmental Protection Agency | | Regulating the use of pesticides and maximum allowable residue levels on food commodities and animal feed |
| Department of the Treasury | Alcohol and Tobacco Tax and Trade Bureau | Enforcing laws covering the production, use, and distribution of alcoholic beverages |
| Department of Homeland Security[b] | | Coordinating agencies' food security activities |
| Federal Trade Commission | | Prohibiting false advertisements for food |

[a]According to USDA, AMS has no statutory authority in the area of food safety. However, the agency performs some functions related to food safety for several foods. For example, AMS graders monitor a shell egg surveillance program that identifies cracked and dirty eggs. In addition, AMS performs functions related to food safety for the National School Lunch Program.

[b]In 2001, by executive order, the president stated that the then Office of Homeland Security, as part of its efforts to protect critical infrastructures, should coordinate efforts to protect livestock, agriculture, and food systems from terrorist attacks. In 2002, Congress enacted the Homeland Security Act of 2002, Pub. L. No. 107-296, 116 Stat. 2135 (2002), setting out the department's responsibility to protect and secure critical infrastructures and transferring several food safety–related responsibilities to the Department of Homeland Security. As a result of the executive order, the Homeland Security Act of 2002 establishing the Department of Homeland Security, and subsequent presidential directives, the Department of Homeland Security provides overall coordination on the protection of the U.S. food supply from deliberate contamination.

*Source:* GAO 2005.

food-processing facilities because these facilities produce multi-ingredient products (e.g., canned or frozen foods) that are covered by various regulations with different jurisdictional authority (GAO 2005). If a product contains meat or poultry ingredients, for example, USDA will inspect the facility daily, and FDA will also inspect the facility at a frequency of every 1 to 5 years. If the product does not contain meat or poultry ingredients, only FDA will inspect the facility.

Sound arguments can be made for and against consolidation of federal agencies responsible for food safety. Consolidation could streamline management and administration, providing better coordination and greater efficiencies of food safety activities. This could save millions of dollars in federal funds and provide greater continuity and oversight of the U.S. food supply (GAO 2005; IOM 2006). For better or worse, consolidation of federal agencies would require an overhaul of the federal laws, which in itself would be extremely challenging. On the flip side, multiple agencies provide complementary expertise and independent scientific views that allow for divergent opinions, forcing reconciliation on complex food safety issues. Agencies with slightly overlapping responsibilities may also provide a system of checks and balances when it comes to oversight of critical infrastructure such as the food supply. But solutions to improving federal food safety functions need not be either complete consolidation or maintaining the status quo. In reports to Congress, GAO has made several recommendations to reduce duplication, leverage resources, and enhance coordination among the federal agencies with responsibility for food safety (GAO 2005). These recommendations include modernization of federal food safety laws, better sharing of information and resources, and updating or establishing interagency agreements, making them more substantive, particularly for overlapping responsibilities and functions.

Federal agencies promulgate regulations to implement the statutory laws passed by Congress (see Appendix A). To do this, federal agencies must interpret the intent of the statute and use technical or scientific expertise to write the regulations, also referred to as administrative rules and standards. Food safety regulations, standards, or rules must be "adopted following proper legal procedures" (Grad 1990). In most cases, regulations are adopted following an informal process called rule making. This usually requires publishing the proposed rule in the *Federal Register* for a period of time. The purpose of publishing the proposed rule before its promulgation is to seek comments from the public, industry, and interest groups. In addition, if required by law, hearings on the proposed rule must be held. Among the comments may be recommendations for changes to the proposed rule. However, the federal agency has the authority to either adopt or reject any recommended changes. After promulgation, the regulation has the full force of law on the basis of the original statute. If cases or disputes arise involving a regulation, the responsible federal agency usually has decision-making authority over it. Decisions by an agency can be subjected to court review, but the courts tend to take a deferential stand with the agency on decisions involving scientific or technical expertise (Grad 1990). The principal concern by the courts is errors in judgment and decisions based on arbitrariness or capriciousness.

With numerous federal statutes and agencies providing safety oversight of the U.S. food supply, it is not surprising that a tremendous number of regulations have been promulgated. The codification and compilation of all federal rules is done in the Code of Federal Regulations (CFR). Regulations are published under titles that typically correspond to the enabling statute (Fortin 2009). The majority of food regulations are found under Titles 7 (Agriculture), 9 (Animal and Animal Products), and 21 (Food and Drugs), though several other titles also contain regulations that affect foods. Finding a specific provision in food safety regulations can be a daunting task for those unfamiliar with CFR organization and legal writing styles. Fortunately, copies of CFR titles are now available on the Internet with multiple modes of retrieval, including searchable text capability (see Useful Resources at the end of this chapter). Table 8-5 is a partial list of relevant CFR titles and parts.

A great many of the federal regulations on food safety are aimed at food processors and manufacturers. Inspections are necessary to enforce these regulations, and FDA and FSIS are the primary agencies responsible for conducting inspections of food processors. Like retail food establishments, but to a lesser degree, FDA and FSIS depend on states and local governments to assist with inspections and regulatory enforcement at food processing plants and other nonretail food facilities. The joint authority for this arrangement is made possible by the similarity of federal and state statutes and regulations. The individual states usually incorporate major provisions of federal statutes, regulations, and model codes into their own laws. By working cooperatively with the states, sometimes under contract, the federal government allows state officials to conduct a large portion of inspections on its behalf (Fortin 2009). Federal agencies still retain the authority to conduct their own inspections and enforcement actions, but if the state programs are deemed at least as strict as federal requirements, the federal agencies often accept state inspections. Nonetheless, jurisdictional issues can arise whenever multiple agencies are involved in food safety. The jurisdiction over a particular problem often depends on the type of food product and its location in the food supply chain, as well as its location in different states and counties (IOM 2003).

A major point of contention among policymakers, industry, interest groups, and the public is the use of regulatory versus voluntary control measures for food safety. Regulations can be a double-edged sword, either hindering or helping individual companies with competition in the marketplace. Regulations add additional costs to food products, possibly making a company's product less competitive. This is particularly true in the global market, where some lesser developed countries do not have a modern regulatory framework and enforcement structure. On the other hand, if regulations are applied evenly to all companies, a level playing field is achieved, and ethical companies can produce high-quality and safe food products at a competitive price. If the regulations are highly restrictive by specifying only certain methods as acceptable, companies have no incentive to develop more cost-effective methods or technologies to achieve compliance. Poorly designed and written regulations stifle innovation and progress in the development of new products and technologies for food safety. Thus, performance-based regulations may be a better approach to managing certain food safety problems.

With some justification, industries complain about the complicated patchwork of food safety regulations and multiple agencies involved with promulgation and enforcement of them. Several economists and policy analysts point out that industry has incentives in the marketplace for self-regulation. Companies linked to a foodborne disease outbreak receive negative media attention, as demonstrated over the past decade with news reports of outbreaks. Such negative attention and the resulting lawsuits can be economically devastating to the company and the industry as a whole. This can provide a strong incentive for voluntarily improving food safety of the product. For example, following an outbreak of *E. coli* O157:H7 in spinach, the sale of spinach dropped drastically (Calvin 2007). Since then, large produce companies have undertaken a multihurdle approach to ensure the safety of their fresh produce products (IOM 2009). Similarly, following

Table 8-5 Selected Code of Federal Regulations (CFR) Titles and Contents

| CFR Title 7 Agriculture | | | CFR Title 9 Animal and Animal Products | | | CFR Title 21 Food and Drugs | | |
|---|---|---|---|---|---|---|---|---|
| Part | Subparts | Contents | Part | Subparts | Contents | Part | Subparts | Contents |
| 42 | .101–.103 | Standards for conditions of food containers | 416 | .1–.17 | Sanitation | 109 | .3–.30 | Unavoidable contaminants in food and food-packaging material |
| 43 | .101–.106 | Standards for sampling plans | 417 | .1–.8 | Hazardous analysis and critical control point (HACCP) systems | 110 | .3–.110 | Current good manufacturing processes in manufacturing, packing, or holding human food |
| 57 | .1–.1000 | Inspection of eggs | 424 | .1–.23 | Preparation and processing operations | 113 | .3–.100 | Thermally processed low-acid (e.g., canned) foods |
| 58 | .1–2827 | Dairy plants and products general specifications and standards | 430 | .1–.4 | Requirements for specific classes of products | 114 | .3–.100 | Acidified foods |
| | | | | | | 115–118 | | Shell eggs |
| 90–98 | .10 | Commodity laboratory testing programs | 441 | .10 | Consumer protection standards: raw products | 120 | .1–.25 | HACCP systems |
| 110 | .1–.9 | Recordkeeping on restricted Use pesticides by certified applicators | 590 | .1–.970 | Inspection of eggs and egg products | 123 | .3–.28 | Fish and fishery products |
| | | | | | | 129–169 | | Product-specific standards |
| 205 | .1 to .691–.699 | National organic program | 592 | .1–.650 | Voluntary inspection of egg products | 170–189 | | Food additives and irradiation |

outbreaks of *E. coli* O157:H7 infection from consuming contaminated hamburgers, several fast-food chains and beef suppliers undertook voluntary measures to reduce hamburger meat contamination and the transmission of pathogens. Among these voluntary measures were the use of clamshell cookers to ensure a thorough "kill" step before serving hamburgers, and negotiated contracts between fast-food chains and beef suppliers who use sophisticated testing programs to control pathogens in hamburger patties (Roberts 2005).

The major difficulty with using industry incentives to implement food safety is rooted in the differences of risk information and risk perceptions (Antle 2001; Segerson 1999). Obviously, if a product has a reputation of being unsafe, consumers will not purchase the product, or they will consciously or subconsciously weigh the risks of harm against the costs. The problem is that risks are not communicated on food product labels. Safety and risk information is imperfect, and consumers unknowingly accept unwanted risks with food products (Antle 2001). Part of the reason for imperfect risk information is lack of sharing. Risk information is often not shared between various levels of the food supply chain. Information about risks from agricultural practices such as pesticide residues may not be shared with food processors, who may not share information about process-related hazards with retailers, ultimately leaving the consumer uninformed of the risks. Differences in risk perception also affect industry incentives. Consumers may be more risk adverse than industry is about certain food hazards. In contrast with consumers, industry may consider certain risks to be minimal and acceptable in terms of product liability. Differences in risk perception and risk taking also exist among individual companies. To the detriment of consumers and the industry, some companies may take greater risks or transfer these risks to others.

All the aforementioned issues (and more) necessitate economic analyses of risk management options during decision making about regulatory versus voluntary controls. Optimal solutions to most food safety problems probably involve a combination of regulations, industry incentives, and education. Regulations should provide the minimum standard of food safety for the consumer, but industry incentives are needed to increase food safety beyond the minimum standards, thus reducing the risks even lower. Several voluntary programs exist within the federal government to assist companies in everything from Trichinae certification (9 CFR 149) to inspections of egg products (9 CFR 952). The strength of industry incentives, however, depends very much on consumer demand, which is related to consumer knowledge and information about foodborne hazards (ERS 2009). Because education helps acquire knowledge, educating consumers about foodborne hazards is an important part of making industry incentives work.

## FOOD DEFENSE

Referred to by several different names over the centuries, terrorism has existed since humans first used violence to influence politics. After the tragic events of the late twentieth century and this current century, it has become clear that catastrophic acts of terrorism can be easily perpetrated by only a few individuals. Events that are burned into the memories of many Americans include the destruction of the Murrah Federal Building in Oklahoma City with a home-made bomb in 1995; the hijacking and crashing of passenger airliners into buildings on September 11, 2001; and anthrax bioterrorism using letters and the U.S. mail in the fall of 2001. A common characteristic of these events and others is that they were carried out by only one or a few individuals, yet they caused death, destruction, and fear on a disproportionate scale. Among the greatest concerns in the future with terrorism are weapons of mass destruction (WMDs) and the disruption of critical infrastructure and key resources (CI/KR). The food supply is a both a potential vehicle for WMDs and a CI/KR, thus making it a high-value target for terrorists.

Federal agencies and various organizations define terrorism slightly differently. Under United States Law Code, *terrorism* is defined as "premeditated, politically motivated violence perpetrated against noncombatant targets by subnational groups or clandestine agents" (U.S. Code Title 22, Ch.38, Para. 2656f(d)). *Food terrorism* is defined as "an act or threat of deliberate contamination of food for human consumption with biological, chemical and physical agents or radionuclear materials for the purpose of causing injury or death to civilian populations and/or disrupting social, economic or political stability" (World Health Organization [WHO] 2008). The terms *agroterrorism* and *agriterrorism* may have slightly different definitions from food terrorism. One definition of agroterrorism is "the deliberate introduction of an animal or plant disease with the goal of generating fear over the safety of food, causing economic losses, and/or undermining social stability" (Monke 2007). Agriterrorism implies contamination of the food supply near the farm end of the farm-to-fork continuum. Whatever terms are used, the collection of measures to protect the food supply against terrorism is called *food defense*.

At several points the food supply is vulnerable to deliberate contamination with biological, chemical, and physical agents. Farms are located in remote and geographically dispersed locations, where observation by the public and law enforcement is infrequent, and where structures are less secure physically, allowing easier access. Animal and zoonotic pathogens are also easy to introduce and transmit within CAFOs compared with traditional grazing operations. Food processing facilities provide opportunities for adding harmful agents to batches of food during mixing, blending, and other operations. During distribution, food in transport vehicles can be deliberately contaminated prior to reaching its final destination. Furthermore, the rapid and long-distance distribution of foods increases the potential for widespread dissemination and impact, no matter where the agents are introduced (International Union of Food Science and Technology [IUFoST] 2007). At the retail level, a great variety of foods is vulnerable to deliberate contamination by the workforce, customers, or unauthorized visitors.

Serious incidents of deliberate food contamination have been documented around the world (IOM 2006; Mohtadi and Murshid 2007). Ironically, most of these malicious acts did not meet the strict definition of terrorism because they were done for revenge, economic competition, or for reasons unrelated to political, religious, or ideological motives. One of the largest incidents occurred in 1984 when restaurant salad bars in Oregon were clandestinely contaminated with *Salmonella* serotype Typhimurium. The resulting salmonellosis outbreak resembled a bimodal distribution over a month-long period, infecting at least 751 people who ate salad bar food from 10 different restaurants (Torok et al. 1997). It is suspected that many more people became infected, including tourists who were traveling through the area. At first, public health investigators could not determine the source of the outbreak because analysis of the outbreak variables did not implicate a typical source of contamination. A subsequent criminal investigation confirmed followers of a religious cult (called Rajneeshees) had spread *S.* Typhimurium from vials onto salad bars and into condiments. The apparent motive was to influence county elections by making citizens too ill to vote. Although inciting terror was not a motive, the incident was aimed at influencing a political outcome. Whatever the motives for deliberate contamination of food, a good food defense plan aims to protect against all types of malicious acts.

From 2005 to 2008, the Federal Bureau of Investigation (FBI), Department of Homeland Security (DHS), USDA, and FDA jointly performed assessments of the U.S. food and agricultural sector. The effort was called the Strategic Partnership Program Agroterrorism (SPPA) Initiative, and its final report was issued in December 2008 (FDA et al. 2008). With voluntary assistance of private industry and state officials, the initiative conducted vulnerability assessments of activities in the food supply chain to identify process "nodes" or "points" of greatest concern for agroterrorism or food terrorism. The SPPA Initiative also identified protective measures and mitigation steps for these nodes and research gaps or needs. A scoring tool called the "CARVER + Shock" program, which is now available as downloadable software (see Useful Resources), was used for the assessments. The acronym and name "CARVER + Shock" represent the following:

> *Criticality:* A measure of impact that a food terrorism attack may have in terms of public health and economic consequences
> *Accessibility:* The relative ease of physical access and egress to and from the node or process point
> *Recuperability:* The ability of the assessed plant or process to recover from a food terrorism attack
> *Vulnerability:* The relative ease of conducting a food terrorism attack at the node or process point, for example, ease of adding sufficient agents at the process point to achieve the terrorist's aims
> *Effect:* Magnitude (percentage) of direct loss in production from a food terrorism attack
> *Recognizability:* The ease of recognizing and identifying an important process point, for example, a highly visible apparatus that requires little or no training to recognize
> *Shock:* A measure of the combined effects of health, economic, and psychological impacts on a national scale

In its final report, the SPPA Initiative identifies general areas of greatest concern in subsectors of the food supply (FDA et al. 2008). Among plant producers/farmers, the greatest concerns are the introduction of plant diseases or persistent toxic substances by human contact (primary contact) or from fertilizers and water (secondary contact). The animal producers/farmers are most concerned about the introduction of highly contagious animal diseases that could result in the destruction of millions of animals. Infectious agents could be introduced to animal agriculture from either human contact (primary contact) or from animal feed and water (secondary contact). Plant and animal producers are principally concerned with the economic consequences, whereas the public health implications are greater at the subsector of food processing/manufacturing. During food processing and manufacturing, large batches of foods could be accessed and contaminated with harmful agents by terrorists or disgruntled employees.

Within the restaurant/foodservice subsector, the node of greatest concern is adulteration of food by humans just prior to consumption or delivery to the consumer. Whereas economic implications are important for restaurants and foodservice, they are overshadowed by the public health implications, particularly among larger establishments or vendors that serve many people. Retail food establishments such as groceries are most concerned about food products not in company control. Unobserved contact by humans (including customers) offers the greatest opportunities for mixing or applying harmful agents to food products in groceries and similar stores. Within the warehousing and logistics subsector, the areas of concern depend very much on the type of food or commodity. Foods stored in bulk for long periods of time are most vulnerable to tampering and adulteration. Holding live agricultural products (animals and plants) is also a concern because contagious animal/plant diseases could be introduced.

The SPPA Initiative report states that the participants did not always achieve consensus about the best mitigation strategies and security practices (i.e., food defense). Therefore, the SPPA Initiative reports only the most agreed upon food defense practices. The topics covered in the report closely parallel those discussed in this chapter for food safety, but the report places greater emphasis on biosecurity procedures in agriculture, physical and personnel security against malicious acts, and source control of materials. An overarching recommendation in the report is the development of dedicated agricultural security and food defense plans for establishments. Both FDA and USDA offer model guidelines and plans for food defense, and the CARVER + Shock computer program and methodology is available for industry use (see Useful Resources at the end of this chapter). Currently, food defense plans and most recommended security practices are voluntary on the part of private industry.

## FOOD SAFETY MANAGEMENT SYSTEM AT THE NATIONAL LEVEL

This chapter provides an overview of safety management of the food supply with a farm-to-fork perspective. To conclude, it is helpful to show the relationships between the components in a food safety management system at the national level. Ideally, safety management of the food supply should be planned and executed in a comprehensive manner to minimize the risks of all foodborne diseases. In reality, the size and complexity of the food supply chain, and the emergence of unforeseen hazards, make planning and execution imperfect at best. Nonetheless, through historical problem solving and the acquisition of knowledge, the national food safety management system has evolved to form a complementary set of activities. This system provides reasonable assurances of food safety and warnings of emerging hazards or threats to the food supply. There is certainly room for improvement, but the basic components of a food safety management system are in place and functioning, at least in the United States and most developed countries. Figure 8-9 provides a conceptual model of a food safety management system at the national level.

One of the most important components of a food safety management system is a robust epidemiologic surveillance and outbreak investigation capability. Epidemiologic surveillance and outbreak investigations are critical to identify new foodborne hazards or threats, mitigate or control outbreaks, and measure the effectiveness of specific food safety programs (ICMSF 2006; IOM 2003). Surveillance systems are categorized by different characteristics. The two most common surveillance systems for foodborne illnesses or diseases are passive and active surveillance systems. Passive surveillance systems have a basic reporting framework and submission forms available for state and local public health officials, but the submission of disease reports is voluntary and not actively solicited by federal officials. Foodborne illness outbreaks are often reported with passive surveillance systems, but sporadic cases of foodborne disease are

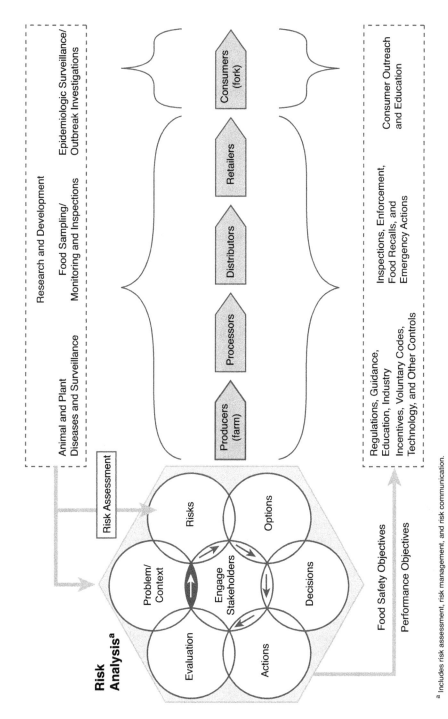

**Figure 8-9** Conceptual Model of a Food Safety Management System at the National Level

[a] Includes risk assessment, risk management, and risk communication.

infrequently reported with passive surveillance systems. State and territorial epidemiologists are generally responsible for conducting disease outbreak investigations in their jurisdictions, and they can share the outbreak data with CDC. The National Outbreak Reporting System (NORS) allows state and territorial epidemiologists to submit data on disease outbreaks via the Internet to CDC (Selman 2010). States and territories also have lists of reportable/notifiable diseases for mandatory case reporting by physician offices, hospitals, and public health laboratories. These reportable/notifiable disease lists include several but not all foodborne diseases (CDC 2010c). Although considered mandatory, reportable/notifiable disease case reporting is a passive surveillance system.

Active surveillance systems are better at capturing data about sporadic foodborne diseases. With active surveillance, the clinical laboratories are contacted by public health authorities to obtain case data on diagnosed diseases (IOM 2003). The Foodborne Disease Active Surveillance Network (FoodNet) is part of the Emerging Infections Program at CDC (Jones, Scallan, Angulo 2007). Initiated in 1996, FoodNet is a laboratory-based network with a catchment area covering approximately 50 million people in 10 states (Patrick 2009). In cooperation with participating states and federal agencies, FoodNet investigators contact more than 650 laboratories to electronically collect information on laboratory-diagnosed cases of diarrheal disease caused by *Campylobacter*, *Cryptosporidium*, *Cyclospora*, *Listeria*, *Salmonella*, shiga-toxin-producing *Escherichia coli* (STEC), *Shigella*, *Vibrio*, and *Yersinia*. The data collected by FoodNet are used to estimate the burden and monitor the trend of foodborne diseases and to identify risky foods and settings associated with foodborne diseases. The results of these analyses can be used to provide input to risk assessments, develop controls and interventions, and measure the effectiveness of food safety programs. A related surveillance system is PulseNet (discussed in Chapter 7), which is an important tool in subtyping pathogens and assisting in outbreak investigations.

Several federal agencies are involved in the systematic and periodic monitoring for hazards of foods and agricultural products (IOM 2003). Monitoring data can come from laboratory sampling and analysis of foods, in-depth surveys, consumer complaints, and inspections. Pesticide residues in raw agricultural products and food commodities are monitored under separate programs by FDA and USDA. USDA monitors antibiotic and chemical residues in animal products and several important pathogens in meat, poultry, and egg products. Food companies frequently monitor their products for contaminants, usually as part of HACCP verification or QC activities, but the data from food companies are not readily available to public health agencies for routine analysis. In theory, monitoring foods for hazards and taking corrective actions when necessary can prevent foodborne illnesses from ever occurring. In reality, several technical issues and challenges, discussed earlier in Chapter 7, make it impractical to rely on food monitoring as a primary prevention tool. Still, monitoring foods for hazards does provide the opportunity of detecting widespread or chronic problems in the food supply chain. Food monitoring also plays an important role in verifying the safety of food processes under HACCP plans. Data from monitoring foods for hazards also permit trend analysis, provide input to risk assessments, and assist in epidemiologic analysis of foodborne illnesses. Several recommendations have been made to improve and expand the utility of monitoring foods for hazards (IOM 2006, 2003).

Research and development (R&D) provides better understanding of foodborne agents and identification of possible solutions to food hazards. Basic research is helpful in understanding the nature of harmful agents, their interactions and persistence in the environment, and their pathogenic mechanisms in humans. Applied research helps to identify high-risk activities and locations in the food supply chain, and it is used to explore new approaches and strategies for controlling food hazards. The data from both basic and applied research also provide essential input to risk assessments of problems. Advanced development (or translational research) and engineering are used to develop new technologies or methods for controlling food hazards. The springboard to R&D is usually the monitoring and surveillance programs because these activities identify problems that require basic science and engineering disciplines to solve.

Introduced earlier in Chapter 6, the risk analysis process consists of risk assessment, risk management, and risk communication. These three elements are particularly applicable to protecting consumers from food hazards. Risks from food hazards are not static—especially with a large and complex food supply chain. New food hazards will likely be encountered in the future. The risks of existing food hazards will change with time and consumer habits. New food technologies will offer the promise of better food controls or, conversely, contribute to the creation of new food hazards. The risk analysis process provides a systematic methodology in which to address the complex technical, social, and legal issues entangled in food hazards and various control options. The hexagon-enclosed circles in Figure 8-9 represent a framework for managing risk problems and highlight the iterative nature of risk analysis (U.S. Presidential/Congressional Commission 1997). Technical activities and inputs to the framework include all the activities listed in the top block of Figure 8-9, whereas the risk management actions are listed in the bottom block. This chapter and/or previous chapters provide detailed discussion of these technical activities and risk management actions.

An adjunct step to some risk management actions is the development of food safety objectives (FSOs) and performance objectives (POs). The United States does not formally designate FSOs and POs in its risk management actions. Conceptually, however, many of the actions taken by U.S. agencies resemble FSOs and POs. According to the International Commission on Microbiological Specifications for Foods (ICMSF 2002), an FSO is the "maximum frequency and/or concentration of a hazard in a food at the time of consumption that provides or contributes to the appropriate level of protection (ALOP)." For some hazards, an FSO is analogous to a tolerance or action level established by FDA or USDA. For other hazards, where cooking of a raw food product by the consumer may reduce the hazard to an ALOP, the tolerance or action level is not equivalent to an FSO. To deal with these situations, a PO is sometimes established for the product earlier in the food supply chain. An analogy to the PO is the *Salmonella* performance standard established by USDA for raw meats and poultry (9 CFR 310.25 and 9 CFR 381.94). Under this performance standard, only a certain percentage of the carcasses or raw food products may test positive for *Salmonella* (e.g., 1.0% of steer/heifer carcasses). The goal of the performance standard is to evaluate process control of the establishment, not to test individual food products for safety.

Finally, evaluation of risk management actions is necessary to ensure that they indeed protect public health. As described previously, the incidence of foodborne illnesses and the frequency and level of food contamination are important metrics to measuring the effectiveness of risk management actions. Ineffective risk management actions may require problem reformulation and revision of the risk assessment. Often, the issues are related to gaps in knowledge about the hazard, and additional research may be necessary to fill these gaps and to gain a better understanding of the hazard. Evaluation of risk management actions also helps to prioritize the most cost-effective actions. In a world with finite resources, prioritization and cost-effectiveness are key considerations to optimizing the safety of the food supply.

## REFERENCES

Acheson DW, Fiore AE. 2004. Preventing foodborne disease—what clinicians can do. *N Engl J Med* 350(5):437–440.

AFSSA (Agence Française de Sécurité Sanitaire des Aliments), CODA-CERVA (Centre d'étude et de recherches vétérinaires et agrochimiques), INRA Clermont-Ferrand (Institut National de la Recherche Agronomique), INRA Toulouse (Institut National de la Recherche Agronomique), IRTA (Institut de Recerca i Tecnologia Agroalimentaries), ISPA (Istituto di Scienze delle Produzioni Alimentari). 2009. *Review of mycotoxin-detoxifying agents used as feed additives: Mode of action, efficacy and feed/food safety.* Report nr Scientific Report submitted to EFSA: CFP/EFSA/FEEDAP/2009/01. Parma, Italy: European Food Safety Authority. Available from: http://www.efsa.europa.eu/en/scdocs/doc/22e.pdf.

Almanza BA, Nesmith MS. 2004. Food safety certification regulations in the United States. *J Environ Health* 66(9):10,4,20.

American Society of Agricultural Engineers. 2003. *Manure production and characteristics.* Report nr ASAE D384.1 FEB03. St. Joseph, MI: American Society of Agricultural and Biological Engineers.

Antle JM. 2001. Economic analysis of food safety. In: *Handbook of agricultural economics.* Gardner BL, Rausser GC, eds. Amsterdam: North-Holland Publishing.

Bach SJ, McAllister TA, Mears GJ, Schwartzkopf-Genswein KS. 2004. Long-haul transport and lack of preconditioning increases fecal shedding of *Escherichia coli* and *Escherichia coli* O157:H7 by calves. *J Food Prot* 67(4):672–678.

Barberis CL, Astoreca AL, Dalcero AM, Magnoli CE. 2010. Food-grade antioxidants and antimicrobials to control growth and ochratoxin a production by *Aspergillus* section nigri on peanut kernels. *J Food Prot* 73(8):1493–1501.

Beuchat LR. 2006. Vectors and conditions for preharvest contamination of fruits and vegetables with pathogens capable of causing enteric diseases. *British Food Journal* 108(1):38–53.

Bhat R, Rai RV, Karim AA. 2010. Mycotoxins in food and feed: Present status and future concerns. *Comprehensive Reviews in Food Science and Food Safety* 9:57–81.

Bleasdale B, Lott PJ, Jagannathan A, Stevens MP, Birtles RJ, Wigley P. 2009. The *Salmonella* pathogenicity island 2-encoded type III secretion system is essential for the survival of *Salmonella enterica* serovar Typhimurium in free-living amoebae. *Appl Environ Microbiol* 75(6):1793–1795.

Boobis AR, Ossendorp BC, Banasiak U, Hamey PY, Sebestyen I, Moretto A. 2008. Cumulative risk assessment of pesticide residues in food. *Toxicol Lett* 180(2):137–150.

Bullerman LB, Bianchini A. 2007. Stability of mycotoxins during food processing. *Int J Food Microbiol* 119(1–2):140–146.

Bureau of Labor Statistics. 2009a. Food services and drinking places. In: *Career guide to industries, 2010–11 edition.* Washington, DC: U.S. Department of Labor. Available from: http://data.bls.gov/cgi-bin/print.pl/oco/cg/cgs023.htm.

Bureau of Labor Statistics. 2009b. Grocery stores. In: *Career guide to industries, 2010–11 edition.* Washington, DC: U.S. Department of Labor. Available from: http://data.bls.gov/cgi-bin/print.pl/oco/cg/cgs024.htm.

Callaway TR, Carr MA, Edrington TS, Anderson RC, Nisbet DJ. 2009. Diet, *escherichia coli* O157:H7, and cattle: A review after 10 years. *Curr Issues Mol Biol* 11(2):67–79.

Callaway TR, Anderson RC, Edrington TS, Genovese KJ, Harvey RB, Poole TL, Nisbet DJ. 2004. Recent pre-harvest supplementation strategies to reduce carriage and shedding of zoonotic enteric bacterial pathogens in food animals. *Anim Health Res Rev* 5(1):35–47.

Calvin L. 2007. Outbreak linked to spinach forces reassessment of food safety practices. *Amber Waves* 5(3):24–31.

Cates SC, Muth MK, Karns SA, Penne MA, Stone CN, Harrison JE, Radke VJ. 2009. Certified kitchen managers: Do they improve restaurant inspection outcomes? *J Food Prot* 72(2):384–391.

Centers for Disease Control and Prevention. 2010a. *Investigation update: Multistate outbreak of human* Salmonella *Enteritidis infections associated with shell eggs.* Atlanta, GA: U.S. Department of Health and Human Services. Available from: http://www.cdc.gov/salmonella/enteritidis/.

Centers for Disease Control and Prevention. 2010b. Preliminary FoodNet data on the incidence of infection with pathogens transmitted commonly through food—10 states, 2009. *MMWR* 59(14):418–422.

Centers for Disease Control and Prevention. 2010c. Summary of notifiable diseases—United States, 2008. *MMWR* 57(54):1–87.

Centers for Disease Control and Prevention. 2007. *Salmonella* Typhimurium infection associated with raw milk and cheese consumption—Pennsylvania, 2007. *MMWR* 56(44):1161–1164.

Cleveland TE, Dowd PF, Desjardins AE, Bhatnagar D, Cotty PJ. 2003. United States Department of Agriculture Agricultural Research Service research on pre-harvest prevention of mycotoxins and mycotoxigenic fungi in US crops. *Pest Manag Sci* 59(6–7):629–642.

Cliver DO. 2009. Disinfection of animal manures, food safety and policy. *Bioresour Technol* 100(22):5392–5394.

Codex Alimentarius Commission. 2004a. *Code of practice on good animal feeding.* Report nr CAC/RCP 54-2004. Geneva: Joint FAO/WHO Food Standards Programme.

Codex Alimentarius Commission. 2004b. *Code of practice for the prevention and reduction of aflatoxin contamination in peanuts.* Report nr CAC/RCP 55 – 2004. Geneva: Joint FAO/WHO Food Standards Programme.

Codex Alimentarius Commission. 2003a. *Code of hygienic practice for fresh fruits and vegetables.* Report nr CAC/RCP 53-2003. Geneva: Joint FAO/WHO Food Standards Programme.

Codex Alimentarius Commission. 2003b. *Code of practice for the prevention and reduction of mycotoxin contamination in cereals, including annexes on ochratoxin A, zearalenone, fumonisins and tricothecenes.* Report nr CAC/RCP 51-2003. Geneva: Joint FAO/WHO Food Standards Programme.

Codex Alimentarius Commission. 2003c. *Recommended international code of practice—general principles of food hygiene.* Report nr CAC/RCP 1-1969, Rev.4- 2003. Rome, Italy: Joint FAO/WHO Food Standards Programme.

Collins JD, Wall PG. 2004. Food safety and animal production systems: Controlling zoonoses at farm level. *Rev Sci Tech* 23(2):685–700.

Crump JA, Griffin PM, Angulo FJ. 2002. Bacterial contamination of animal feed and its relationship to human foodborne illness. *Clin Infect Dis* 35(7):859–865.

Davies PR, Scott Hurd H, Funk JA, Fedorka-Cray PJ, Jones FT. 2004. The role of contaminated feed in the epidemiology and control of *Salmonella enterica* in pork production. *Foodborne Pathog Dis* 1(4):202–215.

Dewell GA, Simpson CA, Dewell RD, Hyatt DR, Belk KE, Scanga JA, Morley PS, Grandin T, Smith GC, Dargatz DA, et al. 2008. Impact of transportation and lairage on hide contamination with *Escherichia coli* O157 in finished beef cattle. *J Food Prot* 71(6):1114–1118.

Doyle MP, Erickson MC. 2008. Summer meeting 2007—the problems with fresh produce: An overview. *J Appl Microbiol* 105(2):317–330.

Drusch S, Ragab W. 2003. Mycotoxins in fruits, fruit juices, and dried fruits. *J Food Prot* 66(8):1514–1527.

Economic Research Service. 2009. *The economics of food, farming, natural resources, and rural America.* Washington, DC: U.S. Department of Agriculture. Available from: http://transcoder.usablenet.com/tt/http://www.ers.usda.gov/Briefing/FoodSafety/private.htm.

Economic Research Service. 2008. *Diet quality and food consumption: Food away from home.* Washington, DC: U.S. Department of Agriculture. Available from: http://www.ers.usda.gov/Briefing/DietQuality/FAFH.htm.

Egger M, Smith GD. 1997. Meta-analysis. Potentials and promise. *BMJ* 315(7119):1371–1374.

Environmental Protection Agency. 2004. *Risk assessment evaluation for concentrated animal feeding operations.* Report nr EPA/600/R-04/042. Washington, DC: U.S. Environmental Protection Agency. Available from: http://www.epa.gov/nrmrl/pubs/600r04042/600r04042.pdf.

Federal Joint Subcommittee on Aquaculture, Working Group on Quality Assurance in Aquaculture. 2007. *Guide to drug, vaccine, and pesticide use in aquaculture.* Available from: http://aquanic.org/jsa/wgqaap/drugguide/drugguide.htm.

Fellows PJ. 2009. *Food processing technology: Principles and practices.* 3rd ed. Cambridge, England: Woodhead Publishing.

Food and Agriculture Organization. 2007. *State of the world fisheries and aquaculture.* Rome: Food and Agriculture Organization of the United Nations.

Food and Agriculture Organization. 2004. *Worldwide regulations for mycotoxins in food and feed in 2003.* Report nr FAO Food and Nutrition Paper 81. Rome: Food and Agriculture Organization of the United Nations. Available from: http://www.fao.org/docrep/007/y5499e/y5499e00.HTM.

Food and Agriculture Organization, Network of Aquaculture Centres in Asia–Pacific, World Health Organization. 1999. Food safety issues associated with products from aquaculture. Report of a joint FAO/NACA/WHO study group. *World Health Organ Tech Rep Ser* 883(i,vii):1–55.

Food and Drug Administration. 2010a. *Guidance for industry: Sanitary transportation of food*. Washington, DC: U.S. Department of Health and Human Services. Available from: http://www.fda.gov/Food/GuidanceComplianceRegulatory Information/GuidanceDocuments/FoodSafety/ucm208199.htm.

Food and Drug Administration. 2010b. *Retail food protection, a cooperative program*. Washington, DC: U.S. Department of Health and Human Services. Available from: http://www.fda.gov/Food/FoodSafety/RetailFoodProtection/default.htm.

Food and Drug Administration. 2009. *Grade "A" pasteurized milk ordinance (2009 revision)*. Rockville, MD: U.S. Public Health Service/U.S. Food and Drug Administration.

Food and Drug Administration. 2004. *Report on the occurrence of foodborne illness risk factors in selected institutional food-service, restaurant, and retail food store facility types (2004)*. Washington, DC: Department of Health and Human Services. Available from: http://www.fda.gov/Food/FoodSafety/RetailFoodProtection/FoodborneIllnessandRiskFactorReduction/ RetailFoodRiskFactorStudies/ucm089696.htm.

Food and Drug Administration, Center for Food Safety and Applied Nutrition. 1998. *Guide to minimize microbial food safety hazards for fresh fruits and vegetables*. Washington, DC: U.S. Department of Health and Human Services.

Food and Drug Administration and Environmental Protection Agency. 2004. *2004 EPA and FDA advice for: Women who might become pregnant; women who are pregnant, nursing mothers; young children*. Report nr EPA-823-R-04-005. Washington, DC: Food and Drug Administration, Environmental Protection Agency.

Food and Drug Administration and Public Health Service. 2009. *Food code 2009*. Washington, DC: Department of Health and Human Services. Available from: http://www.fda.gov/Food/FoodSafety/RetailFoodProtection/FoodCode/ FoodCode2009/default.htm.

Food and Drug Administration, U.S. Department of Agriculture, U.S. Department of Homeland Security, and Federal Bureau of Investigation. 2008. *Strategic Partnership Program Agroterrorism (SPPA) Initiative. Final summary report. September 2005–September 2008*. Washington, DC: Food and Drug Administration, U.S. Department of Agriculture, U.S. Department of Homeland Security, and Federal Bureau of Investigation.

Food Safety and Inspection Service. 1999a. *Generic HACCP model for beef slaughter*. Report nr HACCP-13. Washington, DC: U.S. Department of Agriculture.

Food Safety and Inspection Service. 1999b. *Generic HACCP model for pork slaughter*. Report nr HACCP-14. Washington, DC: U.S. Department of Agriculture.

Food Safety and Inspection Service. 1999c. *Generic HACCP model for poultry slaughter, revision 1*. Report nr HACCP-5. Washington, DC: U.S. Department of Agriculture.

Fortin ND. 2009. *Food regulation: Law, science, policy, and practice*. Hoboken, NJ: John Wiley.

Frost R. 2005, November–December. ISO 22000 is first in family of food safety management system standards. *ISO Management Systems* 16–19.

Glibert PM, Anderson DM, Gentien P, Graneli E, Sellner KG. 2005. The global, complex phenomena of harmful algal blooms. *Oceanography* 18(2):136–147.

Goldman LR, Smith DF, Neutra RR, Saunders LD, Pond EM, Stratton J, Waller K, Jackson RJ, Kizer KW. 1990. Pesticide food poisoning from contaminated watermelons in California, 1985. *Arch Environ Health* 45(4):229–236.

Government Accountability Office. 2009. *Seafood fraud: FDA program changes and better collaboration among key federal agencies could improve detection and prevention*. Report nr GAO-09-258. Washington, DC: U.S. Government Accountability Office.

Government Accountability Office. 2008a. *Concentrated animal feeding operations: EPA needs more information and a clearly defined strategy to protect air and water quality from pollutants of concern*. Report nr GAO-08-944. Washington, DC: U.S. Government Accountability Office.

Government Accountability Office. 2008b. *Federal oversight of food safety: FDA's food protection plan proposes positive first steps, but capacity to carry them out is critical*. Report nr GAO-08-435T. Washington, DC: U.S. Government Accountability Office.

Government Accountability Office. 2005. *Oversight of food safety activities: Federal agencies should pursue opportunities to reduce overlap and better leverage resources*. Report nr GAO-05-213. Washington, DC: U.S. Government Accountability Office.

Government Accountability Office. 2004. *Food safety: USDA and FDA need to better ensure prompt and complete recalls of potentially unsafe food*. Report nr GAO-05-51. Washington, DC: U.S. Government Accountability Office.

Government Accountability Office. 2000. *Food safety: Actions needed by USDA and FDA to ensure that companies promptly carry out recalls.* Report nr GAO/RCED-00-195. Washington, DC: U.S. Government Accountability Office.

Government Accountability Office. 1992. *Food safety and quality: FDA strategy needed to address animal drug residues in milk.* Report nr GAO/RCED-92-209. Washington, DC: U.S. Government Accountability Office.

Government Accountability Office. 1990. *Truck transport: Little is known about hauling garbage and food in the same vehicles.* Report nr GAO/RCED-90-161. Washington, DC: U.S. Government Accountability Office. Available from: http://archive.gao.gov/d23t8/141739.pdf.

Grad FP. 1990. *Public health law manual.* 2nd ed. Washington, DC: American Public Health Association.

Gurian-Sherman D. 2008, April. *CAFOs uncovered: The untold costs of confined animal feeding operations.* Cambridge, MA: Union of Concerned Scientists Publications. Available from: http://www.ucsusa.org/assets/documents/food_and_agriculture/cafos-uncovered.pdf.

Hayward D, Wong J, Krynitsky AJ. 2007. Polybrominated diphenyl ethers and polychlorinated biphenyls in commercially wild caught and farm-raised fish fillets in the United States. *Environ Res* 103(1):46–54.

Hennessy TW, Hedberg CW, Slutsker L, White KE, Besser-Wiek JM, Moen ME, Feldman J, Coleman WW, Edmonson LM, MacDonald KL, et al. 1996. A national outbreak of *Salmonella Enteritidis* infections from ice cream. The investigation team. *N Engl J Med* 334(20):1281–1286.

Hoffert SP. 1997. Meta-analysis gaining status in science and policymaking. *The Scientist* 11(18):1–5.

Hoque A, Sigurdson AJ, Burau KD, Humphrey HE, Hess KR, Sweeney AM. 1998. Cancer among a Michigan cohort exposed to polybrominated biphenyls in 1973. *Epidemiology* 9(4):373–378.

Institute of Food Science and Technology. 2009. *Updated mycotoxins information statement.* London: Available from: http://www.ifst.org/about_ifst/hotspot/index/29514/Updated_Mycotoxins_Information_Statement.

Institute of Medicine. 2010. *Enhancing food safety: The role of the Food and Drug Administration.* Washington DC: National Academies Press.

Institute of Medicine. 2009. *Managing food safety practices from farm to fork: Workshop summary.* Washington, DC: National Academies Press.

Institute of Medicine. 2006. *Addressing foodborne threats to health: Policies, practices, and global coordination (workshop summary).* Washington, DC: National Academies Press.

Institute of Medicine. 2003. *Scientific criteria to ensure safe food.* Washington, DC: National Academies Press.

Institute of Medicine. 1991. *Seafood safety.* Washington, DC: National Academy Press.

Institute of Medicine and National Research Council. 1998. *Ensuring safe food: From production to consumption.* Washington, DC: National Academy Press.

International Commission on Microbiological Specifications for Foods. 2006. Use of epidemiologic data to measure the impact of food safety control programs. *Food Control* 17(10):825–837.

International Commission on Microbiological Specifications for Foods. 2002. *Microorganisms in foods 7. Microbiological testing in food safety management.* New York, NY: Kluwer Academic/Plenum Publishers.

International Union of Food Science and Technology. 2007. *Short summary on food defense.* Report nr IUFoST Scientific Information Bulletin. Ontario, Canada: International Union of Food Science and Technology.

Interstate Shellfish Sanitation Conference and Food and Drug Administration. 2007. *National shellfish sanitation program guide for the control of molluscan shellfish, 2007 revision.* Washington, DC: U.S. Department of Health and Human Services.

Jacob C, Mathiasen L, Powell D. 2010. Designing effective messages for microbial food safety hazards. *Food Control* 21(1):1–6.

Jones TF, Angulo FJ. 2006. Eating in restaurants: A risk factor for foodborne disease? *Clin Infect Dis* 43(10):1324–1328.

Jones TF, Grimm K. 2008. Public knowledge and attitudes regarding public health inspections of restaurants. *Am J Prev Med* 34(6):510–513.

Jones TF, Pavlin BI, LaFleur BJ, Ingram LA, Schaffner W. 2004. Restaurant inspection scores and foodborne disease. *Emerg Infect Dis* 10(4):688–692.

Jones TF, Scallan E, Angulo FJ. 2007. FoodNet: Overview of a decade of achievement. *Foodborne Pathog Dis* 4(1):60–66.

Jouve JL, Stringer MF, Baird-Parker AC. 1998, April. Food safety management tools, report prepared under the responsibility of ILSI Europe Risk Analysis in Microbiology Task Force. Brussels, Belgium: ILSI Europe.

Kabak B, Dobson AD. 2009. Biological strategies to counteract the effects of mycotoxins. *J Food Prot* 72(9):2006–2016.

Kabak B, Dobson AD, Var I. 2006. Strategies to prevent mycotoxin contamination of food and animal feed: A review. *Crit Rev Food Sci Nutr* 46(8):593–619.

Kan CA, Meijer GAL. 2007. The risk of contamination of food with toxic substances present in animal feed. *Animal Feed Science and Technology* 133(1):84–108.

Kendall P, Medeiros LC, Hillers V, Chen G, DiMascola S. 2003. Food handling behaviors of special importance for pregnant women, infants and young children, the elderly, and immune-compromised people. *J Am Diet Assoc* 103(12):1646–1649.

Kiely T, Donaldson D, Grube A. 2004. *Pesticides industry sales and usage: 2000 and 2001 market estimates.* Report nr EPA-733-R-04-001. Washington, DC: Environmental Protection Agency. Available from: http://www.epa.gov/opp00001/pestsales/01pestsales/market_estimates2001.pdf.

LeJeune JT, Wetzel AN. 2007. Preharvest control of *Escherichia coli* O157 in cattle. *J Anim Sci* 85(13 Suppl):E73–80.

Lynch MF, Tauxe RV, Hedberg CW. 2009. The growing burden of foodborne outbreaks due to contaminated fresh produce: Risks and opportunities. *Epidemiol Infect* 137(3):307–315.

Magan N, Aldred D. 2007. Post-harvest control strategies: Minimizing mycotoxins in the food chain. *Int J Food Microbiol* 119(1–2):131–139.

Martens W, Bohm R. 2009. Overview of the ability of different treatment methods for liquid and solid manure to inactivate pathogens. *Bioresour Technol* 100(22):5374–5378.

Mathew AG, Cissell R, Liamthong S. 2007. Antibiotic resistance in bacteria associated with food animals: A United States perspective of livestock production. *Foodborne Pathog Dis* 4(2):115–133.

McEntire JC, Arens S, Bugusu B, Busta FF, Cole M, Davis A, Fisher W, Geisert S, Jensen H, Kenah B, et al. 2009. Traceability (product tracing) in food systems: An IFT report submitted to the FDA, volume 1: Technical aspects and recommendations. *Comprehensive Reviews in Food Science and Food Safety* 9:93.

Mead PS, Slutsker L, Dietz V, McCaig LF, Bresee JS, Shapiro C, Griffin PM, Tauxe RV. 1999. Food-related illness and death in the United States. *Emerg Infect Dis* 5(5):607–625.

Medeiros LC, Hillers VN, Kendall PA, Mason A. 2001. Food safety education: What should we be teaching to consumers? *J Nutr Educ* 33(2):108–113.

Mejia C, McEntire JC, Keener K, Muth MK, Nganje W, Stinson T, Jensen H. 2009. Traceability (product tracing) in food systems: An IFT report submitted to the FDA, volume 2: Cost considerations and implications. *Comprehensive Reviews in Food Science and Food Safety* 9:160.

Mohtadi M, Murshid AP. 2007. Analyzing catastrophic terrorist events with applications to the food industry. In: *The economic costs and consequences of terrorism.* Richards HW, Gordon P, Elliott Moore JE, eds. Northampton, MA: Edward Elgar Publishing.

Molbak K, Olsen JE, Wegener HC. 2005. *Salmonella* infections. In: *Foodborne infections and intoxications.* 3rd ed. Rieman HP, Cliver DO, eds. Amsterdam: Academic Press.

Monke J. 2007. *CRS report for Congress. Agroterrorism: Threats and preparedness.* Report nr Order Code RL32521. Washington, DC: Congressional Research Service.

Morrison RM, Buzby JC, Wells HF. 2010. Guess Who's turning 100? Tracking a century of American eating. *Amber Waves* 8(1):12–19.

Moss MO. 2008. Fungi, quality and safety issues in fresh fruits and vegetables. *J Appl Microbiol* 104(5):1239–1243.

National Advisory Committee on Meat and Poultry Inspection. 2008. *Public health risk-based inspection system for processing and slaughter, technical report.* Washington, DC: U.S. Department of Agriculture. Available from: http://www.fsis.usda.gov/OPPDE/NACMPI/Feb2008/Processing_Slaughter_Tech_Rpt_041808.pdf.

National Agricultural Statistics Service. 2010. Charts and maps by commodity. Washington, DC: U.S. Department of Agriculture. Available from: http://www.nass.usda.gov/Charts_and_Maps/index.asp .

National Agricultural Statistics Service. 2002, updated 2005. *Census of aquaculture (2005), volume 3, special studies part 2.* Report nr AC-02-SP-2. Washington, DC: U.S. Department of Agriculture.

National Oceanic and Atmospheric Administration Aquaculture Program. 2010. *Aquaculture in the United States.* Washington, DC: National Ocean Service, National Oceanic and Atmospheric Administration, Department of Commerce. Available from: http://aquaculture.noaa.gov/us/welcome.html.

National Pollutant Discharge Elimination System. 2010. *Animal feeding operations.* Washington, DC: Environmental Protection Agency. Available from: http://cfpub.epa.gov/npdes/home.cfm?program_id=7.

Natural Resources Conservation Service. 2010. Conservation practice standard: Integrated pest management. Report nr Code 595. Available from: ftp://ftp-fc.sc.egov.usda.gov/NHQ/practice-standards/standards/595.pdf.

Niranjan K, Ahromrit A, Khare AS. 2006. Process control in food processing. In: *Food processing handbook*. Brennan JG, ed. Weinheim, Germany: Wiley-VCH.

Office of Inspector General. 2009. *Traceability in the food supply chain*. Report nr OEI-02-06-00210. Washington, DC: U.S. Department of Health and Human Services.

Office of Inspector General. 1998. *Audit report: Review of departmental actions concerning the Sanitary Food Transportation Act of 1990*. Report nr TR-1998-100. Washington, DC: U.S. Department of Transportation. Available from: http://www.oig.dot.gov/sites/dot/files/pdfdocs/tr1998100.pdf.

Oliver SP, Boor KJ, Murphy SC, Murinda SE. 2009. Food safety hazards associated with consumption of raw milk. *Foodborne Pathog Dis* 6(7):793–806.

Oliver SP, Jayarao BM, Almeida RA. 2005. Foodborne pathogens in milk and the dairy farm environment: Food safety and public health implications. *Foodborne Pathog Dis* 2(2):115–129.

Patil SR, Cates S, Morales R. 2005. Consumer food safety knowledge, practices, and demographic differences: Findings from a meta-analysis. *J Food Prot* 68(9):1884–1894.

Patrick M. 2009. An introduction to FoodNet sites. *FoodNet News* 2(4):1–2.

Pew Commission on Industrial Farm Animal Production. 2008. *Putting meat on the table: Industrial farm animal production in America*. Baltimore, MD: Pew Charitable Trusts and Johns Hopkins Bloomberg School of Public Health. Available from: http://www.ncifap.org/bin/e/j/PCIFAPFin.pdf.

Powers RR. 2007. Captain's corner: Unsafe food transport. *Commercial Motor Vehicle Enforcement Quarterly*. Motor Carrier Division, Michigan State Police. Available from http://www.michigan.gov/documents/msp/CMV_Quarterly_January_2007_205099_7.pdf

Prescott JF. 2008. Antimicrobial use in food and companion animals. *Anim Health Res Rev* 9(2):127–133.

Rahman MS. 1999. Purpose of food preservation and processing. In: *Handbook of food preservation*. Rahman MS, ed. New York, NY: Marcel Dekker.

Redmond EC, Griffith CJ. 2003.Consumer food handling in the home: a review of food safety studies. *J Food Prot* 66(1):130–161.

Reich MR. 1983. Environmental politics and science: The case of PBB contamination in Michigan. *Am J Public Health* 73(3):302–313.

Reilly A, Kaferstein F. 1999. Food safety and products from aquaculture. *J Appl Microbiol* 85(no. suppl. 1):249S–257S.

Roberts T. 2005. Economics of private strategies to control foodborne pathogens. *Choices* 20(2):117–122.

Rogers S, Haines J. 2005. *Detecting and mitigating the environmental impact of fecal pathogens originating from confined animal feeding operations: Review*. Report nr EPA/600/R-06/021. Washington, DC: U.S. Environmental Protection Agency. Available from: http://www.epa.gov/nrmrl/pubs/600r06021/600r06021.pdf.

RTI International. 2005. *Survey of meat and poultry slaughter and processing plants, final report*. Prepared under contract for the U.S. Department of Agriculture. Report nr RTI Project Number 08893.007. Available from: http://www.fsis.usda.gov/PDF/SRM_Survey_Slaughter_&_Processing_Plants.pdf.

Sapkota A, Sapkota AR, Kucharski M, Burke J, McKenzie S, Walker P, Lawrence R. 2008. Aquaculture practices and potential human health risks: Current knowledge and future priorities. *Environ Int* 34(8):1215–1226.

Schroeder CM, Naugle AL, Schlosser WD, Hogue AT, Angulo FJ, Rose JS, Ebel ED, Disney WT, Holt KG, Goldman DP. 2005. Estimate of illnesses from *Salmonella* Enteritidis in eggs, United States, 2000. *Emerg Infect Dis* 11(1):113–115.

Segerson K. 1999. Mandatory versus voluntary approaches to food safety. *Agribusiness* 15(1):53–70.

Selman CA. 2010.Improving foodborne disease prevention. *J Environ Health* 73(2): 28–29.

Singer RS, Cox LA Jr, Dickson JS, Hurd HS, Phillips I, Miller GY. 2007. Modeling the relationship between food animal health and human foodborne illness. *Prev Vet Med* 79(2–4):186–203.

Sofos JN. 2009. ASAS centennial paper: Developments and future outlook for postslaughter food safety. *J Anim Sci* 87(7):2448–2457.

Stewart H, Blisard N, Bhuyan S, Nayga RM. 2004. *The demand for food away from home: Full-service or fast food?* Report nr AER-829. Washington, DC: Economic Research Service, U.S. Department of Agriculture. Available from: http://www.ers.usda.gov/publications/aer829/aer829_reportsummary.htm.

Teplitski M, Barak JD, Schneider KR. 2009. Human enteric pathogens in produce: Un-answered ecological questions with direct implications for food safety. *Curr Opin Biotechnol* 20(2):166–171.

Torok TJ, Tauxe RV, Wise RP, Livengood JR, Sokolow R, Mauvais S, Birkness KA, Skeels MR, Horan JM, Foster LR. 1997. A large community outbreak of salmonellosis caused by intentional contamination of restaurant salad bars. *JAMA* 278(5):389–395.

U.S. Presidential/Congressional Commission on Risk Assessment and Risk Management. 1997. *Framework for environmental health risk management. final report, vol.1.* Available from: http://www.riskworld.com/Nreports/1997/risk-rpt/pdf/EPAJAN.PDF.

Wallace CA. 2006. Safety in food processing. In: *Food processing handbook.* Brennan JG, ed. Weinheim, Germany: Wiley-VCH.

Wittenberger K, Dohlman E. 2010. *Peanut outlook: Impacts of the 2008–09 foodborne illness outbreak linked to* Salmonella *in peanuts.* Report nr OCS-10a-01. Washington, DC: U.S. Department of Agriculture.

World Health Organization. 2008. Food safety issues. *Terrorist threats to food. Guidance for establishing and strengthening prevention and response systems.* Geneva: World Health Organization.

Worm W, Barbier EB, Beaumont N, Duffy JE, Folke C, Halpern BS, Jackson JBC, Lotze HK, Micheli F, Palumbi SR, et al. 2006. Impacts of biodiversity loss on ocean ecosystem services. *Science* 314(5800):787–790.

Yang S, Angulo FJ, Altekruse SF. 2000. Evaluation of safe food-handling instructions on raw meat and poultry products. *J Food Prot* 63(10):1321–1325.

Young KT, Davis LM, Dirita VJ. 2007. *Campylobacter jejuni*: Molecular biology and pathogenesis. *Nat Rev Microbiol* 5(9):665–679.

---

## USEFUL RESOURCES

Association of American Feed Control Officials (AAFCO). http://www.aafco.org/

Electronic Code of Federal Regulations (eCFR). http://ecfr.gpoaccess.gov/cgi/t/text/text-idx?c=ecfr&tpl=%2Findex.tpl

Environmental Health Specialists Network (EHS-Net). http://www.cdc.gov/nceh/ehs/EHSNet/default.htm

FIGHT BAC! Keep Food Safe from Bacteria. Partnership for Food Safety Education (PFSE). http://www.fightbac.org/

Food Safety and Inspection Service. Food Defense & Emergency Response. http://www.fsis.usda.gov/Food_Defense_&_Emergency_Response/Guidance_Materials/index.asp

Food Safety and Inspection Service. Food Safety Education. http://www.fsis.usda.gov/food_safety_education/

FoodSafety.gov, Your Gateway to Federal Food Safety Information. http://www.foodsafety.gov/

History.com. *Modern Marvels* documentary DVD titles. Available from: http://www.history.com/
    "Bread"
    "Cattle Ranches"
    "Cheese"
    "Cold Cuts"
    "Commercial Fishing"
    "Eggs"
    "Fast Food Tech"
    "Fry It"
    "Harvesting"
    "Harvesting 2"
    "Ice Cream"
    "Milk"
    "More Snackfood Tech"
    "Snackfood Tech"
    "The Butcher"

International Organization for Standardization. http://www.iso.org/iso/home.html

Interstate Shellfish Sanitation Conference. http://www.issc.org/

ISO 22000 2005 Food Safety Library. http://www.praxiom.com/22000.htm

National Agricultural Statistics Service. Charts and Maps by Commodity. http://www.nass.usda.gov/Charts_and_Maps/index.asp

National Association of State Departments of Agriculture. *Food Safety: State and Federal Standards and Regulations.* http://www.nasda.org/nasda/nasda/foundation/foodsafety/index.html

National Oceanic and Atmospheric Administration. Aquaculture Program. http://aquaculture.noaa.gov/

Pew Commission on Industrial Farm Animal Production. http://www.ncifap.org/

Recalls.org, a Non-Profit Organization for the Benefit of the Public. Food—2011 Recalls. http://www.recalls.org/food.html

Seafood Network Information Center. http://seafood.ucdavis.edu/index.html

U.S. Environmental Protection Agency. Agriculture. Pesticides. http://www.epa.gov/agriculture/tpes.html

U.S. Environmental Protection Agency. Animal Feeding Operations. http://cfpub.epa.gov/npdes/home.cfm?program_id=7

U.S. Environmental Protection Agency. Animal Feeding Operations: Compliance and Enforcement. http://www.epa.gov/agriculture/anafocom.html

U.S. Environmental Protection Agency. Pesticides and Food: What Integrated Pest Management Means. http://www.epa.gov/pesticides/food/ipm.htm

U.S. Food and Drug Administration. CARVER Software for vulnerability assessments of the food industry. http://www.fda.gov/Food/FoodDefense/CARVER/default.htm

U.S. Food and Drug Administration. *Fish and Fisheries Products Hazards and Controls Guidance*, 3rd ed. http://www.fda.gov/Food/GuidanceComplianceRegulatoryInformation/GuidanceDocuments/Seafood/FishandFisheriesProductsHazardsandControlsGuide/default.htm

U.S. Food and Drug Administration. Food Defense & Emergency Response. http://www.fda.gov/Food/FoodDefense/default.htm

U.S. Food and Drug Administration. Health Educators Food Safety & Nutrition Education Campaigns. http://www.fda.gov/Food/ResourcesForYou/HealthEducators/default.htm

# Principal Federal Laws
# Related to Food Safety

| Law | Agency | Food safety provisions |
|---|---|---|
| Lacey Act of 1900, ch. 553, 31 Stat. 187 (1900) (codified in part at 16 U.S.C. § 3371) | Department of Commerce (NMFS), USDA | The act makes it a federal crime to import, export, sell, or transport in interstate commerce any plant, fish, or wildlife in violation of state law. The act has been used to prosecute individuals who sell plants, fish, or wildlife for human consumption in violation of state law. |
| Federal Meat Inspection Act, ch. 2907, 34 Stat. 1256, 1260 (1907) (codified at 21 U.S.C. § 601) | USDA | The act governs the slaughtering of livestock and the processing and distribution of meat products in the United States, authorizing the Secretary of Agriculture to prescribe the rules and regulations of sanitation covering slaughtering, meat canning, salting, packing, rendering, or similar establishments in which cattle, sheep, swine, goats, horses, mules, and other equines are slaughtered and the meat and meat food products thereof are prepared for commerce. |
| Federal Trade Commission Act, ch. 311, 38 Stat. 717 (1914) (codified at 15 U.S.C. § 41) | FTC | The act prohibits the dissemination of false advertisements for the purpose of inducing the purchase or having an effect upon commerce of foods, drinks, or chewing gum. The act provides for penalties for such false advertisements if the use of the commodity may be injurious to health. |
| United States Grain Standards Act, ch. 313, 39 Stat. 482 (1916) (codified at 7 U.S.C. § 71) | USDA | The act provides for the inspection, weighing, and grading of grain. Under the act, all corn exported from the United States generally must be tested for aflatoxin contamination. |
| Import Milk Act of February 15, 1927, ch. 155, 44 Stat. 1101 (1927) (codified at 21 U.S.C. § 141) | FDA | The act prohibits the importation of milk or cream into the United States without a permit and sets standards for when milk and cream shall be considered unfit for import. |
| Perishable Agricultural Commodities Act, 1930, ch. 436, 46 Stat. 531 (1930) (codified at 7 U.S.C. § 499a) | USDA | The act regulates the sale of perishable agricultural commodities and protects sellers delivering their produce on essentially cash terms. |
| Federal Alcohol Administration Act, ch. 814, 49 Stat. 977 (1935) (codified at 27 U.S.C. § 201) | Treasury | The act requires that alcoholic beverages for sale or distribution in the United States have a warning label. |
| Federal Food, Drug and Cosmetic Act, ch. 675, 52 Stat. 1040 (1938) (codified at 21 U.S.C. § 301) | FDA, EPA | The act and its regulations set forth food and drug labeling requirements, as well as requirements for animal drugs. The act seeks to ensure the purity of the nation's food supply, and accordingly bans "adulterated" and "misbranded" food from interstate commerce. Under the act, EPA regulates the amount of pesticide that may remain on food products. |
| Federal Seed Act, ch. 615, 53 Stat. 1275 (1939) (codified at 7 U.S.C. § 1551) | USDA, DHS | The act establishes seed labeling requirements, including the requirement for a caution statement such as "Do not use for food or feed or oil purposes" on seeds that have been chemically treated when the amount of chemicals remaining with the seeds is harmful to humans or other vertebrate animals. |
| Public Health Service Act, ch. 373, 58 Stat. 682 (1944) (codified at 42 U.S.C. § 201) | FDA, CDC | Under the act, CDC engages in public health activities related to food safety and foodborne diseases. FDA is authorized under the act to promulgate regulations to prevent the spread of communicable diseases, including foodborne illnesses. |
| National School Lunch Act, ch. 281, 60 Stat. 230 (1946) (codified at 42 U.S.C. § 1751) | USDA | The act required the development of a policy and procedures to ensure that schools receive information regarding irradiation technology and any other information necessary to promote food safety in schools. |

*(Continued From Previous Page)*

| Law | Agency | Food safety provisions |
|---|---|---|
| Agricultural Marketing Act of 1946, ch. 966, 60 Stat. 1087 (1946) (codified at 7 U.S.C. § 1621) | USDA, NMFS | The act promotes a scientific approach to the problems of marketing, transporting and distributing agricultural products and authorizes the Secretary of Agriculture to "inspect, certify, and identify the class, quality, quantity, and condition of agricultural products." Under the act, USDA has, among other things, established meat grading and acceptance services. The act also provides authority for the Seafood Inspection Program, which eventually was transferred to the Department of Commerce. |
| Federal Insecticide, Fungicide and Rodenticide Act, ch. 125, 61 Stat. 103 (1947) (codified at 7 U.S.C. § 136) | EPA | The act governs pesticide registration and safe use of pesticides. |
| Poultry Products Inspection Act, Pub. L. No. 85-172, 71 Stat. 441 (1957) (codified at 21 U.S.C. § 451) | USDA | The act governs the slaughtering, processing, and distribution of poultry products. |
| Food Additives Amendment of 1958, Pub. L. No. 85-929, 72 Stat. 1784 (1958) | FDA | The act amended the Federal Food, Drug and Cosmetic Act to prohibit the use in food of additives which have not been adequately tested to establish their safety. |
| Fair Packaging and Labeling Act, Pub. L. No. 89-755, 80 Stat. 1296 (1966) (codified at 15 U.S.C. § 1451) | FDA, FTC | The act prescribes the placement, form, and contents of a label's statement of the quantity of packaged goods. The act supersedes all local regulation that is less stringent or requires different information. |
| Egg Products Inspection Act, Pub. L. No. 91-597, 84 Stat. 1620 (1970) (codified at 21 U.S.C. § 1031) | USDA | The act and its regulations set standards for the quality, condition, weight, quantity, and grade of eggs produced for commercial sale. |
| Safe Drinking Water Act, Pub. L. No. 93-523, § 4, 88 Stat. 1660, 1694 (1974) (codified at 21 U.S.C. § 349) | FDA, EPA | The act, which amended the Federal Food, Drug and Cosmetic Act, and its regulations establish standards for bottled drinking water. |
| Toxic Substances Control Act, Pub. L. No. 94-469, 90 Stat. 2003 (1976) (codified at 15 U.S.C. § 2601) | EPA | Under the act, EPA can regulate the use of certain chemical substances in foods that present an unreasonable risk to health. Under the authority granted by the act, EPA's Toxic Substances Control Act Biotechnology Program regulates microorganisms, such as biofertilizers, intended for commercial use that contain or express new combinations of traits. |
| Infant Formula Act of 1980, Pub. L. No. 96-359, 94 Stat. 1190 (codified at 21 U.S.C. § 350a) | FDA | The act authorizes the Secretary to establish requirements for infant formula for quality factors and good manufacturing practices, including quality control procedures, to assure that an infant formula provides required nutrients and is manufactured in a manner designed to prevent adulteration of the infant formula. The act also authorizes the Secretary to prescribe, by regulation, the scope and extent of recalls of infant formulas necessary and appropriate for the degree of risks to human health. |
| Federal Anti-Tampering Act, Pub. L. No. 98-127, 97 Stat. 831 (1983) (codified at 18 U.S.C. § 1365) | FDA, USDA | The act prohibits tainting a consumer product with intent to cause serious injury to the business of any person where the consumer product affects interstate or foreign commerce. The act also prohibits providing a materially false or misleading label or container for a consumer product. |
| Pesticide Monitoring Improvements Act of 1988, Pub. L. No. 100-418, § 4701, 102 Stat. 1107, 1411 (1988) (codified at 21 U.S.C. § 1401) | FDA | The act requires FDA to have in place computerized data management systems to record, summarize, and evaluate the results of its program for monitoring food products for pesticide residues and requires FDA to provide information to EPA. |
| Sanitary Food Transportation Act of 1990, Pub. L. No. 101-500, 104 Stat. 1213 (1990) (codified at 49 U.S.C. § 5701) | DOT | The act calls for the Department of Transportation to issue regulations prohibiting the transportation of food and food additives in motor or rail vehicles that are used to transport refuse or nonfood products. |
| Nutrition Labeling and Education Act of 1990, Pub. L. No. 101-535, 104 Stat. 2353 (1990) | FDA | The act amended the Federal Food, Drug and Cosmetic Act to prohibit the application of state quality standards to foods moving in interstate commerce and to require labels of food products sold in the United States to display nutritional information. |
| Dietary Supplement Health and Education Act of 1994, Pub. L. No. 103-417, 108 Stat. 4325 (1994) | FDA | The act amended the Federal Food, Drug and Cosmetic Act to allow certain health claims for dietary supplements to be made without petitioning the FDA. These include (1) statements asserting a benefit related to a classical nutrient deficiency disease, (2) claims about the role of a nutrient or dietary ingredient with respect to the structure or function of the human body ("structure/function claims"), and (3) declarations of general well-being from consumption of a nutrient or other dietary ingredient. Under the act such claims are permitted if the manufacturer has "substantiation" that the assertion is truthful and nonmisleading, if the label expressly states that FDA has not evaluated the claim, and if FDA is notified within 30 days of the first marketing of the product that bears the claim. |

| Law | Agency | Food safety provisions |
|-----|--------|------------------------|
| Food Quality Protection Act of 1996, Pub. L. No. 104-170, 110 Stat. 1489 (1996) | EPA, USDA, HHS | The act amended the regulatory scheme under the Federal Insecticide, Fungicide and Rodenticide Act and the Federal Food, Drug and Cosmetic Act to require EPA to reevaluate the safety of pesticide tolerances on a set timetable. |
| Food and Drug Modernization Act of 1997, Pub. L. No. 105-115, 111 Stat. 2296 (1997) | FDA | The act amended the Federal Food, Drug and Cosmetic Act and the Public Health Service Act to authorize health and nutrient claims to be made for foods when certain criteria are met. |
| Animal Health Protection Act, Pub. L. No. 107-171, § 10401, 116 Stat. 134, 494 (2002) (codified at 7 U.S.C. § 8301) | USDA, DHS | The act authorizes the Secretary to prohibit or restrict movements of animals in interstate commerce to prevent the dissemination of any pest or disease of livestock. The act also permits the Secretary to order the destruction or removal of such animals. |
| Public Health Security and Bioterrorism Preparedness and Response Act of 2002, Pub. L. No. 107-188, 116 Stat. 594 (2002) | USDA, FDA | The act expands APHIS's authorities, including activities to enhance methods of protecting against the introduction of plant and animal disease organisms by terrorists. The act also provides FDA with detention authority, expanded recordkeeping provisions, and authorizes FDA to commission other federal officials to conduct examinations and investigations of FDA-regulated foods at jointly regulated facilities. |
| Homeland Security Act of 2002, Pub. L. No. 107-296, 116 Stat. 2135 (2002) | DHS | The act calls for the securing of critical infrastructure and transfers functions relating to the agricultural import and entry inspection activities under certain laws from the Secretary of Agriculture to the Secretary of the Department of Homeland Security. |

Source: GAO analysis of federal laws.

Note: On January 4, 2011, President Obama signed the FDA Food Safety Modernization Act into law. This act sets in motion a number of sweeping changes to federal food laws, including a more risk-based preventive approach to safety from unintentional hazards and defense from deliberate contamination. Furthermore, this act increases the frequency of mandatory inspections for high-risk food facilities, including foreign facilities, and provides the U.S. Food and Drug Administration with mandatory recall authority for unsafe food products.

# Index

Note: Italicized page locators indicate a figure/photo; tables are noted with a *t*.

CPSIA information can be obtained
at www.ICGtesting.com
Printed in the USA
JSHW051455220322
24105JS00001B/5

9 780763 785567